AF730570

Duplex Ultrasound of Superficial Leg Veins

Erika Mendoza • Christopher R. Lattimer
Nick Morrison
Editors

Duplex Ultrasound of Superficial Leg Veins

Springer

Editors
Erika Mendoza, MD, PhD
Venenpraxis Wunstorf
Wunstorf
Germany

Christopher R. Lattimer, MD, PhD
Department of Vascular Surgery
Josef Pflug Vascular Laboratory
Ealing Hospital and Imperial College
London
UK

Nick Morrison, MD
Morrison Vein Institute
Scottsdale, AZ
USA

The book is supplemented with extensive on-line images and videos which can be found at http://extras.springer.com. German references, which were present in the original version, have been removed or replaced with English ones. They can still be found on-line or within an earlier book.

ISBN 978-3-642-40730-7 ISBN 978-3-642-40731-4 (eBook)
DOI 10.1007/978-3-642-40731-4
Springer Heidelberg New York Dordrecht London

Library of Congress Control Number: 2014936597

© Springer-Verlag Berlin Heidelberg 2014
This work is subject to copyright. All rights are reserved by the Publisher, whether the whole or part of the material is concerned, specifically the rights of translation, reprinting, reuse of illustrations, recitation, broadcasting, reproduction on microfilms or in any other physical way, and transmission or information storage and retrieval, electronic adaptation, computer software, or by similar or dissimilar methodology now known or hereafter developed. Exempted from this legal reservation are brief excerpts in connection with reviews or scholarly analysis or material supplied specifically for the purpose of being entered and executed on a computer system, for exclusive use by the purchaser of the work. Duplication of this publication or parts thereof is permitted only under the provisions of the Copyright Law of the Publisher's location, in its current version, and permission for use must always be obtained from Springer. Permissions for use may be obtained through RightsLink at the Copyright Clearance Center. Violations are liable to prosecution under the respective Copyright Law.
The use of general descriptive names, registered names, trademarks, service marks, etc. in this publication does not imply, even in the absence of a specific statement, that such names are exempt from the relevant protective laws and regulations and therefore free for general use.
While the advice and information in this book are believed to be true and accurate at the date of publication, neither the authors nor the editors nor the publisher can accept any legal responsibility for any errors or omissions that may be made. The publisher makes no warranty, express or implied, with respect to the material contained herein.

Printed on acid-free paper

Springer is part of Springer Science+Business Media (www.springer.com)

Foreword

Our understanding of superficial venous anatomy and its often complex haemodynamics have improved considerably during the past 20 years, mainly thanks to the introduction of the duplex ultrasound (DUS) investigation. Nowadays, venous DUS has become an indispensable tool to evaluate and treat our patients with chronic venous disorder (CVD). It is obvious that the introduction of DUS has revolutionized our phlebological practice in several ways. First, DUS has led to a refinement in the description of lower limb venous anatomy in particular, by distinguishing between the saphenous trunks within their fascial compartments and the tributaries situated subcutaneously. Second, DUS has largely improved our insight into venous haemodynamics helping us to move away from dogmatic views about causes and mechanisms of flux and reflux toward a broader insight into the (dys)functioning of the superficial venous system. Third, DUS has become our GPS (global positioning system) for efficacious and safe treatment of patients with varicose veins. Fourth, DUS is the ideal tool for postoperative follow-up after intervention in an individual patient as well as in different patient groups, obviously not as a single tool, but in addition to quality of life assessments and clinical examination of treated patients.

For all practioners who are involved in the diagnosis and treatment of CVD patients, Erika Mendoza's book presents a real treasure, to be discovered little by little. The book has been composed, written and illustrated with a typical German 'Gründlichkeit' (thoroughness). The present English edition was realized in close collaboration with Christopher Lattimer and Nick Morrison, who made an invaluable contribution to the different chapters. The book offers a very comprehensive overview of everything you might want to know about DUS of the superficial venous system. In the first 14 chapters the authors discuss all the details about ultrasound equipment, duplex anatomy, pathophysiology of superficial veins and their detailed examination with DUS during and after treatment. Ultrasound of the deep venous system, including all practical tips and tricks is also examined. The remaining three chapters are of special interest because they address many issues which you usually do not find in most textbooks. These include the examination of superficial veins in the presence of deep venous obstruction or reflux, the DUS examination of leg oedema (venous, lymphatic or lipoedema) and also some incidental, somewhat surprising, sonographic findings. In this book, illustrations are presented in a very didactic way, and these will certainly help you to recognize all the described duplex features more easily in your daily practice. In summary, this book is really worthwhile, from the beginning to the end, and will become your future companion in the diagnosis and treatment of patients with chronic venous disorder.

Marianne De Maeseneer, MD, PhD
Department of Dermatology,
Section Phlebology, Erasmus Medical Centre,
Rotterdam Netherlands and Faculty of Medicine
and Health Sciences, University of Antwerp,
Antwerp, Belgium

Preface

This book was the original idea of Erika Mendoza when it was first published in Germany in 2006 with the help of many leading experts in the discipline of chronic venous disease. It was intended as a practical everyday guide for ultrasound practitioners required to assess and diagnose the haemodynamic abnormalities behind varicose veins. The wealth of high-quality images to illustrate functional anatomy made this work reservedly the most comprehensive book at that time.

The potential for internationalisation into an English version was quickly recognised by Christopher Lattimer (UK) and Nick Morrison (USA). The book was first translated into English by William Barne. It then underwent an extensive process of revision, moderation and improvement by all three authors who have incorporated their experience and accumulated knowledge directly into the book. Collectively we hope that this will maintain its position as the definitive guide on the use of duplex ultrasound in assessing superficial leg veins.

We acknowledge the work of the following contributors:

1. Hans-Peter Weskott (Chaps. 1 and 17)
2. Alberto Caggiati (Chap. 2)
3. Renato Murena-Schmidt (Chap. 2)
4. Claude Franceschi (Chap. 3)
5. Birgit Kahle (Chap. 3)
6. Thomas M. Proebstle (Chap. 12)
7. Achim Mumme (Chaps. 12 and 13)
8. Franz Xaver Breu (Chap. 12)
9. Andreas Hildebrandt (Chap. 13)
10. Hans-Joachim Kruse (Chap. 14)
11. Helmut Kopf (Chap. 17)

The book is supplemented with extensive on-line images and videos which can be found at http://springer.duplexofsuplegveins.com. Non english references, which were present in the original version, have been moved into the appendix "foreign literature" or replaced with English ones.

Wunstorf, Germany — Erika Mendoza, MD, PhD
London, UK — Christopher R. Lattimer, MD, PhD
Scottsdale, AZ, USA — Nick Morrison, MD
February 2014

Acknowledgements

Our gratitude is given to Sigvaris GmbH (D-87700, Memmingen, Germany) and STD Pharmaceutical (Hereford, HR4 0EL, UK) for their help in funding the translation to make this project possible.

Erika Mendoza, Christopher R. Lattimer and Nick Morrison

SIGVARIS

STD Pharmaceutical

Contents

Contributors

Franz Xaver Breu, MD Praxis für Gefäßmedizin am Tegernsee, Rottach-Egern, Germany

Alberto Caggiati, MD Department of Anatomy, Universita di Roma, Rome, Italy

Claude Franceschi, MD Angiologist Consultant, Hopital Saint Joseph, Paris, France

Andreas Hildebrandt, MD Ullsteinhausklinik GmbH, Berlin, Germany

Birgit Kahle, MD, PhD Klinik für Dermatologie, Allergologie und Venerologie, UKSH Campus Lübeck, Lübeck, Germany

Helmut Kopf, MSc Institut für diagnostische und interventionelle Radiologie Wilhelminenspital Wien, Wien, Austria

Hans-Joachim Kruse, MD, PhD Praxis für Gefäßmedizin, Zschopau, Germany

Christopher R. Lattimer, MD, PhD Department of Vascular Surgery, Josef Pflug Vascular Laboratory, Ealing Hospital and Imperial College, London, UK

Erika Mendoza, MD, PhD Venenpraxis Wunstorf, Wunstorf, Germany

Nick Morrison, MD Morrison Vein Institute, Scottsdale, AZ, USA

Achim Mumme, MD, PhD Klinik für Gefäßchirurgie, St. Josef-Hospital, Universitätsklinikum, Bochum, Germany

Renate Murena-Schmidt, MD Praxis für Gefäßerkrankungen, Köln, Germany

Thomas M. Proebstle, MD, PhD Hautklinik und Poliklinik, Universitätsmedizin der Johannes Gutenberg-Universität Mainz, Mainz, Germany

Hans-Peter Weskott, MD Klinikum Siloah – Zentrale Sonographie, Hannover, Germany

1 The Ultrasound Scanner

Hans-Peter Weskott, Erika Mendoza, and Christopher R. Lattimer

Chapter Summary

This chapter explains the basic information on how images are generated and how the machine should be configured. The probe or duplex transducer is so called because it converts electrical energy into sound by exciting piezoelectric crystals. The resulting acoustic wave is a pressure wave which propagates into the tissues by compression and expansion. Reflected waves are received, processed and projected onto a screen.

H.-P. Weskott, MD (✉)
Klinikum Siloah – Zentrale Sonographie,
Roesebeckstr. 15, 30449 Hannover, Germany
e-mail: hans-peter.weskott@krh.eu

E. Mendoza, MD, PhD
Venenpraxis Wunstorf,
Speckenstraße 10, 31515 Wunstorf, Germany
e-mail: erika.mendoza@t-online.de

C.R. Lattimer, MD, PhD
Department of Vascular Surgery,
Josef Pflug Vascular Laboratory,
Ealing Hospital and Imperial College, London, UK

1.1 Physical Principles of Duplex Ultrasound

1.1.1 Creation of an Ultrasound Image

Images are generated through the transmission and reception of three types of ultrasound wave characteristics: the frequency, phase and amplitude. The **frequency** used for diagnosis is in the megahertz range (MHz) and is defined by the wavelength (λ). The phase is controlled by switching between (+) and (–). The change of its amplitude reflects the acoustic pressure dictated by the amplitude (Fig. 1.1).

The **amplitude** provides information about the reflective properties of tissue. The stronger the amplitude of the reflected echo, the brighter the corresponding pixel within the image point in the image. It can be likened to the contrast of the image.

Spatial **resolution** describes the ability to discriminate between two neighbouring points in the image. There are two types of spatial resolution. Axial resolution means the separate representation of two neighbouring points in the direction of the sound wave. It represents depth resolution. Lateral resolution means the separate representation of reflecting points at right angles to the sound wave. It represents the minimum distance between points at the same depth. Temporal resolution means discrimination of the same point between 2 time points.

E. Mendoza et al. (eds.), *Duplex Ultrasound of Superficial Leg Veins*,
DOI 10.1007/978-3-642-40731-4_1, © Springer-Verlag Berlin Heidelberg 2014

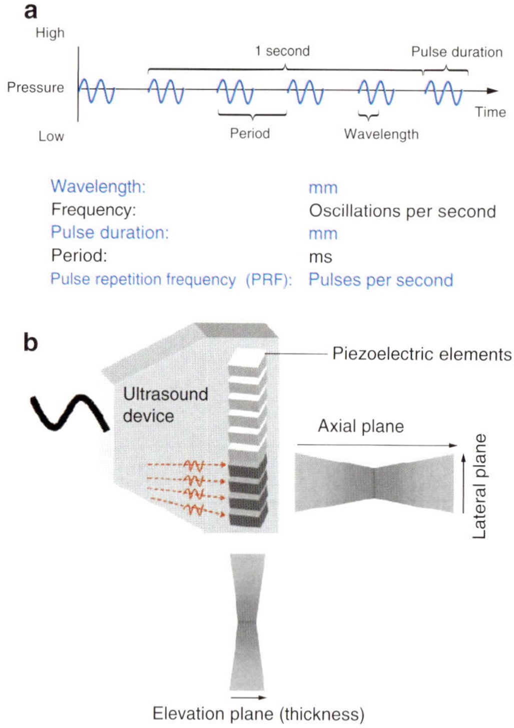

Fig. 1.1 (**a**) Important characteristics of sound waves. (**b**) The resolution depends also on the width of the sound wave front entering the tissues. This is determined by the depth adepth of the entering column of sound travelling along the *z*-axis (elevation plane, perpendicular to the surface of the transducer). The focus is normally set at a fixed depth by a rigid acoustic lens Copyright: [Author]

The **z-plane** or elevation plane refers to the width of the sound wave front going into the tissues along the *z*-axis (Fig. 1.1b).

The transmit frequency controls the resolution of the image. With low transmit frequencies, blood appears to be echo-free and black. With increasing frequencies, aggregates of erythrocytes become visible as flowing, echogenic reflections. This is called spontaneous natural contrast.

The higher the transmission frequency, the shorter the wavelength and the better the spatial resolution. However, a higher transmit frequency is at the cost of a greater attenuation. This limits the penetration depth both for B scan ultrasound and especially for Doppler ultrasound, since the latter uses higher frequencies. Thus, the higher the frequency, the better the resolution, but the less the penetration.

When examining peripheral veins, it is advisable to use probes with different frequencies. In general, transmission frequencies between 5 and 15 MHz cover most eventualities. Frequencies between 5 and 7.5 MHz are the most popular.

Image resolution depends also on **focusing of the sound waves**, just like a torch. Adjusting the focus improves the brightness and clarity of the region of interest.

Sound waves are propagated by compression and expansion of the molecules in the medium through which the sound is transmitted. When the acoustic properties of the tissue change as the acoustic wave front advances, sound waves are reflected back as echoes. This process takes energy away from the advancing front (Fig. 1.2a). Consequently, the sound loses intensity exponentially as it progresses deeper into the tissues. This can be compensated to a certain degree by amplifying the receive signal strength by the machine (Fig. 1.2b).

B scan (B = brightness) is imaging of the acoustic boundary surfaces or interfaces. Fluids are echo-free and thus appear black. Different tissues appear in distinguishable shades of grey depending on their different acoustic properties. Bone tissue is echo-dense and therefore reflects all the sound wave. Therefore, bone contours appear as a white line behind which everything is black since no further echoes can penetrate. This is called the acoustic shadow.

Changes to echoes along a scan line over time can be shown in **M mode** (M = motion). Here the screen is split. Half is used for the B scan along the scan line, and the other half shows a continuous recording of the changes in echo amplitude over time. This mode is recommended for moving objects, particularly for examining the heart muscle and its valves. In the venous system it has been used for assessing the compressibility of a vein segment (Fig. 5.10).

B-Mode artifacts

The brighter the dots in the image, the greater the amplitude of the echo reflected by the tissue and the less the energy available to insonate the tissues behind. With complete reflection, there is no onward penetration. For example, no acoustic information can be seen behind calcifications (Fig. 1.3a) and **weakened** behind complex echogenic structures (Fig. 1.3b). As almost no energy is lost in fluids, the sound energy distal to cystic spaces is higher than in the surrounding tissues. This explains the paradox of an apparent **strengthening** of the signal (Fig. 1.3c, d).

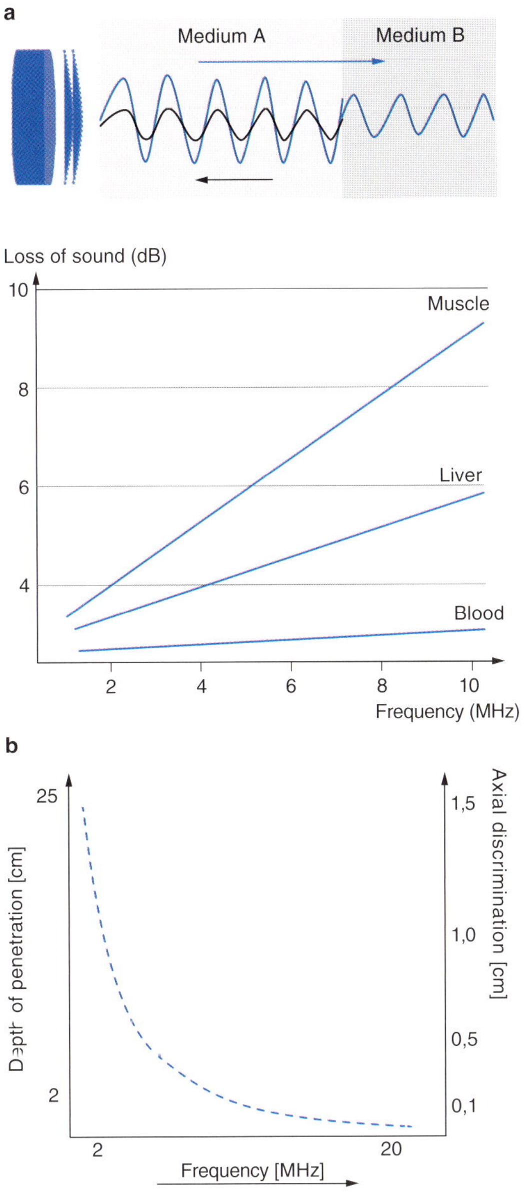

Fig. 1.2 (**a**) Loss of sound energy due to changes in the acoustic properties of tissue (*medium A*, *B*). The transmitted sound wave is shown in blue and its partial reflection in black. The graph shows that the loss of sound in muscle tissue is significantly higher than that of liver or blood. (**b**) Diagram showing the inverse relationship between the transmission frequency and the penetration depth achievable. It also shows the direct relationship between frequency and point-to-point resolution Copyright: [Author]

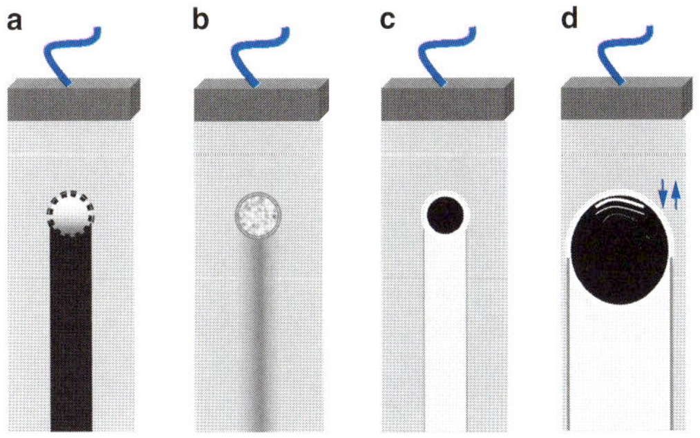

Fig. 1.3 Diagram of the important behavioural characteristics of ultrasound: (**a**) Acoustic shadow behind a calcified artery due to the complete lack of sound wave penetration. (**b**) Weakening of the sound wave behind a strongly echogenic tissue such as a lipoma. (**c**) Strengthening behind a small vein or cyst. (**d**) Strengthening behind a large vein or cyst with sound elimination at the lateral margins due to a deflection artefact (*arrows*). These are shown as *grey vertical lines*. The anterior vessel wall echo is projected into the lumen to give a false impression of intraluminal pathology. These reflections are seen as white lines in the upper part of the vein/cyst Copyright: [Author]

In larger cysts or vessels, the signal may be eliminated deeper when the sound wave front breaks against the lateral cyst or lateral vein borders. This is known as a **reflection artifact** (lateral edge shadow). Repeated mirroring originating the layers of the anterior vein wall often causes a **reverberation artifact**. This happens when the anterior echogenic wall is projected in the lumen. This may be confused with intraluminal pathology (Fig. 1.3d).

1.1.2 Measurement of Flow Velocities

Doppler ultrasound assessments of blood flow are based on frequency and phase analysis. To reach the required signal strength, lower frequencies are used in pulsed and colour Doppler than those in B scans. For a B scan frequency of 7.5 MHz, the frequency used for colour Doppler ultrasound is usually 5 MHz.

Detection of blood flow is based on the **Doppler principle**. Sound waves are reflected from moving intraluminal echoes, namely, the red blood cells. Just as the frequency of the siren of an ambulance increases as it approaches, and diminishes after it has passed, the frequency of the echo from the flowing blood alters according to its velocity and direction. The faster the blood is flowing, the greater the difference between the transmitted and received frequency.

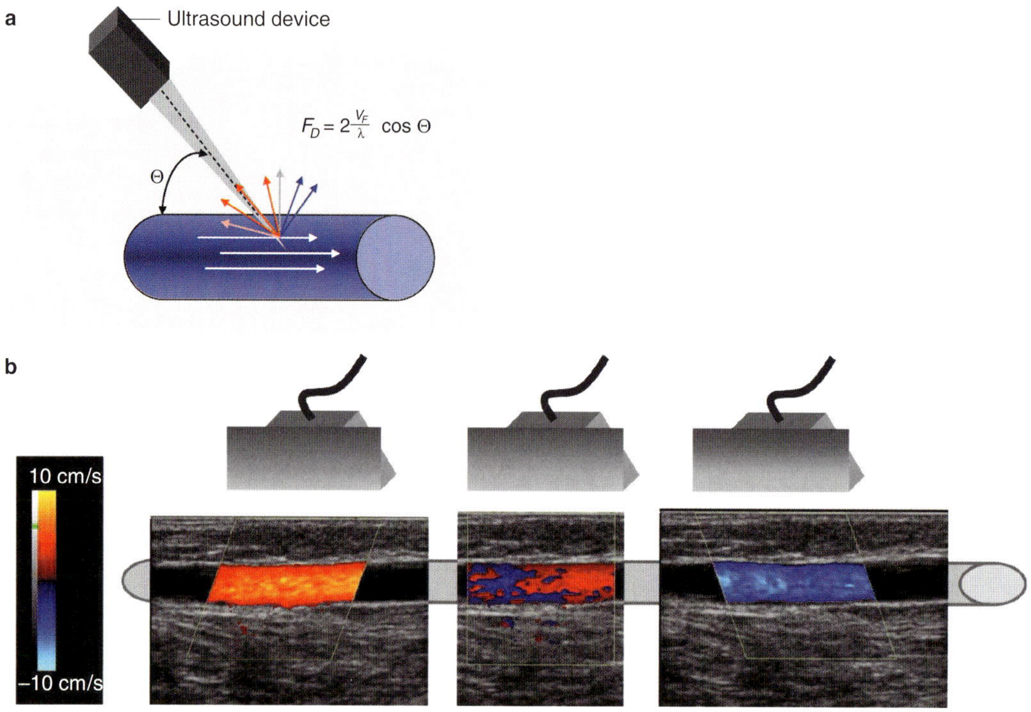

Fig. 1.4 (**a**) The Doppler equation of frequency shift. The Doppler angle or angle of insonation Θ is the angle between the axis of the direction of flow in a vein and the angle of incidence. The formula for the frequency shift F_D is shown where λ = wavelength and V_F = transmission frequency. (**b**) The direction of flow is represented by a colour. This depends on the position of the probe and the direction selected which is identified by the colour bar. The colour at the *top* of the colour bar shows the code for flow towards the probe (*red*). The example shows a longitudinal examination of a great saphenous vein refluxing from left to right. Blood flows towards the probe (*red*), past the probe (*mixed*) and away from the probe (*blue*) Copyright: [Author]

This difference is known as the **Doppler shift frequency**. The frequencies of the change in signal can be displayed graphically as a spectral curve against time. If the angle between the vein or more correct the vector of the moving blood cells and the axis of the sound is known, the machine can calculate the flow velocity (Fig. 1.4).

The sensitivity for detecting blood flow depends on three factors: (1) the emitted acoustic **energy**; (2) the **frequency** where the lower the frequency, the greater the penetration but the poorer the resolution; and (3) mainly the angle of insonation and the blood vessel (Fig. 1.4a). The accuracy of the velocity measurement depends on the angle of insonation. Angles > 60° do not produce an accurate velocity measurement. If the sound waves meet the blood stream at right angles with a Doppler angle of 90°, then the machine will not be able to detect any movement because the shift frequency will in theory be zero (Fig. 1.4b). The closer the angle is to 0°, the more reliable the velocity measurement will be.

The loss of energy with depth (Fig. 1.2b) is one of the factors hampering **sensitivity**. This is especially important when measuring slow flow or small volume flows. The sensitivity at greater depths can be improved by increasing the gain, by changing to a lower frequency probe or by switching to power Doppler. The sensitivity can be improved greatly by administering an contrast agent.

1.1.3 Continuous, Pulsed and Power Modes

If a continuous Doppler signal is transmitted and received, the movements of blood corpuscles can be detected along the transmission axis. This is

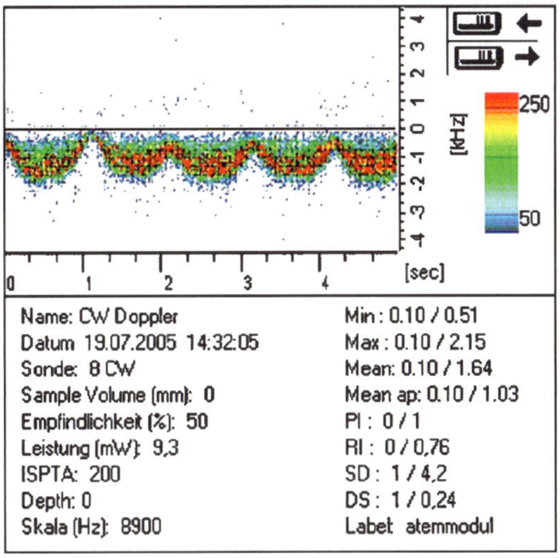

Fig. 1.5 Spectral curve with CW Doppler measuring flow in the common femoral vein of a lying patient. The pen-probe is held at an angle with the head pointing upwards and therefore away from the direction of flow. The sound can be heard on the online material, together with an example of reflux and turbulence in the great saphenous vein of a standing patient (Manfred Stimal, Reinfeld; by kind permission) Copyright: M. Stimal

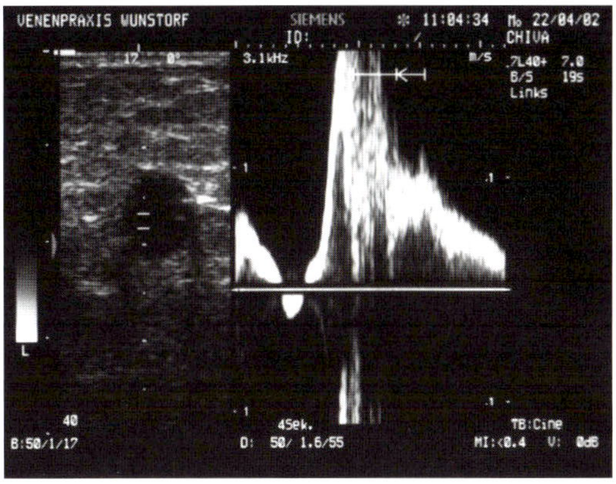

Fig. 1.6 Transverse view through the left thigh demonstrating PW duplex of the great saphenous vein. The probe is held at a slight angle upwards. The *left half* shows the echo-free lumen in B scan with the sample volume between the parallel cursor lines. The *right half* shows the spectral curve consisting predominantly of reflux Copyright: [Author]

represented graphically as a frequency analysis. The depth cannot be determined in continuous mode. This continuous wave (**CW**) Doppler is used in pen-probes or pocket Doppler machines (Fig. 1.5).

Unlike CW, the pulsed wave (**PW**) Doppler uses intermittent transmission of sound waves. The reflected waves are received in the interval between two pulse transmissions and then compared with the transmission frequency. The signals are analyzed in a defined window of time corresponding to a specific depth. This interval is defined in advance by the examiner and corresponds to the sample volume in the vessel. In B scan this measurement area is shown between two parallel cursor lines (Fig. 1.6). The distance between these cursor lines is termed the gate.

In **colour duplex ultrasound**, the Doppler shift frequency is measured by PW at every point selected within the colour box. The colour coding defines the direction of flow in relation to the position of the probe. Red indicates flow towards the probe while blue indicates flow away from the probe (Figs. 1.4b and 1.7). Although the colour coding can be changed by the operator, standard convention dictates that red is flow towards the probe. The colour in the upper half of the colour bar on the screen always defines the colour of flow towards the probe. The brighter the colour, the higher the frequency shift, the greater the flow velocity.

In **power Doppler mode**, neither direction nor velocity information is shown (Lamboul et al. 2009). Instead the power of the Doppler shift frequencies is shown in monochrome. The advantage is greater sensitivity in visualising slow velocities with an unfavourable angle of insonation (Fig. 1.8a). The power is derived from a greater sensitivity at recording the amplitude of the echoes. Consequently flow looks brighter and it is the best way of imaging vascularity. It is not prone to aliasing because it only indicates the presence of flow and cannot measure velocity. Some equipment suppliers combine information on the amplitude of the Doppler signal with its frequency, so as to combine the advantages of direction recognition with the high sensitivity of the power Doppler (Fig. 1.8b).

1.1.4 Aliasing

With the exception of CW Doppler, which transmits and receives sound waves continuously,

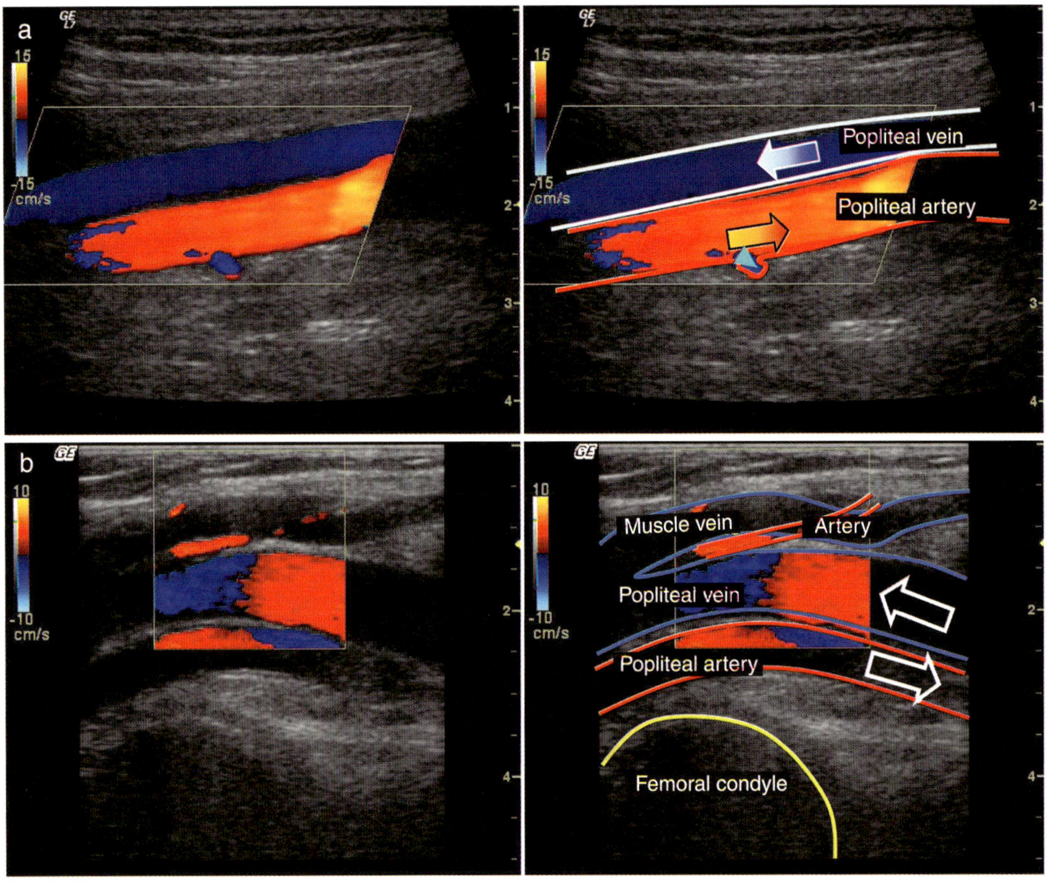

Fig. 1.7 Direction or phase. The colour bar in the *top left* of the screen codes the flow direction. The *red* (+) indicates flow towards the probe. The *blue* (–) indicates flow away from the probe. (**a**) Longitudinal view through the popliteal region with the popliteal artery and vein. The flow in the vein is going away from the probe and is therefore coloured *blue*. The flow in the artery is coming towards the probe and is therefore shown *red*. There is a minor artery branching upwards in which the flow is away from the probe and which therefore also appears blue (*light blue arrow head*). (**b**) Colour switch in an artery and vein where the vessel curves. Longitudinal view with the knee partially flexed. The popliteal artery and vein come to the surface, towards the probe, as they leave the calf, and run deeper again, away from the probe, as they enter the thigh. There is therefore a switch in the colour on ultrasound in both vessels. There is typically a thin black line between the colours where no velocity is measured because the blood runs parallel to the probe. Occasionally its *dark blue* or *dark red* indicating a slow flow in relation to the probe. Furthermore, the filter frequently excludes the perpendicular flows typical in a colour switch when the Doppler angle is about 90°. This is in contrast to the rapid flow of aliasing (Fig. 1.9b), when the colour in the area of the switch is *yellow*, *white* or *light blue* (see accompanying online material) Copyright: [Author]

sound transmission and reception is noncontinuous in all other Doppler modes, including PW Doppler and colour Doppler. In order to reconstruct the correct wavelengths from the reflected echoes, at least one measurement point must be assigned for each trough and crest of the transmission frequency sine curve. The Doppler shift frequency is only correctly recorded when the sampling pulse repetition frequency (PRF) is at least twice the Doppler shift frequency. This boundary is called the **Nyquist frequency**. For example, if the PRF is 11 kHz, then the highest Doppler shift frequency which can be calculated correctly is 5.5 kHz. The Nyquist theorem states that the sampling frequency should be at least twice the highest frequency contained in the signal to be analysed.

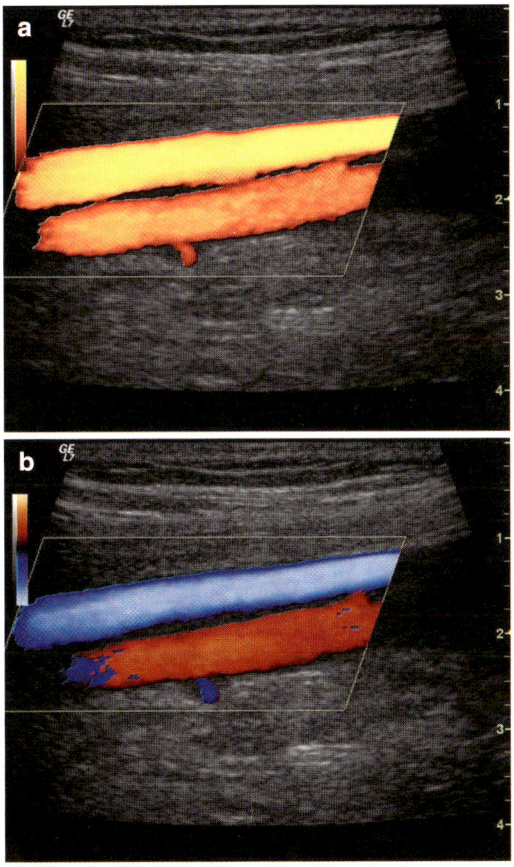

Fig. 1.8 Power Doppler. (**a**) Power Doppler of the same popliteal region as in Fig. 1.7a without information on flow direction. Flow is visualised as a brighter image. (**b**) Bidirectional power Doppler. The increased sensitivity of the power Doppler is complemented by information on flow direction Copyright: [Author]

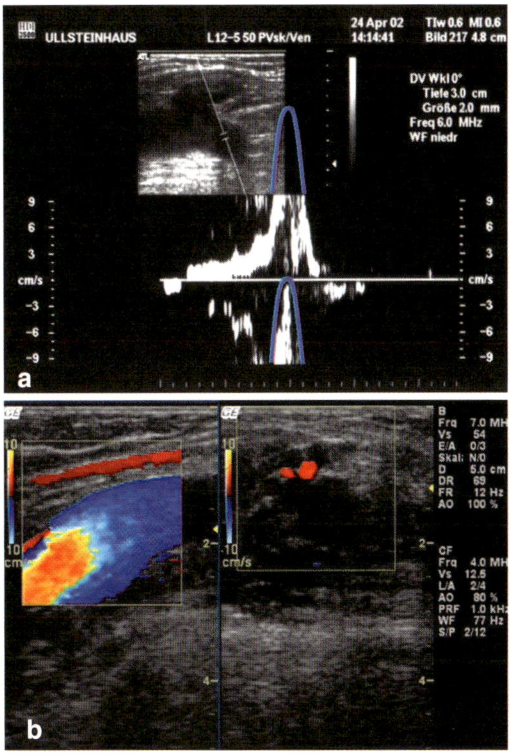

Fig. 1.9 Aliasing. (**a**) PW measurement in the popliteal vein. With fast flow the velocity is shown in the opposite direction. The flow is so fast that it "slips out of the measurement window" and reappears in the negative zone below. The "upside down" flow curve is outlined in *blue*. (**b**) Colour-coded measurement in the popliteal region. Slow reflux from the vein of Giacomini is seen as *red* in the *upper part* of the image. However, aliasing is seen in the faster-flowing popliteal vein. Note that a *white or yellow border* is typically visible between the *red and blue areas* when the colours are reversed from aliasing Copyright: [Author]

Transmission frequency, pulse repetition frequency and penetration depth determine the accuracy of recording the receiving echoes at a set velocity band. With slow venous blood flow, a low PRF must be set to ensure that slow reflux phenomena are not overlooked. In the arterial system, the PRF must be set higher to record the faster velocities without aliasing.

Aliasing can easily be recognised in the graphic representation of the Doppler spectrum. Frequencies higher than the Nyquist sampling limit, which should be above the baseline when flowing towards the probe, appear in the *reverse* direction. This is known as **overfolding** or the **wrap-around** effect. As a result velocities in PW mode are shown with the opposite direction (Fig. 1.9a), while in colour mode they appear in the wrong colour (Fig. 1.9b). A white or yellow border is typically visible between the red and blue areas when the colours are reversed from aliasing.

With aliasing, "black holes" appear when the colours are reversed if the resulting bright interface colours are eliminated by the colour filter settings on the scanner. If the blood is in fact flowing in different directions, a black line will be seen between the two coloured areas where there is no measurable flow (Figs. 1.4b and 1.7b).

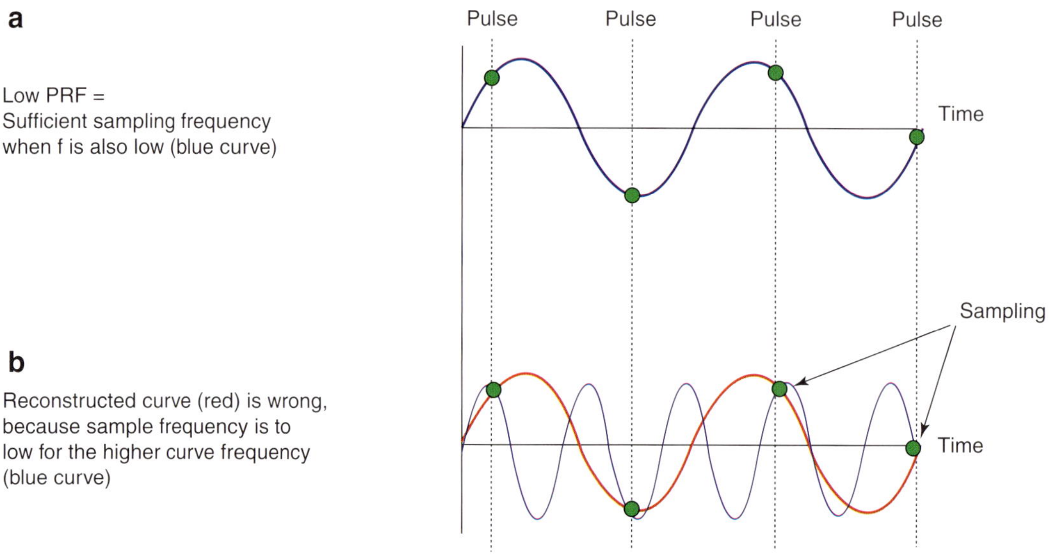

Fig. 1.10 Aliasing. (**a**) A PRF just sufficient to sample more than 2 points on the wave. The curve is generated correctly. (**b**) The wave is too fast for the PRF. Fewer than 2 points are sampled per cycle (crest and trough), and a false curve is generated (*red line*) Copyright: [Author]

A simple model for aliasing is analogous to the second hand of a clock. If you look at the clock at intervals of 15 s, the second hand appears to be moving clockwise. If this sampling interval is extended to 30 s, it is no longer possible to determine the direction of movement. If the interval is extended to 45 s, the second hand appears to be going anticlockwise. Thus, the sampling frequency is critical for accurate analysis. If the clock frequency (Doppler shift frequency) is 1 revolution per minute, then a correct assessment of the direction of rotation can only be made if the sampling frequency (pulse repetition frequency) is greater than 2 per minute (Fig. 1.10).

The aliasing effect is well known from old Western films. At a slow frame rate or fast wheel revolution, the spokes of the wagon wheels apparently start to turn backwards.

1.1.5 Blooming

Another clinically significant artefact is called blooming (McDicken and Anderson 2002). It results in an overestimation of the vessel boundaries, venous valves and small thrombi from propagation. This underlines the value of compression ultrasound in diagnosing thrombosis.

Reducing the colour gain and increasing the Doppler frequency are measures which will reduce blooming.

1.2 Probe Selection

The choice of transducer head dictates the range of transmit frequencies and therefore the penetration and resolution. The probe selected depends on the anatomical circumstances. It should offer sufficient image quality for diagnostic purposes combined with acceptable image repetition rate and maximum sensitivity for the detection of slow flow.

There are three different **types of probe**:

- The *linear probe* is characterised by the linear arrangement of the crystals which transmit parallel sound waves. This is a rectangular image format. This arrangement gives the best spatial resolution. However, the width of the image is limited by the length of the probe. A linear probe is especially suitable for showing tissue in its close vicinity (Fig. 1.11a, b).
- A technical variant of the linear probe is the virtual convex configuration. The outer elements of this probe can be deflected allowing an increase of approximately 20 % in image size (Fig. 1.11b).

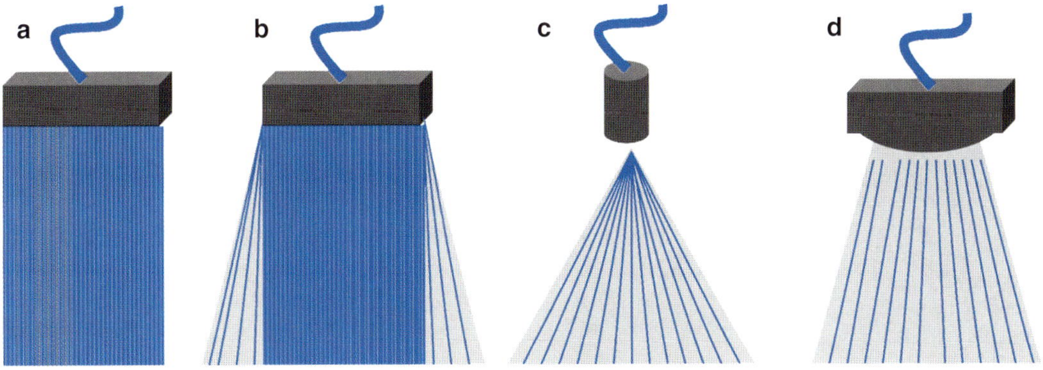

Fig. 1.11 Probes. (**a**) Linear probe. (**b**) "Virtual" curved array. (**c**) Sector probe. (**d**) Curved array Copyright: [Author]

- In small contact areas the *sector probe* transmits sound waves radially which emanate from a point (Fig. 1.11c) thus achieving maximum image width at depth. The principal disadvantage is its poor spatial resolution especially at greater depth. This probe is especially suitable for cardiac imaging.
- The *curved array* is a linear probe with a convex shape (Fig. 1.11d). Its imaging properties make it a compromise between linear and sector probes. It is particularly suitable for ultrasound of the abdomen and deep leg veins. Single flow direction usually gives a composite image of blue and red. This is because straight flow can be both towards one end of the probe and away from the other end.

As venous flows need to be shown sufficiently accurately both in the superficial region and at depth behind thick layers of muscle, it is a good idea to have a wide range of probes available. A high-frequency linear probe is ideal for superficial vessels (5–10 MHz) with a low-frequency linear probe or curved array for the deep leg veins (3.5–5 MHz).

1.3 Technical Developments

1.3.1 Tissue Harmonic Imaging

Sound waves are propagated in a medium by molecular compression and decompression. This fluctuation in pressure also has the effect of compressing and decompressing the tissue itself. The speed of sound depends on the density of the tissues. This is subject to periodic alteration because the sound causes a transient state of compression. The speed of sound accelerates in compressed tissues, and it is correspondingly slower in decompressed tissues (Fig. 1.12).

On the receive side, the echo separates into two frequency components. These are termed the **fundamental frequency** (f_0) and the **harmonic frequency** ($2f_0$), which is twice the basic frequency (Fig. 1.12) and is produced by the tissue itself. The magnitude of the compression or decompression depends on the acoustic (mechanical) properties of tissue. Modern transducers have a sufficient bandwidth capable of a transmission of 2 MHz which allows a harmonic frequency of 4 MHz to be received.

Harmonic frequencies can be detected in all solid tissues but not in fluids like cysts or blood. The energy of the harmonic frequencies is always lower than the fundamental. While the transmitted sound wave is weakened twice as it travels through the tissue and back, the harmonic sound wave is weakened only once on its single journey because it arises from the tissue. An image which is generated using only the reception of the harmonic frequency is therefore known as **tissue harmonic imaging** (THI) (Simpson et al. 1999).

The image is richer in contrast and cystic volumes are shown more clearly thanks to the elimination of disturbance echoes.

1.3.2 Compound Scanning

This technique reduces image artefacts and thus helps to improve B scan quality. Every image

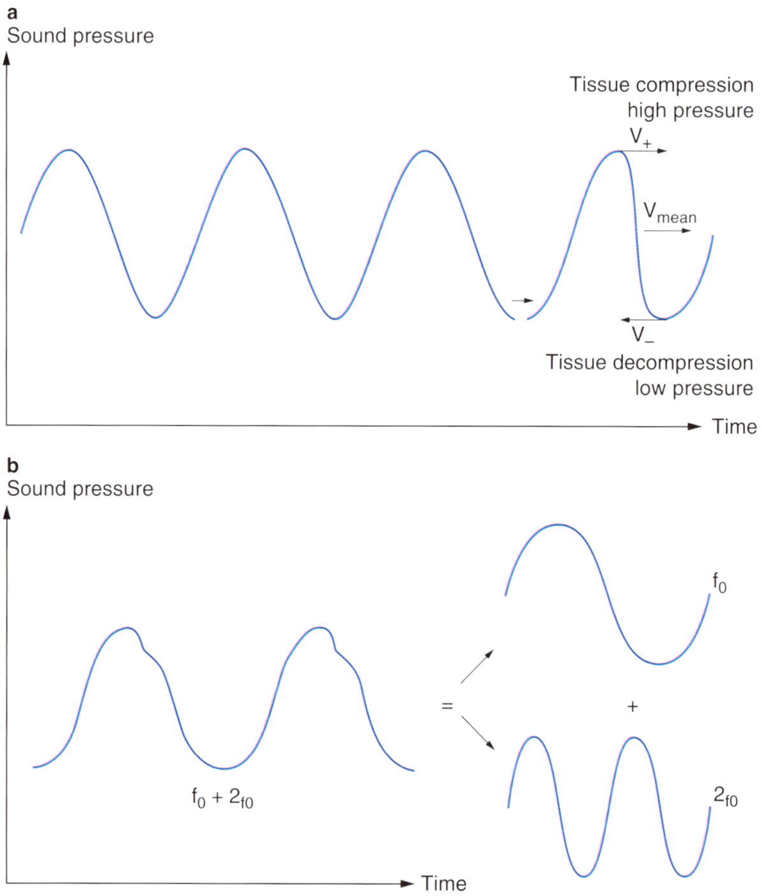

Fig. 1.12 (**a**) In compressed tissue the speed of sound accelerates. In decompressed tissue it decelerates. V_+ Relative acceleration, V_- relative deceleration, V_{mean} mean speed. (**b**) Composite sound wave reflected out of the tissue. The wave breaks down into a fundamental frequency (f_0) and a harmonic frequency ($2f_0$) Copyright: [Author]

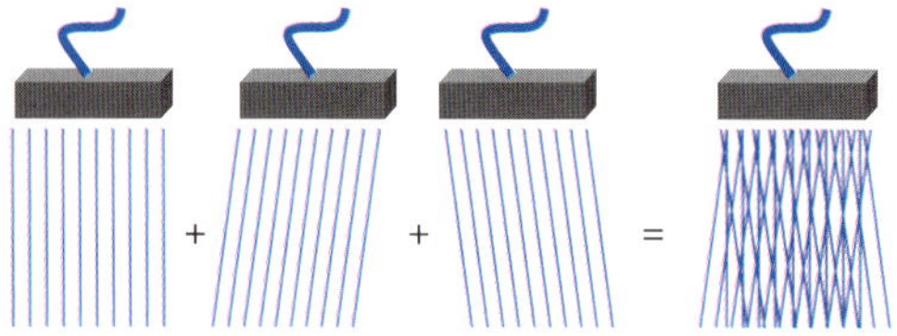

Fig. 1.13 Compound scan using cross beams. The information from 3 to 9 individual images is taken at different angles and matched to create a compound image Copyright: [Author]

point in the echo field is insonated from several angles. The echoes from an image point are then matched together. Discrepant information is interpreted as artefacts and deleted. Only identical data are accepted for image generation (Fig. 1.13). Numerous noise or reflection artefacts, as sketched in Fig. 1.3d, should be reduced by this technique.

The disadvantage of the technique is the extensive elimination of artefacts which may be helpful for diagnosis, such as acoustic shadows behind small calcifications.

1.3.3 Transmission Frequency Coding

Transmission of coded frequencies helps to optimise image quality and reduce artefact, especially with low amplitude signals. In Coded Excitation Mode, frequencies are transmitted into the tissue in coded form called digital frequency coding. The transmission frequency is coded by changing the polarity or the time lapse between individual pulses (Tranquart et al. 1999).

When the reflected echoes are received, only those which correspond to the mirror image of

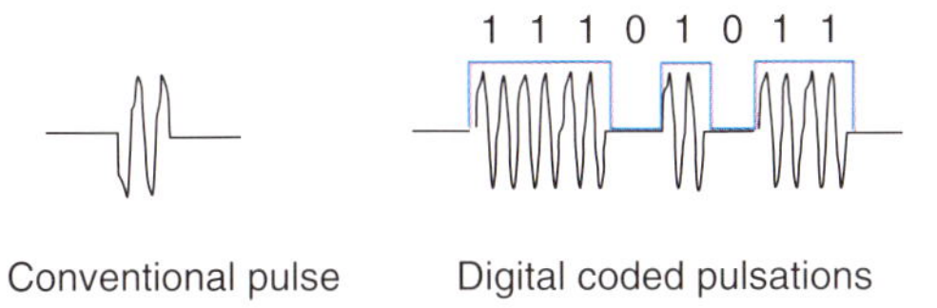

Fig. 1.14 Transmission frequency coding. If the frequency transmission is coded by pauses and phase-inverted pulses, this coding is recognised in the echoes received and all other noise signals can be eliminated Copyright: [Author]

the transmission code are used for image construction. This is similar to a cash register in a supermarket recognising a bar code. The bar code reader validates the received frequency by comparing the received frequencies of the reversed bar code with the bar code. Only the recognised echo signals have the right frequency and are used for image generation. Any echoes which are not correctly coded are recognised as artefacts and eliminated (Fig. 1.14).

1.3.4 B Flow

For a long time, only Doppler based techniques like power and colour Doppler were available for imaging blood flow in real time fashion. Both image blood flow indirectly by the detection of acoustic scatter from the movement of blood corpuscles.

The B flow technique has been available since early 1999 and detects echoes reflected of blood particles. In B flow, the echo amplitudes of two to four sound pulses, transmitted at a short interval, are subtracted from one another. This allows stationary echoes to be distinguished from moving echoes.

As with power Doppler, B flow demonstrates the amplitude of the moving reflectors but is unable to measure their velocity or direction of flow. The flowing blood is shown as a light grey, moving, reflective cloud.

The advantages are relative independence of the angle of insonation and the absence of overvisualisation of vessel boundaries or small thrombi due to the blooming effect which occurs with colour duplex (Fig. 1.15).

1.3.5 Panoramic Imaging

This is also known as extended field-of-view imaging. With this technique the probe is moved at a constant speed in the direction of its longitudinal axis over a long segment. The moving image information is added together to produce an overview or panoramic image (Fig. 1.16).

The advantage of this technique is that it provides a better overview of an anatomical region.

1.3.6 Three-Dimensional Ultrasound

Large amounts of data can be acquired when a 3-D probe is moved over an area of tissue at a regular speed. This data can be reconstructed to produce a three-dimensional image. This allows sections of varying depths and angles to be visualised, which is not jet possible in a real time fashion. The section level parallel to the skin surface is called a **C level**.

In this way, oedemas, scars and their relationship to neighbouring structures can be shown more clearly (Fig. 1.17).

1.3.7 Contrast-Enhanced Ultrasound (CEUS)

Air is much more reflective than soft tissue or fluid. This is the principle of using air as a contrast medium which is based on the interaction between sound and air bubbles (Fig. 1.18a). Ultrasound contrast media consist of tiny bubbles of air or gas which are one-third of the size of an erythrocyte. These can pass through capillary beds and are not dangerous to the tissues (Weskott 2000). The bubbles are surrounded by a flexible coating in order to stabilise them and prevent them from coalescing into larger bubbles. They act as sound wave reflectors with echoes significantly stronger than blood or tissue.

When contrast microbubbles are injected into peripheral veins, they can be used for diagnosis for several minutes. The bubbles are very fragile

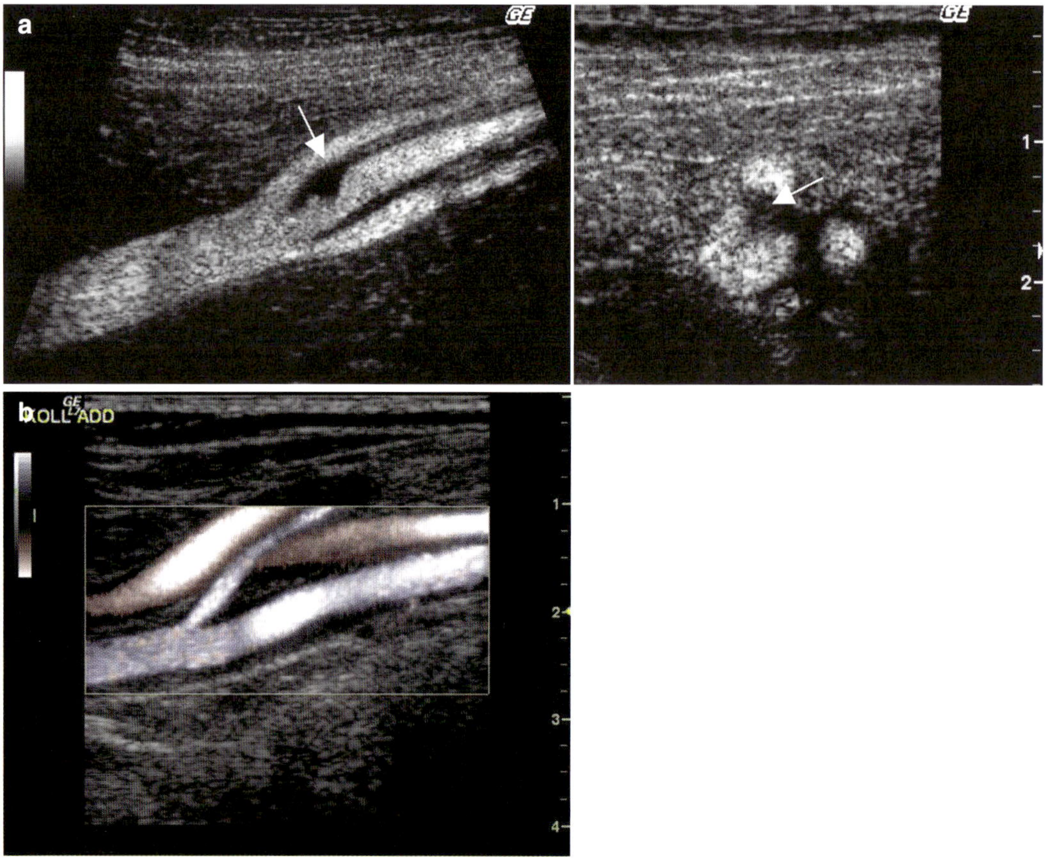

Fig. 1.15 B flow. (**a**) *Left*: longitudinal section through the popliteal fossa demonstrating the formation of the popliteal vein from the calf veins. *Right*: transverse view. In both longitudinal and transverse views, a small filling defect is seen resulting from a thrombus (*arrowed*). This could not be seen in colour Doppler due to blooming artefacts. (**b**) B flow with added colour coding for flow direction. The colour bar indicates that *red* is away from the probe and *blue* is towards Copyright: [Author]

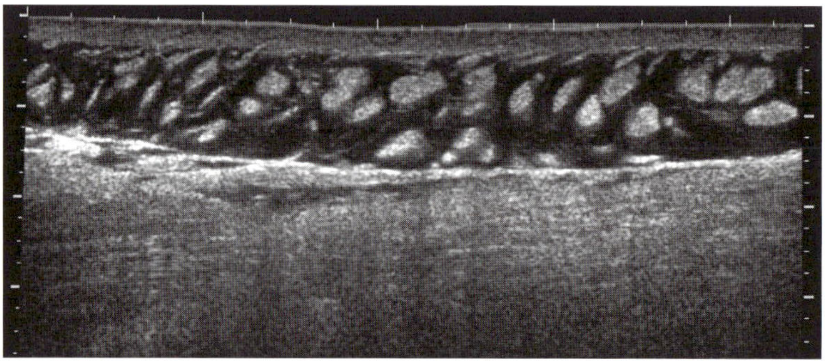

Fig. 1.16 Panoramic image over a length of 22 cm. Longitudinal view through the thigh in a patient with lymphoedema Copyright: [Author]

so they must be imaged using a weak acoustic transmission setting. However, the ultrasound scanner has a microbubble-friendly transmission mode called **pulse inversion** (Wilson et al. 2009).

Ultrasound contrast media increase the signal strength of flowing and stationary bubbles in organs and in the lumen of abdominal and peripheral vessels. Their greatest clinical value in venous diseases lies in the improved imaging of

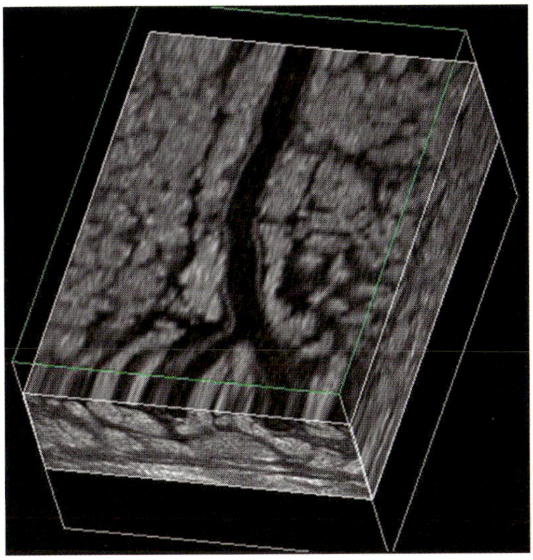

Fig. 1.17 Three-dimensional image of lymphoedema with a vein passing through it at C level. This level is parallel to the skin surface Copyright: [Author]

flow in deep veins to exclude thrombosis and in differentiating tumor thrombi from clots (Fig. 1.18b, c).

1.4 Choice of Scanner and Transducer

The selection of the correct ultrasound machine is an important decision in the planning of a vascular practice. The detection of deep vein thrombosis is especially important as well as increasing the diagnostic possibilities of venous pathology. In hospitals a good machine is usually available and it is only a question of deciding upon a suitable probe (see below). All the duplex scanners sold by current companies are suitable for use on veins and are now at affordable prices. However, if a better resolution and a higher image quality

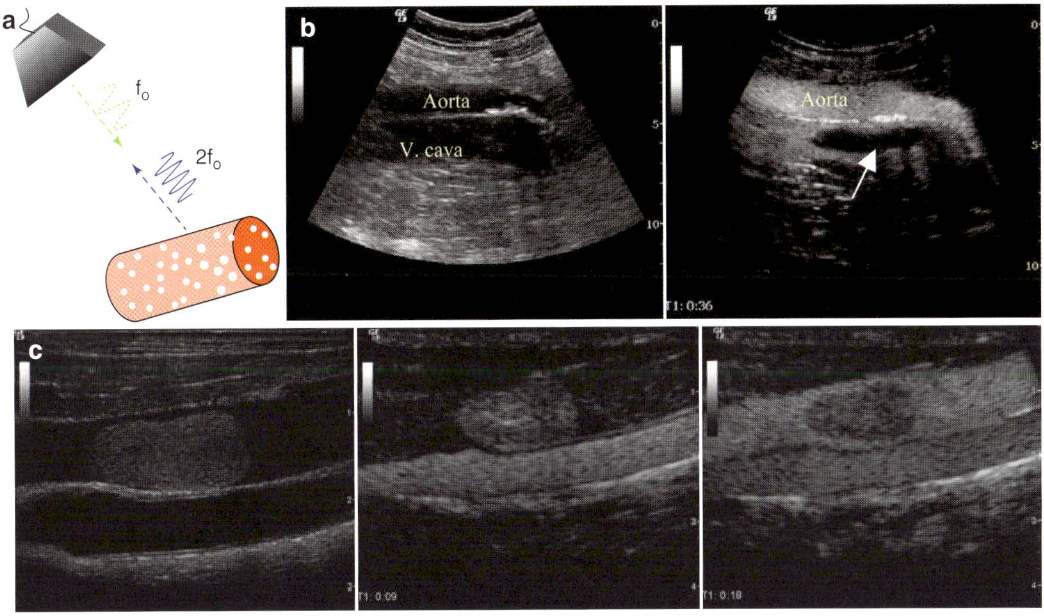

Fig. 1.18 Contrast-enhanced ultrasound (CEUS). (**a**) The principle is a low-energy insonation of a sound wave (f_0) to start a resonance vibration in the bubbles. This then generates harmonic frequencies. The second harmonic frequency ($2f_0$) is used in the image construction. The low sound intensity emitted from the B scan is too poor to provide tissue information which increases the relative visualisation of the vessels containing the microbubbles. (**b**) Thrombus in the inferior vena cava not visible in B scan (*left*). After administration of contrast (*right*), it can be recognised as a thrombus with surrounding flow. The contrast does not enter the thrombus (*Arrow*). (**c**) *Left*: thrombus in the internal jugular vein. *Middle*: 9 s after administration of i.v. contrast, it appears in the common carotid artery. The signal from the thrombus is strengthened by a supply from the carotid. This is typical behaviour of a vascular tumour. *Right*: after 17 s the contrast medium fills the internal jugular vein whilst it has been largely washed out of the tumour. This patient had a neoplastic thrombus from a thyroid metastasis of a renal cell carcinoma Copyright: [Author]

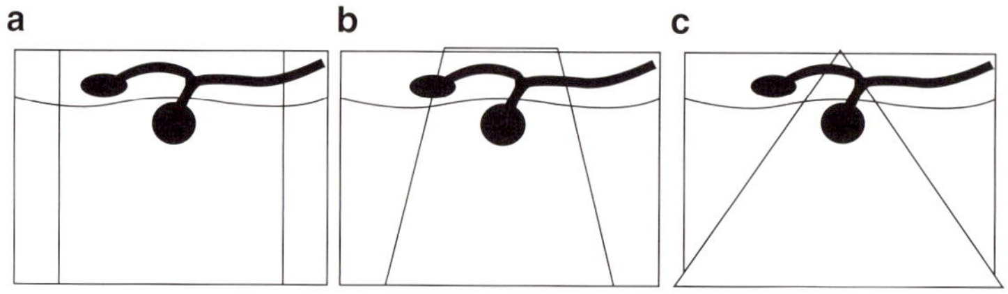

Fig. 1.19 Diagram of a subcutaneous vein with a tributary. The field projected by the B scan from top to bottom is shaded *grey* and the veins are shown in *black*. (**a**) The linear probe demonstrates the entire vein. (**b**) The curved array probe conceals the left and right parts. (**c**) A sector probe narrows the field further and confines the view to the central region (From Mendoza E (2002) Handbuch CHIVA. Arrien, Wunstorf; by kind permission of Arrien GmbH) Copyright: Arrien, Wunstorf

are required, the capital investment is much greater.

High-end machines offering even better resolution with all the new imaging modalities described above are not necessary for most practices. They are reserved for hospitals and specialist centres.

Make sure the scanner provides good resolution in the near field in **B scan**. It is important to be able to distinguish structures without difficulty from only 1–2 mm under the skin. The machine must provide adequate resolution in B scan, so that even healthy perforating veins like the thigh perforating veins can be seen.

Almost all the duplex machines offered for sale have the colour Doppler option. However, the alternative of purchasing a second-hand **black-and-white machine** would be very tedious. The examination is more time-consuming than with a machine which has colour-coded duplex. Furthermore, visualisation of perforating veins and the saphenofemoral tributaries in the groin is hindered by a lack of colour coding.

Some machines are offered for sale with only a colour-coded duplex facility. However, **PW mode** is indispensable for examining veins making these machines unsuitable for this task. Recording in PW mode can be carried out in either frozen or moving B scan. The advantage of recording in frozen B scan is the better time resolution of the frequency spectrum. The advantage of active B scan is the continuous control of the location of the sample volume. Modern devices do not lose PW quality when recording simultaneously with B scan.

Ideally the machine should also include an 8 MHz **CW probe**. The **Doppler pen-probe** in addition helps to investigate very superficial tributaries.

In **colour mode**, the image in B scan is usually displayed on a window which covers an area of approximately 1.5 by 2 cm. This must not be slowed down when a colour window is used. Movements generated by the examination can be filtered out, so a sea of colour does not flood the image every time the probe moves. If the probe is moved, the flow should be visible only in the vein without colour artefact in the surrounding tissue. However, slow flows may be missed if the filter setting is too high.

A **7.5 MHz probe** is indispensable for examining the superficial veins. Today probe frequencies are adjustable so the ideal range to include all possibilities should be 6–8 MHz. The probe achieves its highest resolution at the centre of this range. A linear probe is best because the near field is the commonest requirement of the examination. Curved array or convex probes are poor at demonstrating veins which appear blurred or absent (Fig. 1.19a–c).

The **3.5 MHz probe** is ideal for examining deep leg veins in obese subjects and for examining the iliac and caval veins. The use of a **5 MHz probe** is a poor compromise because it is inadequate for deep veins or subcutaneous tributaries.

The high-resolution ability of a **10 MHz probe** is not essential for varicose veins. Veins which can only be seen using this probe and are missed with a 7.5 MHz probe are too small to cause significant pathology.

Interestingly, some insurance companies have a list of machines/probes which they will only recognise for reimbursement purposes. It is advisable to check on this before investing in duplex equipment.

1.5 Choice of Examination Mode

The commonest modes in the examination of superficial leg veins are **B scan**, **pulsed wave duplex** (**PW**) and **colour duplex**. The other options described, using high-end machines, are unnecessary for a routine assessment. B flow or power duplex mode may be helpful in revealing a very slow flow. However, these flows should also be recognisable in PW mode. The advantage of B flow and power duplex is in recognising slow flows in deeply situated veins.

The morphology and compressibility of veins are examined in B scan and blood flow overview and direction in colour duplex, and a detailed assessment of individual vessels is examined in PW mode.

Colour coding allows a good, rapid overview of the course of the vein and its blood flow and direction. Colour is especially helpful for detecting deep veins in the calf. Aliasing must be taken into account during stimulation manoeuvres and in the presence of fast reflux because it often gives the misleading impression of coexisting reflux and antegrade flow. The setting should remain for the detection of slow reflux with the operator ignoring fast velocity artefacts caused by aliasing. This strategy avoids having to alter the pulse repetition frequency (PRF) constantly.

Unfortunately colour coding has its limitations and false-negative results may occur. If the filter is set too high in order to exclude surrounding movement artefacts, slow blood flows may be masked (Sect. 1.6). If there is turbulence or aliasing in the perforating veins, it may be difficult to obtain a clear flow direction using colour. Furthermore, colour is totally unsuitable for measuring and documenting the reflux volume in a vein. Differentiating between drained and poorly drained systems is also impossible using colour duplex (Sect. 3.2.3).

The diagram in Fig. 1.20 shows the flow curve as it appears in colour and PW duplex in three different drainage conditions. In an undrained system (Fig. 1.20d), the selection choice of PW mode is decisive because it can detect very slow reflux. Otherwise the examination in morphological terms may be unremarkable because these veins do not appear significantly dilated either externally or in B scan.

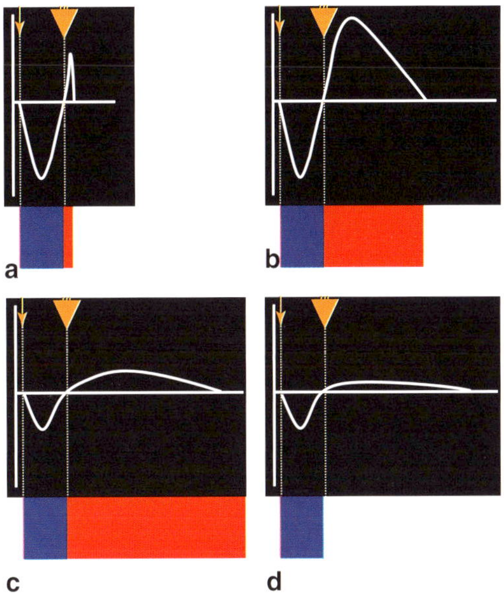

Fig. 1.20 Schematic diagram of the flow curve in a superficial leg vein. The PW duplex is shown above on the black background. The colour mode is paralleled below this result. The first thin arrow corresponds to the moment the toes are raised. The second broader arrow corresponds to their relaxation. (**a**) Flow in a healthy vein is antegrade when the toes are raised and retrograde until the valves close. (**b**) Flow in a well-drained refluxive vein has a sharp rise to the reflux which ends relatively quickly. (**c**) Flow in a poorly drained refluxive vein has a slower, long-lasting reflux. (**d**) Flow in an undrained refluxive vein has a very slow reverse flow which does not register in colour mode (From Mendoza (2002); by kind permission of Arrien GmbH) Copyright: Arrien, Wunstorf

1.6 Configuring the Ultrasound Scanner

New machines leave the factory with a standard preset configuration. The ideal settings for superficial veins have been preprogrammed by the manufacturer. These include the penetration depth, gain (in B scan and duplex), contrast, PRF, filter and blood flow measurement window size. These settings can be altered and saved into a profile according to the user's personal preferences.

Each parameter has an optimum setting. If these settings are changed, it may take up more of the working memory used for generating the image. With several changes, the end result is that this can make image generation so slow that real-time ultrasound is no longer possible. Therefore, the optimal overall configuration is a compromise between the benefits of a parameter adjustment against the image generation speed. This is less applicable to modern machines with faster processors and more memory.

The optimal setting is when the veins are shown in black in **B scan** and that the fascias in the subcutaneous tissue stand out as white against their surroundings. In high-resolution machines, erythrocytes can be identified in the vein. This means that the lumen is not completely black but contains tiny, bright, moving elements. The scale of greys (gain) can be adjusted with sliding controls on the machine for individual areas and with the B scan knob for the whole image.

The **penetration depth** of the sound pulse sometimes needs to be altered. This depends on the region examined (thigh or calf) and the thickness of the fat layer. Ideally, the great saphenous vein should lie in the central area of the image in the thigh. In the lower leg, a penetration depth of 3–4 cm is generally sufficient.

The **focus** must be set with particular care. The narrower the focus, the greater the resources of the machine are used up in the calculation leaving them less available for other tasks. The optimal adjustment is to set the focus at the depth of the vein under examination or a little deeper to allow perforating veins to be seen clearly.

The **measurement window** in **PW duplex** must be adjusted to the diameter of the vein. It should not be any bigger than the vein; otherwise, a large number of artefacts will be shown. In dilated, refluxive veins, it can be set significantly smaller than the diameter and does not always have to be adjusted.

The **colour window** selected must not be too big; otherwise, colour recognition will be slow. In the groin a window big enough to show the deep veins and the saphenofemoral junction in colour is sufficient. The smaller the window, the faster the computer can generate the image.

Since the flow velocity in the veins is slower than the arteries, the **PRF** must be set lower. The value is normally found at the edge of the image near the colour scale. It is displayed indirectly as a flow velocity and not as a direct PRF value. The optimum for veins is between 5 and 15 cm/s.

The **filter** is an important instrument for eliminating artefacts created by the vein wall and the tissue from the flow curve. The filter simply eliminates very slow flow velocities from the analysis. It is especially difficult to adjust the filter when working in colour duplex. This is because the system recognises the movement of the probe along the leg as flow. If the probe is moved along the vein in colour mode, the surrounding tissue will flicker with colour. This colour signal can be eliminated by the filter. However, if the filter is set too high, slow flows may be missed (Fig. 1.21).

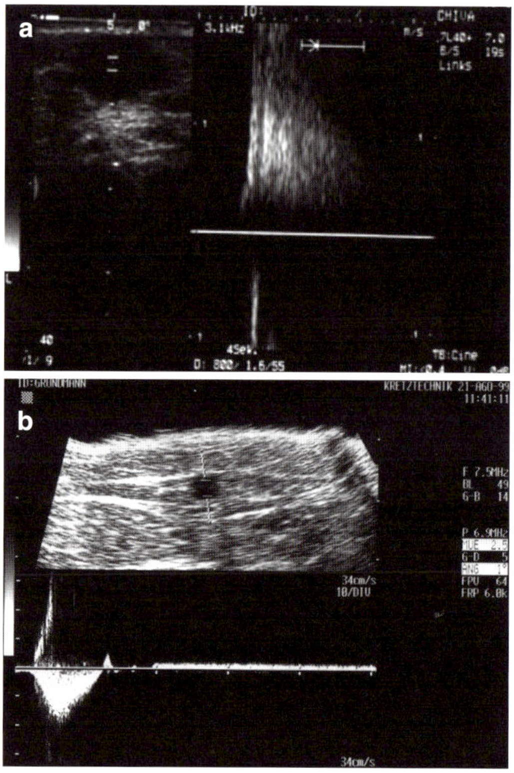

Fig. 1.21 (**a**) PW scan of a refluxive vein in the leg in transverse view. The filter is set high and there is no signal present around the zero line. (**b**) Very slow refluxive flow demonstrated in the great saphenous vein. If the filter was set slightly higher, this flow would be missed Copyright: [Author]

References

Lamboul B, Bennett MJ, Anderson T, McDicken NW (2009) Basic considerations in the use of coded excitation for color flow imaging applications. IEEE Trans Ultrason Ferroelectr Freq Control 56(4): 727–737

McDicken WN, Anderson T (2002) The difference between colour Doppler velocity imaging and power Doppler imaging. Eur J Echocardiogr 3(3):240–244

Simpson DH, Chin CT, Burns PN (1999) Pulse inversion Doppler: a new method for detecting nonlinear echoes from microbubble contrast agents. IEEE Trans Ultrason Ferroelectr Freq Control 46(2):372–382

Tranquart F, Grenier N, Eder V, Pourcelot L (1999) Clinical use of ultrasound tissue harmonic imaging. Ultrasound Med Biol 25(6):889–894

Weskott HP (2000) B-flow – a new method for detecting blood flow. Ultraschall Med 21:59–65

Wilson SR, Greenbaum LD, Goldberg BB (2009) Contrast-enhanced ultrasound: what is the evidence and what are the obstacles? AJR Am J Roentgenol 193(1):55–60

Wu CY, Lo MT, Tsao J, Chu A, Chou YH, Tiu CM (2004) Factor analysis in both spatial and temporal domains of color blooming artifacts in ultrasound investigations utilizing contrast agents. Comput Med Imaging Graph 28(3):129–140

Anatomy of the Superficial Veins

2

Alberto Caggiati, Erika Mendoza,
Renate Murena-Schmidt,
and Christopher R. Lattimer

Chapter Summary
Veins arise from capillaries and transport blood away from the tissues towards the heart. In contrast to arteries which divide into smaller parts, veins form a network which merges repeatedly to form larger veins. They are named according to their calibre and position as venous capillaries, venules, tributaries and saphenous trunks.

A. Caggiati, MD (✉)
Department of Anatomy, Universita di Roma,
Via Borelli, 50, 00161 Rome, Italy
e-mail: alberto.caggiati@uniroma1.it

E. Mendoza, MD, PhD
Venenpraxis Wunstorf,
Speckenstraße 10, 31515 Wunstorf, Germany
e-mail: erika.mendoza@t-online.de

R. Murena-Schmidt, MD
Praxis für Gefäßerkrankungen,
Hansaring 102-104, 50670 Köln, Germany
e-mail: renate.murena@netcologne.de

C.R. Lattimer, MD, PhD
Department of Vascular Surgery,
Josef Pflug Vascular Laboratory,
Ealing Hospital and Imperial College, London, UK

2.1 General Appearance and Nomenclature

The venous system has two functionally distinct parts. The first is the **superficial** or **epifascial system** which courses under the skin and is responsible for carrying the blood away from the subcutaneous tissue. The second is the **deep or subfascial system** which is responsible for draining the muscles and bones. These two systems are separated anatomically by the muscle fascia. The veins between the muscle and the skin are assigned to the superficial system and all those inside the muscles to the deep system.

Whilst the arterial system resembles a tree with a trunk (arteries) which divides into branches (arterioles) down to the smallest twig (arterial capillaries), veins resemble an interconnecting drainage network. All the segments are interlinked with several communications between venules, tributaries and saphenous veins which form numerous connections between the superficial and deep veins.

In the superficial venous system, blood is carried from the capillaries and venules which drain into tributaries, arch veins or, according to international terminology, accessory saphenous veins. These deliver blood into the great and small saphenous veins or directly into the deep veins through perforating veins. The great and small saphenous veins also drain into the deep veins through various perforating veins along their length or through their junctions. These are called the saphenofemoral junction at the groin

E. Mendoza et al. (eds.), *Duplex Ultrasound of Superficial Leg Veins*,
DOI 10.1007/978-3-642-40731-4_2, © Springer-Verlag Berlin Heidelberg 2014

and the saphenopopliteal junction in the popliteal fossa. The deep venous system drains the leg.

Venules and smaller tributaries form a network under the skin. The connections between these smaller tributaries are very variable in location. Consequently, they do not have anatomical names. In health, they are invisible to the naked eye, but on ultrasound, they can be demonstrated using a high-resolution probe. They can only be seen through the skin when they are pathologically filled. The anatomy-based consensus document has divided them into *tributaries* (over 3 mm diameter) and *reticular veins* (less than 3 mm diameter) (Caggiati et al. 2002). Reticular veins have a profile and are palpable, whereas thread veins or telangiectasia are only visible. Usually, epifascial veins of the medial part of the thigh and leg and the dorsal part of the calf drain into the great and small saphenous veins, respectively, and are therefore called tributaries of these veins. The epifascial veins of the lateral aspect of the leg have no major vein to drain in and are called lateral plexus of the leg (Caggiati et al. 2002).

The veins of the leg, in comparison to other veins, must carry blood against gravity and overcome a height of up to 1.5 m. To help this process, the largest veins have valves. These are wings of intraluminal connecting tissue which are anchored to the vein wall and look like a swallow's nest (Fig. 2.1).

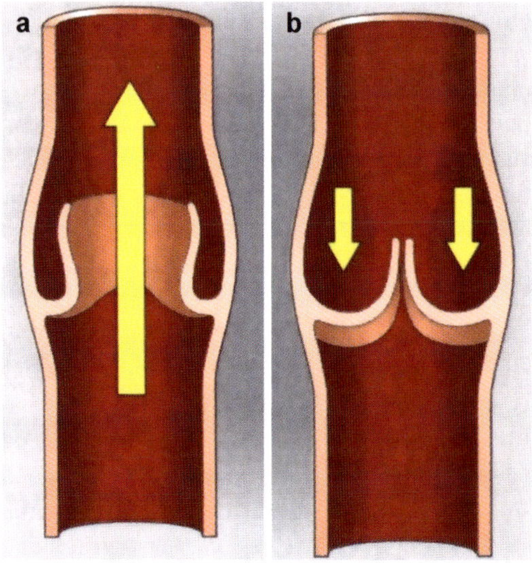

Fig. 2.1 The venous valves in the leg. (**a**) With upward flow, the valve opens. (**b**) When there is return flow, the blood flows back into the "swallow's nest" (*small arrows*) and closes the valve Copyright: [Author]

The nomenclature used follows international convention. The saphenous trunks are the "great saphenous vein" (GSV) (Latin: *V. saphena magna*) and the "small saphenous vein" (SSV) (Latin: *V. saphena parva*). In international use, the **accessory veins** are called anterior (formerly lateral), superficial and posterior (formerly medial) accessory saphenous veins (Caggiati et al. 2002).

This chapter describes the anatomy of the superficial veins (Askar 1963; Dodd and Cockett 1976; Bergan 1999; Caggiati and Mendoza 2004; Cavezzi et al. 2006; Kubik 1985 in Appendix 2). To avoid duplication, anatomical variants important for diagnosis will be discussed in the relevant chapters. The deep venous system is described in Chap. 14.

2.2 The Fascial Compartment of the Saphenous Veins

In addition to the **subfascial** and **epifascial** veins, the perforating veins are described as **transfascial**. The muscle fascia or deep fascia is regarded as the border. According to this description, all the veins which lie between the muscle fascia and the dermis are called superficial with no further differentiation. However, the great saphenous vein, small saphenous vein and the proximal section of the accessory saphenous veins run in their own intermediate fascial compartment with the tributaries remaining truly epifascial.

2.2.1 Membranous Layer

The subcutaneous tissue is constructed around a skeleton of connective tissue, which is filled with fat (Fig. 2.2). On ultrasound, this connective tissue is visible as white, echogenic layers which blend irregularly into the grey fat tissue in widely differing patterns (Fig. 2.3a). In the deeper zone of the subcutaneous tissue, the connective tissue fibres thicken to form a membrane which usually lies directly on the muscle fascia. This is called the membranous layer or pseudofascia. This membranous layer is not a duplication of the **muscle fascia** as described in the anatomy book by Tillaux in 1897, because their embryological origin is differ-

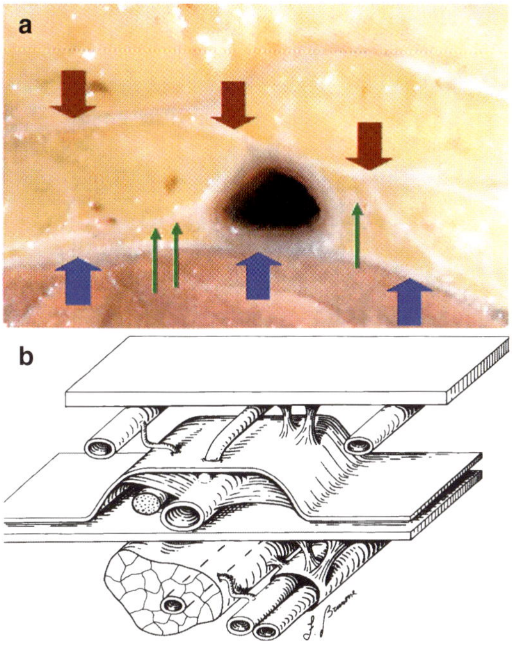

Fig. 2.2 (**a**) Section through the thigh in an anatomical preparation demonstrating layers of connective tissue separating cushions of fat around the great saphenous vein. (**b**) Sketch depicting the anatomical section with the muscle fascia and immediately above it the great saphenous vein in the fascial compartment. A connecting tributary is seen in the subcutaneous fatty tissue (Prof. A. Caggiati, Rome; by kind permission) Copyright: A. Caggiati, Rome

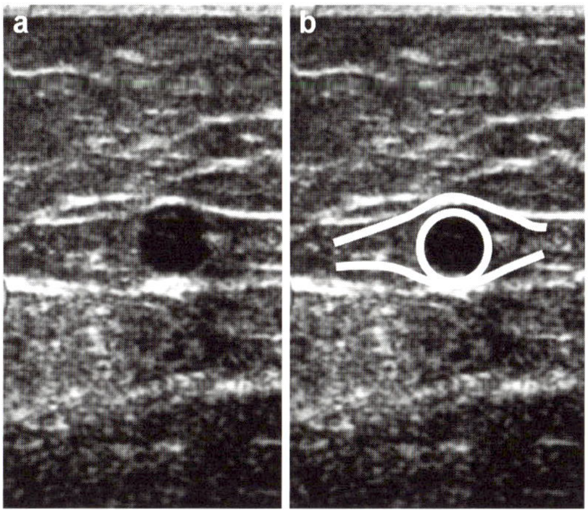

Fig. 2.3 (**a**) Transverse view through the thigh showing the great saphenous vein. (**b**) Overlay highlighting the "saphenous eye" where the upper lid is the saphenous fascia, the lower lid is the muscle fascia and the iris is the great saphenous vein. In the upper half of both images, the structure of the lax subcutaneous connective tissue can be seen as a white pattern in the grey fatty tissue Copyright: [Author]

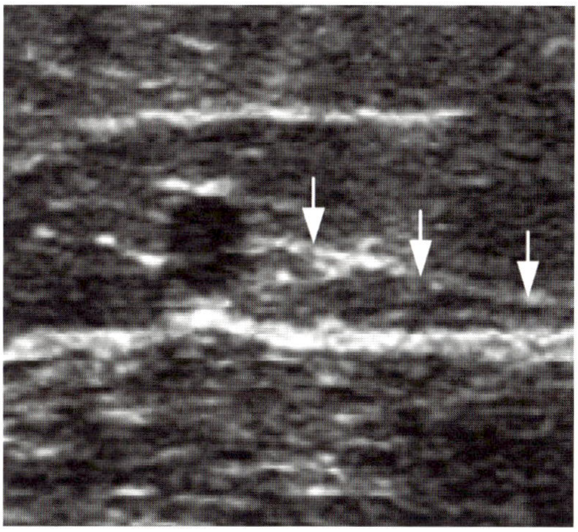

Fig. 2.4 Transverse view through the thigh in an obese patient showing the great saphenous vein within its fascial compartment surrounded by fat. The *arrow* demonstrates the saphenous ligament Copyright: [Author]

ent. Muscle fascia arises from the mesoderm, while the membranous layer arises from the ectoderm (Tillaux 1897 in Appendix 2).

The muscle fascia and the membranous layer form a structural unit of connective tissue separating the muscle from the subcutaneous fatty tissue. In some parts of the leg, the two fasciae separate to form a tunnel for the veins and their accompanying arteries, nerves and lymphatic vessels. This tunnel is called the **compartment** of the great and small saphenous veins. In the upper part of the leg, it also contains the accessory saphenous veins. Within the fascial compartment, there are varying amounts of fat cushioning the vein (Figs. 2.3 and 2.4). Fascial compartments are found surrounding the following structures within the leg:

- Great and small saphenous veins.
- Vein loops on the dorsum of foot connecting the great and small saphenous veins.
- Proximal section of the anterior accessory saphenous vein.
- Proximal section of the posterior accessory saphenous vein and occasionally along its entire course up to the confluence with the small saphenous vein.
- In the region of the greater trochanter, mentioned for completeness. The principal content in this compartment is fat and it is only surgically important in the context of liposuction.

The membranous layer along the saphenous veins is seen as a white layer on ultrasound and can be distinguished easily from the surrounding echo-poor fat and muscle fascia. The fascia enveloping the saphenous trunks is important as a landmark for diagnosis and treatment and has only recently been discovered by duplex ultrasound. The characteristic ultrasound image of the saphenous veins between the two fasciae led to the description of the saphenous eye (Bailly [1995]) (Fig. 2.3b).

2.2.2 Saphenous Compartment

The saphenous veins lie directly on the muscle fascia. At some point along their course, the membranous layer separates from the muscle fascia to form a cover over the vein. These fasciae form an enclosed volume called the "**saphenous compartment**" (Caggiati and Ricci 1999; Caggiati 2001). In lean legs, this saphenous compartment is limited and contains very little fat (Fig. 2.3). The saphenous veins are tightly enclosed. However, in legs swollen by lipoedema, the saphenous compartment appears enlarged and stretched on ultrasound (Fig. 2.4). Here, a layer of fat is usually seen separating the vein from its enveloping fascia.

The membranous layer along the course of the saphenous vein was given the name **saphenous fascia** and has since been adopted into anatomical nomenclature.

2.2.3 Anchoring of the Saphenous Veins

In transverse view, two echogenic connective tissue streaks are visible which appear to anchor both sides of the saphenous trunks. They connect the adventitia of the saphenous vein, run relatively parallel to the membranous layer and the muscle fascia and finally merge into them (*white arrows* in Fig. 2.4). This was confirmed by anatomical dissection where two layers of connective tissue were identified connecting the saphenous adventitia to the membranous layer and the muscle fascia (*green arrows* in Fig. 2.2). Using ultrasound, they are easier to see in the thigh for the great saphenous vein and in the upper calf for the small saphenous vein. Caggiati called them the "**saphenous ligament**" (Caggiati and Ricci 1999).

The envelopment of the saphenous veins by the saphenous compartment between the membranous layer and the muscle fascia and their anchorage by the saphenous ligament appear to be responsible for the lack of tortuosity observed when they become refluxive and dilated. This is in direct contrast to the behaviour of their refluxing tributaries.

2.3 The Foot Veins

For each toe, there are four veins, two dorsal and two ventral, which drain into the metatarsal veins. These in turn drain into the dorsal vein loop. The medial extension of this dorsal vein loop forms the origin of the great saphenous vein (Fig. 2.5), while

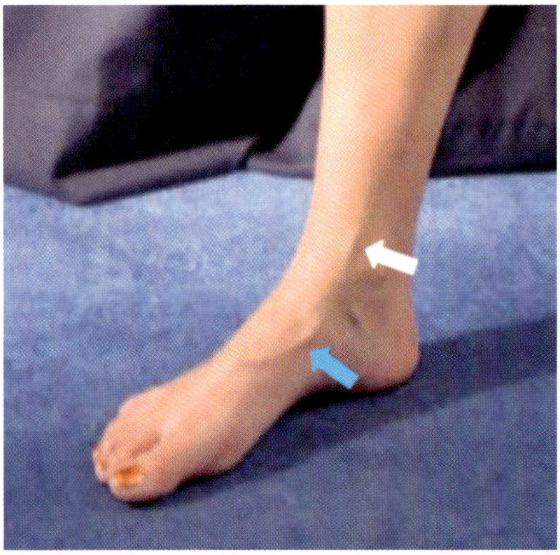

Fig. 2.5 The medial part of the dorsal vein loop of the right foot (*blue arrow*) and its junction with the great saphenous vein. It is visible in front of the medial malleolus (*white arrow*) Copyright: [Author]

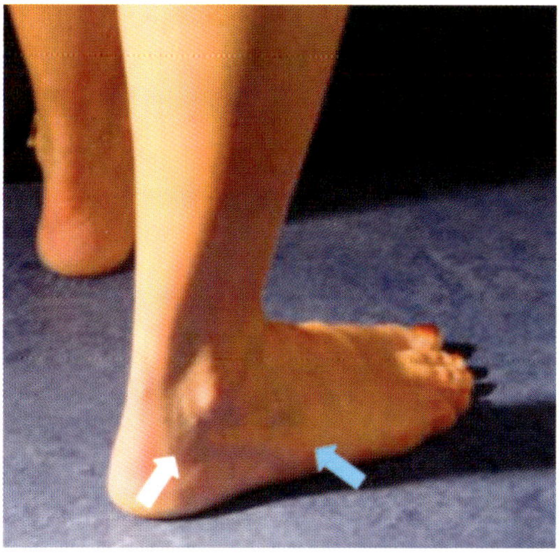

Fig. 2.6 The lateral part of the dorsal vein loop of the right foot (*blue arrow*) and its junction with the small saphenous vein. It is visible behind the lateral malleolus (*white arrow*) Copyright: [Author]

the lateral extension forms the small saphenous vein (Fig. 2.6). The two veins are therefore haemodynamically connected by this loop. The dorsal vein loop on the foot also receives the marginal veins which connect the ventral and dorsal foot veins on the instep and lateral side of the foot.

2.4 The Great Saphenous Vein

2.4.1 Course of the Great Saphenous Vein

The great saphenous vein is the longest vein in the body. It originates from the confluence of the dorsal foot veins on the medial side of the dorsal vein loop and runs consistently along the front of the medial malleolus where it can be seen or felt when standing (Fig. 2.5).

It continues medial to the edge of the tibia up to the knee. At first, it runs in a slightly posterior position, but at about a hand's-breadth below the knee, it curves further posterior behind the medial femoral condyle (Fig. 2.7).

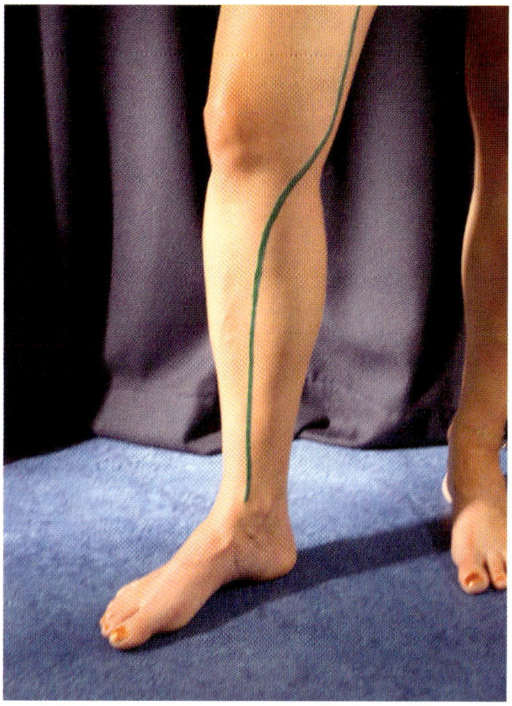

Fig. 2.7 Course of the great saphenous vein in right lower leg and knee Copyright: [Author]

In its course along the thigh, it returns to a more ventral position reaching the inner third of the groin where it drains into the femoral vein (Figs. 2.8 and 2.9). Throughout its course, it rests on the muscle or deep fascia. It lies deep to the arch of the saphenous fascia (Sect. 2.4.2).

At its upper end, the great saphenous vein drains into the common femoral vein at the **saphenofemoral junction**. Here, it curves down towards the deeper femoral vein where its path has been described as the "**crosse**" which is French for a bishop's crook. The junction is located in the groin and is always distal of the inguinal ligament (Fig. 2.10).

The **saphenofemoral junction** is the confluence of the great saphenous vein with the common femoral vein. As shown in Figs. 2.10 and 2.11, the "crosse" refers to the region of the saphenofemoral junction rather than the point of entry into the common femoral vein.

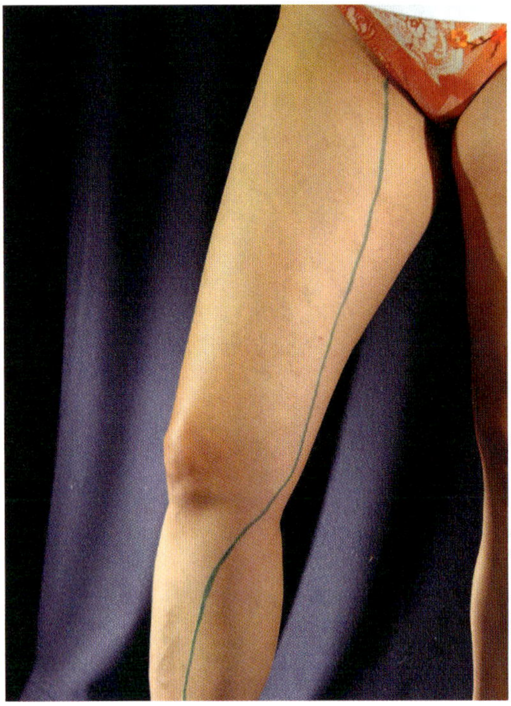

Fig. 2.8 Course of the great saphenous vein in the right thigh Copyright: [Author]

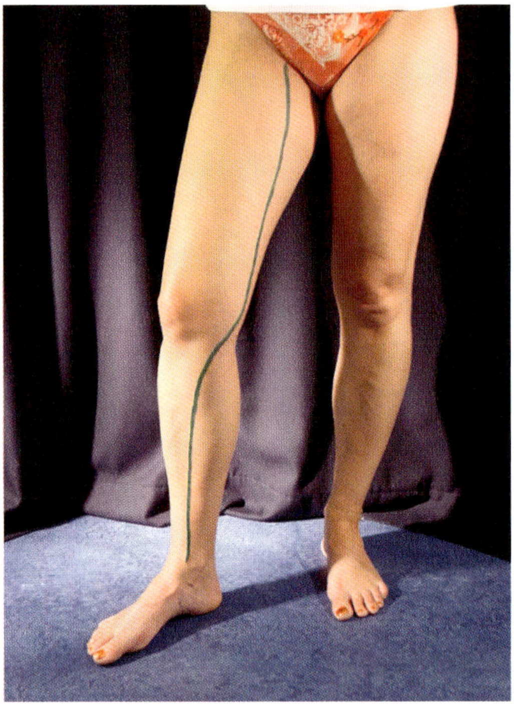

Fig. 2.9 Course of the great saphenous vein in the whole right leg Copyright: [Author]

The common femoral vein is a deep vein which runs below the deep fascia, while the great saphenous vein runs above the fascia. There is therefore an opening in the deep fascia, called the saphenous hiatus or oval foramen, through which the great saphenous vein passes immediately before it joins the deep vein. This saphenous hiatus allows the confluence of the great saphenous vein with the deep leg vein to be distinguished from confluences of other tributaries with the great saphenous vein when the saphenofemoral junction region is surgically exposed (Figs. 2.10 and 2.11).

A variable number of tributaries drain into the great saphenous vein in the groin, forming the **confluence of superficial inguinal veins**. Starting medial of the left great saphenous vein and going clockwise, these are the superficial external pudendal, superficial epigastric, superficial circumflex iliac, anterior accessory saphenous and posterior accessory saphenous veins (Figs. 2.10 and 2.11). The presence and form of the confluence of the individual veins are very variable and are described in more detail in Sect. 7.1.

In 88.5 % of cases, the great saphenous vein has a terminal valve in the region of its confluence. The distance of the terminal valve from the saphenofemoral junction varies between 0.0 and 1.4 cm. A preterminal valve is present in 89.2 % of cases, 1.4–8.2 cm from the saphenofemoral junction (in Mühlberger et al. 2009).

In the saphenofemoral junction region, the superficial external pudendal artery usually crosses the great saphenous vein from lateral to medial (Fig. 2.11).

2.4.2 Fascial Compartment of the Great Saphenous Vein

The membranous layer covers the great saphenous vein over its whole course, creating a tunnel from ankle to groin known as the

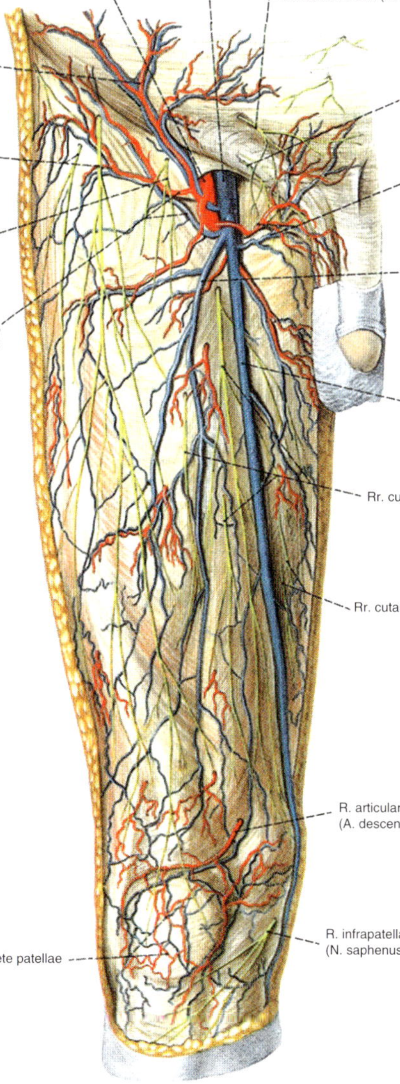

Fig. 2.10 Diagram of the saphenofemoral junction in the groin and its relation to the inguinal ligament. (*) Anterior accessoric saphenous vein. (**) Common femoral artery and vein. (With kind permission from Paulsen, Waschke, Sobotta Atlas der Anatomie des Menschen, 23. Auflage 2010 © Elsevier GmbH, Urban & Fischer, München)

saphenous compartment (Caggiati and Ricci 1999). In the distal part of the leg, the great saphenous vein is closely attached to both fasciae forming a compartment with a narrow tunnel. This broadens at the knee, and the distance over which the membranous layer is separated from the muscle fascia continues to broaden in the thigh (Figs. 2.12, 7.32 and 7.40). With normal amounts of fat, the great saphenous vein remains in constant contact with the two membranes. In this situation, the tunnel becomes broader with the corners of the eye further apart but the eye is no "wider open". The broadening continues to increase up to the inguinal

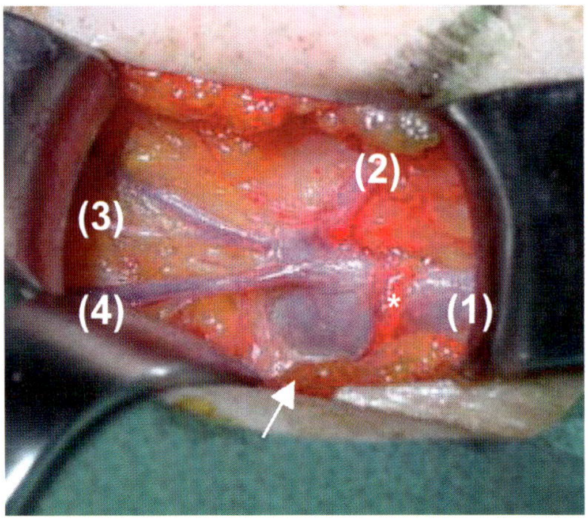

Fig. 2.11 Intra-operative picture of the saphenofemoral junction with the exposed saphenofemoral junction of the left leg (right = distal). The great saphenous vein (1) passes downwards through the saphenous hiatus (*black arrow*), a hole in the fascia, to join the common femoral vein. The region of the saphenofemoral junction contains the confluence of the anterior accessory saphenous vein (course marked on the skin in black *2*), as well as those of the superficial circumflex iliac (*3*) and superficial epigastric veins (*4*). Also in the saphenofemoral junction region, the external pudendal artery (*) crosses the great saphenous vein Copyright: [Author]

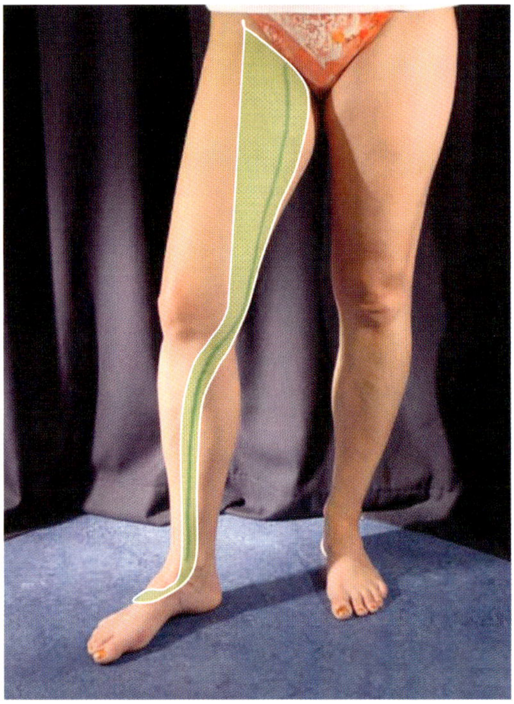

Fig. 2.12 The fascial compartment of the great saphenous vein. The course of the great saphenous vein is drawn on the inner side of the leg. The green hatching shows the width of the saphenous compartment starting on the dorsal foot. It is very narrow along the lower leg, grows broader in the thigh and ends at the inguinal ligament where the two fasciae (muscle fascia and saphenous fascia) are joined Copyright: [Author]

ligament, where the two membranes (membranous layer and muscle fascia) terminate, closing the upper end of the compartment.

In the knee region, the membranous layer is poorly defined. Using ultrasound, it appears to be composed of several layers which are loose and open in places. This disruption may result from the forces placed on the knee joint.

The saphenous fascia in an anatomical preparation can be seen in Fig. 2.13.

2.4.3 Duplication of the Great Saphenous Vein

From descriptions and from the histology of the veins in the saphenous compartment as compared with tributaries (Sect. 2.6), it may be concluded that only veins which course through the saphenous compartment really correspond to the great saphenous vein. Duplication of the great saphenous vein is therefore only present when both vessels course through the compartment (Fig. 2.14). Using this criterion, duplication of the great saphenous vein is only found in 1 % of patients (Table 2.1) (Ricci and Caggiati 1999). This is in contrast to the considerably higher figures published previously for duplication (27 %, Kubik 1985 in Appendix 2).

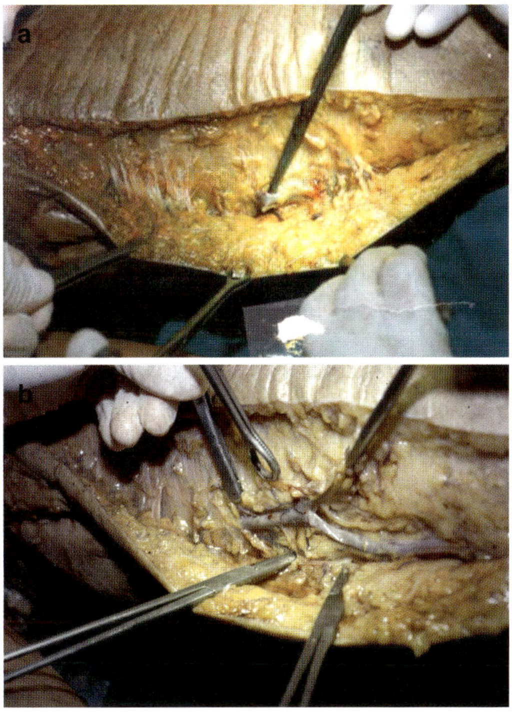

Fig. 2.13 The inner thigh of an anatomical preparation. (**a**) Inside of the left thigh where the skin and fat layers have been incised lengthwise and roughly separated from the saphenous fascia. The saphenous fascia has been opened at this point and the great saphenous vein lifted with a hook. (**b**) The saphenous fascia has been removed in the middle region revealing the great saphenous vein. To the left of the picture, the great saphenous vein disappears under the unopened tunnel of saphenous fascia (Prof. A. Caggiati, Rome; by kind permission) Copyright: A. Caggiati, Rome

Table 2.1 Classification of the courses of the great saphenous vein and its principal tributaries in the thigh as seen in ultrasound in 676 legs (Ricci and Caggiati 1999)

Type	Description	%
A	One longitudinal vein visible running through the saphenous compartment	52
B	Two longitudinal veins visible both in the saphenous compartment (true duplication)	1
C	Two longitudinal veins visible, the saphenous vein in the compartment and one parallel to this which joins the great saphenous vein proximally	26
D	Two longitudinal veins, one in the classic saphenous compartment and the other further ventral in the thigh, also in its own fascial eye. Proximally, these two saphenous eyes unite together	10
E	Aplastic/hypoplastic segment of the great saphenous vein. A large vein in the subcutaneous fatty tissue pierces the saphenous fascia somewhere in the thigh and then continues as the great saphenous vein proximally	11

True Duplication?

Epifascial, lengthwise tributaries can be distinguished clearly from saphenous veins by ultrasound. Ricci and Caggiati found these veins (superficial accessory veins) in 26 % of legs. They run parallel to the saphenous vein, but in the subcutaneous fatty tissue (Fig. 2.15). This is not duplication of the great saphenous vein. This

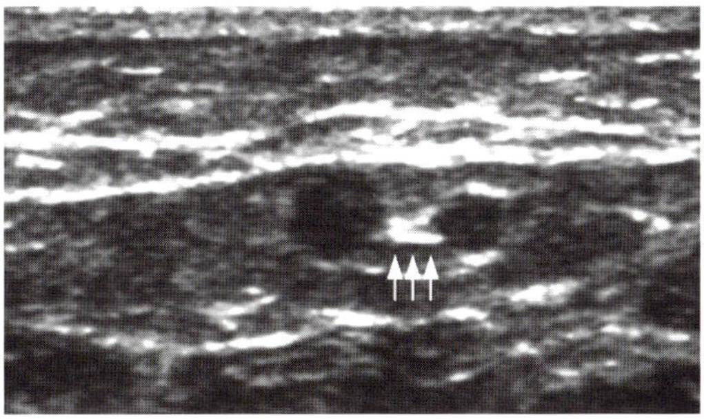

Fig. 2.14 Ultrasound view through the thigh showing a duplicated great saphenous vein. The two saphenous veins are bound together by the saphenous ligament (*arrowed*). It may be noted that the "eye" here is very wide; the corners are not visible in the transverse image because it is taken quite high up the thigh Copyright: [Author]

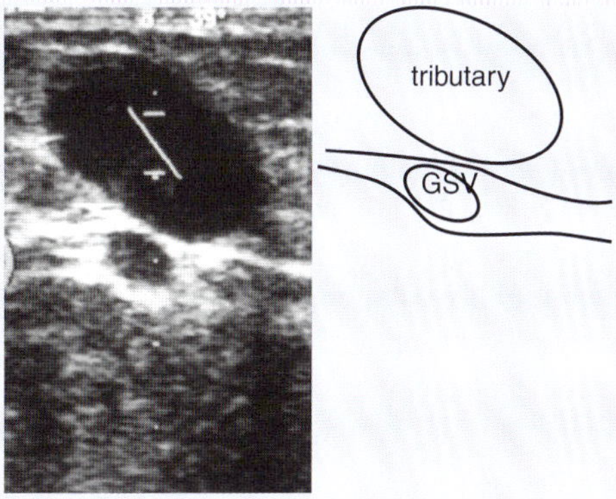

Fig. 2.15 Ultrasound view through the inner thigh showing the great saphenous vein and a parallel epifascial tributary. The sample volume cursor is seen in the epifascial refluxing tributary Copyright: [Author]

configuration was previously evaluated as duplication before the discovery using duplex ultrasound of the difference between the great saphenous vein and other parallel veins on the basis of the saphenous fascia. If the 1 % of true duplication in the fascial compartment is added to the 26 % of great saphenous veins and superficial accessory saphenous veins with parallel courses, the result is the 27 % duplication rate given in the literature.

2.4.4 Hypoplasia and Aplasia of the Great Saphenous Vein

In the groin region and proximal thigh, the great saphenous vein is fairly constantly seen in the fascial compartment. However, between the mid thigh and knee, the saphenous vein is absent from the saphenous eye in 15 % of legs: 12 % of patients with healthy veins and 24 % of patients with reflux (Caggiati and Mendoza 2004). This condition is described as a segmental aplasia of the great saphenous vein since histologically this vein is always present in the saphenous eye in rudimentary form (Caggiati 2000; Caggiati and Ricci 2000). In legs with segmental aplasia of the great saphenous vein, a large straight venous tributary is always visible in the subcutaneous fatty tissue, parallel to the empty saphenous eye. This joins the distal and proximal sections of the great saphenous vein and maintains the flow between them. Since this vein loop replaces the great saphenous vein functionally, it may be termed a **functional great saphenous vein**.

Great saphenous vein hypoplasia was defined by Caggiati when a segment of less than 3 mm in luminal diameter was found (Caggiati 2000).

Aplasia and Hypoplasia of the Great Saphenous Vein in the Literature

Ricci and Caggiati (1999) found that in 11 % of the 676 legs examined, there was no great saphenous vein in stretches of the fascial compartment. Instead, there was a vein running through the subcutaneous fatty tissue parallel to the expected course of the great saphenous vein. In these cadavers, Caggiati showed that a histologically rudimentary great saphenous vein with the same wall properties was present in the fascial compartment (Sect. 2.6; Caggiati et al. 1998). In a further survey (Caggiati and Ricci 2000), they found a reduction of >30 % of the calibre of the great saphenous vein in some segments in 20 % of legs. They conjectured that the aplasia/hypoplasia variants were associated with the formation of varicose veins because they were frequently found in legs with a refluxive great saphenous vein compared to legs with healthy veins.

Subsequent examinations by Mendoza and Mahdy (in Caggiati and Mendoza [2004]) showed that hypoplasia, defined as a reduction in the luminal calibre of the great saphenous vein to below 3 mm, has no statistical correlation with the occurrence of varices. This is in contrast to segmental aplasia wher e there is a weak relationship. Furthermore, in 15 % of patients and volunteers, the great saphenous vein between the knee and the mid thigh is not found in the fascial compartment under ultrasound. Instead, continuity between the proximal and distal parts of the aplastic segment is maintained by an extrafascial great saphenous vein which has pierced the fascia to become subcutaneous (Figs. 2.16 and 2.17).

Segmental aplasia of the great saphenous vein is found in only 12 % of healthy legs. However, in legs with a refluxive great saphenous vein, an aplastic segment occurs in 24 %. The difference is statistically significant. This would indicate that segmental aplasia of the great saphenous vein is related with venous insufficiency, while hypoplasia is not (Caggiati and Mendoza 2004).

The classification of vein courses in the lower leg is difficult because they are more variable with many more tributaries. Interestingly, the great saphenous vein itself sometimes disappears completely. True duplications were not found in this region (Caggiati and Ricci 1999).

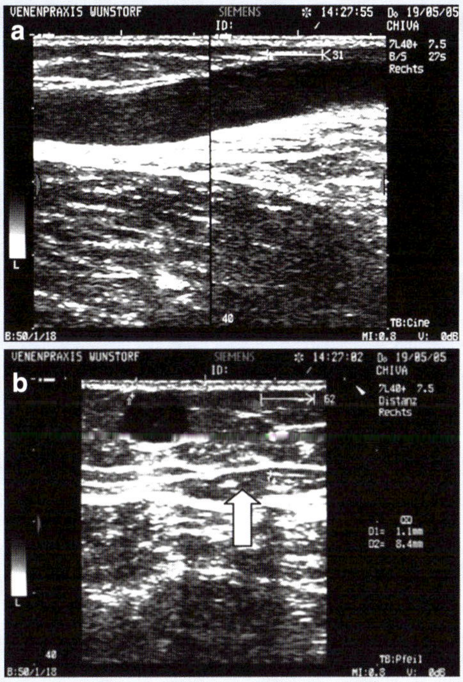

Fig. 2.16 (**a**) Longitudinal view of the inner thigh demonstrating the junction of the great saphenous vein with a tributary in segmental aplasia of the great saphenous vein. (**b**) Transverse view distal of this junction where the tributary runs in the subcutaneous fatty tissue and the saphenous eye is empty (*arrow*) Copyright: [Author]

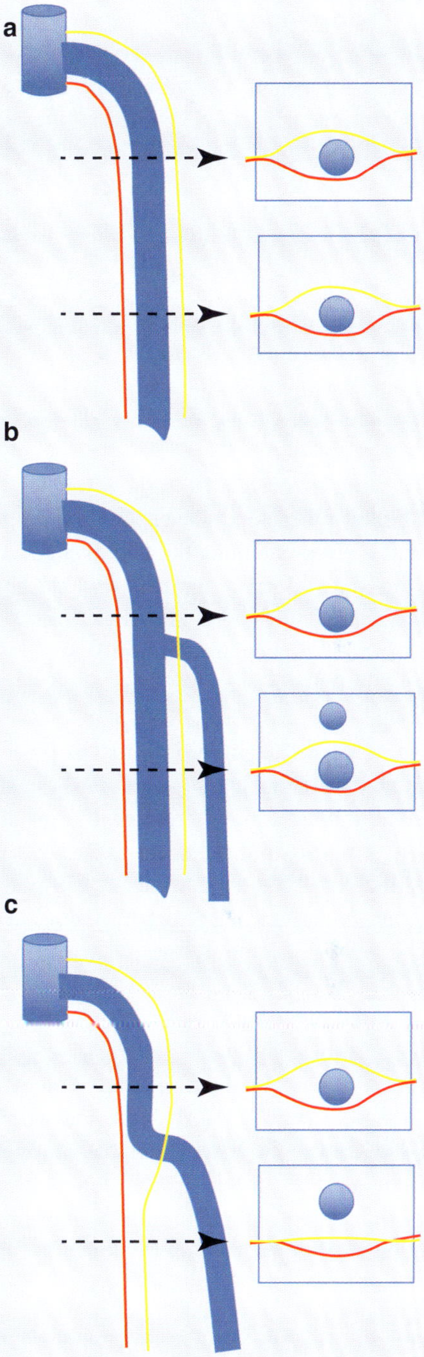

Fig. 2.17 The great saphenous vein and the variation in the connection of its tributaries. (**a**) The vein has a straight course within the saphenous fascia which is confirmed at bot h ultrasound points in the thigh. (**b**) A parallel extrafascial tributary is seen at the distal ultrasound point. (**c**) An aplastic segment is seen at the distal ultrasound point with the absence of a lumen in the fascia, "empty saphenous eye" and a replacement epifascial lumen Copyright: [Author]

2.4.5 Tributaries of the Great Saphenous Vein

The great saphenous vein does not have very many described tributaries visible on ultrasound. However, in a pathological vein, more tributaries can be seen on ultrasound or contrast phlebography. It is also known from saphenous vein harvesting that a healthy vein has few tributaries (Caggiati 2000).

The **tributaries** are known as anterior and posterior **arch veins** in the lower leg region and as the anterior and posterior accessory saphenous veins in the thigh. These named veins are fairly constant in position.

The **anterior arch vein** in the lower leg runs from the lateral region of the foot via the lateral malleolus, proximal along the lateral edge of the tibia, and crosses the tibia at a variable height between halfway and one-third from the top. It joins the great saphenous vein in the upper third of the calf. Two anterior arch veins are occasionally found in the calf (Fig. 2.18).

The **posterior arch vein** originates posterior to the medial malleolus and runs fairly straight proximally along Linton's line on the inside of the leg. It drains into the great saphenous vein below the medial femoral condyle. Most of the important pathological perforating veins in the calf lie along Linton's line (Fig. 2.19 and Sect. 2.4.7).

An **inter-saphenous** vein arising from the small saphenous vein meets the great saphenous vein in the region of the termination of the posterior arch vein (Fig. 2.19). Its junction with the great saphenous vein is very variable which may occur below the posterior arch vein where it enters the upper section of the posterior arch vein. Alternatively, it may drain above the knee directly into the great saphenous vein.

Two or three more tributaries join in the mid-thigh region, in very variable locations. In the lower thigh, an anterior and posterior tributary may be seen joining the great saphenous vein. These appear dilated and tortuous in venous reflux pathology. In the middle third, a vein may join from the lateral side linking the great saphenous vein with the anterior accessory saphenous vein. A more detailed anatomical description of these variable tributaries is superfluous. If they are small, they are usually competent. They become easily identifiable if they are pathologically dilated and refluxive (Sect. 7.4).

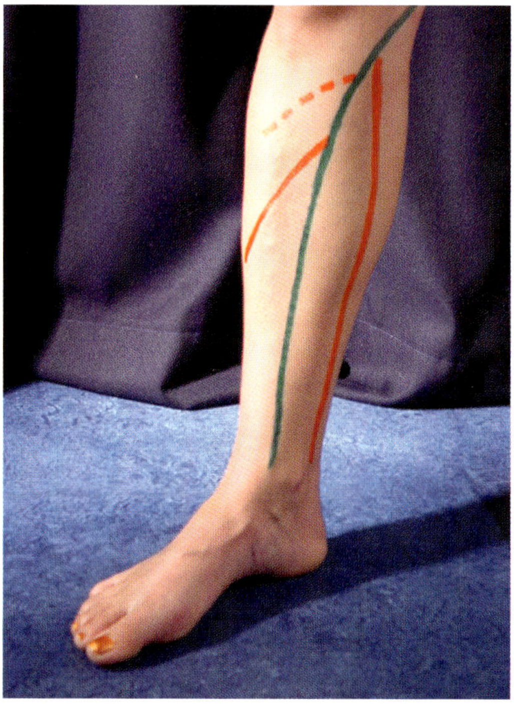

Fig. 2.18 Arch veins with a view of the inner side of the right calf. The course of the great saphenous vein is marked *green*. The anterior arch vein, marked in *orange*, enters just after it crosses the tibia. The *dotted line* is a frequent alternative and/or additional course of the arch vein. The posterior arch vein is marked medially, also in *orange*, along Linton's line Copyright: [Author]

2.4.6 Anterior and Posterior Accessory Saphenous Veins

The anterior and posterior accessory saphenous veins join the upper section of the great saphenous vein in an almost constant position (Fig. 2.20).

The **anterior accessory saphenous vein** is an axial vein which originates from the lateral part of the calf. Then, it ascends to the posterior knee running medially along the thigh to drain into the great saphenous vein in the groin. The anterior

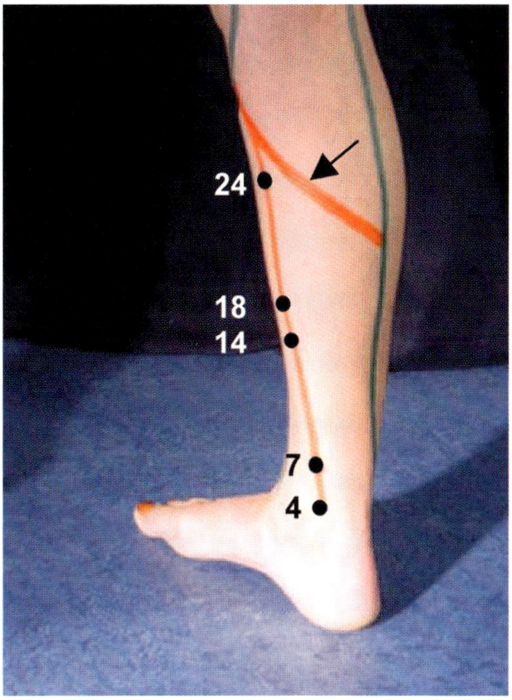

Fig. 2.19 Postero-medial view of the calf demonstrating the inter-saphenous vein between the small and great saphenous veins in the calf (*arrow*). The posterior arch vein arises behind the medial malleolus and travels straight up to the great saphenous vein. The *black dots* represent the locations of the perforating veins. The *numbers* by the perforating veins show their distance in cm from the ground in a standing patient (*4* medial ankle perforating vein, formerly Kuster perforating vein; *7* lower posterior tibial perforating vein, formerly Cockett 1, C1; *14* middle posterior tibial perforating vein, formerly Cockett 2, C2; *18* upper posterior tibial perforating vein, formerly Cockett 3, C3, *24* medial paratibial perforating vein in the mid lower leg, formerly Sherman perforating vein) Copyright: [Author]

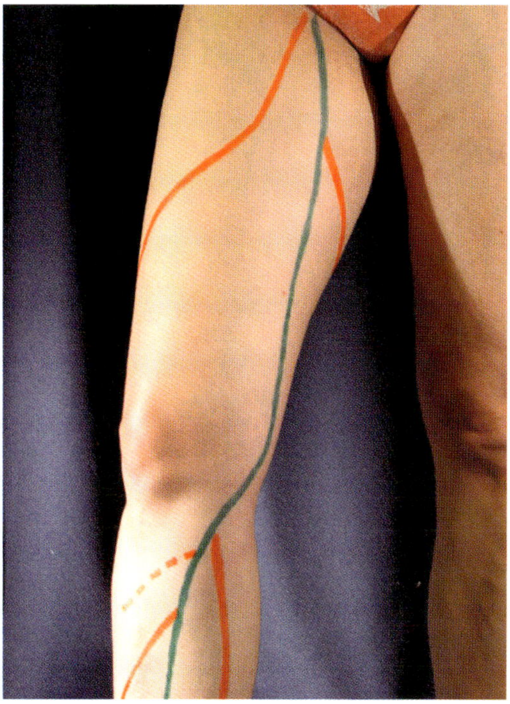

Fig. 2.20 Anterior and posterior accessory saphenous veins. The usual configuration is that the anterior accessory saphenous vein joins the great saphenous vein directly within the confluence of superficial inguinal veins. The posterior accessory saphenous vein joins further down the thigh Copyright: [Author]

accessory saphenous vein almost always connects directly with the great saphenous vein in the confluence of superficial inguinal veins as a saphenofemoral tributary. Rarely, it drains into the great saphenous vein in the upper thigh or directly into a deep vein in the groin.

The proximal part runs inside the compartment of the great saphenous vein where it is often separated by a layer of connective tissue (Sect. 10.2). In healthy veins, its course along the thigh is only visible on ultrasound from the groin to where it leaves the fascia (Fig. 2.21) or slightly distal of that point. If the vein is refluxive it can be seen varicosed directly beneath the skin in several places along its length. As with the thigh tributaries, the exact anatomical course of this vein is superfluous, as it forms part of a venous network. If the anterior accessory saphenous vein is refluxive, it is easily identified because of its superficial location.

In the middle third of the thigh, a connecting vein is often found between the anterior accessory saphenous vein and the great saphenous vein. If one of these veins becomes incompetent, the other may become overloaded with reflux from this vein.

The **posterior accessory saphenous vein** arises from the back of the leg, generally from the cranial extension of the small saphenous vein. It then runs around the inside of the thigh where it joins the great saphenous vein about 5–10 cm distal to the groin. This kind of confluence is also called the *femoral type* (Figs. 2.20 and 2.21).

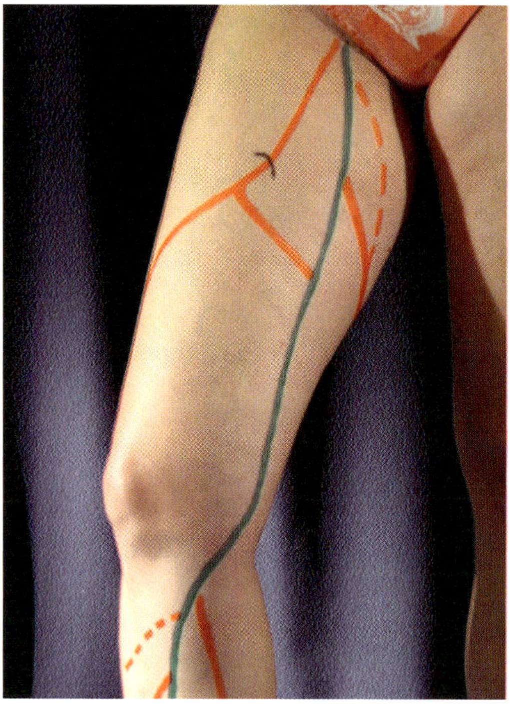

Fig. 2.21 Anterior and posterior accessory saphenous veins (*orange*) demonstrating variations in their termination with the great saphenous vein (*green*). The *dotted line* marks the alternative course of the posterior accessory saphenous vein into the confluence of superficial inguinal veins. The *black mark* indicates where the anterior accessory saphenous vein leaves the fascial compartment of the great saphenous vein and becomes epifascial. Distal of this point, there is very often a connecting vein between the anterior accessory saphenous vein and the great saphenous vein Copyright: [Author]

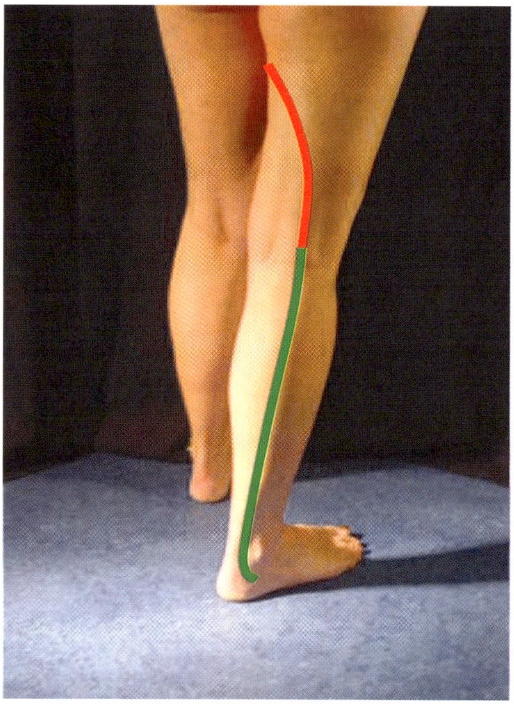

Fig. 2.22 Dorsal view of the Giacomini anastomosis on the back of the leg demonstrating the connection between the small saphenous vein (*green*, arising from the calf) and the proximal part of the anastomoses leading into the great saphenous vein (Fig. 2.21) Copyright: [Author]

Like the anterior accessory saphenous vein, the posterior accessory saphenous vein in its proximal section also runs between the muscle and saphenous fascia within the saphenous compartment. In some cases, the whole thigh course of the posterior accessory saphenous vein is inter-fascial.

Frequently, the posterior accessory saphenous vein forms a connection between the small saphenous vein and the great saphenous vein (Fig. 2.22) where it may acquire haemodynamic importance. This connection receives different names in different textbooks. The following three variants can be described:

1. The posterior accessory saphenous vein can be followed from the great saphenous vein in the lower leg until it turns posteriorly in the thigh leaving the fascia to course freely in the subcutaneous fatty tissue. Here, it separates into a few smaller vessels which cannot be followed further.
2. The posterior accessory saphenous vein connects the great saphenous vein with the small saphenous vein as an entirely subfascial structure. On ultrasound, it can easily be seen running cranially from the small saphenous vein beneath the muscle fascia as far as the middle third of the thigh. Here, it runs fairly exactly in the middle of the back of the thigh. It then pierces the muscle fascia and courses medially under the membranous layer around to the inner thigh to join the great saphenous vein usually below the groin.

3. As an extrafascial structure, the posterior accessory saphenous vein connects the great saphenous vein with the small saphenous vein. Its upper course is similar to that of the first variant described except that one of the subcutaneous branches is visible as a large vein in the back of the thigh. It may meet the small saphenous vein in the popliteal region or pierce the muscle fascia posteriorly in the lower part of the back of the thigh to join a cranial extension of the small saphenous vein.

A direct connection between small saphenous vein and great saphenous vein is called the **femoro-popliteal** vein. On ultrasound or contrast phlebography, it runs subfascially or epifascially as in variants 2 and 3. Its physiological flow is upwards and it should therefore be called the popliteofemoral vein. This connecting vein is often also called the **vein of Giacomini** or **Giacomini anastomoses**. However, other authors reserve Giacomini for the extrafascial connection between the cranial extension of the small saphenous vein and the mid/lower third of the great saphenous vein.

Whichever nomenclature is used, this connection between the great saphenous vein and the small saphenous vein is of great significance in vein pathology.

2.1.7 Perforating Veins of the Great Saphenous Vein

Perforating veins are veins which connect the superficial veins to the deep veins. The great saphenous vein connects with the deep vein through the saphenofemoral junction as well via a series of perforating veins along its course.

These are divided into direct and indirect perforating veins:

- **Direct** perforating veins are those which connect the superficial vein system, principally the saphenous trunks or their important tributaries, directly with the deep veins.
- **Indirect** perforating veins are those which first connect the saphenous trunk veins with muscle veins which only later in their course join the deep veins. The most commonly found muscle veins are the gastrocnemius vein and the soleus vein.

Most perforating veins do not join the saphenous trunks directly after they pierce the fascia. Instead, they connect first to saphenous tributaries. However, the perforating veins of the adductor canal in the thigh (formerly Dodd) and the paratibial perforating veins in the proximal lower leg (formerly Boyd) usually join the below-knee great saphenous vein directly.

The non-junctional perforating veins of the great saphenous vein from groin to foot are as follows:

Connection with the deep femoral vein

In rare cases, a connection is seen in the groin between the great saphenous vein and the deep femoral vein. It is only noticed if it is refluxive which occurs in approximately 2 legs per 1,000. It joins the great saphenous vein posteriorly approximately 5 cm below the saphenofemoral junction.

Perforating veins of the adductor [femoral] canal

In the thigh region, there are direct perforating veins which connect the great saphenous vein with the femoral vein. Occasionally, there is a perforating vein in the upper third of the thigh, but most are found in the middle third and occasionally a little lower (Fig. 2.23). The mid-thigh perforating vein plays a greater role in venous pathology than those lower down. Both were described by Dodd and were formerly called Dodd perforating veins. However recently, they have been renamed as perforating veins of the adductor canal in accordance with the new international nomenclature (Caggiati et al. 2002).

Other perforating veins of the adductor canal

In the distal third of the thigh, a perforating vein, formerly known as the Hunter perforating vein, is found. This is rarely within the adductor canal itself, but below. Surprisingly, today, this is also termed correctly as a perforating vein of the

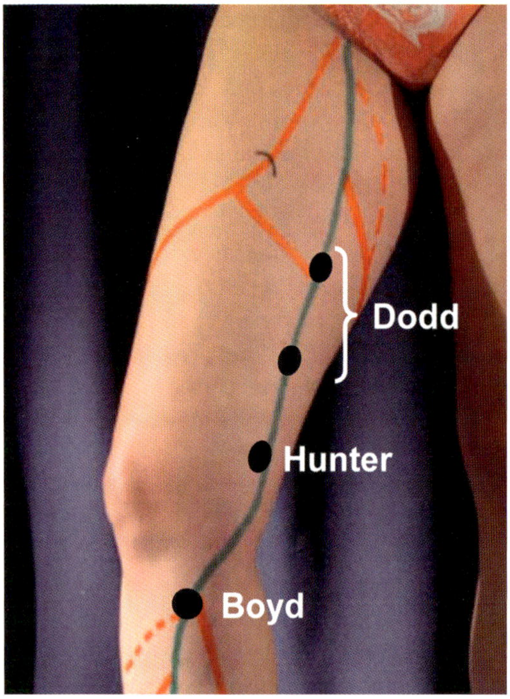

Fig. 2.23 Location of the perforating veins of the adductor canal (formerly Dodd and Hunter) in the above-knee great saphenous vein. Location of the paratibial perforating veins (formerly Boyd) in the below-knee great saphenous vein Copyright: [Author]

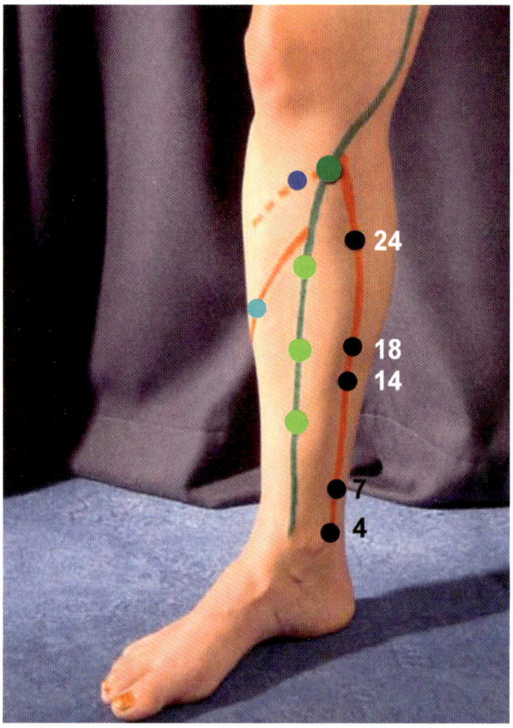

Fig. 2.24 Location of the perforating veins on the front and inner sides of the calf (*Blue*, perforating veins of the anterior arch vein; *light blue*, outflow into the arch vein lateral of the edge of the tibia and drainage into the anterior tibial veins; *dark blue*, outflow into the arch vein medial of the edge of the tibia and drainage into the posterior tibial veins; *green*, perforating veins of the great saphenous vein; *dark green*, Boyd perforating vein; *light green*, paratibial perforating veins with drainage into the posterior tibial veins; *black*, perforating veins of the posterior arch vein; see Fig. 2.19) Copyright: [Author]

adductor canal. At this point, the great saphenous vein is often dilated and palpable and therefore can be easily mistaken for a fascial defect from an incompetent perforating vein (Sect. 7.4).

Other perforating veins in the thigh are:

- Anterior thigh perforating veins, which pierce the quadriceps femoris muscle
- Sciatic perforating veins, which lie along the midline on the posterior side of the thigh
- Posterior-lateral perforating veins, which break through the biceps femoris and the semitendinosus muscles (formerly Hach perforating veins)
- Lateral thigh perforating veins, which pierce the lateral thigh muscles

Paratibial and tibial perforating veins in the proximal leg

The paratibial perforating vein (formerly Boyd perforating vein) is found fairly constantly in the proximal leg immediately below the knee. It is a direct perforating vein connecting the great saphenous vein with the posterior tibial veins. The paratibial perforating vein in the proximal lower leg usually connects the deep wall of the great saphenous vein to the posterior tibial vein (Figs. 2.23 and 2.24).

The upper posterior tibial perforating veins (formerly called Sherman perforating veins) connect the posterior arch vein with the posterior tibial veins or the calf muscle veins. They usually join at a height of approximately 24 cm from the ground.

Connections with the posterior tibial veins

Perforating veins of the distal calf great saphenous vein are described rarely in anatomical and phlebological publications. However, they are observed frequently in both patients and healthy subjects. An inconstant number of connections of the great saphenous vein with the posterior tibial veins occur. They originate in the great saphenous vein, course laterally up to the edge of the tibia where they go deeper and meet the group of posterior tibial veins. The course of these perforating veins is S-shaped (Figs. 2.24 and 9.1).

Posterior tibial perforating veins (perforating veins of the posterior arch vein)

They connect the posterior arch vein with the posterior tibial veins and are classified into the lower medial posterior tibial perforating vein (formerly Cockett I), the middle medial posterior tibial perforating vein (formerly Cockett II) and the upper medial posterior tibial perforating vein (formerly Cockett III). They are of great significance in vein pathology. These perforating veins are located generally at 7, 14 and 18 cm from the ground; however, these figures may vary depending on the stature of the subject (Figs. 2.19 and 2.24).

Anterior leg perforating veins

The anterior leg perforating veins connect the anterior tributaries of the great saphenous vein with the anterior tibial veins by piercing the fascia of the anterior tibial compartment (Fig. 2.24).

Ankle perforating veins (malleolar perforating veins)

The anterior and medial ankle perforating veins (formerly Kuster perforating veins) belong to the great saphenous vein. The medial ankle perforating veins (formerly Kuster) are found fairly constantly at 4 cm from the ground immediately behind the medial malleolus at the distal end of the posterior arch vein.

Foot perforating veins

The medial plantar and dorsal foot perforating veins belong to the great saphenous vein territory.

2.4.8 Accompanying Structures of the Great Saphenous Vein

The accompanying structures of the great saphenous vein course together in the saphenous compartment. The **anterior cutaneous branches** of the **femoral nerve** accompany the great saphenous vein along the thigh. The fascial compartment is ample in this region leaving a space between it and the vein.

In the knee region, the great saphenous vein is accompanied by a branch of the **descending genicular artery**. This artery may assume an important collateral function in distal femoral and popliteal arterial occlusions.

In the lower leg, the **saphenous nerve** runs immediately beside the vein. The fascial compartment is very narrow especially in the middle and distal thirds of the lower leg. Occasionally, the nerve is incorporated into the vein wall where it becomes inseparable. There is therefore a danger of damage to this nerve during great saphenous vein surgery. The saphenous nerve is responsible for the sensitivity of the distal inner calf and the inside of the foot.

Throughout its length, the great saphenous vein is surrounded by **lymphatic vessels** which drain the dorsal foot and the anterior and medial parts of the leg and thigh. They end in the superficial group of the groin lymph nodes which are also found in the great saphenous compartment in the region of the saphenous hiatus (Fig. 2.10).

2.4.9 Topographical Anatomy of the Great Saphenous Vein

In the groin, the common femoral artery and vein lie in a recess formed by the iliopsoas muscle antero-lateral and the adductor muscles (brevis, longus, minimus and magnus) which are postero-medial (Fig. 2.25). The deep fascia tightly surrounds the muscles of the whole thigh. There is an opening in the groin, the

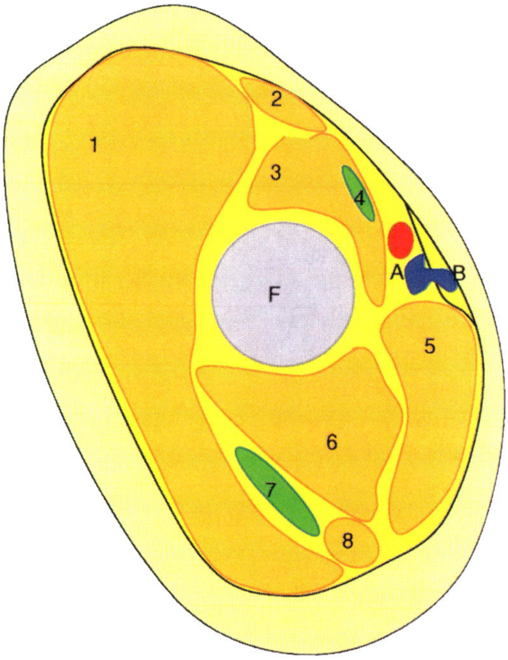

Fig. 2.25 Transverse view through the thigh from medial distal to lateral proximal, parallel to the inguinal ligament (*F* femur, *A* common femoral vein and artery, *B* saphenofemoral junction, *1* gluteus muscles, *2* sartorius muscle, *3* iliopsoas muscle with *4* femoral nerve, *5* adductor muscles: magnus, brevis, longus and minimus, *6* quadratus femoris muscle, external and internal obturator muscles and superior and inferior gemelli muscles, *7* sciatic nerve, *8* semimembranosus, semitendinosus and biceps femoris muscles, *violet* deep fascia) Copyright: [Author]

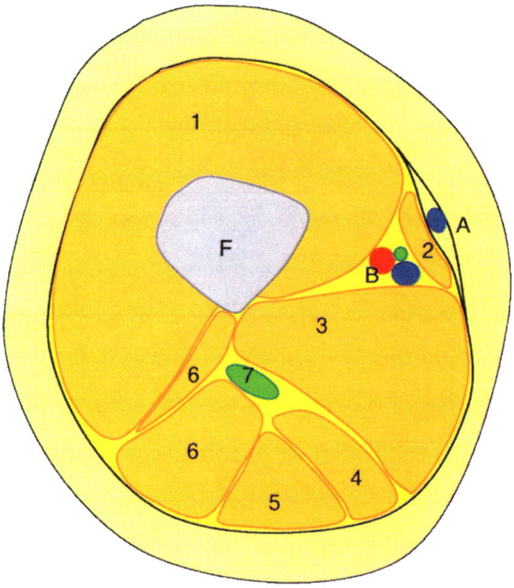

Fig. 2.26 Transverse view through the mid thigh (*F* femur, *A* great saphenous vein, *B* common femoral artery and vein with saphenous nerve, *1* quadriceps femoris muscle, *2* sartorius muscle, *3* longus and magnus adductor muscles and gracilis muscle, *4* semimembranosus muscle, *5* semitendinosus muscle, *6* biceps femoris muscle (long and short heads), *7* sciatic nerve) Copyright: [Author]

saphenous hiatus, through which the great saphenous vein passes deep to join the common femoral vein. It is covered by the cribriform fascia, which merges with the saphenous fascia.

In its further course down the thigh, the great saphenous vein lies close to the adductor muscles and later the sartorius muscle (Fig. 2.26). In the mid thigh, sartorius separates the saphenous vein from the femoral artery and vein. The great saphenous vein accompanies the muscle to below the knee where it inserts into the medial side of the tibia.

Below the knee, the great saphenous vein runs between the popliteus muscle and the medial gastrocnemius head (Fig. 2.27). Then, it descends between the edge of the tibia and the soleus muscle (Fig. 2.28) to the ankle where it lies anteromedial to the tibia (Fig. 2.29).

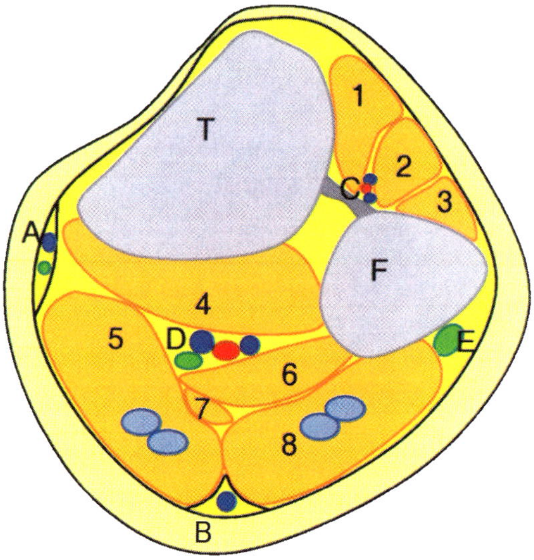

Fig. 2.27 Transverse view through the proximal third of the right thigh (*T* tibia, *F* fibula, connected by the interosseous membrane, *A* great saphenous vein and saphenous nerve, *B* small saphenous vein, *light blue* muscle veins (very variable arrangement), *C* anterior tibial artery and veins, *D* tibiofibula trunk with tibial nerve, *E* common peroneal nerve, *1* anterior tibial muscle, *2* long digital extensor muscle, *3* long peroneal muscle, *4* popliteus muscle, *5* medial gastrocnemius muscle, *6* soleus muscle, *7* plantaris muscle, *8* lateral sgastrocnemius muscle) Copyright: [Author]

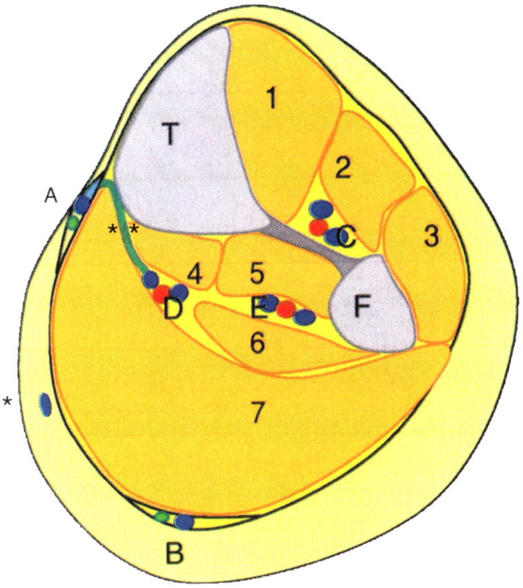

Fig. 2.28 Transverse view through the proximal third of the right leg (*T* tibia, *F* fibula, connected by the interosseous membrane, *A* great saphenous vein and saphenous nerve, *B* small saphenous vein and sural nerve, * posterior arch vein, ** paratibial perforating vein, *C* anterior tibial artery and veins, *D* posterior tibial artery and veins, *E* fibular artery and veins, *1* anterior tibial muscle, *2* long digital extensor muscle, *3* long and short peroneal muscles, *4* long digital flexor muscle, *5* posterior tibial muscle, *6* long hallucis flexor muscle, *7* soleus muscle) Copyright: [Author]

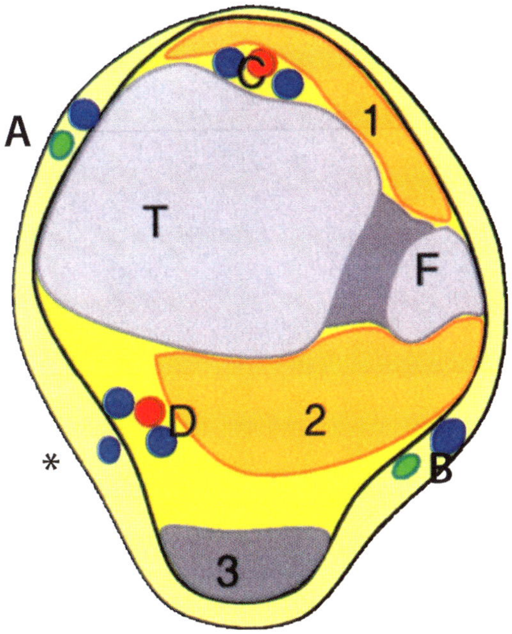

Fig. 2.29 Transverse view through the distal third of the right leg (*T* tibia, *F* fibula, connected by the interosseous membrane, *A* great saphenous vein and saphenous nerve, *B* small saphenous vein and sural nerve, * posterior arch vein, *C* anterior tibial artery and veins, *D* posterior tibial artery and veins, *E* fibular artery and veins, *1* muscle tendon group comprising anterior tibial muscle and foot extensors, *2* muscle tendon group comprising peroneal muscles and foot flexors, *3* Achilles tendon) Copyright: [Author]

Figures 2.25, 2.26, 2.27, 2.28, and 2.29 show sections through the right leg (seen from above). Those structures which are visible on ultrasound are highlighted as grey, bones and tendons; blue, veins; red, arteries; green, nerves; and orange, muscle tissue.

2.5 The Small Saphenous Vein

2.5.1 Course of the Small Saphenous Vein

The small saphenous vein originates from the lateral foot vein loop and becomes visible as an independent vessel posterior to the lateral malleolus. Here, it can often be seen and felt in healthy subjects when standing. In its course upwards, it passes lateral to the Achilles tendon, over the lateral edge of the soleus muscle to the midline of the back of the calf. It then runs between the two bellies of the gastrocnemius muscle to enter the popliteal fossa where it typically joins the popliteal vein (Fig. 2.30).

The connection between the small saphenous vein and the deep vein system, or saphenopopliteal junction, is very variable. There are seven different configurations which may be seen on ultrasound in the popliteal fossa (Fig. 2.31).

In 1926, Kosinski published a classification on the varieties of termination of the small saphenous vein (Table 2.2). In 2001, Caggiati investigated likewise the termination of the small saphenous vein in 300 legs with duplex ultrasound and classified them into three groups (Table 2.3). The results were similar as seen from the frequencies in the right-hand columns of the table. The first variant described by Kosinski, of a final termination into the great saphenous vein via an inter-saphenous vein, is shown in Figs. 2.19, *arrow* and 2.31g.

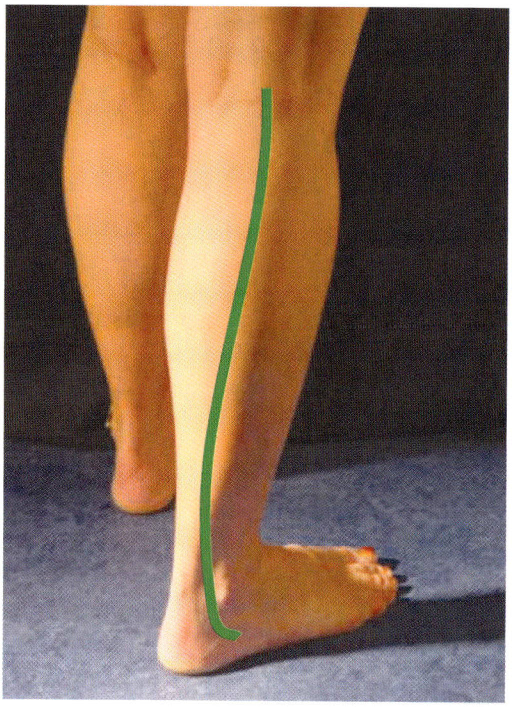

Fig. 2.30 View of the back of the calf. The course of the small saphenous vein is drawn on the skin Copyright: [Author]

Meta-analysis showed that the height of the termination of the small saphenous vein may vary and depends on venous pathology. A high confluence (>7 cm above the popliteal skin crease) is more frequent in subjects with healthy veins. In contrast, the majority of patients with insufficiency (57–93 %) have a confluence within the popliteal fossa (0–7 cm above the popliteal skin crease) (Creton 2005).

Caggiati classified the different confluence heights as follows:

- 1 % below the popliteal fossa (Fig. 8.6)
- 7 % in the popliteal fossa, below the knee crease (Fig. 2.31a, c)
- 54 % in the popliteal fossa, above the knee crease (Fig. 2.31a, c)
- 14 % above the upper apex of the popliteal fossa into the deep veins of the back of the thigh (Fig. 2.31d)
- 24 % in the proximal part of the thigh above the femoro-popliteal vein (Fig. 2.31e, f)

An upward extension of the small saphenous vein to a femoro-popliteal vein, independent of a connection to the popliteal vein, was found by Caggiati in 65 % of legs (Fig. 2.31c, e, f).

The terminal section of the small saphenous vein contains two valves: the terminal valve in the immediate vicinity of the popliteal vein and the preterminal valve generally found below the departure point of the vein of Giacomini or the cranial extension. Gastrocnemius veins may drain into the popliteal vein, the small saphenous vein or the saphenopopliteal junction directly.

In 10–30 % of cases, a confluence of the gastrocnemius veins with the small saphenous vein was found below the saphenopopliteal junction (Cavezzi et al 2002 in Appendix 2).

2.5.2 Fascial Compartment of the Small Saphenous Vein, Duplication, Aplasia

The small saphenous vein runs from behind the lateral malleolus to the popliteal region. Just like the great saphenous vein, this occurs in a fascial compartment which envelops the vein (Fig. 2.32). Towards the ankle, in cross-section, where the small saphenous vein runs along the soleus muscle, it looks like a half-moon (Figs. 2.28 and 2.33).

Further upwards, the small saphenous vein enters the recess between the two gastrocnemius heads. The saphenous fascia at this region is thicker, and in transverse view, it forms a triangle with one corner pointing inwards (Figs. 2.27 and 2.34). In the popliteal region, both gastrocnemius heads and accompanying muscle fascia turn down away from the subcutaneous fat. The

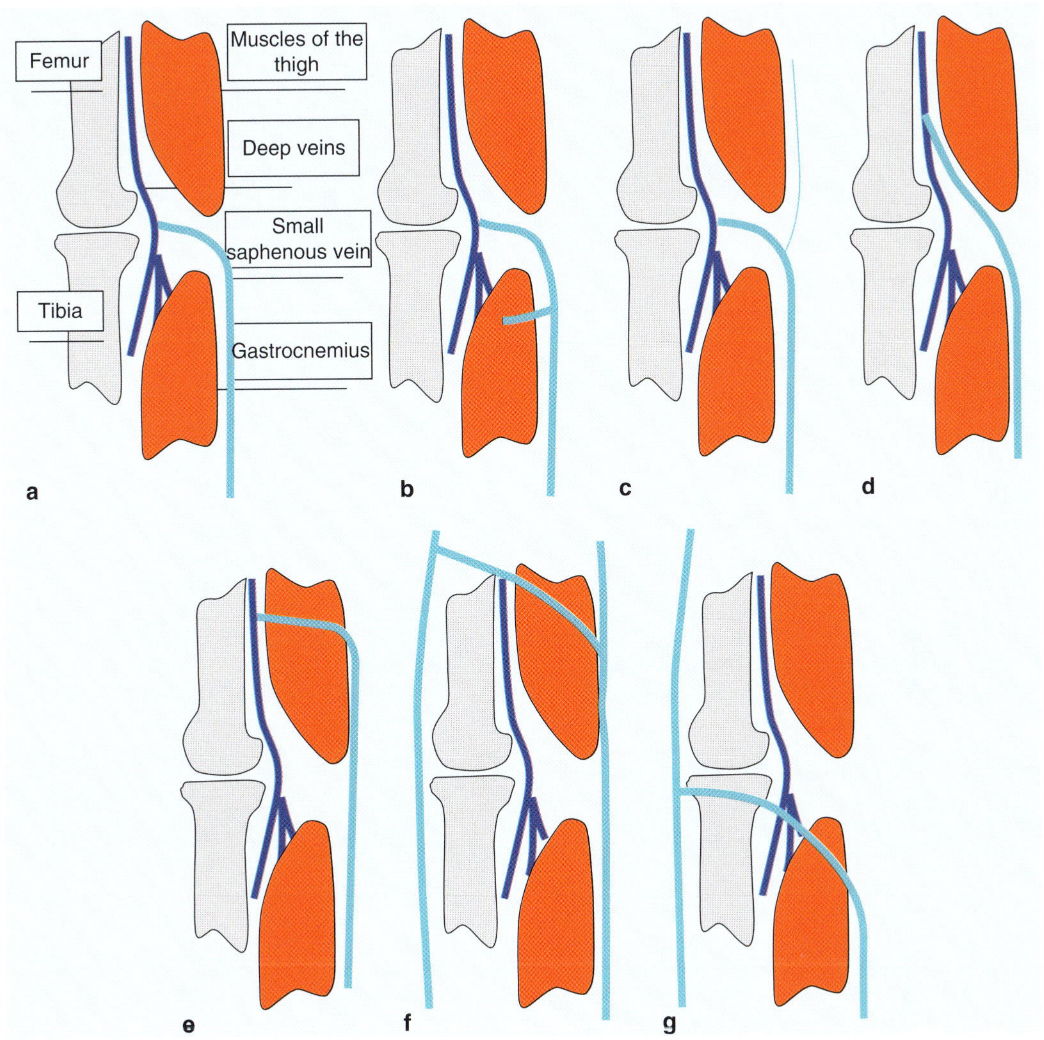

Fig. 2.31 Variations of the termination of the small saphenous vein: (**a**) Termination of the small saphenous vein (SSV) in the popliteal fossa. (**b**) Termination of the SSV in the popliteal fossa with an additional connection to the deep vein through the gastrocnemius veins. The terminal part of the SSV is often very thin in these cases. (**c**) Termination of the SSV in the popliteal fossa with an additional connection to the femoro-popliteal vein or vein of Giacomini. (**d**) Termination of the SSV above the popliteal fossa without piercing the muscle fascia. (**e**) Termination of the SSV above the popliteal fossa where it also pierces the muscle fascia and the muscles of the back of the thigh. (**f**) Termination of the SSV with the vein of Giacomini or femoro-popliteal vein with drainage into the great saphenous vein or the gluteal veins. (**g**) Termination of the SSV via an inter-saphenous vein into the great saphenous vein below the knee. The true terminal segment of the SSV is absent and there is no saphenopopliteal junction present in the popliteal fossa Copyright: [Author]

saphenous fascia stretches across the popliteal fossa, with the saphenous compartment, as if it was the boundary of the deep compartment. The calf muscle fascia turns deeper and inwards on the gastrocnemius heads and the muscle fascia of the hamstrings does likewise with the muscles of the *pes anserinus* in the medial region and the biceps femoris muscle in the lateral region. This leaves a region devoid of deep fascia and explains why there is no fascia present between

Table 2.2 Classification of the small saphenous vein terminations according to Kosinski (1926)

Type	Description	Kosinski [%]
Normal confluence	**Confluence in the popliteal fossa, a few centimetres above the popliteal skin crease**	**57.3**
Variants	Direct confluence with no further tributaries	42.0
	A tributary leaves the small saphenous vein before the termination in the popliteal fossa forming a cranial extension of the small saphenous vein (femoro-popliteal vein)	15.3
High confluence	**Confluence of the small saphenous vein above the popliteal fossa**	**33.0**
Variants	Small saphenous vein passes above the popliteal fossa and joins the deep veins in the distal third of the thigh	13.7
	Small saphenous vein passes above the popliteal fossa and joins the great saphenous vein in the proximal third of the thigh with no further tributaries	12.9
	Small saphenous vein has its confluence in the distal third of the thigh. A tributary leaves it beforehand which continues to the great saphenous vein as the femoro-popliteal vein	6.4
Low confluence	**Small saphenous vein has its confluence below the popliteal fossa**	**9.7**
Variants	Small saphenous vein joins the great saphenous vein at the height of the popliteal skin crease	8.1
	Small saphenous vein terminates via muscle veins in the middle third of the calf	1.6

Table 2.3 (c.f. Table 2.2) Classification of small saphenous vein terminations according to Caggiati (2001)

Type	Description	Caggiati [%]
A	Confluence in the popliteal fossa into the popliteal vein or via a gastrocnemius vein into the popliteal vein (Fig. 2.31a–c)	**62.0**
Variants	Confluence in the popliteal fossa above the posterior knee crease	54.0
	Confluence in the popliteal fossa below the posterior knee crease	7.0
	Principal drainage through a muscle perforating vein. A thin, barely visible small saphenous vein continues to the confluence in the popliteal fossa (Fig. 2.31b)	1.0
B	Small saphenous vein joins a deep vein above the popliteal fossa (deep femoral vein, superior genicular vein or a persisting sciatic vein). It runs above the popliteal fossa under the muscle fascia (Fig. 2.31d)	**14.0**
C	Small saphenous vein has no confluence in the popliteal fossa but joins the femoro-popliteal vein (Fig. 2.31e, f)	**24.0**
Variants	Confluence with the great saphenous vein through the Giacomini anastomosis (ventral variant) (Fig. 2.31f)	19.0
	Confluence with the deep femoral vein through a perforating vein. In 2 patients, Caggiati found an upward extension to the gluteal fold (0.6 % of all subjects) (Fig. 2.31e)	5.0

the termination of the small saphenous vein and the popliteal vein (Fig. 2.35). This is in direct contrast to the situation at the saphenofemoral junction.

The compartment of the small saphenous vein is particularly wide at its junction (Fig. 2.32). With a high junction in the back of the thigh (Fig. 2.31e), the fascial compartment continues upwards from the popliteal fossa.

In the popliteal region and the upper two-thirds of the calf, the saphenous fascia is so thick that it could be mistaken for the muscle fascia. Thus, it is often described incorrectly that the small saphenous vein pierces the muscle fascia in the distal third of the lower leg to run extrafascially down to the ankle. Anatomical and histological preparations (Fig. 2.36) as well as systematic examination of the course of the small saphenous vein in numerous subjects have confirmed that this is not the case. The small

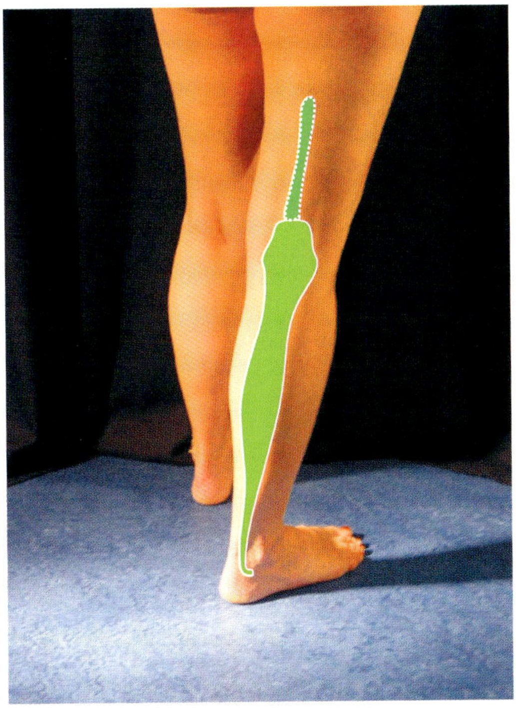

Fig. 2.32 Rear view of the leg demonstrating the compartment of the small saphenous vein as a *green area*. The *dotted line* shows the position of the proximal extension, if present Copyright: [Author]

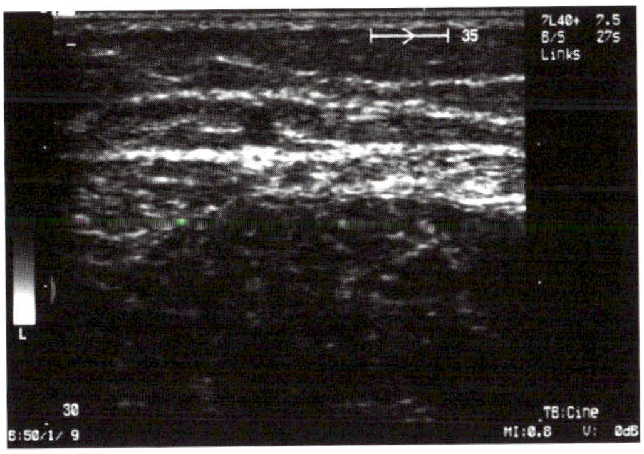

Fig. 2.33 Ultrasound image through the middle third of the calf. The fascial compartment of the small saphenous vein is visualised with saphenous ligament Copyright: [Author]

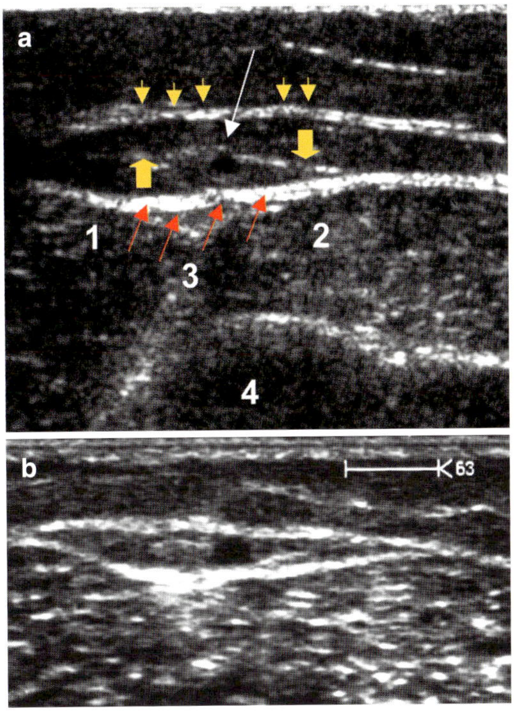

Fig. 2.34 (**a**) Ultrasound image through the upper third of the calf in an obese leg. The fat helps to delineate the structures in the fascial compartment. (**b**)Ultrasound image through the upper third of the calf in a normal leg. The saphenous and muscle fasciae are touching the small saphenous vein with a vague appearance of the saphenous ligament (*1* medial gastrocnemius muscle, *2* lateral gastrocnemius muscle, *3* fascia between the two bulges of the gastrocnemius, *4* soleus muscle, *white arrow* small saphenous vein, *narrow yellow arrows* saphenous fascia, *broad yellow arrows* saphenous ligament, *red arrows* muscle fascia) Copyright: [Author]

saphenous vein runs from the ankle to the popliteal region on top of the muscle fascia and beneath the saphenous fascia.

Duplication of the small saphenous vein occurs in 4 % of subjects which is more frequent than with the great saphenous vein (Caggiati 2001). Duplication occurs principally in the middle third. As with the great saphenous vein, true duplication only occurs when both veins are connected by a band of connective tissue over the whole length of the duplication (Fig. 2.37).

Hypoplasia of the small saphenous vein occurs in only 1 % of legs. This **reduction in calibre**, if present, appears at its terminal segment. In these cases, the small saphenous vein drains the majority of its blood into a muscle vein (gastrocnemius or soleus vein) via a perforating vein in the upper third of its course. Therefore, its calibre is reduced for the final part into the saphenopopliteal region (Fig. 2.31b).

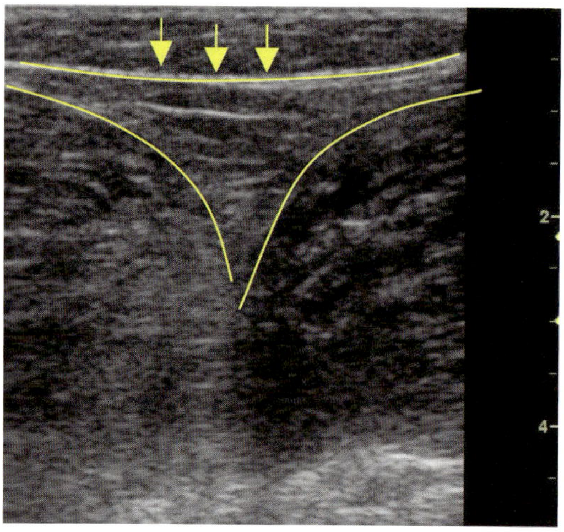

Fig. 2.35 Longitudinal view through the popliteal fossa slightly lateral of the confluence of the small saphenous vein with the popliteal vein. The bulge of the lateral gastrocnemius in the distal region (*right*) and the biceps femoris muscle in the proximal region (*left*) meet deep within the popliteal fossa creating a deep valley because their fasciae run directly on the muscle. The compartment of the small saphenous vein becomes very wide and its superficial fascia can be seen very clearly in the image (*arrows*). It separates the popliteal fossa from the subcutaneous fatty tissue. The muscle and superficial fascias are not indicated Copyright: [Author]

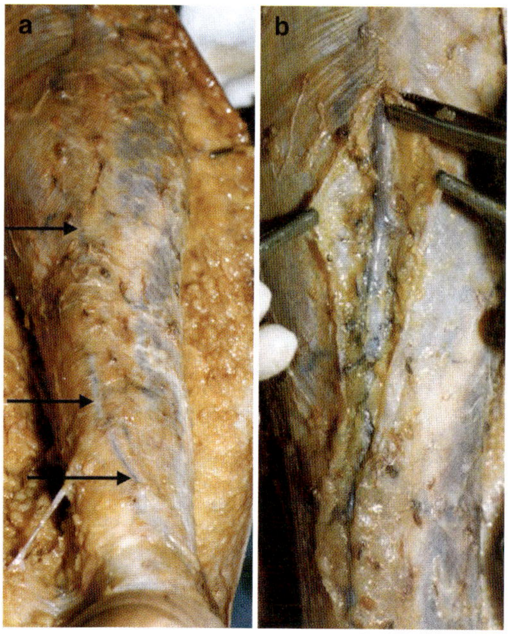

Fig. 2.36 Anatomical preparation of the back of the leg. (**a**) The skin was opened and the subcutaneous fat was separated. The small saphenous vein can be seen beneath the saphenous fascia (*arrows*). (**b**) The saphenous fascia is being opened to reveal the small saphenous vein (Prof. A. Caggiati, Rome; by kind permission) Copyright: A. Caggiati, Rome

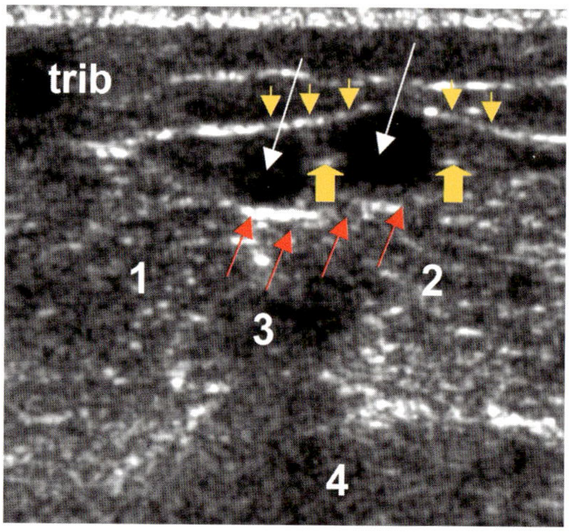

Fig. 2.37 Ultrasound image through the back of the calf with a true duplication of the small saphenous vein (explanation Fig. 2.34a). Copyright: [Author]

Aplasia has not been described in the small saphenous vein. The rare cases where the small saphenous vein drains via an inter-saphenous vein into the great saphenous vein may have been caused by aplasia of the terminal segment of the small saphenous vein. This extremely rare finding has not yet been researched histologically so it is not known whether a rudiment of the small saphenous vein exists in these cases.

2.5.3 Cranial Extension of Small Saphenous Vein and Giacomini Anastomosis

In 65 % of cases, there is a cranial extension of the small saphenous vein. It runs beneath the muscle fascia up the back of the thigh to the point where the bulge of the semitendinosus muscle meets the long head of the biceps femoris muscle. This point is the apex of the popliteal fossa and is in the midline. Here, it may stay subfascial or emerge from the fascia and run epifascial. This vein may drain posteriorly into a deep vein (a) or through a connection into the great saphenous vein (b).

(a) The cranial extension joins the deep leg vein through a posterior-lateral perforating vein (formerly Hach) (Fig. 2.31e), or it emerges from the muscle fascia to continue its course upwards under the membranous layer or freely in the subcutaneous fatty tissue (Fig. 2.31c). In rare cases, it may join a persisting sciatic vein in the gluteal fold.

(b) The cranial extension joins a sub- or epifascial tributary from the great saphenous vein at mid thigh or the accessory posterior saphenous vein more cranially, draining its blood into the great saphenous vein. It may also emerge from the muscle fascia and veer medially and anteriorly around the inner thigh to join the great saphenous vein (Sect. 2.4.6). This anastomosis is called the Giacomini anastomosis.

2.5.4 Tributaries of the Small Saphenous Vein

The tributaries of the small saphenous vein are very variable making classification pointless. Like the great saphenous vein tributaries, it is only when they are pathologically altered they become visible.

The tributaries which have an important haemodynamic function are those which connect the small saphenous vein with the great saphenous vein, namely, the **inter-saphenous veins**. In the mid-calf, this vein often arises from the small saphenous vein coursing upwards to join the great saphenous vein (Fig. 2.19, arrow). However, this connection can be horizontal or even downwards.

Furthermore, a tributary may be seen coursing from the posterior arch vein just below the medial malleolus to join the small saphenous vein. It either crosses over the Achilles tendon to join the small saphenous vein just posterior to the lateral malleolus or meets the small saphenous vein directly over the Achilles tendon itself. If the small saphenous vein is refluxive, then these tributaries may become varicose and easily identified.

2.5.5 Perforating Veins of the Small Saphenous Vein

The small saphenous vein has four fairly constant connections with the deep veins (Fig. 2.38):

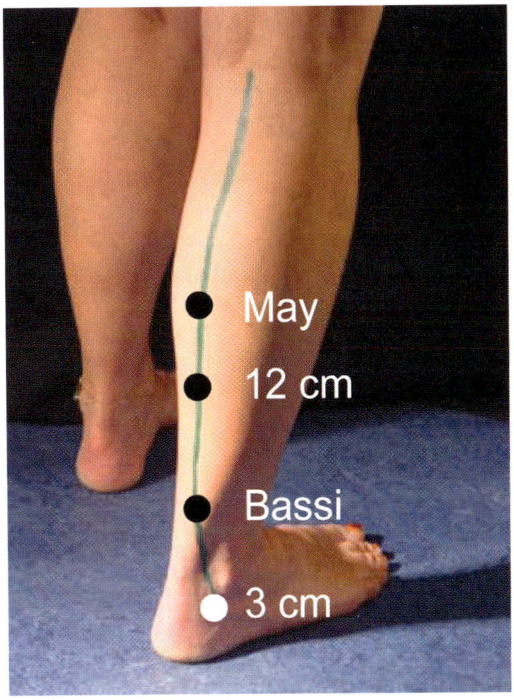

Fig. 2.38 Location of the soleal perforating vein (formerly May) Copyright: [Author]

1. Soleal perforating vein (formerly May). This connects the small saphenous vein with the muscular veins of gastrocnemius and soleus in the middle of the calf at the so-called gastrocnemius point. It may depart directly from the small saphenous vein or from a tributary when it runs in a medial direction. It is around 15 cm from the ground in a standing subject.
2. A perforating vein at a height of 12 cm connecting the small saphenous vein with the fibular veins.
3. A para-Achillean perforating veins (formerly Bassi). Like the perforating vein at 12 cm, this connects the small saphenous vein with the fibular (peroneal) veins at a height of 8 cm.
4. Below the lateral malleolus, there is a direct connection between the small saphenous vein and the fibular (peroneal) veins at a height of 3 cm.

Also in the popliteal fossa is the confluence of the *popliteal fossa perforating veins* which were first described by Dodd (1958, 1964). One of these veins may run subcutaneously along the back of the calf often parallel to the small saphenous vein. It joins the popliteal vein separately and usually lateral to the SSV.

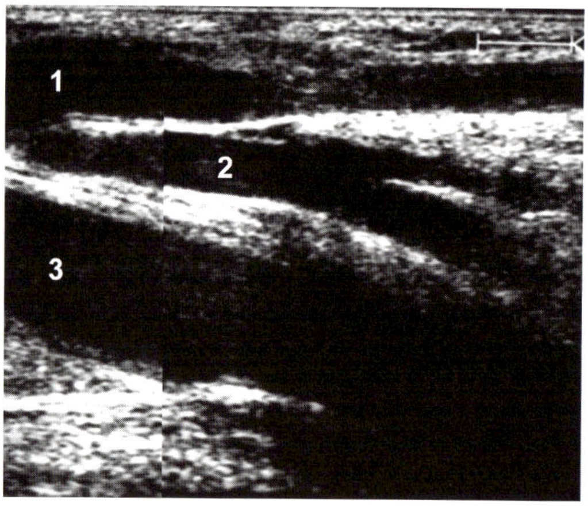

Fig. 2.39 Longitudinal image through the lower part of the popliteal fossa demonstrating a connection between the small saphenous vein (1) and a muscle vein (2). To the left, the small saphenous vein joins the popliteal vein (3) Copyright: [Author]

Numerous Posterior-Lateral Lower Leg Perforating Veins

There are numerous, unclassified, possible connections of the small saphenous vein and/or its tributaries with the muscular veins. In the popliteal region, the small saphenous vein may connect with the muscular veins of gastrocnemius. Here, this can be easily confused with the saphenopopliteal junction (Fig. 2.39 and Sect. 8.5).

Perforating Veins Overview

- The lateral calf perforating veins connect the veins of the lateral plexus with the fibular (peroneal) veins.
- The posterior calf perforating veins also include the medial gastrocnemius perforators on the medial side of the calf and the lateral gastrocnemius perforators on the lateral side of the calf.
- Perforating veins in the knee region or popliteal fossa. There are medial and lateral knee perforating veins as well as supra- or infra-patellar perforating veins.

2.5.6 Accompanying Structures of the Small Saphenous Vein

Above the popliteal fossa, the sciatic nerve divides into the common peroneal nerve and the tibial nerve. The **common peroneal nerve** runs laterally along the biceps femoris muscle and distally immediately behind the head of the fibula. In cases of a high lateral termination of the small saphenous vein with the common femoral vein, the small saphenous vein lies very near to this nerve. Damage to this during surgery may lead to a frequent and serious neurological complication called foot-drop with **paralysis of the foot extensors**.

The **tibial** nerve runs deep within the popliteal fossa accompanying the artery and vein. They all exit the popliteal fossa beneath the gastrocnemius heads (Sect. 17.6).

The medial sural cutaneous nerve is a branch of the tibial nerve which accompanies the small saphenous vein distally. In the lower third, it joins the peroneal communicating branch to form the sural nerve. This is responsible for the sensitivity of the back of the distal calf and the outer side of the foot. Inadvertent injury may occur during open surgery or thermal endovenous procedures. Therefore, it is advisable to identify this nerve preoperatively by ultrasound (Sect. 17.6).

Like the great saphenous vein, the small saphenous vein is accompanied by **lymphatic vessels**. However, there are no lymph nodes in the small saphenous compartment.

2.5.7 Topographical Anatomy of the Small Saphenous Vein

In its upper segment, the small saphenous vein runs in the recess between the medial and lateral gastrocnemius (Fig. 2.27) and further down directly on the soleus muscle (Fig. 2.28). In the ankle region, it runs lateral of the Achilles tendon and posterior to the lateral malleolus (Fig. 2.29).

2.6 Histology of the Saphenous Trunk Veins and the Epifascial Branches

Like the arteries, the larger veins consist of three layers (Caggiati et al. 1998). From inside to outside, they are the **intima**, **media,** and **adventitia**. The intima is coated with an endothelium where the cells are orientated longitudinally and in direct contact with the blood. The valve cusps develop from horizontally orientated endothelial cells which arise from the intima in both the deep veins and the saphenous trunks.

Histologically, the saphenous trunks can be differentiated from the tributaries (epifascial branches).

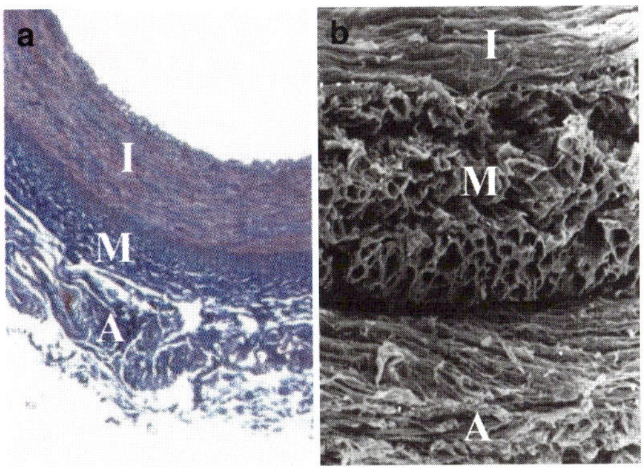

Fig. 2.40 Histology of the juvenile great saphenous vein. (**a**) Light microscopy of a transverse section (haematoxylin and eosin, ×10). (**b**) Electron microscopy of a longitudinal section. At the *top* of each picture, the intima (*I*) is coated with a layer of endothelium on the luminal surface. In the *centre*, the media (*M*) is seen with its circular muscle fibres. The adventitia (*A*) is at the *bottom* (Prof. A. Caggiati, Rome; by kind permission) Copyright: A. Caggiati, Rome

2.6.1 Saphenous Trunks

The saphenous trunks consist of smooth muscle cells in all three layers of the vein wall. They are orientated longitudinally in the intima and adventitia with a circular orientation in the media (Fig. 2.40). The thickness of the wall reduces from the foot upwards. There is a higher collagen content and a higher number of muscle cells in all three layers at the foot.

The thickness of the saphenous wall increases with age. In the elderly, there are more smooth muscle cells and collagen fibres present, but fewer elastic fibres. The longitudinal musculature of the adventitia also increases (Fig. 2.41).

The adventitia of the saphenous vein contains very small supply vessels called vasa vasorum as well as terminal fibres of the sympathetic system.

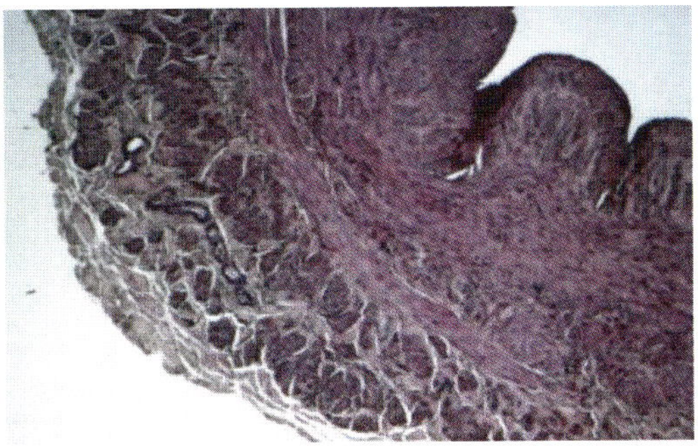

Fig. 2.41 Light microscopy of a transverse section through a senile great saphenous vein (Masson-Färbung, ×10). There is marked hypertrophy of the intima which has developed an undulating surface. There is significantly more smooth muscle in the adventitia as compared to the juvenile vein (c.f. Fig. 2.40) (Prof. A. Caggiati, Rome; by kind permission) Copyright: A. Caggiati, Rome

2.6.2 Extrafascial Veins

Caggiati separated the extrafascial veins into those with a diameter 2–3 mm and those less than 1 mm because they have different histological features.

2.6.2.1 Veins with Diameter 2–3 mm

The intima and adventitia of the larger epifascial tributaries have scarcely any longitudinal smooth muscle cells. Under the endothelium, there is only a thin layer of collagen, and in the media, a thin layer of muscle. The thickness of these walls does not vary from their distance up the leg. They are significantly thinner than those of the saphenous veins of the same diameter, irrespective of their height (Figs. 2.42 and 2.43).

2.6.2.2 Veins with Diameter 1 mm or Less

The intima and adventitia do not have any smooth muscle cells. There is only a thin layer of smooth muscle in the media.

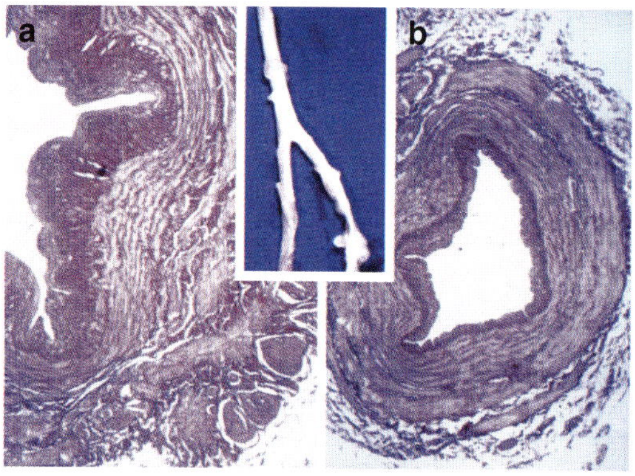

Fig. 2.42 Histology (haematoxylin and eosin ×10) of the great saphenous vein (**a**) and a tributary (**b**) at the same height from the ground. The vein preparation is shown in the centre. The wall of the great saphenous vein is unmistakably and significantly thicker than that of the tributary (Prof. A. Caggiati, Rome; by kind permission) Copyright: A. Caggiati, Rome

2.6.3 Aplasia of the Great Saphenous Vein

In an empty saphenous eye on ultrasound (Fig. 2.16b), a histological rudiment of a saphenous vein is always found. There are smooth muscle cells in all three layers of the wall but the lumen is absent (Fig. 2.44). Further studies are needed to determine whether this vein was

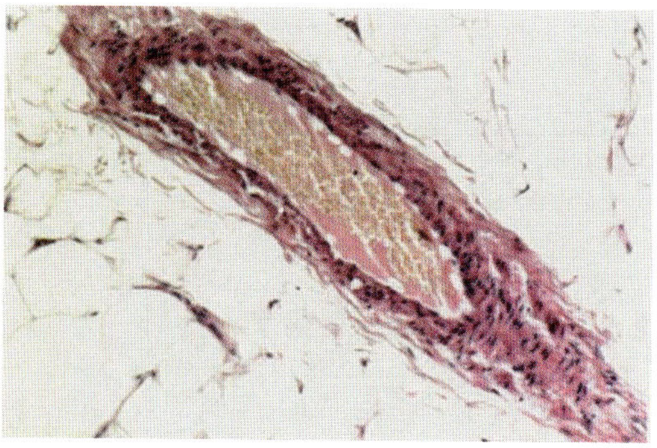

Fig. 2.44 Histology of a remnant of great saphenous vein in an empty saphenous eye (haematoxylin and eosin, ×10) (Prof. A. Caggiati, Rome; by kind permission) Copyright: A. Caggiati, Rome

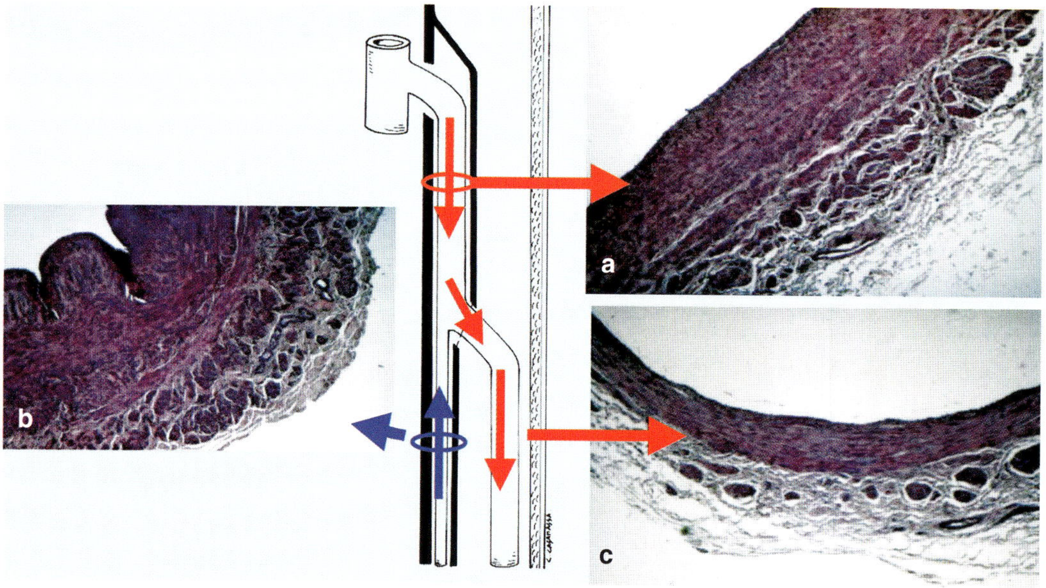

Fig. 2.43 Histology of a refluxing great saphenous vein (**a**) compared to a healthy great saphenous vein in the same leg (**b**) (c.f. Fig. 2.41) and a refluxive tributary (**c**) (Masson-Färbung, ×10) (Prof. A. Caggiati, Rome; by kind permission) Copyright: A. Caggiati, Rome

originally functional and later atrophied or whether it was aplastic from the outset.

Saphenous trunk veins differ from their tributaries in their course and histology (Caggiati 2000; Caggiati et al. 1998).

References

Askar O (1963) The short saphenous vein. J Cardiovasc Surg 4:126–137

Bergan JJ (1999) Common anatomic patterns of varicose veins. In: Goldmann MP, Weiss RA, Bergan JJ (eds) Varicose veins and telangiectasias. Quality Medical Publishing Inc, St Louis, pp 70–86

Caggiati A (2000) Fascial relations and structure of the tributaries of the saphenous veins. Surg Radiol Anat 22:1–4

Caggiati A (2001) Fascial relationships of the short saphenous vein. J Vasc Surg 34:241–246

Caggiati A, Mendoza E (2004) Segmental hypoplasia of the great saphenous vein and varicose disease. Eur J Vasc Endovasc Surg 28:257–261

Caggiati A, Ricci S (1999) The long saphenous vein compartment. Phlebology 12:107–111

Caggiati A, Ricci S (2000) The caliber of the human long saphenous vein and its congenital variations. Ann Anat 182:1–7

Caggiati A, Macchiarelli G, Familiari G (1998) Topographical structural variations of the human long saphenous vein and its age-related remodelling as revealed by correlated light and scanning electron microscopy. Phlebology 13:156–162

Caggiati A, Bergan JJ, Gloviczki P, Jantet G, Wendell-Smith CP, Partsch H (2002) Nomenclature of the veins of the lower limbs: an international interdisciplinary consensus statement. J Vasc Surg 36:416–422

Cavezzi A, Labropoulos N, Partsch H, Ricci S, Caggiati A, Myers K, Nicolaides A, Smith CP (2006) Duplex ultrasound investigation of the veins in chronic venous disease of the lower limbs-UIP Consensus Document. Part II. Anatomy. Eur J Vasc Endovasc Surg 31:288–299

Creton D (2005) Saphenopopliteal junctions are significantly lower when incompetent. Phlebolymphology 48:347–354

Dodd H (1958) Persistent varicose veins with special reference to the varicose tributaries of the superficial femoral and popliteal veins. Proc R Soc Med 51:817–820

Dodd H (1964) The varicose tributaries of the popliteal vein. Proc R Soc Med 57:394–396

Dodd H, Cockett FB (1976) The pathology and surgery of the veins of the lower limb. Churchill Livingstone, Edinburgh/London/New York

Kosinski C (1926) Observations on the superficial venous system of the lower extremities. J Anat 60:131–138

Mühlberger D, Morandini L, Brenner E (2009) Venous valves and major superficial tributary veins near the saphenofemoral junction J Vasc Surg 49:1562–1569

Ricci S, Caggiati A (1999) Does a double long saphenous vein exist? Phlebology 14:59–64

Pathophysiology of the Superficial Venous System

3

Erika Mendoza, Claude Franceschi, Birgit Kahle, and Christopher R. Lattimer

Chapter Summary
The previous chapter described venous anatomy. Duplex ultrasound demonstrates both the blood flow inside the veins and their structures. To analyse this flow, an understanding of normal flow and the significance of pathological flow is essential.

3.1 Anatomical and Physiological Basics

Anatomical landmarks like muscle fascia are not the only distinction between the superficial and deep veins. Superficial veins unlike deep veins have **muscle cells** in their wall. This enables them to adapt in size as a reaction to cold, heat, external stimuli like being pinched with tweezers, fear and medication. Cold and ergotamine cause contraction and venospasm. Warmth and hypotensive drugs cause their relaxation.

Venous behaviour varies depending on whether the subject is standing or lying. In the lying subject, the blood flows towards the heart slowly and continuously driven by arterial flow from behind, called *vis a tergo*. After flowing through the capillaries, the blood has lost most or all of its pulsatility. In addition, respiration has the effect of augmenting the venous return. During inhalation, the negative intrathoracic pressure encourages venous flow upwards into the chest (see also Sect. 6.2.1).

When the subject stands up, the muscle veins in the calf fill with a reserve of around 350 ml of blood (Dodd and Cockett 1976), meaning that at first no blood flows out of the leg. If the subject continues to stand still, the venous return resumes due to *vis a tergo*. This is enhanced substantially by the activity of the calf **muscle pump**. The combined action of the calf muscle pump and the valves propels the blood towards the heart during muscular contraction. The blood is forced in *one* direction through the openings of the venous valves which prevent retrograde flow towards the feet or outwards into the superficial veins. When the muscles relax, the blood cannot flow back because the venous valves close. This action results in a pressure drop in the deep veins which draws blood in from the superficial and muscle veins.

E. Mendoza, MD, PhD (✉)
Venenpraxis Wunstorf,
Speckenstraße 10, 31515 Wunstorf, Germany
e-mail: erika.mendoza@t-online.de

C. Franceschi, MD
Angiologist Consultant, Hopital Saint Joseph,
21, quai Alphonse Le Gallo, 92000 Paris, France
e-mail: claude.franceschi@gmail.com

B. Kahle, MD, PhD
Klinik für Dermatologie, Allergologie und Venerologie,
UKSH Campus Lübeck, Ratzeburger Allee 160,
23538 Lübeck, Germany
e-mail: birgit.kahle@uksh.de

C.R. Lattimer, MD, PhD
Department of Vascular Surgery,
Josef Pflug Vascular Laboratory,
Ealing Hospital and Imperial College, London, UK

E. Mendoza et al. (eds.), *Duplex Ultrasound of Superficial Leg Veins*,
DOI 10.1007/978-3-642-40731-4_3, © Springer-Verlag Berlin Heidelberg 2014

This pumping action can be compared to the heart using the terms **muscular systole** for muscle contraction and **muscular diastole** for muscle relaxation. Muscular systole pumps blood out of the deep veins, while muscular diastole fills them by draining the superficial veins.

3.1.1 Flow Behaviour of Liquids in Rigid Tubes

The principles of blood flow are derived experimentally from the behaviour of liquids in rigid tubes. However, blood vessels are not ideal tubes as they are collapsible and the flow within them is not exposed to a constant pressure (Kamm and Pedley 1989).

Flow through a straight rigid tube depends on two factors:

1. The pressure difference between the ends of the tube.
2. The resistance of the tube to flow. This is influenced by the viscosity of the liquid, the properties of the wall and the diameter of the tube.

If the tube is smooth, the liquid inside will flow in an orderly way, within a certain range of velocities. The layer in immediate contact with the wall flows very slowly due to friction. The next layer flows faster over the first and so progressively towards the centre of the pipe where the flow is the fastest (Fig. 3.1). This is known as **laminar flow** which is a property of a Newtonian fluid.

If bends are introduced into the tube, impediments like venous valves are found in the wall, the pipe diameter is very small or the velocity is very high, then **turbulence** occurs. This causes the blood to divert from its parallel path and flow in all directions, even towards the wall. This results in an increase in friction and resistance. Consequently, the forward velocity is reduced and pressure on the wall increases.

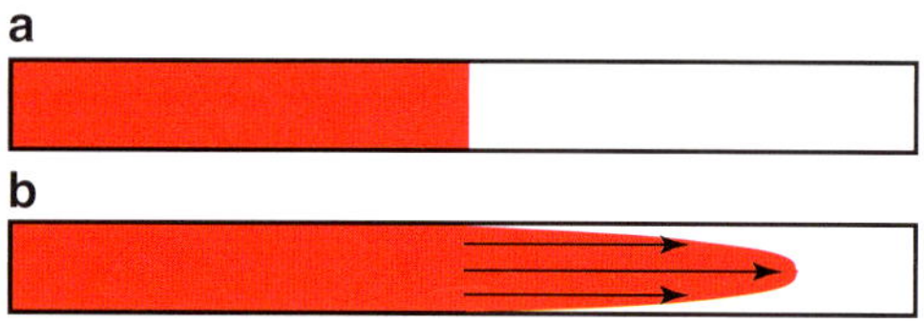

Fig. 3.1 Diagram of a tube containing two different coloured fluids to demonstrate laminar flow: (**a**) no flow at rest; (**b**) a velocity profile is created as the red fluid begins to flow. Flow is faster and occurs further at the centre compared to the periphery Copyright: [Author]

3.1.2 Relative Pressures in Veins

Veins are expandable adapting their diameter and length to volume and pressure. This adaptability is called **compliance**. If the vein walls were rigid, the intravenous pressure would rise in direct proportion to an increase in volume. However, veins are able to contain differing amounts of blood without these pressure increases. The compliance of veins is much greater than that of arteries making them an ideal blood reservoir for the body. In fact, 70–85 % of the circulating blood volume is in the post-capillary veins, including the deep and superficial leg veins (Dodd and Cockett 1976).

The hydrostatic **pressure differences** within veins are generally predetermined by gravity. The pressure in the right atrium of a healthy person is equal to 0 mmHg. After 30 s standing still, the pressure in both the deep and superficial veins in the region of the foot, regardless of whether the venous system is healthy or pathological, is 90–100 mmHg. This is determined by the hydrostatic pressure of the blood column from the right atrium to the foot. In this way, a hydrostatic pressure difference is created by the force of gravity. This needs to be exceeded before antegrade flow can resume.

When the calf muscles contract during muscular systole, the pressure in the deep veins rises to up to 235 mmHg. This is higher than systolic blood pressure. Pressures of up to 115 mmHg are found in the thigh. This increased pressure exceeds that of the hydrostatic column, thereby driving blood upwards towards the heart. After muscle contraction, venous valves prevent the volume expelled from flowing backwards. The valves close during diastole and divide the hydrostatic column into sections. This process is called fractionation. During calf diastole, very low pressures of about 25 mmHg are generated in the deep veins. This leads to a new pressure difference between the deep and superficial veins causing drainage of the superficial veins inwards into the deep veins.

The frequently described condition of **venous hypertension** occurs in the superficial veins when the system decompensates. In this situation, calf muscle systole is not longer able to cope with the excess recirculating volume. This excess of volume is caused by reflux down the superficial veins. Varicose veins then begin to appear with stretching of the vein walls before any noticeable increases in pressure. When the patient is standing still, the pressure in the deep and superficial veins approximates to hydrostatic pressure. If the perforating veins are incompetent, they reflux during muscular systole causing blood to flow outwards into the superficial veins.

The **flow pattern** influences the pressure transmitted onto the vein wall. Turbulent flow is more likely to cause higher pressures than laminar flow. The properties of the wall are also important in resisting dilatation. Interestingly, unlike superficial tributaries, the great saphenous vein almost never becomes varicose, irrespective of whether it is used as an arterial bypass or is subjected to venous pressures considerably higher than arterial.

3.2 Recirculation

In healthy veins, blood flows from superficial to deep veins, from tributaries into the saphenous or deep veins directly and from the saphenous trunks into the deep veins (Fig. 3.2). Venous blood flows upwards generally leaving the leg through the deep system. As shown in Fig. 3.2, saphenous blood in the standing patient during muscle diastole has a brief duration of retrograde flow between a perforating vein and the next higher valve. In healthy veins, the quantity of blood flowing in superficial veins is very small. The venous reservoir in health consists almost entirely of the deep and muscle veins.

Recirculation can cause varicose veins which is dependent on two conditions:

1. The flow direction must be reversed so that blood flows from the deep to the superficial veins or from a saphenous vein into tributaries. The starting point of reverse flow is called the *reflux source*. The receiving vessel is not adapted to receive this flow and therefore dilates.
2. This reflux volume must re-enter the deep veins at some point further down the leg; otherwise, the blood column would thrombose. Re-entry occurs through perforating veins or healthy saphenous veins. They may become secondarily dilated because they carry the same extra volume as the dilated superficial veins which are pathologically filled. This may lead to secondary incompetence.

In isolated **saphenous vein incompetence**, without the participation of any tributaries, recirculation occurs between the deep veins and the

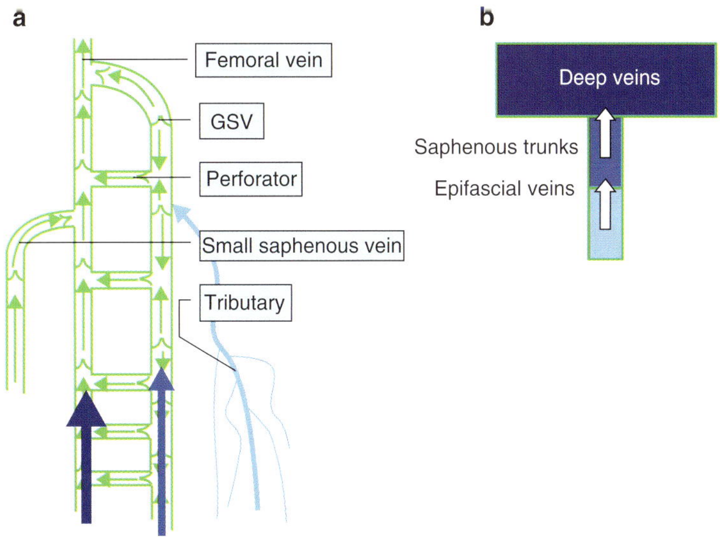

Fig. 3.2 (**a**) Diagram of the blood flow in healthy veins, standing; (**b**) diagram of the total blood volume in the veins of a healthy subject. The *arrows* indicate that the blood in the leg flows from the superficial to the deep veins from where it leaves the leg (From Mendoza (2002); by kind permission of Arrien GmbH) Copyright: Arrien, Wunstorf

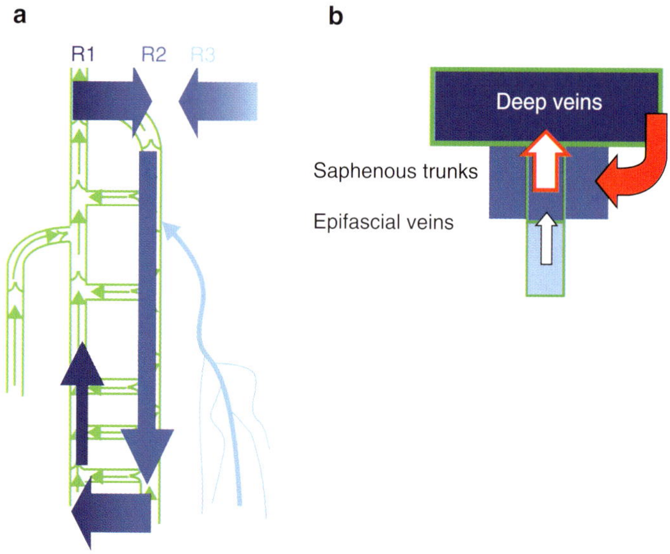

Fig. 3.3 (**a**) Blood flow with reflux confined to the great saphenous vein. Recirculation starts from the deep veins and enters the great saphenous vein where it refluxes down until it re-enters back into the deep veins; (**b**) diagram of the total blood volume in the leg veins in the recirculation loop shown in (a). The healthy veins are shown in green (cf. Fig. 3.2b) (From Mendoza (2002); by kind permission of Arrien GmbH) Copyright: Arrien, Wunstorf

saphenous veins (Fig. 3.3a). The saphenous vein therefore becomes volume overloaded (Fig. 3.3b). Despite this, it still continues to drain the normal tributaries with blood flowing from the tributaries through the refluxive saphenous vein and into the deep veins. Eventually, the net blood flow is out of the leg through the deep veins, but this is constantly hampered by the recirculation.

With **saphenous vein incompetence and additional refluxive tributaries**, the situation is more complex. The tributaries may also become overloaded by participating in the recirculation loop (Fig. 3.4). Assuming healthy deep veins, this results in an extra volume load through a perforating vein as well as the deep veins. The volume burden caused by recirculation may result in secondary deep venous insufficiency. This is because the blood volume which flows refluxively into the superficial veins must be transported inwards in addition to the blood normally present in the deep veins (Fig. 3.4b; note the wider profile of the dark blue box)

Only those **perforating veins** which have suffered secondary dilatation from refluxive outward flow will serve as re-entry points for a recirculation. Undilated perforating veins are present but do not participate in recirculation. This can be demonstrated by measuring the flow in a varicose vein, without compressing the perforating vein, and then measuring the flow in the re-entry perforating vein under compression. In the first case, there is a typical reflux curve. In the second case, there is no retrograde flow during muscular diastole. This is termed the reflux elimination test (Zamboni et al. 2010) (see Sect. 4.2.9).

3.2.1 Analysis of the Flow Curve in PW Mode

In B scan with colour duplex ultrasound, it is easy to see the flow direction. However, this information is often not sufficient (Fig. 1.20), and important information can be lost. Therefore, when investigating venous insufficiency, it is recommended to analyse the PW curve at a minimum of one point at least, since this is the easiest way of confirming a diagnosis of reflux.

Unlike an arterial examination, flow curve analysis is only a **semi-quantitative assessment**. Flows may differ in the same vein during the same examination, so flow velocities and blood volumes should not be regarded as absolute values. They depend on how long the patient has been standing, how long it is since the last stimulation manoeuvre, how much force was used or even the size of the examiner's hand.

The PW Doppler mode measures the **velocities** of the erythrocytes per unit of time in the measurement window. The PW curve records these velocities as white points along the time axis. If the velocities of the individual erythrocytes are similar, as in laminar flow, a curve will

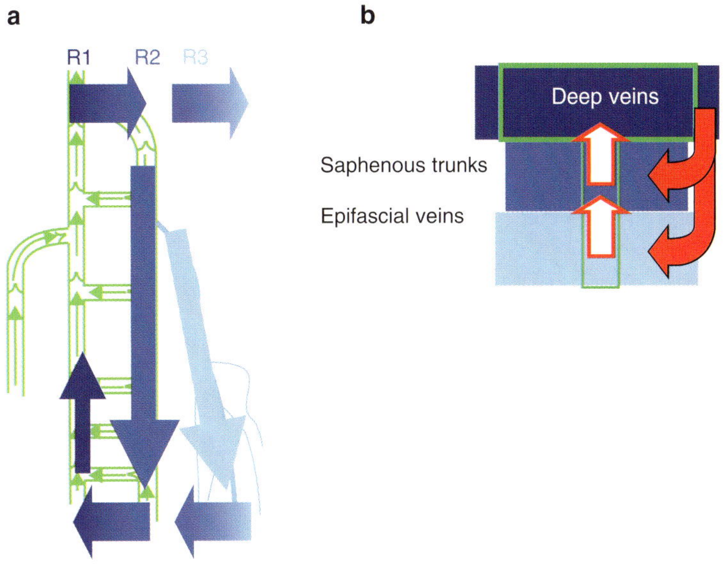

Fig. 3.4 (**a**) Diagram of recirculation in the great saphenous vein and its tributaries with re-entry through perforating veins at the ankle; (**b**) diagram of the blood volumes in the three vein systems. The epifascial and saphenous systems are completely overloaded. However, blood will only leave the leg through the deep veins (From Mendoza (2002); by kind permission of Arrien GmbH) Copyright: Arrien, Wunstorf

be formed with a white contour and a black space under the curve. If different velocities are recorded (turbulent flow), the whole curve will be filled in with white points.

The following data are important (Fig. 3.5):

- Velocity of retrograde flow (curve height).
- Duration of retrograde flow (curve length).
- Evolution or change in velocity – velocity profile (curve contour).
- Area under the flow curve with reflux as compared to area under the flow curve with antegrade flow. This estimates the blood volume ejected upwards during the stimulation manoeuvre as compared to the blood volume which finally flows towards the foot.
- Filling of the area under the flow curve – black with laminar or white with turbulent flow.

Flow curve analysis in the following veins is particularly important:

- Saphenofemoral junction tributaries (Sect. 7.3.6)
- Flows into the great saphenous vein from healthy tributaries or through perforating veins (Sect. 7.5.2)
- Examination of perforating veins (Sect. 9.3)

As a rule, a **high reflux velocity** is associated with a sharp rise and a short reflux duration (Fig. 3.5a, b). This is typical in large-calibre venous insufficiency from reflux sources with large lumina. These are generally saphenous vein junctions which permit fast filling of the incompetent vein from a large blood reservoir of deep veins and in large-calibre re-entry perforating veins which allow a fast drainage of the recirculation volume.

There are four possible causes of slow **reflux** which is usually long-lasting (Fig. 3.5d, f and Sect. 3.2.3):

1. Small blood reservoir as a source of reflux (e.g. reflux from a healthy saphenous vein into a refluxive tributary)
2. Small-calibre link between reflux source and refluxive vessel (e.g. reflux from the pelvis through the pudendal or epigastric veins)
3. Lack of compliance in the refluxive vein so that it cannot receive large blood volumes (e.g. due to sclerosis or irradiation)
4. Small-calibre drainage (e.g. through re-entry perforating veins)

3.2.2 Definitions of Reflux

Recirculation

The pathological situation in varicose vein disease is recirculation. The blood which should flow towards the heart leaks out of the deep veins at some point to enter the superficial veins where it overloads a segment. Then usually further down the leg, this re-enters the deep system

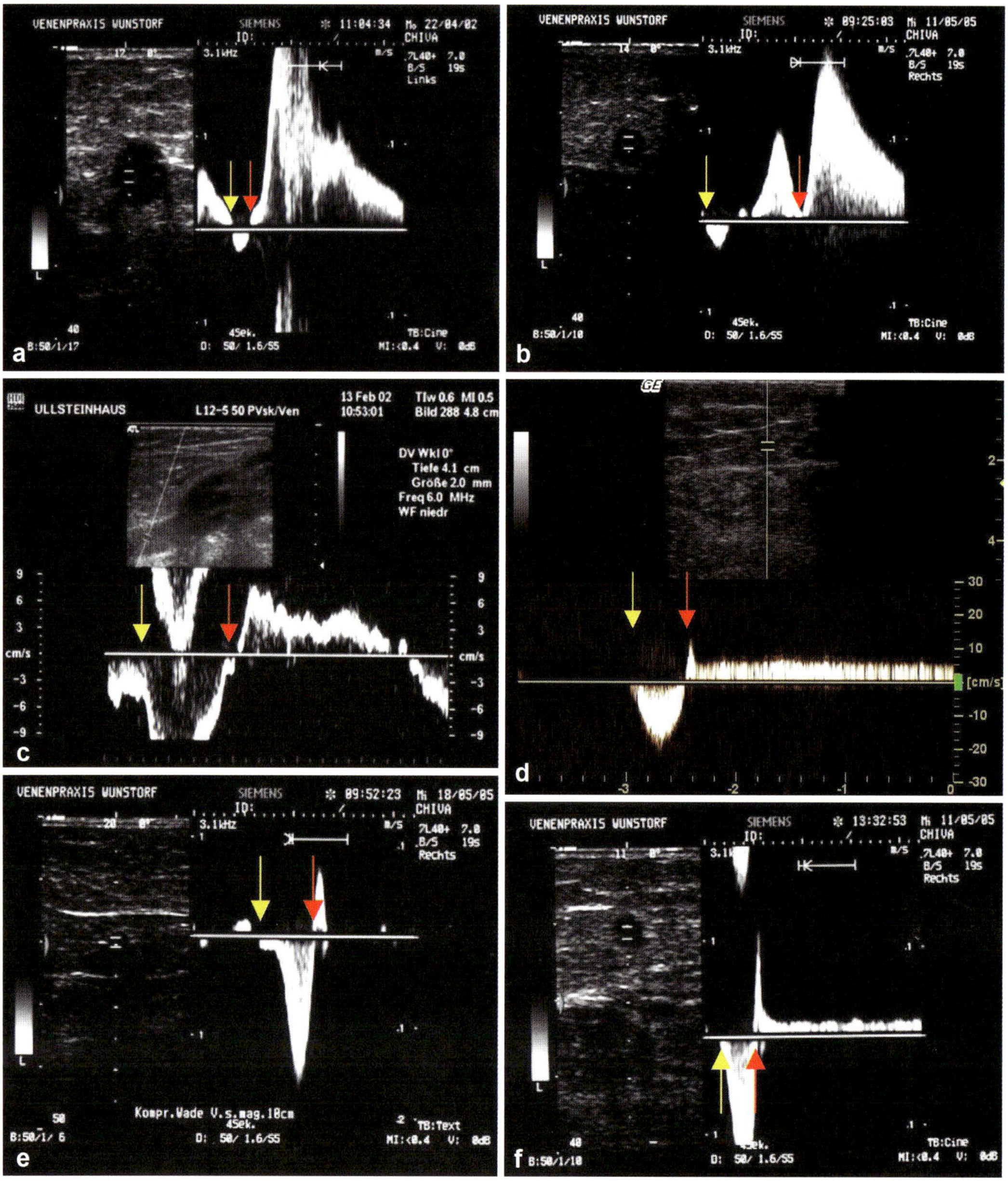

Fig. 3.5 Flow curve analysis. All measurements except (**c**) were taken from the great saphenous vein in the mid thigh. The *yellow arrow* indicates the beginning of muscular systole, and the *red arrow* the beginning of diastole. (**a**) Sharp rise, high reflux velocity. The area under the curve is not filled indicating that the flow is not very turbulent. Length of reflux is approximately 4 s which is clearly stronger than antegrade flow. (**b**) Short antegrade flow with reflux in two phases: one short, not very rapid curve during the period of muscular contraction (explanation Fig. 6.15) and one longer-lasting, faster curve. The flow is turbulent as the area under the curve is almost completely filled with *white*. This indicates the wide range of different velocities being measured which are typical of turbulence. (**c**) Flow in the popliteal vein just above an incompetent saphenopopliteal junction. Almost laminar flow as the curve contour is thin. The blood volume which flows in an antegrade direction during muscular systole is much greater than the volume which flows back during diastole. This blood flows in a retrograde direction from the popliteal vein into the refluxive small saphenous vein. The popliteal vein itself is not incompetent (explanation Fig. 6.12c). (**d**) Slow, long-lasting reflux. (**e**) Antegrade flow during muscle contraction with a short reflux until the valve closes. There is a sharp rise lasting <0.5 s confirming the vein is competent. (**f**) Short, steep reflux at first until valve closure, as in (e), but followed by a slow, long-lasting reflux. The saphenofemoral junction is competent. The short retrograde flow indicates the closure of the first subterminal valve. The long-lasting reflux which follows is from the epigastric vein draining into a refluxing great saphenous veinCopyright: [Author]

where it flows upwards once more towards the heart. This recirculation is the pathophysiology behind varicose vein disease. It describes the superfluous blood circuit in a varicose vein which has been termed a **repetition** or **private circuit** (Trendelenburg 1891). These terms are also applied when blood from a competent saphenous vein fills an incompetent tributary.

Volume Overload of the Superficial Venous System

The affected veins in the superficial venous system are filled with more blood by the recirculation than the veins were originally supposed to contain. In response to this volume overload, the vein walls dilate.

Reflux

This is defined as pathological blood flow following normal, antegrade flow. Blood which flows normally towards the heart during muscular systole then flows in a retrograde direction towards the foot to become reflux. Reflux is the part of the recirculation loop which occurs in incompetent veins during diastole. It includes blood already within the vein from antegrade flow as well as blood which originally entered another vein like the deep veins and then passed through an incompetent valve into the refluxive superficial vein. The reflux fills the incompetent vein with an additional volume of blood.

Drainage

This is defined as blood in retrograde flow, which physiologically belongs to the vessel. It is not extra blood and therefore does not overload the vein. An example of drainage occurs in the venous tributaries draining into the vein of Giacomini after closure of the proximal reflux source. Another example is in the great saphenous vein after ligation of the saphenofemoral junction or crossectomy. The saphenofemoral tributaries normally drain into the proximal great saphenous vein. After closure of an incompetent junction, this blood is diverted retrograde down the great saphenous vein during muscular diastole to the next perforating vein further down through which it enters the deep veins. The great saphenous vein is the correct drainage for this blood, which is neither a pathological volume nor part of a recirculation loop.

3.2.3 Drained and Poorly Drained Systems

The rate of recirculation depends on two main variables:

- The compliance of the refluxive vein
- The calibre of the re-entry perforating vein

Compliance is the capacity of the vein wall to stretch (Sect. 3.1.2). It can receive different volumes of blood by varying its diameter. Indirect measurements of venous compliance can be achieved by measuring venous diameter standing and then lying. If there is little variation in the diameter, the elasticity of the wall is slight and its compliance is poor. Poorly compliant veins fill when the patient stands and are more likely to remain full if they have reduced venous elastic recoil. Patients with venous disease have an increased venous volume, increased rate of filling and reduced venous elastic recoil. These can be measured using air plethysmography.

If the patient has been standing for some time, the veins become quite full regardless of their compliance. The **calibre of the re-entry perforating veins** then has a considerable influence on the flow curve. During muscular diastole, only so much blood will flow towards the foot as can pass back into the deep veins through the perforating vein. Thus, the perforating vein acts like a gatekeeper throttling the rate of recirculation.

These two variables determine how well varicose veins drain. In general, good compliance is associated with large perforating veins (drained system), while poor compliance is associated with narrow re-entry points (poorly drained system).

3.2.3.1 Drained System

Because of their capacity to stretch, varicose veins receive more blood than their diameter at rest allows. This excess of blood then flows down to drain through the large-calibre perforating veins, allowing the vein to collapse. The flow curve in PW mode will rise steeply and then fall again over a few seconds during a stimulation manoeuvre. These patients generally have large-calibre, very winding varicose tributaries but little distress.

3.2.3.2 Poorly Drained System

If however the vein wall is rigid and stiff, with no stretch capacity, only a small amount of blood will be received proximally at the start of muscular diastole. Small-calibre perforating veins also hamper drainage. Only so much blood will be able to enter the vein as can be drained distally. A further cause of a poorly drained system is an impaired muscle pump. If the deep veins are not properly emptied during systole, no pressure drop can be generated during diastole to allow the superficial veins to empty.

The blood will flow very slowly in the varicose vein demonstrated by the curve in PW duplex which is long and flat. In many instances, the flow may be too slow to measure even after adjusting the machine settings (Sects. 1.6 and 6.9). Slow flow results in higher transparietal pressure leading to the formation of an oedema. This group often includes patients with scarcely visible varices but suffers the distress associated with chronic venous insufficiency (Lattimer et al. 2012a).

3.2.4 Duration of Reflux

Various investigations have been carried out to establish the duration of reflux standing which correlates with venous disease (Evans et al. 1998; Labropoulos et al. 2003; Lurie et al. 2012). In general, no difference was found between durations of 0.5 and 1 s. In other words, the number of legs determined to suffer from reflux did not alter significantly depending on whether the duration of reflux was set at 0.5 or 1 s. Although the cut-off value was set at 0.5 s, a definition of reflux set at 1 s may avoid diagnosing pathology at borderline values when there are no clinical signs.

Reflux duration can also be measured during an elevation-dependency manoeuvre (see Sect. 6.8). Reflux duration decreases with severity of disease and has been described as the time taken for the anti-gravitational mechanisms of the leg to fail (Lattimer et al. 2013, 2014).

3.3 Reflux Sources

As described in Sect. 3.2, the basic cause of varicose veins is a circuit with two main points: the **reflux source**, where recirculation starts, and the **re-entry point**, where the refluxive segment ends. The segment between these points has retrograde flow.

Precise identification of the reflux source(s) of a recirculation is the most important prerequisite for good treatment decisions. The point at which the blood starts to flow retrograde, unphysiologically, "the wrong way", is the reflux source. This is the point at which the blood leaves the physiological network to flow from a deeper to a more superficial venous network (Figs. 3.2, 3.3 and 3.4; Sect. 4.2.1). Network in French is "réseau", abbreviated to R. The level of the network, from deep to superficial, is designated by R1, R2 and R3. Several other recirculations may coexist downstream of this **principal recirculation**, which finally carries blood back to the deep veins through other tributaries (Fig. 3.6). If a collateral vessel is filled from an already incompetent vein (as in Fig. 3.6 the tributary is filled from the saphenous trunk), this does not represent a new reflux source. The reflux source is exclusively the point at which the blood flowing physiologically in a healthy vein first starts to flow in a pathological direction.

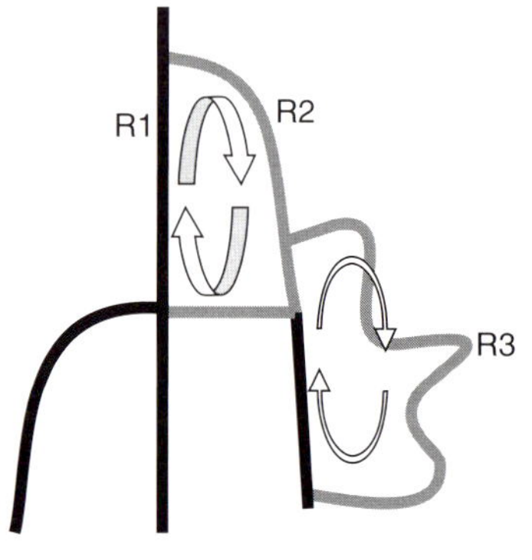

Fig. 3.6 Diagram of a principal recirculation from the deep system into the great saphenous vein and through a paratibial perforating vein (formerly Boyd perforating vein) back into the deep vein system (R1–R2–R1) with recirculation downstream through a tributary (R3) Copyright: [Author]

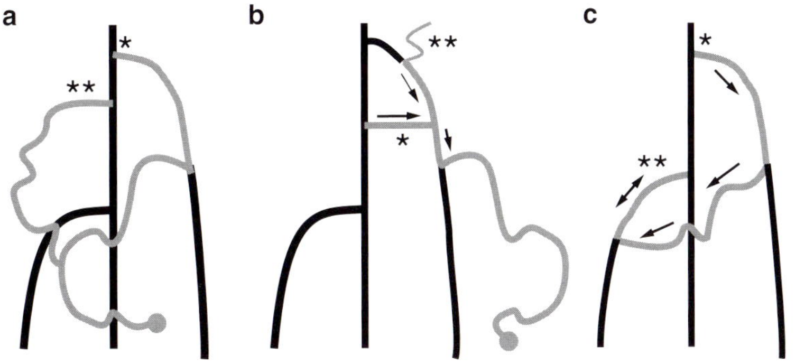

Fig. 3.7 (**a**) Diagram of coexisting reflux sources in recirculation (principal reflux source*), with an additional recirculation (reflux source marked**). Both recirculations flow through a common perforating vein. The refluxive segments are shown in *grey*, and the single re-entry perforating vein is marked with a *dot*. (**b**) Slight reflux from the pelvis (**) with the principal recirculation from a perforating vein in the adductor canal (formerly Dodd) (*). (**c**) Reflux in the great saphenous vein with drainage through a tributary into the small saphenous vein. The proximal section of the small saphenous vein is dilated but not significantly refluxive at first (**). Instead there is an oscillating flow pattern refluxing upwards on calf muscle diastole. Later, tributaries may also carry some of the reflux and offer a drainage route from the great and small saphenous veins. Thus, both veins are refluxive, even though the small saphenous vein was not refluxive at the start. Nevertheless, the principal reflux source is from the great saphenous vein (*) Copyright: [Author]

More than one reflux source may occasionally be found in a leg when there is retrograde flow from the deep veins at several independent points, or two independent tributaries are filled refluxively from a saphenous vein with antegrade flow. In these cases, the higher reflux source is generally more important, for example, a refluxive saphenofemoral junction and a refluxive perforating vein in the back of the thigh (Fig. 3.7a). However, the reverse may occur, for example, if there is minor reflux from the pelvis through the pudendal vein which fills the great saphenous vein in retrograde flow, but the latter is only really dilated and refluxive from a perforating vein in the adductor canal (formerly Dodd) (Fig. 3.7b). Evaluation of the flow curves in PW mode is particularly important in prioritising the relative importance and contribution of a reflux source.

It is also possible for two independent disconnected recirculation circuits to occur. One principal source may be reflux through an incompetent terminal valve into the great saphenous vein with drainage through a dilated perforating vein in the adductor canal (formerly Dodd) with no refluxive tributary. The additional principal source may be reflux into the small saphenous vein with drainage through a perforating vein further down.

Diagnostic problems arise when **both saphenous junctions are refluxive** and the saphenous trunk veins are connected by a tributary (ramus communicans). In this case, it cannot always be clearly established whether the small saphenous vein suffered the primary incompetence or if it started as the drainage route of the great saphenous vein and at some point was so volume overloaded that it subsequently became incompetent (Fig. 3.7c).

3.3.1 Reflux Sources from Deep Veins into Saphenous Trunks

Blood flow may be observed arising directly from a deep vein into a saphenous vein:

- From the femoral vein into the great saphenous vein through the saphenofemoral junction (Fig. 4.1 and Sect. 7.3)
- From the popliteal vein into the small saphenous vein through the saphenopopliteal junction (Fig. 4.19 and Sect. 8.3)
- From the deep veins into the great saphenous vein through perforating veins (Fig. 4.9 and Chap. 9)
- From the deep veins into the small saphenous vein through muscle veins or perforating veins (Fig. 4.15a, c and Chap. 9)

The further down the leg a perforating vein is located, the less likely it is to act as a reflux source, and the more likely it is to act as a re-entry point.

3.3.2 Reflux Sources from Deep Veins into Varicose Tributaries

This refers to the flow of blood from the deep veins, through a perforating vein and thence directly into a tributary, without a saphenous trunk being involved as a reflux source. In its subsequent course downwards, the saphenous vein can of course form part of the recirculation. Such a primary reflux source is frequently observed in the **back of the thigh** where the dorsal thigh perforating vein originates (Fig. 4.9b).

In athletes, especially footballers, it is not unusual to find several refluxive muscle veins which fill the lower leg tributaries through perforating veins (Fig. 4.8c). Thus, these patients may have various reflux sources. It may be that the pressure on muscle veins or perforating veins is so high from trauma to damage the valves leaving these veins permanently incompetent.

3.3.3 Reflux Sources from Saphenous Trunks into Tributaries

This occurs when blood flows out of a competent saphenous trunk vein into a varicose tributary. In these cases, reflux is confined to the varicose veins. The saphenous vein carries blood upwards from its healthy tributaries which then reflux from the saphenous trunks into pathologically dilated ones. The saphenous trunks in this case are not filled from the deep veins or from pathologically refluxive pelvic or superficial inguinal veins (Fig. 4.24).

Varicose veins without saphenous reflux are generally a cosmetic problem. They do not cause any chronic venous incompetence, since they do not increase the total volume flowing through the leg. Many phlebologists advocate treatment for these because they could be precursors of saphenous reflux (Sect. 3.3.4).

3.3.4 Retrograde Flow with No Upstream Reflux Source

In many patients with saphenous reflux, the examiner is unable to find a reflux source from the deep vein on duplex ultrasound (Labropoulos et al. 1997). The junctions and tributaries are competent as are the perforating veins and the proximal saphenous vein. Further down, a discreet reflux may be found as successive healthy tributaries join together. The volume of this reflux towards the foot increases with each joining tributary. This reflux starts in a tributary, and **by definition**, the **reflux source** is therefore **at the confluence of the tributaries**. These then drain into the great saphenous vein. Occasionally, there is retrograde flow in the saphenous vein above this tributary, but in physiological terms, the blood belongs to the tributaries, and the refluxive saphenous vein above the tributary is a secondary phenomenon.

Reverse flow without a prior reflux source is very often found by chance in the contralateral leg which has minimal or no signs of clinical venous disease.

Ascending and Descending Theories of Varicose Vein Progression

Whether reflux originates near the foot and progresses upwards or arises from an incompetent junction and progresses downwards is important. If the direction of progression can be predicted, then treatments can be more focused. If an ascending pathology is interrupted, this may prevent subsequent incompetence of the upper end of the great saphenous vein and the saphenofemoral junction (Bernardini et al. 2002). In a standing patient, a refluxive vein is constantly refilled with blood by the force of gravity. Suction into the deep veins caused by calf diastole will suck blood out of the varicose vein. This in turn will result in a downward **suction** force in the tributary in addition to the effect of gravity. If these forces continue, then the valves in the upper saphenous vein may begin to fail leading to the slow development of a retrograde flow. When the suction reaches the saphenofemoral junction, this may create a reflux source and the formation of a recirculation loop now involving the deep veins (Fig. 3.8). Interestingly, the saphenous veins of many patients can regain competency after interruption of refluxive tributary. This can be observed after saphenous conservation approaches like CHIVA (Zamboni et al. 2010) (Sect. 12.2) and ASVAL (Pittaluga et al. 2010).

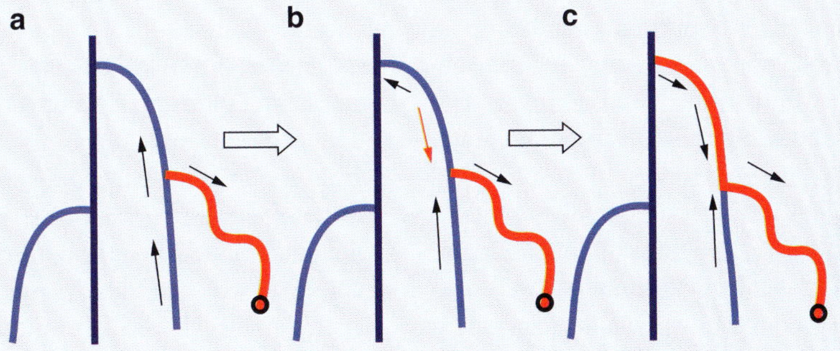

Fig. 3.8 Ascending progression theory. (**a**) Varicose tributary with a competent great saphenous vein; (**b**) varicose tributary with a suction (siphon) effect on the proximal saphenous vein causing the start of a retrograde flow out of part of the saphenous vein and into the varicose tributary; (**c**) further ascending progression to complete incompetence of the great saphenous vein and the saphenofemoral junction Copyright: [Author]

3.3.5 Reflux Sources Above the Inguinal Ligament

Occasionally, the reflux source is above the inguinal ligament. The leg veins become filled via an incompetent vein from higher up. The following variants have been observed.

Refluxive saphenofemoral tributaries, especially the pudendal vein from medial and the epigastric or circumflex vein from above, can be filled by a:

- Refluxive network over the labia in the inner thigh.
- Refluxive network on the abdominal wall with flow into the subcutaneous venous network on the front of the thigh.
- Connection from a varicocele via a scrotal venous network to the thigh.
- A refluxive vein which comes to the surface of the skin below the breast. This is visible where it runs down the lateral abdomen towards the feet filling the great saphenous vein with retrograde flow below the groin.

A common element in all these variants is that the refluxive blood **does not come from the leg** but from the abdominal skin, from the scrotum/labia or from organs in the pelvis. The various forms of varicose veins which result from this reflux are described in Sects. 4.1.3, 7.3.4, 7.3.5 and 7.3.6.

In clinical practice, recirculation from reflux sources above the inguinal ligament is a frequent source of **recurrence** after treatment of the leg veins. This is because the actual reflux point is not eliminated by normal interventions for varicose veins. They are usually treated from higher up using radiological interventions. After crossectomy, these patients often suffer recurrence in the groin at sites unconnected with the common femoral vein (Sect. 13.4).

Pelvic venous reflux can be demonstrated using transvaginal ultrasound and a Valsalva manoeuvre which should be mandatory in all women suspected of having this condition. Gross engorgement of veins is a better sign of pathology than reverse flow which is ubiquitous. Interestingly, the internal iliac vein tributaries are often a pelvic reflux source as well as ovarian vein reflux. Nutcracker syndrome is another possibility detectable in a thin patient using transabdominal duplex ultrasound. The contribution of venous reflux to haemorrhoids is more common than originally proposed.

Supra-inguinal reflux is frequently observed after pregnancy, gynaecological intervention, hernia operations and prostatectomies and also after the use of endovenous catheters in young infants and premature babies in intensive care.

3.3.6 Point P and Point I According to Franceschi

According to Rouviere (1975 in Appendix 2), there are no valves in any visceral or genital veins in the female pelvis except for those present in 50 % of the ovarian veins. The veins in the pelvis have multiple interconnections. There are ipsilateral and contralateral anastomoses through many different venous plexi (rectal, uterine, vaginal, vesical and periurethral). They can be regarded as a large venous **network** which is incompetent because it has no valves. These are not superficial veins or deep veins in the sense of collecting vessels like the femoral or iliac veins. They are **post-capillary vessels** which form a valve-free network enclosed by the wall of the pelvis. In contrast, the perineal and labial veins are superficial possessing valves which prevent blood from refluxing into the superficial venous network of the leg.

Pregnancy causes haemodynamic alterations in the pelvis and the legs in three ways. Firstly, there is a slight increase in the pressure of the pelvic venous network because the veins act as arteriovenous fistulae and may become grossly dilated. Secondly, there is an increase in outflow resistance with the rise in intra-abdominal pressure from the developing foetus. Thirdly, the high hormone levels have a relaxant effect on the vein wall which increases venous compliance and precipitates incompetence when the valve cusps no longer meet. This gives rise to vulval and leg varices. These usually reduce after delivery.

An engorged pelvic venous plexus may communicate with the superficial venous network of the perineum, the vulva or the legs. There are two points at which this may occur (Fig. 3.9):

1. The perineal point (P point), which is filled from the internal pudendal vein. It is located in the posterior region of the labia majora at the junction between the posterior quarter and anterior three-quarters. Vaginal varices meet at this point where their reflux passes to the inner leg. It acts like the narrow part of an hourglass.
2. The inguinal point (I point), which is filled from the vein of the round ligament. This vein can be seen on ultrasound where it leaves the inguinal canal carrying refluxive blood to the confluence of superficial inguinal veins or the front of the leg.

These reflux sources function exactly like incompetent perforating veins filling the superficial veins with reflux.

The dilated intrapelvic network of veins normally persists after birth. They rarely produce symptoms. Treatment by embolisation or stripping is unnecessary because they are part of a complex venous network which is incompetent as a whole. However, occasionally there are refluxing veins like the ovarian vein and tributaries from the internal iliac vein which feed the intrapelvic veins causing pelvic congestion syndrome.

In the absence of a definitive reflux source feeding the intrapelvic network, reflux which exits from the pelvis into the leg may be interrupted at the P or I points (Franceschi and Bahnini 2005).

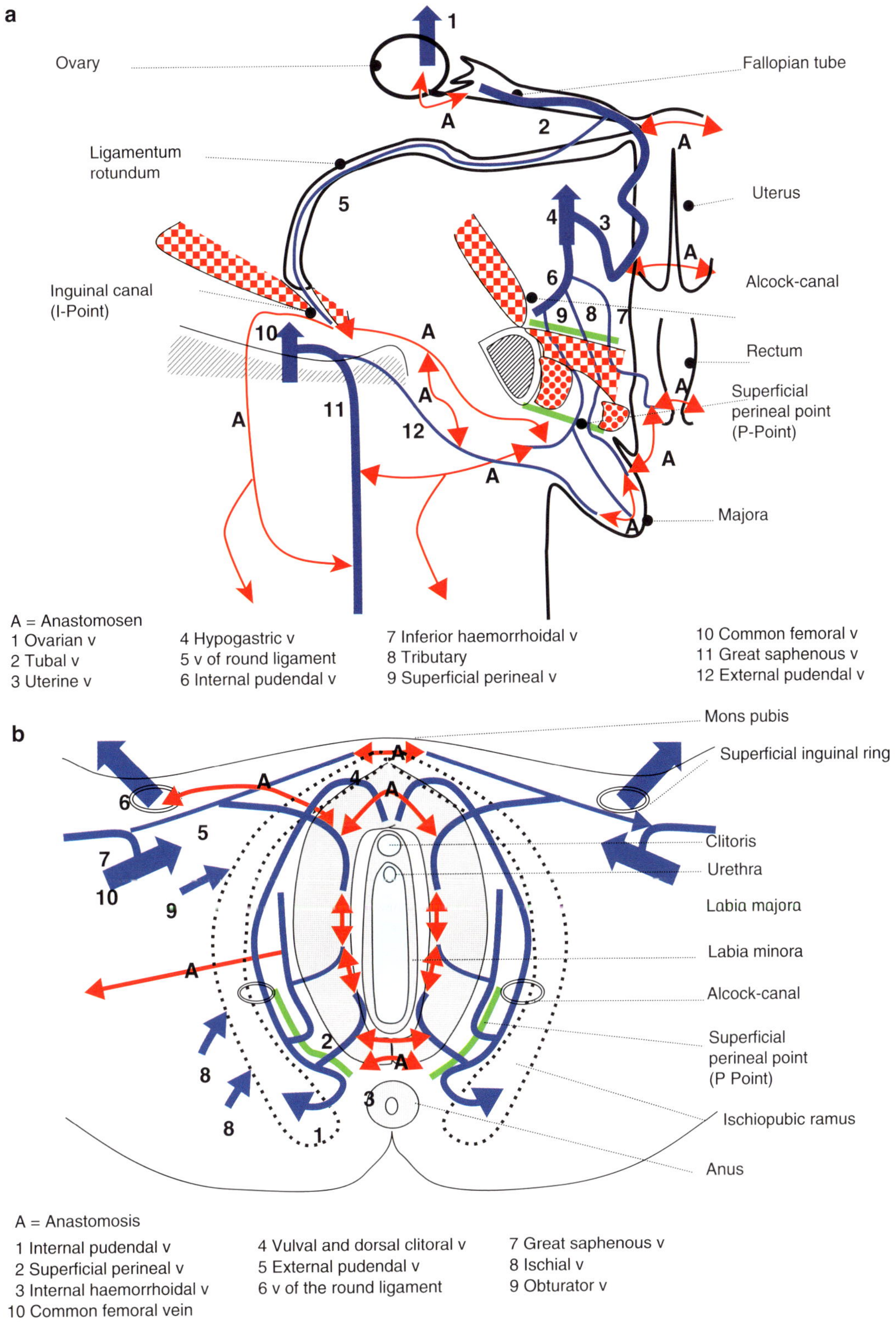

Fig. 3.9 Diagram of the alterations to the venous system due to pregnancy described by Franceschi. (**a**) Axial section through the pelvis and right thigh; (**b**) transverse section through the pelvic floor (Dr. Claude Franceschi, Paris; by kind permission) Copyright: Dr. Claude Franceschi, Paris

3.4 Re-entry Points

Re-entry points occur when the blood recommences physiological antegrade flow. Examples include from tributary to saphenous vein, from saphenous to deep vein or from tributary to deep vein. Re-entry points complete the recirculation circuit (Sect. 3.2). Whilst there is normally only one reflux source for every recirculation loop, the number of re-entry points is generally greater than one. Different types of re-entry points may occur in the same leg.

The furthest distal re-entry point in the circuit is the **terminal perforating vein** (Zamboni et al. 1998). When varicose veins are clinically visible and dilated, there is always a terminal perforating vein marking the point where reflux terminates.

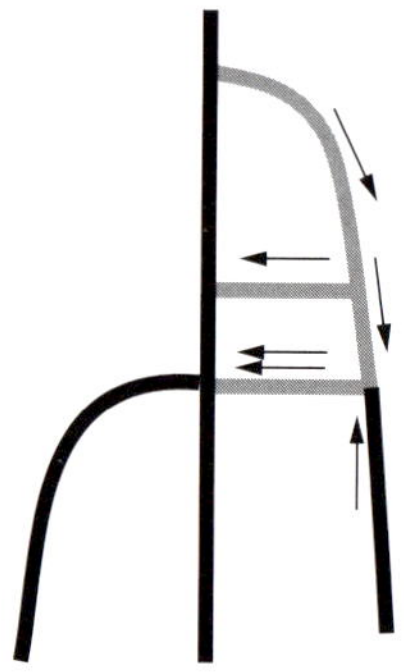

Fig. 3.10 Re-entry from the saphenous vein into the deep veins. Perforating veins are seen draining the great saphenous vein. There is entire above-knee incompetence of the great saphenous vein with 2 re-entry perforating veins: The lower one (*two arrows*) is a terminal perforating vein through which the below-knee part of the competent great saphenous vein drains in antegrade flow Copyright: [Author]

3.4.1 Re-entry from Saphenous Trunks

Perforating veins draining reflux from an incompetent great saphenous vein must be sufficiently wide for the blood volume involved. Therefore, perforating veins which are not visible in B scan are unable to accommodate this drainage and are not significant. It is also known from phlebography studies that not all incompetent perforating veins can be visualised in this way because recirculating blood dilutes the contrast and the flow is inwards in a competent direction.

The re-entry point from the refluxive saphenous vein may be a perforating vein in the middle of its course (Fig. 3.10) or a terminal perforating vein below which the flow in the great saphenous vein is antegrade (see Fig. 3.10, double arrow). The terminal perforating vein is also the drainage for the distal part of the great saphenous vein, through which the blood flow is antegrade. In addition to this draining perforating vein, there are usually refluxive tributaries which carry the recirculation volumes from the great saphenous vein to the deep veins through other perforating veins.

Terminal perforating veins at the ankle and those which carry reflux into the posterior arch vein of the foot into the deep veins are difficult to visualise on ultrasound.

3.4.2 Re-entry from Refluxive Tributaries

The blood from refluxive tributaries can find various drainage routes. It may drain into a competent saphenous vein (Sect. 3.4.3); however, the following variants are the most common drainage routes into deep veins.

The tributary:

- Winds for a long stretch until it finally joins a terminal perforating vein (Fig. 3.11a)
- Winds without dividing and drains through several perforating veins (Fig. 3.11b)
- Divides into further refluxive tributaries drained by the possibilities described above (Fig. 3.11c)

These three variants are common in the region of the posterior accessory vein in the calf (formerly posterior arch vein) and the posterior tibial perforating veins (formerly Cockett perforating veins).

3.4.3 Re-entry from a Tributary into a Saphenous Vein

There are several possible variants:

- A tributary drains into the *same saphenous vein* from which it has received the reflux higher up. The intervening segment of saphenous vein is usually refluxive (not always) as well

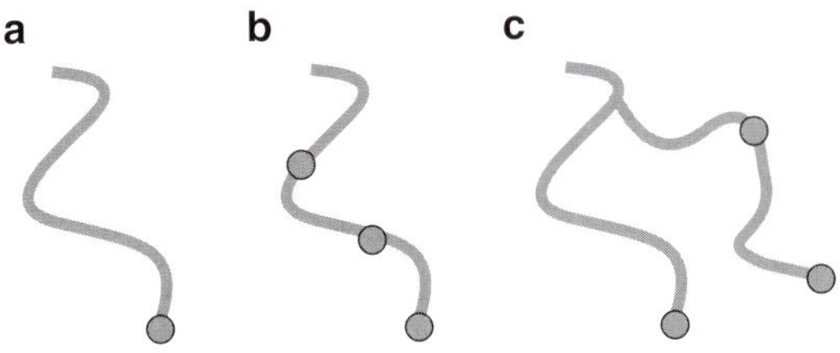

Fig. 3.11 Varicose tributary showing the different drainage possibilities via the perforating veins (shown as a *dot*): (**a**) through a single terminal perforating vein, (**b**) through several perforating veins, and (**c**) through several tributariesCopyright: [Author]

as its distal part (Fig. 4.11a). Another possibility is that the saphenous vein carries the refluxive blood antegrade to a higher perforating vein or junction.

- A tributary drains into the other saphenous vein (usually the small saphenous vein) which is not the original source of the reflux. In this case, the draining saphenous vein may itself become incompetent (Fig. 4.16a, b), but it may also carry the reflux volume antegrade into the deep veins through its junction. This may be the precursor of the situation described above with reflux through both saphenous junctions (Sect. 3.3).

Refluxive connections between the saphenous trunks are confusing when trying to assess haemodynamics. Special attention must be paid to these ramus communicans during examination.

3.4.4 Re-entry from a Tributary Through a Poorly Drained Venous Network

Occasionally, a dilated perforating vein cannot be identified at the end of a varicose tributary. This is common with **reticular varices** which are remote from the anatomical distribution of the saphenous trunks, for example, the lateral and posterior sides of the thigh and the lateral side of the calf.

Reticular varices are partially intradermal and minute and form an unsightly venous network. They drain into perforating veins which are not visible either clinically or on ultrasound. Flow/reflux in reticular veins is very slow and barely measurable on ultrasound (Sect. 3.2.3).

3.5 Venous Arterial Flow Index (VAFI)

Determining the degree of haemodynamic severity of venous disease can be helpful for planning treatment and documentation. The first non-invasive option for a quantitative measurement of haemodynamic parameters is **duplex ultrasound**. This can measure the velocity of blood flow in a vein. This parameter can be used to calculate the volume flow (l/min) by multiplying the average blood flow velocity (cm/s) by the cross-sectional area of the vein. Cross-sectional area $= \pi \times r^2$ or $\pi \times d^2/4$. Once the diameter ($d = 2r$) is measured by positioning the cursors on the machine, the time-averaged mean velocity (TAMV) and volume flow (VF) are automatically calculated and displayed on the screen.

The common femoral vein can be taken as a representative vessel from which the volume flow can be measured. Volume flow can also be measured in the saphenous vein (Lattimer et al. 2012a). Conclusions can then be made on the venous haemodynamics draining the affected leg.

Arterial parameters should be included in the quantitative assessment since they influence venous haemodynamics. For this reason, a ratio can be calculated for the venous and arterial volume flow in the common femoral vein and the common femoral artery, respectively. This ratio is called the venous arterial flow index (VAFI).

Volume flow (VF) is measured in the relaxed, lying patient, with the leg rotated slightly outwards and the head supported on a pillow. While the measurements are taken, it is important that the patient should breathe calmly and that the vein should not be compressed by excessive pressure of the probe on the skin.

The diameters of the common femoral artery and common femoral vein are then measured in transverse view. Volume flow is measured in longitudinal view.

Artery

It is recommended to measure the flow over several pulses to calculate the time-averaged mean velocity (TAMV). This function is usually configured in the machine (Fig. 3.12a).

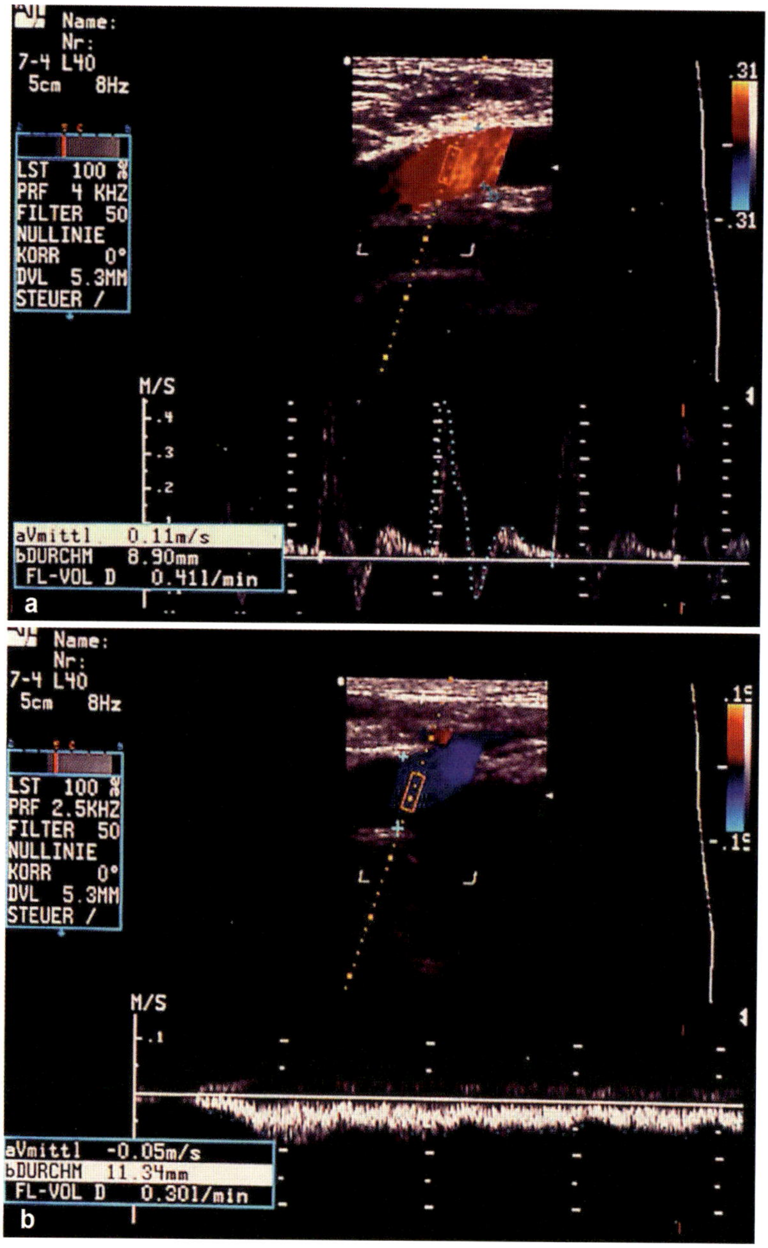

Fig. 3.12 Longitudinal view of the groin with measurement of the time-averaged mean velocity in the lying patient in order to calculate the VAFI. The diameter was measured longitudinally for the sake of clarity. This should normally be measured in transverse view. (**a**) Common femoral vein, (**b**) common femoral artery (*VAFI* venous arterial flow index) Copyright: [Author]

Vein

The typical flow pattern is slow and relatively constant, modulated by respiration. It should be measured over several seconds and then the average calculated as with the artery (TAMV, Fig. 3.12b).

Since the artery and the vein flow in opposite directions, the flow in the vein appears as a negative value. It must be treated as positive for calculating the VAFI. The flow velocity is given in m/s, m/min or cm/s, at the site of the measured vessel diameter (d). The volume flow (VF) in each vessel is calculated from the diameters and flow velocities using the following formula:

$$\mathrm{VF}\left[\mathrm{cm}^3/\mathrm{s}\right]=\mathrm{TAMV}\left[\mathrm{cm/s}\right]\times\pi\times d^2/4\left[\mathrm{cm}^2\right]$$

$$1\ \mathrm{cm}^3=1\ \mathrm{ml}\ \text{Area is}\ \pi\times r^2\ or\ \pi\times d^2/4$$

If the volume flow in the common femoral vein and common femoral artery are designated VFa and VFv, respectively, then

$$\mathrm{VAFI} = \mathrm{VFv}[\mathrm{ml/min}] / \mathrm{VFa}[\mathrm{ml/min}]$$

Example

For example, the VAFI of the leg in Fig. 3.12 is calculated as follows:

Volume flow in the common femoral vein (CFV, Fig. 3.12b): Diameter (d) = 11.34 mm (1.13 cm). The cross-sectional area ($\pi \times r^2$ or $\pi \times d^2/4$) = 1.00 cm^2. The time-averaged mean velocity = 0.05 m/s (5 cm/s).

$$\mathrm{VFv}(\mathrm{CFV}) = 5\ \mathrm{cm/s} \times 1.00\ \mathrm{cm}^2 = 5.00\ \mathrm{ml/s}$$

Volume flow in the common femoral artery (CFA, Fig. 3.12a): Diameter (d) = 8.9 mm (0.89 cm). The cross-sectional area ($\pi \times d^2/4$) = 0.64 cm^2. The time-averaged mean velocity = 0.11 m/s (11 cm/s).

$$\mathrm{VFa}(\mathrm{CFA}): 11\ \mathrm{cm/s} \times 0.64\ \mathrm{cm}^2 = 7.04\ \mathrm{ml/s}$$

$$\mathrm{VAFI} = 5.00\ \mathrm{ml/s} / 7.04\ \mathrm{ml/s} = 0.71$$

In subjects with healthy veins, the VAFI is ≤1.0. In patients with haemodynamically significant impairment, the VAFI increases >1.2. It can even increase up to 2.0 (Kahle et al. 2003). This means that the flow in the femoral vein is much higher than the arterial inflow into the leg. This occurs when there is a recirculation loop.

The VAFI is also very useful for measuring the haemodynamic situation before and after intervention. The influence of intervention on haemodynamics is seen after only a few days when the high preoperative values return to normal.

The non-invasive nature of ultrasound in measuring VF is a clear advantage compared to invasive measurement techniques.

Validation of the VAFI

To clarify how suitable VAFI is for measuring the haemodynamic severity of a venous disease, the index was measured in patients with different venous diseases under different conditions. It was shown that with primary varicose veins, significantly higher values were measured than those found in healthy subjects (Kahle et al. 2003). A similar pattern was found in patients with post-thrombotic syndrome compared to healthy subjects (Kahle et al. 2003) and that the level of the VAFI values correlated with the clinical severity of the disease. In the above studies, subjects with healthy veins were found to have an average VAFI ≤1.0. This may be interpreted to mean that there is a point of equivalence between arterial inflow per unit of time and the corresponding venous outflow per unit of time.

The high VAFI values found in varicose patients may be an index of recirculation which normalises after intervention.

With respect to the reliability of the measurement results, it was shown that the VAFI remained stable both during uninterrupted examination for 1 h and over 3 consecutive days (Kahle et al. 2003). The VAFI is a repeatable, sensitive parameter for venous haemodynamics which has been confirmed with modern phase-contrast MR techniques (Rudolphi 2012 in Appendix 2).

References

Bernardini E et al (2002) Development of primary superficial venous insufficiency: the ascending theory. Observational and hemodynamic data from a 9 year experience. Ann Vasc Surg 24:709–720

Dodd H, Cockett FB (1976) The pathology and surgery of the veins of the lower limb. Churchill Livingstone, Edinburgh/London/New York

Evans CJ, Allan PL, Lee AJ, Bradbury AW, Ruckley CV, Fowkes FGR (1998) Prevalence of venous reflux in the general population on duplex scanning: the Edinburgh Vein Study. J Vasc Surg 28:767–776

Franceschi C, Bahnini A (2005) Treatment of lower extremity venous insufficiency due to pelvic leak points in women. Ann Vasc Surg 19:1–6

Kahle B, Hennies F, Bolz S, Pritsch M (2003) The Reproducibility of the Ratio of volume flow in the common femoral vein and artery (VAFI) for quantification of the severity of venous insufficiency. Vasa 32:199–203

Kamm RD, Pedley TJ (1989) Flow in collapsible tubes: a brief review. J Biomech Eng 111(3):177–179

Labropoulos N, Giannoukas AD, Delis K, Mansour MA, Kang SS, Nicolaides AN et al (1997) Where does venous reflux start? J Vasc Surg 26(5):736–742

Labropoulos N, Tiongson J, Pryor L, Tassiopoulos AK, Kang SS, Mansour A, Baker WH (2003) Definition of venous reflux in lower-extremity veins. J Vasc Surg 38:793–798

Lattimer CR, Azzam M, Kalodiki E, Geroulakos G (2012a) Hemodynamic changes at the saphenofemoral junction during the application of a below-knee graduated compression stocking. Dermatol Surg 38(12):1991–1997

Lattimer CR, Kalodiki E, Azzam M, Geroulakos G (2012b) Varicose veins and severity of chronic venous disorder. Acta Phlebologica 13(2):93–99

Lattimer CR, Kalodiki E, Azzam M, Geroulakos G (2013) Reflux time estimation on air-plethysmography may stratify patients with early superficial venous insufficiency. Phlebology 28(2):101–108

Lattimer CR, Azzam M, Kalodiki E, Geroulakos G (2014). Venous filling time using air-plethysmography correlates highly with great saphenous vein reflux time using duplex. Phlebology 29(2):90–97

Lurie F, Comerota A, Eklof B, Kistner RL, Labropoulos N, Lohr J, Marston W, Meissner M, Moneta G, Neglen P, Neuhardt D, Padberg F, Welsh HJ (2012) Multicenter assessment of venous reflux by duplex ultrasound. J Vasc Surg 55:437–445

Mendoza E (2013) Diameter reduction of the great saphenous vein and the common femoral vein after CHIVA long-term results. Phlebologie 42:65–69

Pittaluga P, Chastanet S, Locret T, Barbe R (2010) The effect of isolated phlebectomy on reflux and diameter of the great saphenous vein: a prospective study. Eur J Vasc Endovasc Surg 40(1):122–128

Trendelenburg F (1891) Ueber die Unterbindung der Vena saphena magna bei Unterschenkelvaricen. Beiträge zur Klinischen Chirurgie (Tübingen) 7:195–210, Translated to be found on www.chiva.info/Informationenfürärzte

Zamboni P, Marcellino MG, Cappelli M, Feo CV, Bresadola V, Vasquez G, Liboni A (1998) Saphenous vein sparing surgery: principles, techniques and results. J Cardiovasc Surg 39:151–162

Zamboni P, Gianesini S, Menegatti E, Tacconi G, Palazzo A, Liboni A (2010) Great saphenous varicose vein surgery without saphenofemoral junction disconnection. Br J Surg 97(6):820–825

Ultrasound-Based Classifications of Varicose Veins

4

Erika Mendoza and Christopher R. Lattimer

Chapter Summary

Varicose disease presents a remarkable variety of forms and clinical expressions. The morphological expression of the disease especially in patients with very large, visible tributaries seldom correlates with their clinical significance. Similarly, ulceration can occur without any visible varicose veins and just a refluxing saphenous trunk.

Many systems for classifying varicose veins have been published (Eklöf et al. 2004; Hach and Hach-Wunderle 1994 in Appendix 2; Nicolaides 2000). Some consider the clinical results, others the morphology and some both. Classification is advisable for clinical assessment and epidemiological studies on the severity and progression of the disease. It is also required for comparisons between different treatment modalities and phlebology practices.

This chapter examines the morphological, anatomical and physiological classifications where duplex ultrasound is necessary in the evaluation process.

E. Mendoza, MD, PhD (✉)
Venenpraxis Wunstorf,
Speckenstraße 10, 31515 Wunstorf, Germany
e-mail: erika.mendoza@t-online.de

C.R. Lattimer, MD, PhD
Department of Vascular Surgery,
Josef Pflug Vascular Laboratory,
Ealing Hospital and Imperial College, London, UK

4.1 Hach Classification of Primary Saphenous Incompetence

The classification system for saphenous vein incompetency proposed by Hach and Hach-Wunderle (1994 in Appendix 2) has become established in the German-speaking world. If used in combination with Widmer's CVI classification, it has improved clinical significance and helps guide prognosis. This is because the clinical appearance of the number and distribution of varicose veins has little relationship with the expression of the disease in the saphenous trunks (Lattimer et al. 2012). The classification has many merits and is as good as many other existing classifications.

Hach originally based his proposal on the evaluation of a **phlebogram**. This classification refers only to **primary incompetence** of the saphenous veins. It is not a classification that should be used for varicose veins occurring as a result of a deep vein thrombosis and the post-thrombotic syndrome. Since phlebography has been replaced by **duplex ultrasound**, the classification system was updated to accommodate the advancement in diagnosis (Mendoza 2013). This is presented below.

4.1.1 Recirculation Circuit

Hach defines four sections for the recirculation circuit (Hach and Hach-Wunderle 1994). They are explained by way of example in the great saphenous vein (Fig. 4.1).

E. Mendoza et al. (eds.), *Duplex Ultrasound of Superficial Leg Veins*,
DOI 10.1007/978-3-642-40731-4_4, © Springer-Verlag Berlin Heidelberg 2014

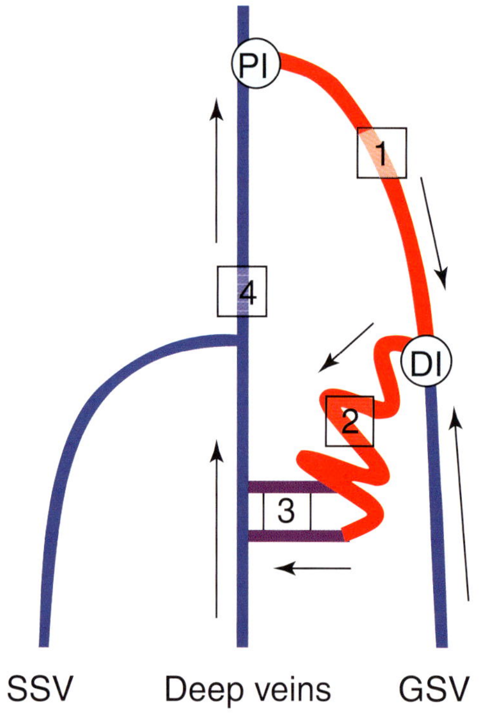

Fig. 4.1 The recirculation circuit. Veins with antegrade flow are shown in *blue*, refluxive superficial veins in *red* and perforating veins affected by recirculation in *violet*. The direction of recirculation flow is marked with *arrows* (*PI* proximal reflux point, *DI* distal reflux point, *GSV* great saphenous vein, *SSV* small saphenous vein). The recirculation sections are *1* incompetent great saphenous vein, *2* incompetent tributaries, *3* drainage through perforating vein(s) and *4* deep veins Copyright: [Author]

First Section

Extends from the proximal to the distal reflux point and therefore consists of the refluxive section of the great saphenous vein. The **proximal reflux source** is the point where the saphenous vein starts to fill refluxively. It is the highest reflux point in the saphenous vein (Fig. 4.1). The **distal reflux point** is where the refluxive flow of blood leaves the saphenous vein. Distal to this point, the great saphenous vein is competent (Fig. 4.1).

Second Section

In older phlebology studies, it was believed that the blood always entered a varicose tributary at the distal reflux point. This is the second section of the recirculation circuit. These tributaries are most often found at the end of the refluxive part of the saphenous vein. They are called **incompetent varicose tributaries**. However, in duplex studies, this is not always the case because reflux may drain to deep veins through perforators without an intervening refluxive tributary.

Third Section

The blood from the incompetent varicose tributaries flows through the different perforating veins into the deep veins.

Fourth Section

This is where the deep veins complete the circuit. Antegrade flow occurs back to the beginning of the recirculation loop.

Hach distinguished different forms of incompetence on **proximal reflux source**:

Complete Incompetence

If the reflux passes directly through the saphenofemoral junction, from the common femoral vein into the great saphenous vein or the popliteal vein into the small saphenous vein, the situation is one of complete incompetence (Fig. 4.2). Here the saphenous veins are filled by retrograde flow through an incompetent terminal and preterminal valve.

Incomplete Incompetence

If the terminal valve is competent and the saphenous vein fills from another refluxive source, the incompetence is described as incomplete (Fig. 4.3).

Hach divided recirculation into compensated and uncompensated. The distinction depends on the condition of the **deep veins**:

Compensated Recirculation

If the deep leg veins, especially the femoral and the popliteal, are competent and not dilated, then there is compensated recirculation.

Uncompensated Recirculation

If the deep leg veins, especially the femoral and the popliteal, are dilated and incompetent, then there is uncompensated recirculation. In this situation, there is secondary popliteal and femoral vein incompetence.

Secondary incompetence of the deep veins requires a precise definition. A distinction must be made between return flows from deep veins through an incompetent terminal valve into the superficial veins (see Fig. 4.2) and a genuinely

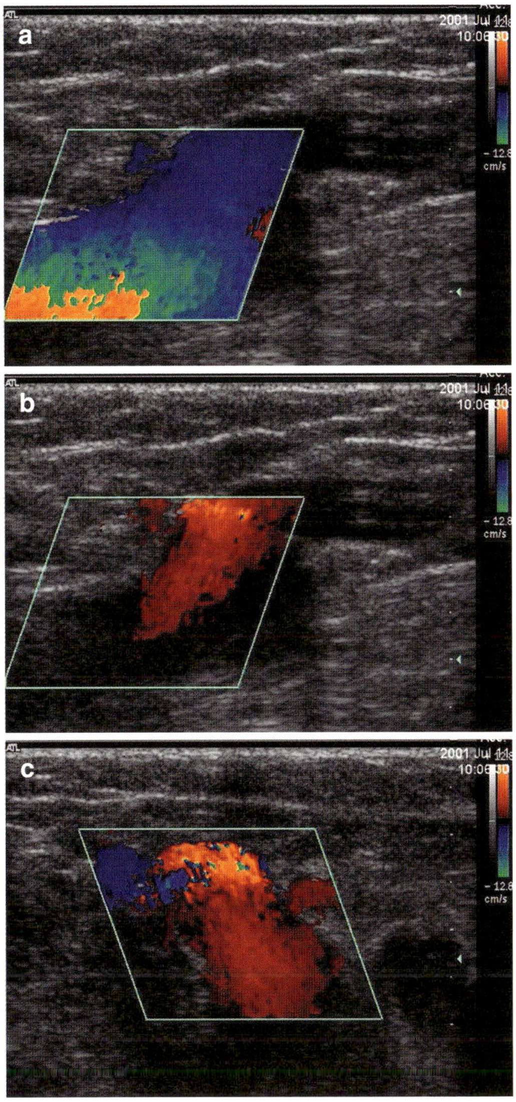

Fig. 4.2 Reflux from the deep veins into a complete incompetence of the great saphenous vein. (**a**) Longitudinal view through the left groin of a standing patient. The common femoral vein is on the left with the saphenofemoral junction in the centre. During muscular systole, there is antegrade flow in the great saphenous vein, the saphenofemoral junction and the common femoral vein. (**b**) Identical view 2 s later during muscular diastole. The saphenofemoral junction is refluxive with an incompetent terminal valve. The source of the reflux filling the great saphenous vein is the femoral vein. In the standing patient, blood flows from the femoral vein above the saphenofemoral junction into the great saphenous vein. These findings are similar with a Valsalva manoeuvre. (**c**) Transverse view through the groin in muscular diastole. There is reflux from the femoral vein through the saphenofemoral junction and into the great saphenous vein. Again, this is similar to the appearances following a Valsalva manoeuvre Copyright: [Author]

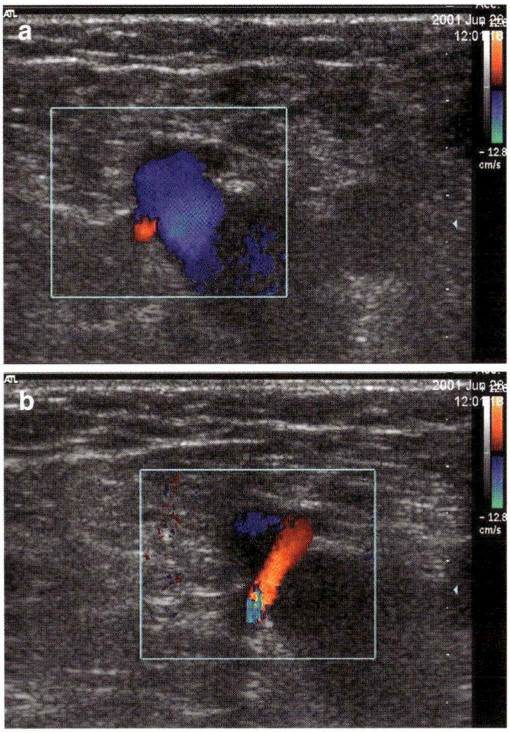

Fig. 4.3 Incomplete incompetence of the great saphenous vein. (**a**) Transverse view through the left groin. During muscular systole, there is antegrade flow in the great saphenous vein. (**b**) During muscular diastole, there is no reflux from the femoral vein because the terminal valve is competent. In this case, the pudendal vein is the source of the reflux with retrograde filling of the great saphenous vein Copyright: [Author]

incompetent deep vein, with valves which have become secondarily incompetent due to volume overloading.

4.1.2 Great Saphenous Vein

4.1.2.1 First Section, Proximal Reflux Source

Hach distinguishes between complete and incomplete incompetence based on the reflux source. With reflux from the deep veins through the saphenofemoral junction and incompetent terminal valve, the incompetence is complete. With a competent terminal valve and reflux further down the great saphenous vein, the incompetence is incomplete. Depending on the source of the refluxive blood, these are classified into tributary type (55 %), perforating vein type (28 %) when the source of the reflux is from refluxive perforating veins and posterior (dorsal) type (17 %) with a reflux source from the femoropopliteal vein or the posterior accessory saphenous vein.

Based on duplex ultrasound criteria, the reflux source in incomplete incompetence can be differentiated according to:

- Reflux source
- Course of the reflux into the great saphenous vein bypassing the competent terminal valve

The following are the possible **sources of reflux** in cases of incomplete incompetence:

Pelvic veins	Pelvic type (see. Fig. 4.4)
Perforating veins	Perforating type (see Fig. 4.5)
Small saphenous vein	Small saphenous vein type (see Fig. 4.6)
Healthy tributaries	Reticular type (see Fig. 4.7)

Reflux from these sources can reach the great saphenous vein through the following **connections**:

Direct	Perforating vein in the adductor canal (formerly Dodd, Hunter) or a paratibial perforating vein (Boyd)
Through a tributary of the saphenofemoral junction	Pelvic type (Fig. 4.4)
Posterior through the posterior accessory saphenous vein	Pelvic type Perforating type (dorsal thigh perforators, formerly Hach perforating vein) Small saphenous vein type through the cranial extension of the small saphenous vein or Giacomini anastomosis
Anterior through the anterior accessory saphenous vein	Pelvic type
Distal through a tributary in the calf	Small saphenous vein type Perforating type
Through many healthy tributaries in the course of the vein	Reticular type

4.1.2.2 First Section: Course of the Great Saphenous Vein

In 16.6 % of cases, analysis of refluxing great saphenous veins has revealed that at least one competent segment may exist between two refluxing segments. The competent segment is situated between the proximal and distal reflux point (Mendoza 2002 in Appendix 2). In these cases, the reflux leaves the great saphenous vein by a tributary and re-enters the great saphenous vein further down (Fig. 4.8). This variant is called segmental incompetence. It may occur two or three times along the course of the great saphenous vein.

4.1.2.3 First Section: Distal Reflux Point

The distal reflux point determines the Hach class (I–IV). This is the point where the reflux leaves the interfascial great saphenous vein and fills a varicose tributary. Alternatively, it may enter the deep veins through a perforating vein. The great saphenous vein distal to this point is competent in its extension down to the ankle (Fig. 4.9):

I	The reflux fills the great saphenous vein and then immediately flows down one of the tributaries of the saphenofemoral junction. The great saphenous vein is therefore refluxive only at the junction region. The reflux then leaves the great saphenous vein in the groin where it remains competent further down
II	The distal reflux point is in the thigh. The great saphenous vein is competent in the lower leg
III	The distal reflux point is below the knee. The reflux leaves the great saphenous vein at some point in the lower leg
IV	The whole great saphenous vein is refluxive down to the ankle

The frequency of the various classes has been investigated by Hach using phlebography (Table 4.1, left) and by Mendoza using duplex ultrasound (Table 4.1, right). The latter was from an evaluation in 547 legs with complete saphenous incompetence from an incompetent terminal valve.

Recognition of the refluxive great saphenous vein from a refluxive tributary may be difficult.

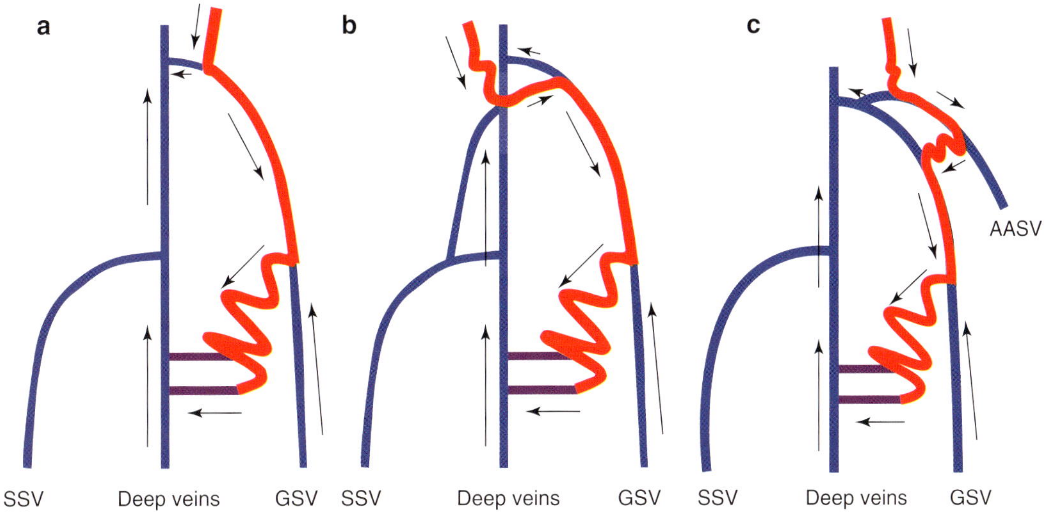

Fig. 4.4 Incomplete incompetence of the pelvic type. (**a**) Junction tributary type demonstrating reflux from the superficial epigastric vein with a competent saphenofemoral junction, (**b**) incomplete incompetence of the posterior pelvic type, (**c**) incomplete incompetence of the anterior pelvic type (*AASV* anterior accessory saphenous vein, *GSV* great saphenous vein, *SSV* small saphenous vein) Copyright: [Author]

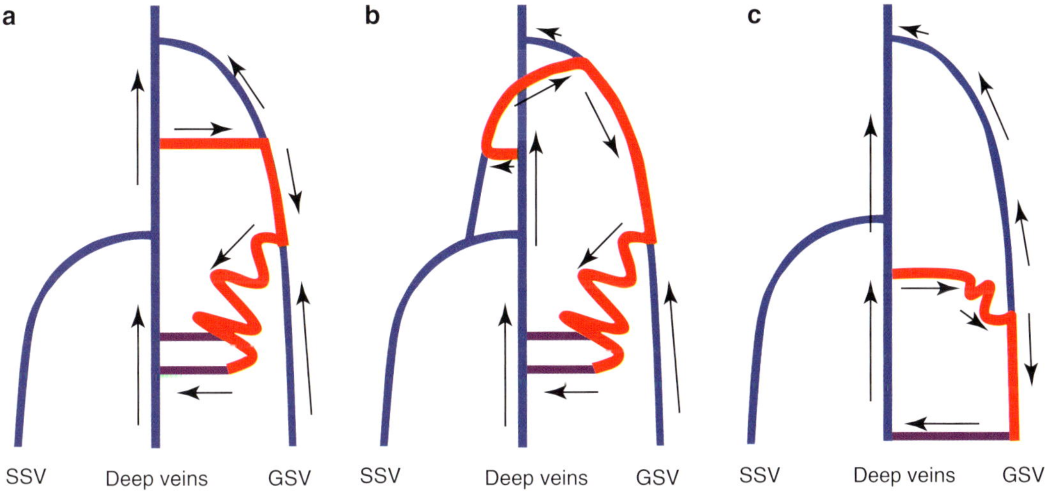

Fig. 4.5 Incomplete incompetence of the perforating type. (**a**) Direct perforating type demonstrating a direct connection with the perforating vein in the adductor canal (formerly Dodd), (**b**) posterior perforating type, (**c**) distal perforating type Copyright: [Author]

Therefore, the following **criteria** may help to define the distal reflux point:

- The refluxive great saphenous vein runs a straight classic course in the fascial compartment where the "saphenous eye" is visible in transverse view (Fig. 7.32).
- The refluxive tributary is often tortuous until it pierces the fascia and connects with the great saphenous vein.
- Distal from this point, the great saphenous vein is not refluxive and may have a sudden reduction in calibre on the ultrasound image (Fig. 7.34).
- The tributary is not protected by a fascia. It remains epifascial throughout its downward course.

The distal reflux point established using the duplex ultrasound criteria given above is

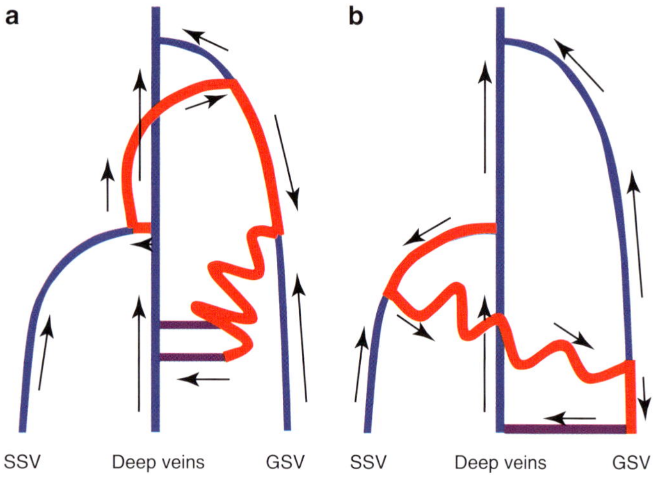

Fig. 4.6 Incomplete incompetence of the small saphenous vein type. (**a**) Posterior, (**b**) distal Copyright: [Author]

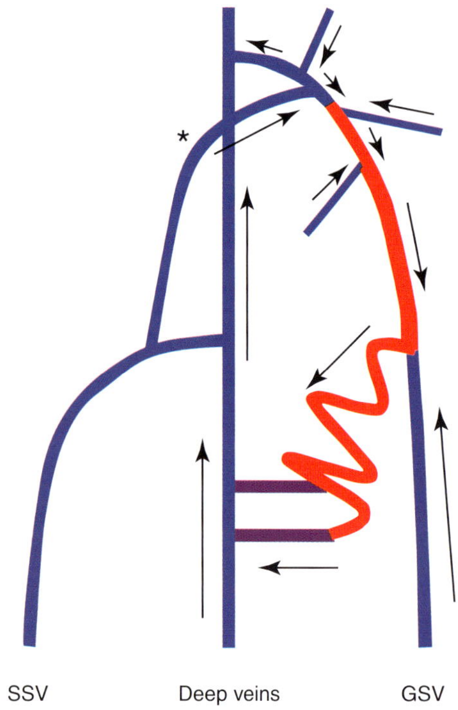

Fig. 4.7 Competent saphenofemoral junction. Antegrade blood from healthy tributaries (*blue*) and the posterior accessory saphenous vein (*) drains into the great saphenous vein which then refluxes downwards. There is no pathologically refluxive connection with the deep vein system Copyright: [Author]

sufficient to determine the Hach class for a report to the primary physician and for a general evaluation. Additional information on the course of the great saphenous vein is only relevant for planning treatment.

4.1.2.4 Second Section

The second recirculation section relates to the **incompetent varicose tributaries**. It is described by Hach but not yet divided into classes. The morphology and presence of tributaries may have influence on the treatment of saphenous vein incompetence. Their removal has been shown by some authors to render competence in saphenous trunks (Pittaluga et al. 2009; Zamboni et al. 2010).

The second component of recirculation is not always apparent. Reflux may flow directly from the first section (saphenous vein) to the third (perforating vein). If incompetent varicose tributaries exist, they are often at the distal reflux point. If there is complete incompetence of the great saphenous vein with reflux to below-the-knee draining through the paratibial perforating vein (formerly Boyd), then a varicose tributary may be found in the thigh (Fig. 4.10). Sometimes the incompetence of the great saphenous vein does not end with the passage of the blood from the great saphenous vein to the tributary in the thigh. It may continue down the great saphenous vein beyond the visible incompetent tributary. In this case, the drainage through the perforator defines the Hach class.

4.1.2.5 Third Section

The re-entry perforating veins comprise the third section. Hach assigns particular significance to the posterior tibial perforating vein (formerly Cockett), without further definition.

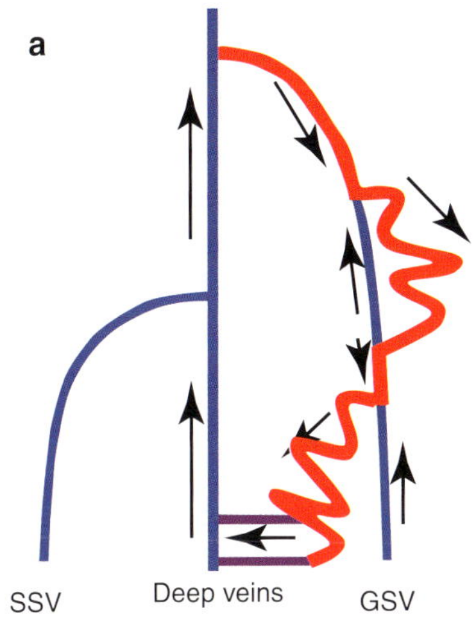

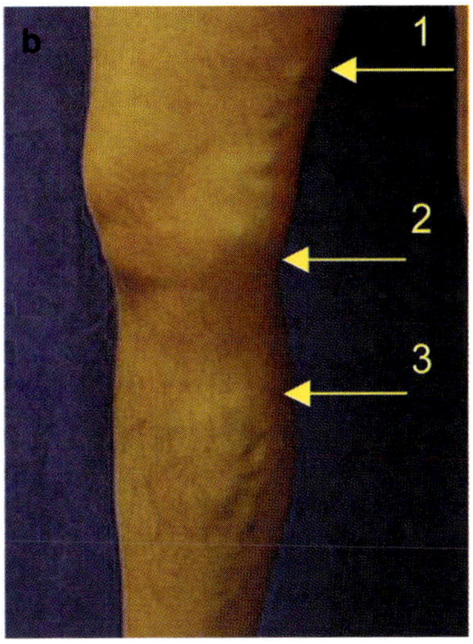

Fig. 4.8 (**a**) Segmental incompetence of the great saphenous vein with reflux arising initially through the saphenofemoral junction. From there, the reflux enters a tributary in the thigh leaving a competent segment of the great saphenous vein between the knee and the mid thigh. It is then refluxively refilled from the tributary below the knee and then redelivers this reflux to a cluster of varicose veins further down. (**b**) This situation may be deduced clinically when there are two varicose clusters along the course of the great saphenous vein as seen in the illustration. The great saphenous vein is refluxive above *arrow 1*, competent between *arrows 1* and *2*, refluxive between *arrows 2* and *3* and competent once more below *arrow 3* Copyright: [Author]

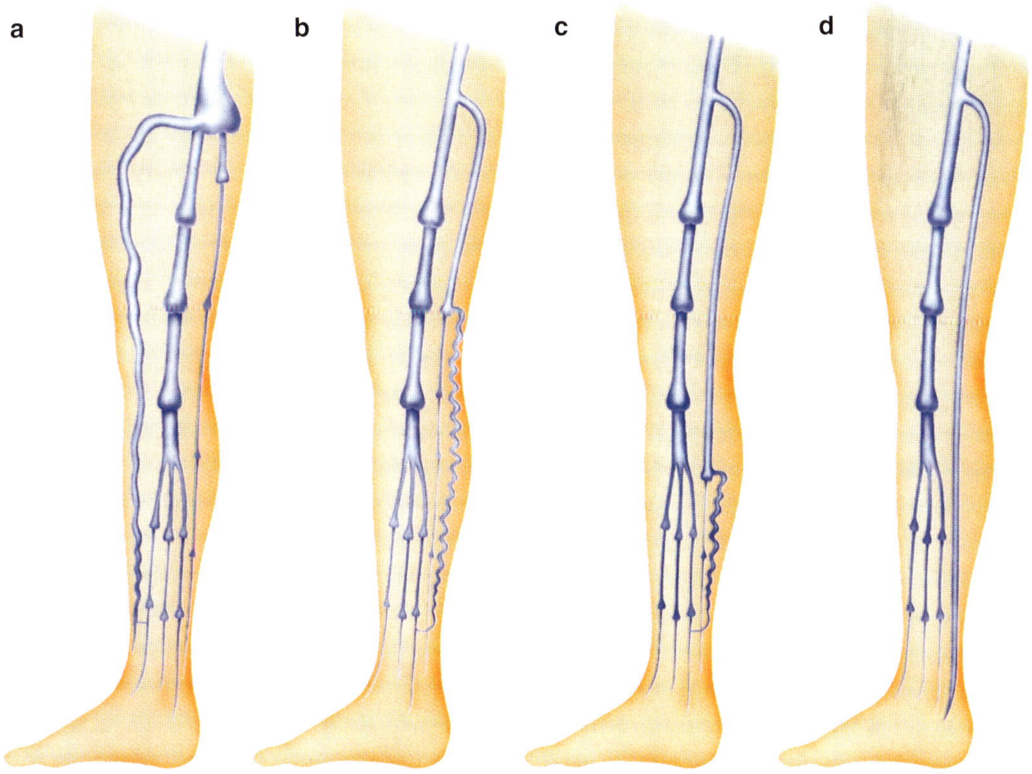

Fig. 4.9 Diagram of the four classes of reflux of the great saphenous vein according to the location of the distal reflux point (source). (**a**) Distal reflux source within an abnormally dilated termination of the great saphenous vein. In this example, the distal reflux point is the termination of the anterior accessory saphenous vein (Hach I). (**b**) Distal reflux source in the thigh region (Hach II). (**c**) In the lower leg (Hach III). (**d**) In the foot (Hach IV) (From Hach and Hach-Wunderle 1994 in Appendix 2) Copyright: Springer

Table 4.1 Frequencies of the Hach classes established by phlebography and ultrasound

Hach class	Frequency using phlebography (%)	Frequency using duplex ultrasound (%)
I	30	6.5
II	30	22.5
III	40	43.4
IV	<1	1

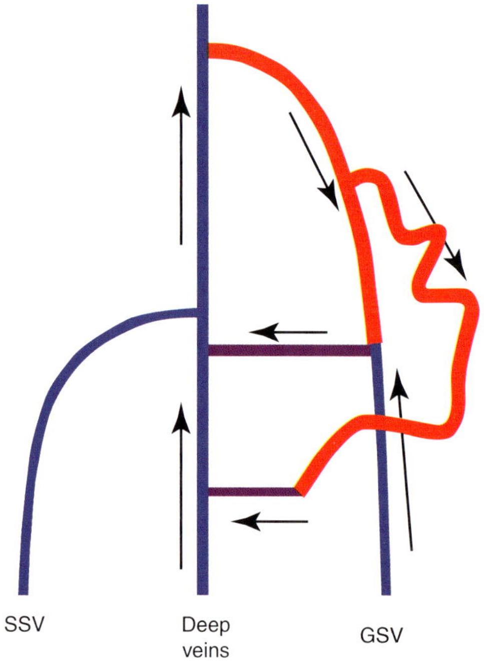

Fig. 4.10 Complete incompetence of the great saphenous vein in Hach class III. The reflux fills an incompetent tributary in the thigh. The great saphenous vein is refluxive to the paratibial perforating vein (formerly Boyd), where the reflux flows into the deep system Copyright: [Author]

The re-entry process is defined as the perforating veins which drain blood from the superficial refluxive veins into the deep veins during muscular diastole (Chap. 9).

In the early stages of venous insufficiency, the perforating vein in the calf serves as a re-entry point for the recirculating blood. As the volume of reflux increases, so does the calibre of the perforating vein.

With a large recirculation volume, the perforating vein becomes very dilated and can no longer be closed by muscular contraction. This causes an outward flow during muscular systole which drains inwards again during muscular diastole (Sects. 3.4 and 9.3.2). This situation can cause dilatation with secondary reflux in the deep veins termed an **uncompensated recirculation**.

If there is only an **outward flow** through a perforating vein, then this is either the proximal reflux source or secondary to a deep venous obstruction caused by the post-thrombotic syndrome (PTS). In either case, the perforating vein does not form the third component of the recirculation circuit. Secondary varicose veins caused by the post-thrombotic syndrome are rarely part of a recirculation.

4.1.2.6 Fourth Section

The deep leg veins comprise the fourth section of the recirculation circuit. The blood recirculating through the incompetent superficial veins must be transported by the deep veins in addition to its native blood flow. If there is a large recirculation volume, the veins become dilated to form secondary deep venous incompetence (see Chap. 14).

4.1.3 Small Saphenous Vein

The same principles apply as for the great saphenous vein. There are four sections, with proximal and distal reflux sources in the first section.

4.1.3.1 First Section: Proximal Reflux Source

As described above, complete and incomplete incompetence may be defined on the type of the proximal reflux source. **Complete** forms of recirculation are those in which the reflux from the popliteal vein enters the small saphenous vein through an incompetent terminal valve (see also Sect. 2.5.1 and Fig. 2.31a–d).

Incomplete incompetence occurs when the reflux source bypasses the competent terminal valve of the small saphenous vein and enters further down. The possible reflux sources correspond to those described for the great saphenous vein.

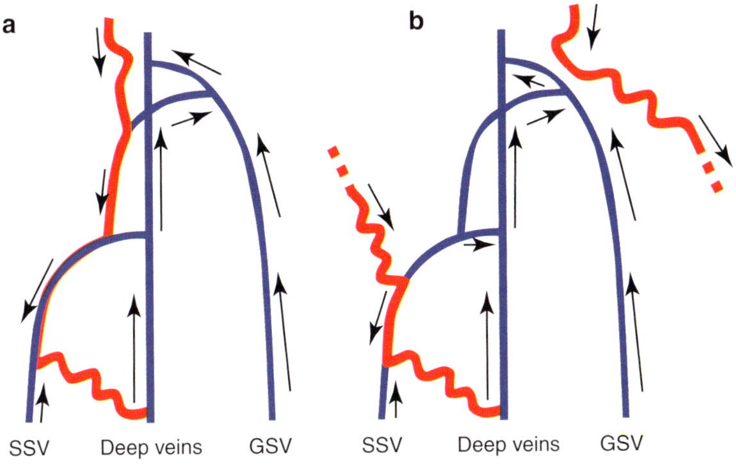

Fig. 4.11 Incomplete incompetence of the small saphenous vein of the pelvic type. (**a**) In the posterior pelvic type, the reflux from the pelvis flows down through veins on the inner side of the thigh and labia to meet the posterior accessory saphenous vein. (**b**) In the lateral pelvic type, the reflux from the pelvis flows down through veins in the anterior part of the thigh to meet the anterior accessory saphenous vein. This winds around the lateral side of the leg (interrupted line to the *right* and re-entering the illustration from the *left*) to fill the small saphenous vein Copyright: [Author]

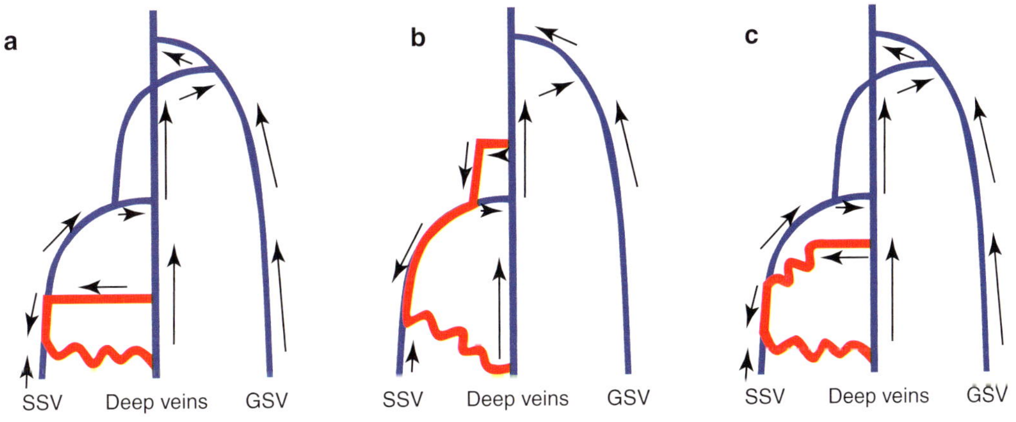

Fig. 4.12 Incomplete incompetence of the small saphenous vein of the perforating type. (**a**) The direct perforating type is from the soleus perforating vein (formerly May). (**b**) The posterior perforating type from the back of the thigh (Hach). (**c**) The distal perforating type where the perforating vein fills the small saphenous vein in the calf through intermediate tributaries Copyright: [Author]

Under the assumption that the saphenopopliteal junction is competent and that the small saphenous vein is refluxive in its course, the following classification of incomplete incompetence of the small saphenous vein is suggested which is based on the:

- Reflux source
- Course of reflux into the small saphenous vein bypassing the competent terminal valve

The following are possible **original sources** of reflux with incomplete incompetence:

Pelvic veins	Pelvic type (see Fig. 4.11)
Perforating veins	Perforating type (see Fig. 4.12)
Great saphenous vein	Great saphenous vein type (see Fig. 4.13)

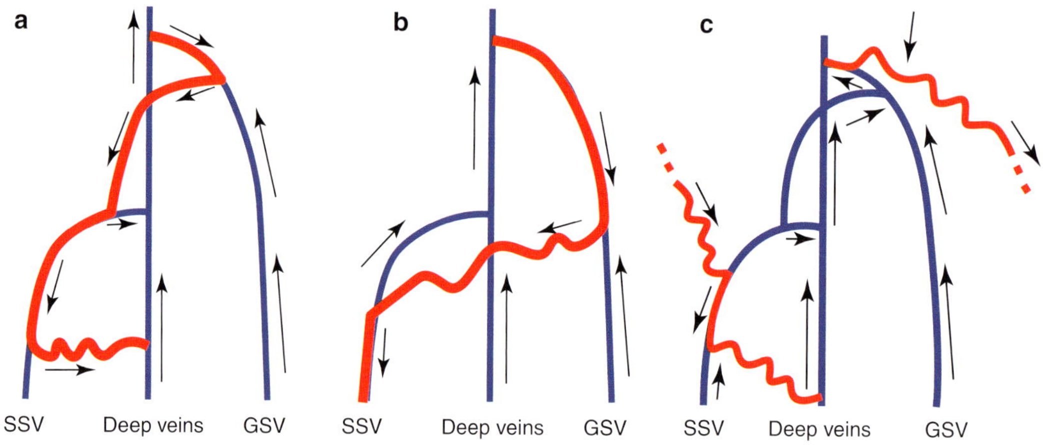

Fig. 4.13 Incomplete incompetence of the small saphenous vein of the great saphenous vein type. (**a**) In the posterior (dorsal) great saphenous vein type, the great saphenous vein fills the small saphenous vein through the posterior accessory saphenous vein and the cranial extension of the small saphenous vein (Giacomini anastomosis). (**b**) In the distal great saphenous vein type, the great saphenous vein fills the small saphenous vein through a tributary in the calf. (**c**) In the lateral great saphenous vein type, the great saphenous vein fills the small saphenous vein through the anterior accessory saphenous vein laterally Copyright: [Author]

Reflux from these sources can reach the small saphenous vein through the following **connections**:

Direct	Soleus perforating veins (formerly May)
Dorsal through the cranial extension of the small saphenous vein (vein of Giacomini)	Pelvic type Perforating type (Hach perforating vein) Great saphenous vein type
Lateral through the anterior accessory saphenous vein	Pelvic type Great saphenous vein type
Distal through a tributary in the calf	Great saphenous vein type (tributary from medial) Perforating type

If reflux from the pelvic veins reaches the small saphenous vein through a recirculation from the great saphenous vein, then the leg will have incompetence in both saphenous trunks. This is called "incomplete incompetence of the great saphenous vein, tributary type with incomplete incompetence of the small saphenous vein, distal great saphenous vein type" (Fig. 4.14).

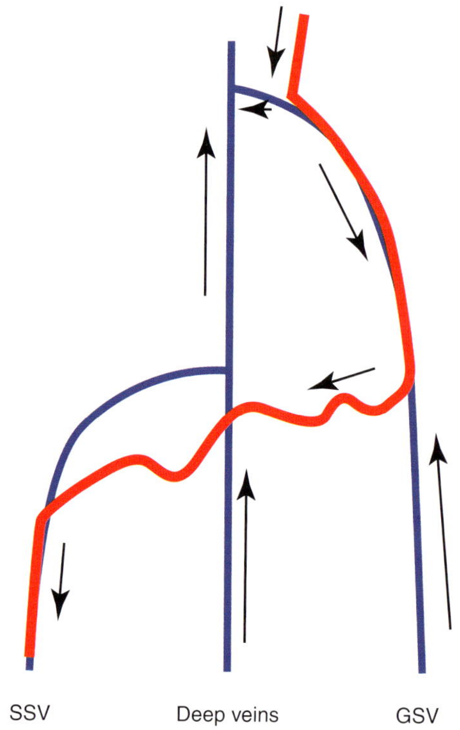

Fig. 4.14 Incomplete incompetence of the great saphenous vein, tributary type with incomplete incompetence of the small saphenous vein, distal great saphenous vein type Copyright: [Author]

4.1.3.2 First Section: Course of the Small Saphenous Vein

Normally, there are no extrafascial or aplastic segments in the course of the small saphenous vein. It is entirely intrafascial. Only in very rare cases is the proximal section hypoplastic or aplastic. In this situation, any incompetence of the distal section would be an incomplete incompetence.

4.1.3.3 First Section: Distal Reflux Point

Hach classified incompetence of the small saphenous vein into three classes, according to the position of the distal reflux source (Fig. 4.15).

I The reflux leaves the small saphenous vein in the immediate area of the saphenopopliteal junction
II The reflux leaves the small saphenous vein in its course down the calf
III The whole small saphenous vein is refluxive

Occasionally, duplex ultrasound may reveal refluxive tributaries which break through the fascia in the popliteal fossa. This is a direct tributary reflux from the refluxive upper part of the small saphenous vein. This pattern of extrafascial **incompetent varicose tributaries** is also a Hach class I (Fig. 4.16).

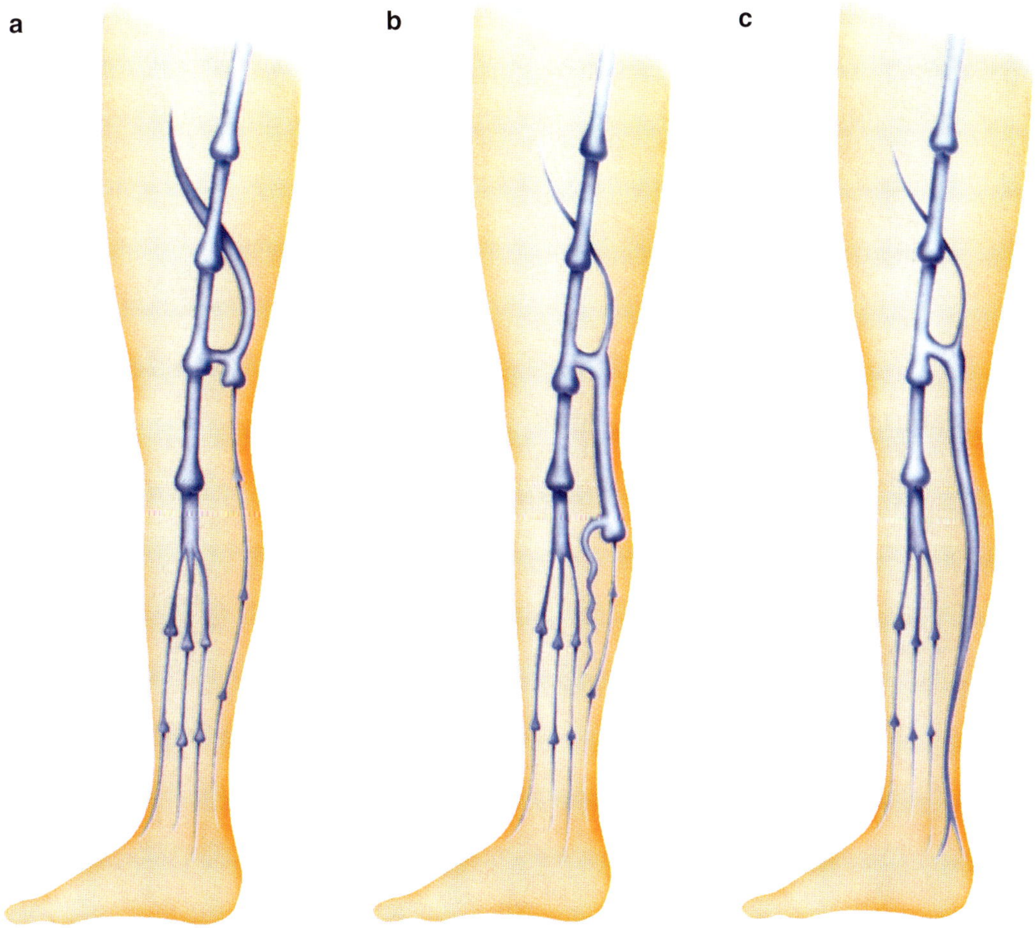

Fig. 4.15 Recirculation routes in the small saphenous vein. (**a**) Reflux leaving from the small saphenous vein in the saphenopopliteal region (Hach I). (**b**) Reflux leaving the small saphenous vein further down the calf (Hach II). (**c**) The whole small saphenous vein is refluxive (Hach III) (From Hach and Hach-Wunderle 1994 in Appendix 2) Copyright: Springer

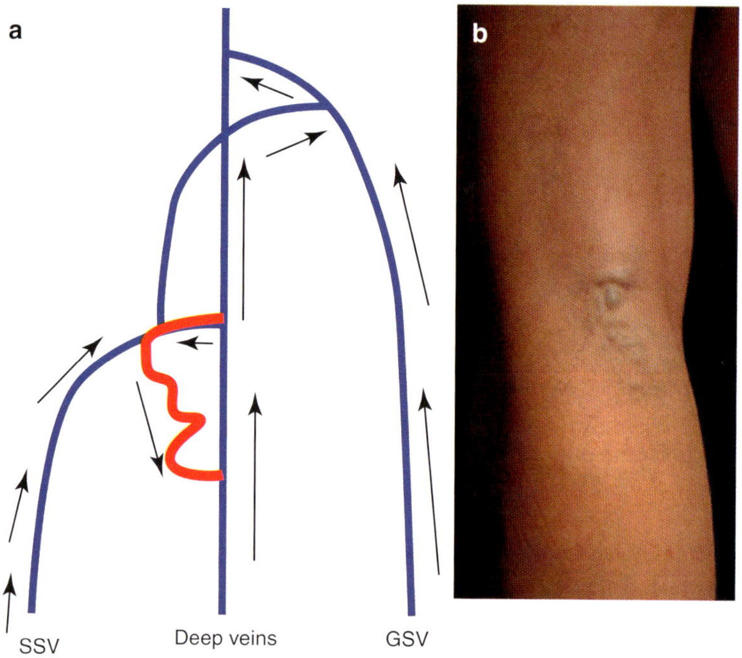

Fig. 4.16 (**a**) Hach class I with extrafascial tributary; (**b**) these are seen clinically as a small cluster of varicose veins in the popliteal fossa Copyright: [Author]

4.2 Franceschi Shunt Classifications

In 1988, Franceschi published the **CHIVA method** for leg vein treatment. It is based on an analysis of the recirculation circuit using **haemodynamic–physiological criteria**. This differs from Hach which principally describes a morphological classification (Franceschi 1993 for the English version).

To apply the CHIVA method of treatment, it is essential to understand the classification of recirculation routes into the so-called shunt types (Mendoza 2002 in Appendix 2). These were last revised at the 2002 Annual Conference in Teupitz.

4.2.1 Venous Networks

Franceschi divided the superficial leg veins into two morphologically and functionally distinguishable systems, the saphenous veins and the tributaries. The different systems were termed by the French word "réseaux", meaning networks: R1, R2 and R3 (Fig. 4.17). The saphenous fascia is the boundary between R2 (saphenous veins) and R3 (tributaries).

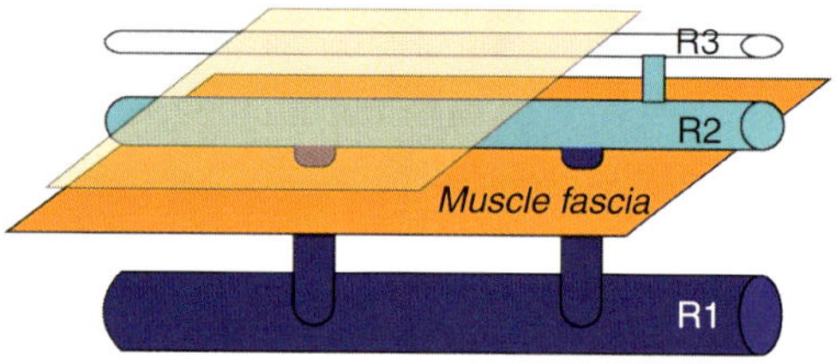

Fig. 4.17 Diagram of the venous networks R1, R2 and R3. R1 are the deep leg and perforating veins (*dark blue*) which run below the muscle fascia. R2 are the "interfascial" veins (*medium blue*) which run between the muscle fascia (*orange*) and the saphenous fascia (semi-transparent). R3 are the veins (*light blue*) running through the epifascial region (From Mendoza (2002 in Appendix 2); by courtesy of Arrien GmbH) Copyright: Arrien, Wunstorf

The **R1 network** consists of the deep vein system and the perforating veins which are all the veins running beneath the muscle fascia.

The **R2 network** consists of the superficial veins, running between the muscle fascia and the saphenous fascia. They are interfascial. The great and small saphenous veins belong to the R2 network. Since the proximal segments of the anterior and posterior accessory saphenous veins always run interfascially, they also belong in part to the R2 network. In many patients, the distal extension of the posterior accessory saphenous vein, the femoropopliteal vein and the cranial extension of the small saphenous vein, with or without the Giacomini anastomosis, run in the fascial compartment as far as the popliteal fossa. In that case, they also belong to the R2 network.

The **R3 network** consists of all the tributaries which run epifascially, in the subcutaneous fatty tissue, regardless of their diameter.

In a healthy leg, the blood always flows **from a higher R to** a lower one, for example, from a tributary to a saphenous vein (R3 → R2) or directly to a perforating vein (R3 → R1) or from a saphenous vein into a deep vein (R2 → R1). Thereafter, blood remains in the R1 network flowing up to the heart.

4.2.2 Shunt Principles

A varicose vein indicates the presence of **recirculation**. This was originally described by Trendelenburg in 1891. Franceschi divided these recirculations into shunt types according to the vein segments involved (Franceschi 1993).

Selection of the word "shunt" as a term describing a venous recirculation circuit is somewhat misleading in English because it is not a true shunt defined as a short circuit between arterial and venous vessels or vascular systems. In France, Italy and Spain, the short circuit is called a "deviation" so it seemed appropriate at the time to reserve the word shunt to describe recirculation in varicose veins. This term was later adopted internationally to comply with consensus statements. However, we must be aware that this is a recirculation and not a classic shunt.

The shunt types distinguish which R networks are involved in the recirculation and in what order. In other words, it is necessary to define the origin of the blood, through which venous network the reflux runs and especially to the connections of the re-entry perforating veins. Only dilated re-entry perforating veins are taken into consideration in defining shunt types. For example, it is known that there is a series of perforating veins along the great saphenous vein. However, if they are not dilated, they are not involved to accommodate to the extra blood volume from the refluxive vein. Therefore, they are irrelevant for recirculation and shunt classification.

In complex forms of recirculation with nested, repeating circuits, shunt classification is based on the **principal recirculation**. This is the point at which the greatest proportion of the recirculating blood passes from a lower to a higher R. This is usually the highest reflux source and therefore likely to be the saphenofemoral junction or a perforating vein.

Shunts may be divided in closed and open shunts. A closed shunt represents the classical recirculation situation: a reflux source, a superficial refluxing path, a re-entry point and an upward circulation in the deep vein to come back to the start of the recirculation, to the reflux source. One erythrocyte could repeat this recirculation more than one time without leaving the leg.

An open shunt occurs when the path with the upward circulation is not bringing the blood back to the origin of the recirculation. This may be found in case of refluxive tributaries of one saphenous vein with drainage through the other saphenous vein (see Fig. 4.24c). In case of deep vein obstruction, we find open shunts as bypass for the deep veins (see Fig. 15.1b). Blood from the deep vein (R1) changes the level into R2 (reflux source) via a perforator and flows upwards in the R2 just to enter the deep vein upwards. According to the R levels, we have a shunt (R1–R2–R1) – but no recirculation, just a bypass for the deep venous system. Franceschi called this shunt "open vicarious shunt", derived from the Latin word *vicarius* which means substitute.

A review of the different shunt types is shown in Table 4.2, with their frequency in Table 4.3. In the revised version (Mendoza 2002), shunt type "0" was introduced for the reticular type (Fig. 4.7) of incomplete incompetence of the great saphenous vein described above. Although there is downward refluxive flow in the lower part of the great saphenous vein, this does not represent a classic recirculation because the circuit is incomplete. Apart from this, the revision only affects shunt types IV–VI. A complete, detailed description of the shunt types can be found online and in Fig. 4.24.

Table 4.2 Description of the various shunt types (see also Fig. 4.24)

Shunt type	Principal recirculation	Description
I	R1–R2–R1	The principal recirculation occurs in the saphenous veins with re-entry through a perforating vein directly from the saphenous vein. Refluxive tributaries may also be present, but their ligation will not prevent recirculation
II	R2–R3–R2 or R1	Varicose tributary filled refluxively from the saphenous vein. Tributary drainage may be into the same saphenous vein, the other saphenous vein or directly into a deep vein
III	R1–R2–R3–(R2–)R1	The principal recirculation of the saphenous vein drains into a deep vein only through one or more tributary(ies). There is no saphenous drainage directly through a perforating vein. Ligation of the tributary(ies) interrupts the recirculation
IV	R1–R3–R2–R1	Reflux enters the saphenous vein from a pelvic or perforating vein. The principal drainage is into a deep vein through a perforating vein directly from the saphenous vein. The re-entry is analogous with shunt I
V	R1–R3–R2–R3–R1	Reflux enters the saphenous vein from a pelvic or perforating vein. Drainage is into a deep vein through a tributary. The re-entry is analogous with shunt III
VI	R1–R3–R1	Rare forms of recirculation with no involvement of the saphenous veins

4.2.3 Shunt Type I

This recirculation always affects the **saphenous veins (R2)**. Its source is the deep system (R1–R2). The saphenous vein is filled directly from the saphenofemoral or saphenopopliteal junction (Fig. 4.18a) or through a perforating vein (Fig. 4.19b). The principal recirculating blood drains into the deep system directly from the saphenous vein through a perforating vein without being diverted through a tributary. The R3 network is not involved in the principal recirculation. The principal circuit is therefore deep vein (R1), saphenous vein (R2) and deep vein (R1).

Table 4.3 Frequency of the different shunt types in the literature

Authors	Zamboni et al. (1998)[a]	Cappelli et al. 2000	Mendoza (2006)[b]
Shunt type I	186/357 (53 %)	33 %	338/989 (34 %)
Shunt type II	–	N. D.	154/989 (16 %)
Shunt type III	171/357 (47 %)	60 %	384/989 (39 %)
Shunt types IV–VI	–	N. D.	113/989 (11 %)

N. D. no data

[a]This study included only patients with reflux through the saphenofemoral junction. Shunt types II and IV–VI did not occur

[b]Characteristics of 989 legs prior to intervention between 1999 and 2000. The small saphenous vein was included in the analysis

Usually, **R3 tributaries** are also filled from the refluxive R2 vein which may themselves become refluxive and varicose (Fig. 4.19b). An important point defining shunt type I is that the drainage from the saphenous vein occurs irrespective of additional tributary drainage (see also Sect. 4.2.9). Shunt type I with refluxive tributaries is called shunt type I+II by some authors. A pure shunt type I with no refluxive tributaries is rare.

The most important criterion is that blood is transported directly from the dilated saphenous vein by a dilated **perforating vein** back into the deep system. Deep vein (R1)–junction/perforator to saphenous vein (R2)–perforating vein to deep veins (R1).

In summary:

1. Reflux source from the deep veins directly into the saphenous vein
2. Reflux down the saphenous vein
3. Re-entry through a perforating vein directly from the saphenous vein

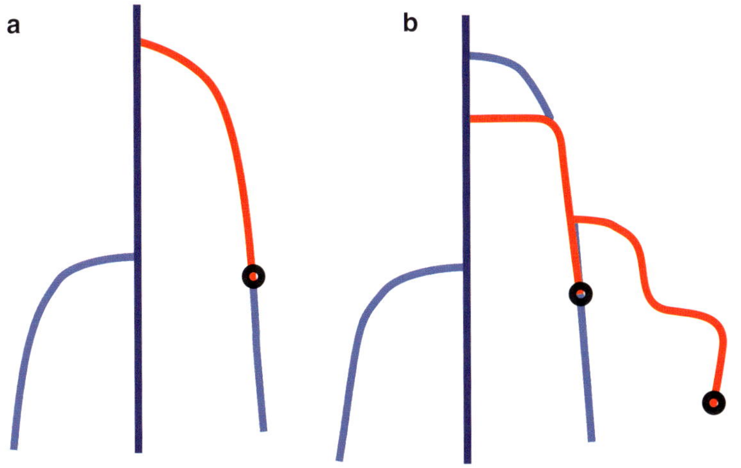

Fig. 4.18 In the following figures, the haemodynamically relevant re-entry perforating veins are shown as a *red point* in a *black circle* on the vein which they drain. The R1 network is *dark blue*, the R2 network is *medium blue* and the R3 network is *light blue*. The refluxive segments are shown in *red*. Shunt type I. (**a**) R1–R2–R1. (**b**) Competent saphenofemoral junction with reflux originating from the perforating vein in the adductor canal. The R3 network is involved in the form of a refluxive tributary, but this is not the principal drainage. It is also called shunt type I+II by some authors Copyright: [Author]

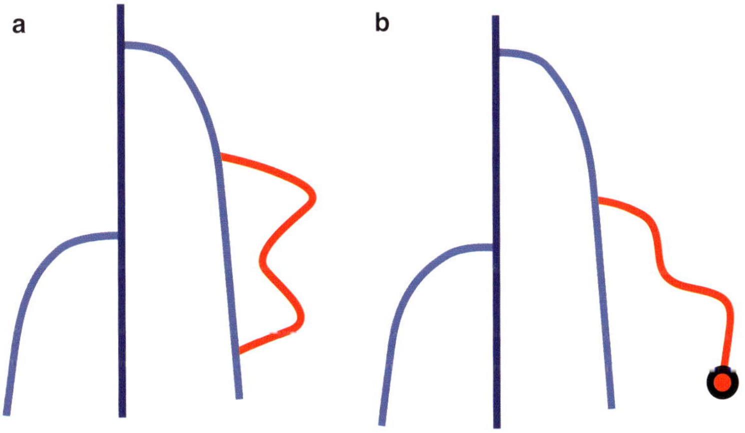

Fig. 4.19 Shunt type II. (**a**) R2–R3–R2. (**b**) Drainage through a perforating vein. This is an "open shunt" because there is no recirculation. R2–R3–R1 Copyright: [Author]

4.2.4 Shunt Type II

The deep veins are not involved in shunt type II. The recirculation occurs only in the superficial veins. Consequently, a smaller volume of blood is involved in the recirculation. The general clinical appearance is of mildly dilated tributaries which are only cosmetically undesirable. The reflux source is from an R2 saphenous vein with normal antegrade flow. This fills an R3 tributary which then drains back into the saphenous vein (Fig. 4.19a) or directly into a perforating vein (Fig. 4.19b). The latter is termed an "**open shunt**" because there is no recirculation. The blood does not flow back to its source.

In type II open shunts, the system is **not overloaded by volume** because of the absence of a recirculation circuit. However, the tributary may be cosmetically undesirable. This is because it dilates to accommodate the blood from the relatively larger-diameter saphenous vein.

Regardless of whether there is an open or closed type II shunt, a **reversal of saphenous flow** may occur above the outflow point of the incompetent tributary. This can be detected with duplex ultrasound as a weak signal over a variable distance upwards (Fig. 4.24e, f). The source of this reflux is not easily identified. It is not from a proximal reflux source arising from a junction with the deep veins. Instead, the blood leaking into the saphenous vein is from healthy tributaries further up. The flow direction in the saphenous vein between the healthy tributaries and the refluxive tributary is retrograde for a stretch until it flows out into the refluxive tributary. One or two incompetent valves in the saphenous vein facilitate this process (see also Fig. 7.49) (Fig. 4.24e, f and additional material online).

In summary:

1. Reflux source from a saphenous vein into a tributary
2. Reflux in tributary
3. Re-entry through a perforating vein or competent saphenous vein

4.2.5 Shunt Type III

As with shunt type I, the primary reflux source in shunt type III is a connection between the deep veins and the R2 network (R1–R2). The saphenous vein is filled directly from the deep vein, either through a saphenous junction or a perforating vein. In contrast to shunt type I, the whole refluxive volume then passes to one or more tributaries (R3). It is the R3 tributaries which return the blood to the deep veins. This may occur in different ways, either directly through a perforating vein (Fig. 4.20a) in which case the tributary may split and lead the blood to several perforating veins or alternatively back into a saphenous vein (Fig. 4.20b). The small saphenous vein may also act as a drainage pathway (Fig. 4.24h) and become incompetent as a result (Fig. 4.16b)

It is important to note that only those perforating veins which are dilated on ultrasound may be considered in shunt classification. A strategy to differentiate between shunt types I and III is described below (Sect. 4.2.9).

In shunt type III, the reflux begins in the saphenous vein having originated from the deep veins. Thereafter, it does not flow from the saphenous vein into the deep system directly but through an intermediate tributary. This varicose tributary is a key player in the recirculation circuit. Without it, there would be no recirculation.

In summary:

1. Reflux source from a deep vein directly into the saphenous vein
2. Reflux through the saphenous vein and a tributary
3. Re-entry through a tributary into a perforating vein or saphenous vein

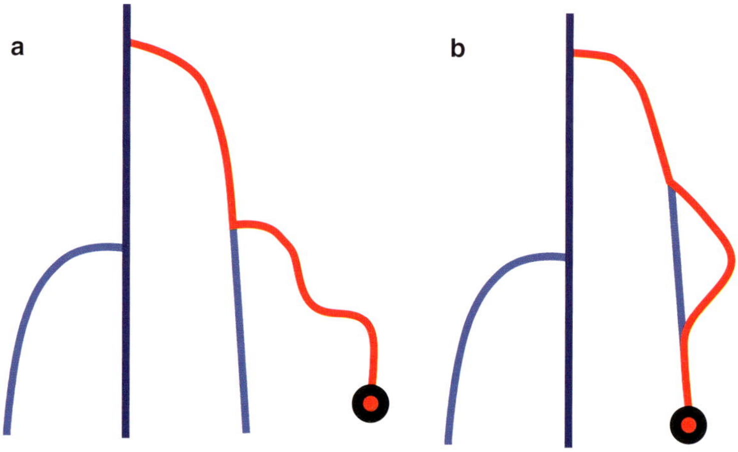

Fig. 4.20 Shunt type III. (**a**) R1–R2–R3–R1, (**b**) R1–R2–R3–R2–R1 Copyright: [Author]

4.2.6 Shunt Type IV

In shunt type IV, the recirculation involves the saphenous vein. However, the reflux source is not R1–R2. There is no reflux through the junction or a direct perforating vein. Instead the reflux source is from the pelvic veins (pelvic shunt type IV, the most common, Fig. 4.21a) or from a perforating vein, which fills the saphenous vein through a tributary (perforating shunt type IV, less common, Fig. 4.21b). The principal re-entry point of the recirculation is through a perforating vein, directly from the saphenous vein, irrespective of whether there are further re-entry points from a distal varicose tributary. The shunt type IV re-entry corresponds to the re-entry in shunt type I.

In summary:

1. Reflux source from a pelvic or perforating vein into the saphenous vein
2. Reflux down the saphenous vein
3. Re-entry through a perforating vein directly from the saphenous vein

4.2.7 Shunt Type V

The reflux source into the saphenous vein is the same as shunt type IV. There is also the pelvic shunt type V (the most common, Fig. 4.22a) or a perforating shunt type V (less common, Fig. 4.22b). However, re-entry is different. The

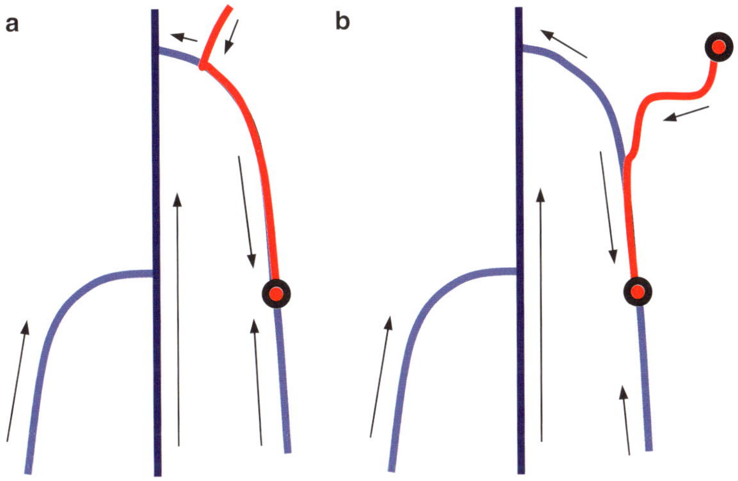

Fig. 4.21 Shunt type IV. (**a**) Pelvic type R1–R3–R2–R1, (**b**) perforating type R1–R3–R2–R1 Copyright: [Author]

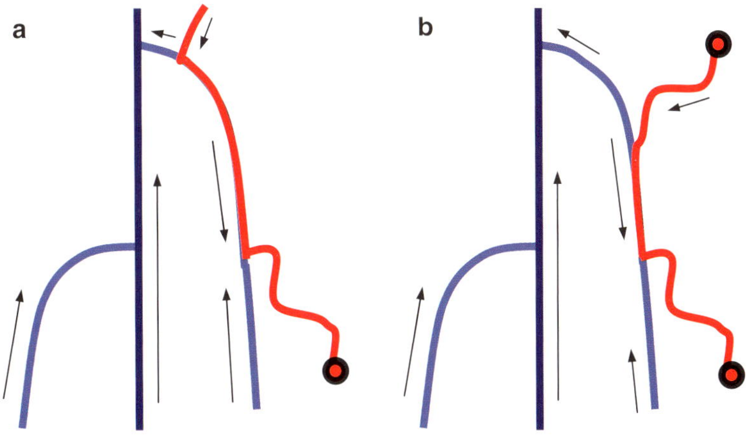

Fig. 4.22 Shunt type V. (**a**) Pelvic type R1–R3–R2–R3–R1, (**b**) perforating type R1–R3–R2–R3–R1 Copyright: [Author]

re-entry volume flows into a tributary at the lower end of the refluxive segment of saphenous vein. In contrast to shunt type IV, there are no draining perforating veins on the saphenous vein.

In summary:
1. Reflux source from a pelvic or perforating vein into the saphenous vein
2. Reflux down the saphenous vein and a tributary
3. Re-entry through a tributary perforating vein

There are many possible **reflux sources** in pelvic shunt types IV and V (Fig. 4.7):

- The reflux enters the great saphenous vein through the junction tributaries. The reflux starts just below the saphenofemoral confluence (Fig. 4.7a).
- Recirculation through the labia into a reticular network in the inner thigh which leads into the posterior accessory saphenous vein and then the great saphenous vein. This may result in a varicose reticular network on the inner and posterior thigh (Fig. 4.7b).
- The reflux from a junction tributary fills the anterior or posterior accessory saphenous veins which lead into one of the two saphenous trunks. The great saphenous vein is the most common trunk involved (Fig. 4.7c).

4.2.8 Shunt Type VI

All other possibilities of a recirculation circuit can be defined as a shunt type VI. Shunt type VI is thus a conglomeration of refluxes from the pelvic or perforating veins. The saphenous veins (R2) are not involved (Fig. 4.24l).

In summary:
1. Reflux source from a pelvic or perforating vein
2. Reflux through tributaries
3. Re-entry into a perforating vein or healthy saphenous vein

4.2.9 Differentiating Between Shunt Types I and III and IV and V

Differentiating between the two most common shunt types (I and III) and the less common shunt types (IV and V) has clear therapeutic implications. This is because of the importance of the tributary (shunt types III and V) as a re-entry point. The differentiation is performed using duplex ultrasound (Fig. 4.23) (Mendoza 2002 in Appendix 2; Zamboni et al. 2010).

Shunt type III can be recognised if there is no further reflux in the saphenous vein when the tributary is occluded. This is because the whole **recirculating volume is drained via the tributary**. In practice, this is achieved by direct digital compression over the refluxive tributary(ies). If there is a perforating vein, which drains directly from the saphenous vein, the reflux continues because there is a drainage path further down into the deep system. Recirculation unaffected by tributary occlusion defines shunt type I (Zamboni et al. 2010).

Studying the details of the R1–R3 venous networks and shunt types clarifies the mechanisms of venous insufficiency and facilitates treatments based on the different shunt types. This is the principle behind the CHIVA method of treatment which corrects the underlying haemodynamic disorder. A summary of shunt types is illustrated in Fig. 4.24 and with additional material online.

4.3 CEAP Classification

In 1994, a commission was set up under the leadership of A. Nicolaides to seek for a way of stratifying venous disease for comparative studies.

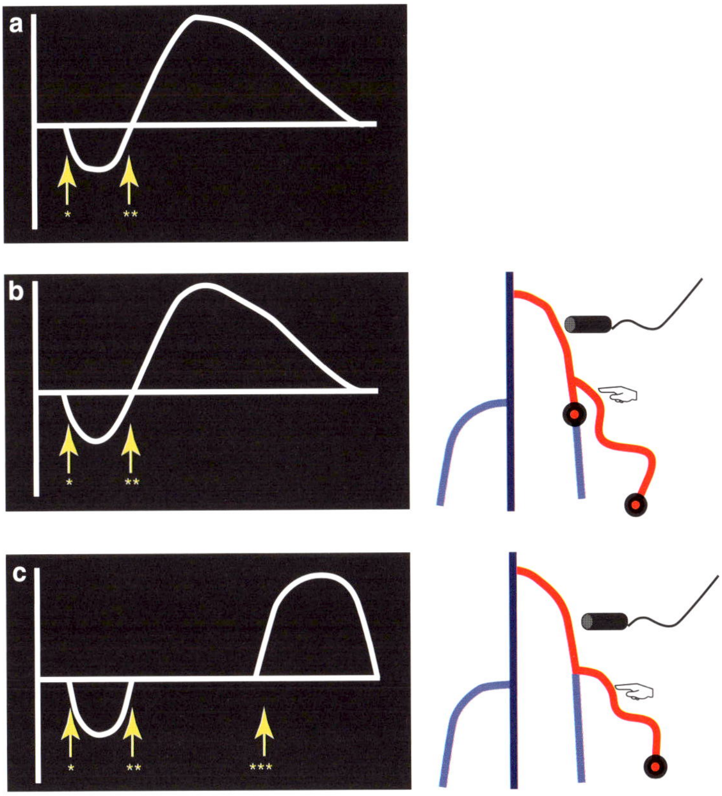

Fig. 4.23 Differentiating between shunt types I and III using duplex ultrasound (see also Fig. 7.52). (**a**) Flow profile in the proximal refluxive segment of the saphenous vein in both shunt types demonstrating antegrade flow (*under the line*) and reflux (*above the line*). * Manual compression of the calf – or raising the toes by the patient in the Wunstorf manoeuvre (Sect. 6.7); ** decompression of the calf – or relaxing the toes. (**b**) Flow profile at the same point as in (a) with digital compression of the tributary in shunt type I. The reflux profile remains unchanged occurring at the point of calf diastole. (**c**) Flow profile at the same point as in (a) with digital compression of the tributary in shunt type III. Reflux is eliminated by digital compression until the point of digital release. *** Digital compression relaxed (From Mendoza (2002); by courtesy of Arrien GmbH) Copyright: [Author]

They developed a descriptive classification of the disease called the CEAP classification (C clinical picture, E aetiology, A anatomy and P pathophysiology). The classification was published internationally and quickly became widely known (Nicolaides 2000).

The clinical part of CEAP is the most widely used, having undergone extensive validation, and it is a component of nearly all clinical trials on venous disease. It is intended as a severity classification, but it is not strictly progressive from C_0 to C_6. It continues to undergo revision in light of earlier recommendations (Antignani et al. 2004; Lattimer et al. 2013). The CEAP classification can be separated into a basic section for practical work and a more complex section for clinical studies. Despite these initiatives, the definitive CEAP classification has not yet been reached (Eklöf et al. 2004).

4.3.1 Descriptive Section

This very complex approach to the classification of chronic venous diseases is presented here in its latest version (2004).

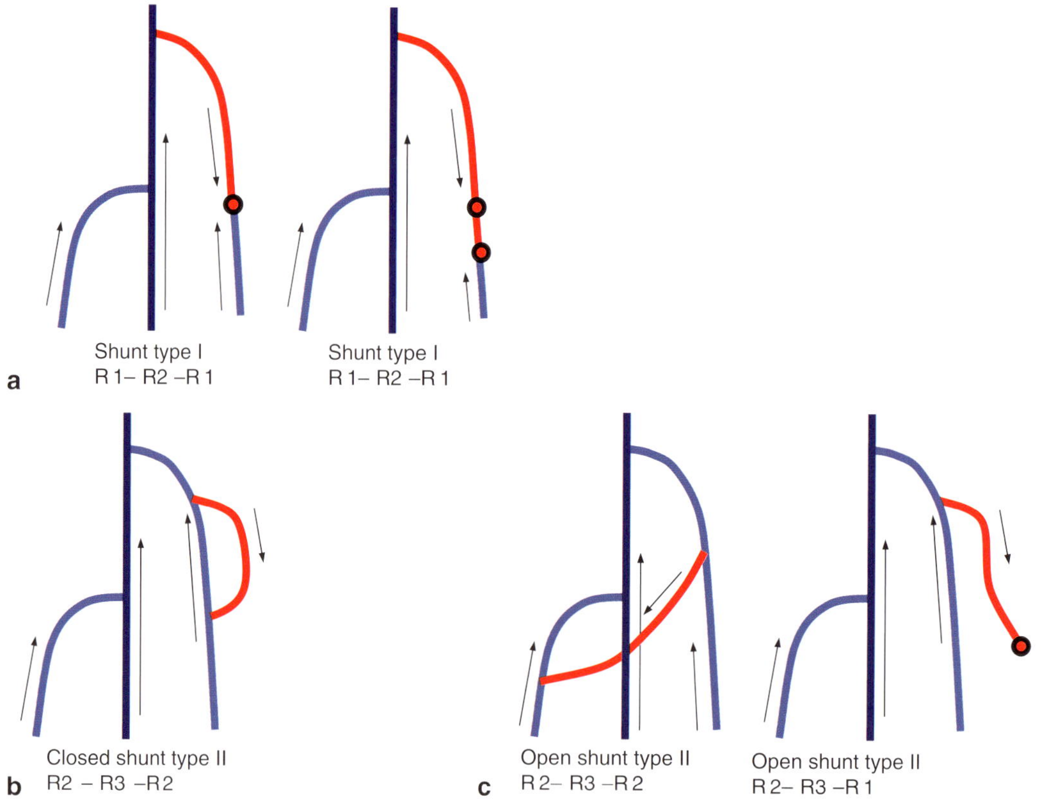

Fig. 4.24 (**a**) Shunt type I: The reflux originates in the deep veins and fills a saphenous vein directly through the saphenofemoral or saphenopopliteal junction, as shown, or through perforating veins (R1–R2). At least one dilated perforating vein is found draining the refluxive section of the saphenous vein (R2–R1) (Sect. 4.2.3). (**b**) Closed shunt type II: Reflux originates from the saphenous vein and re-enters the same saphenous vein (R2–R3–R2). (**c**) Open shunt type II: Reflux originates from the saphenous vein and re-enters the other saphenous veins (R2–R3–R2) or via a perforating vein (R2–R3–R1). (**d**) Shunt type II A: The saphenous vein remains competent. (**e**) Shunt type II B: The saphenous vein is incompetent just above the refluxive tributary. It is important to note that there are no reflux sources from deep veins and the saphenofemoral junction remains competent. The reflux results from the blood that enters the great saphenous vein retrograde from healthy proximal tributaries. (**f**) Shunt type II C: The great saphenous vein is incompetent just above the refluxive tributary, but re-entry is from the great saphenous vein to the deep vein through a perforator (Sect. 4.2.4). (**g**) Shunt type I+II: There is recirculation in the saphenous vein from the deep vein (R1–R2) with drainage directly back into the deep vein (R2–R1) and via a tributary (R3–R1). (**h**) Shunt type III: The saphenous vein is filled from the deep vein (R1–R2), and the reflux is drained through a tributary (R3). The saphenous vein is devoid of a dilated perforating vein to drain the reflux before it enters into this tributary (Sect. 4.2.5). (**i**) Shunt type IV: Reflux fills the saphenous vein through a tributary (R3) and flows directly out of the saphenous vein through a perforating vein. This is analogous to the drainage path of shunt I, but the reflux source is from a pelvic or perforating vein (R1–R3–R2–R1) (* R1 refers to the deep pelvic veins and * R3 to the conduit down to the leg). Re-entry is directly from R2 into R1 (Sect. 4.2.6). (**j**) Shunt type IV with refluxive tributaries: As above, but the principal drainage remains directly from the saphenous vein (R2–R1) irrespective of other refluxive tributary drainage points. (**k**) Shunt type V: Reflux fills the saphenous vein through a tributary (R3) and leaves the saphenous vein through a tributary. There are no intervening saphenous perforating veins to drain the reflux. This drainage is the same as shunt type III (R1–R3–R2–R3–R1) (Sect. 4.2.7). (**l**) Shunt type VI: Reflux originates from a tributary to drain into deep veins via a tributary (R1–R3–R1) or into a competent saphenous vein (R1–R3–R2–R1) (Sect. 4.2.8) Copyright: [Author]

Fig. 4.24 (continued)

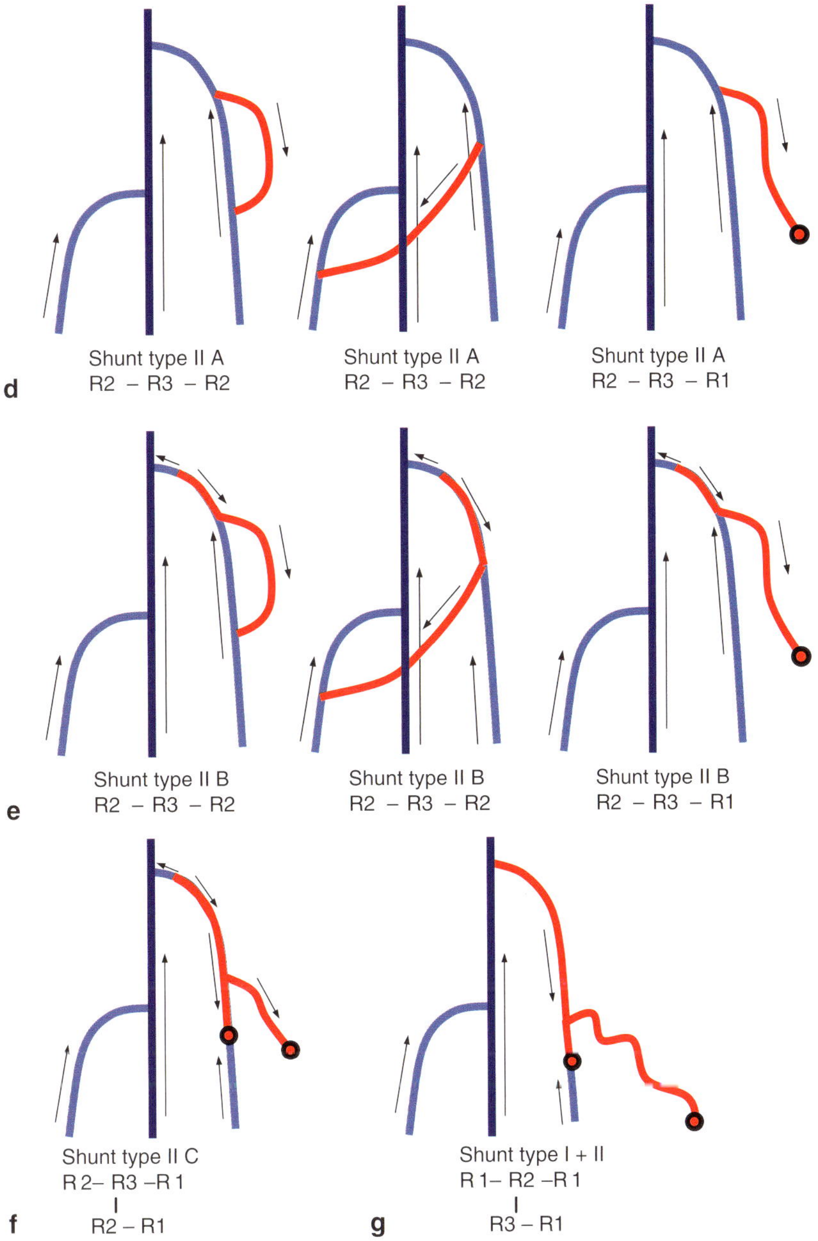

Fig. 4.24 (continued)

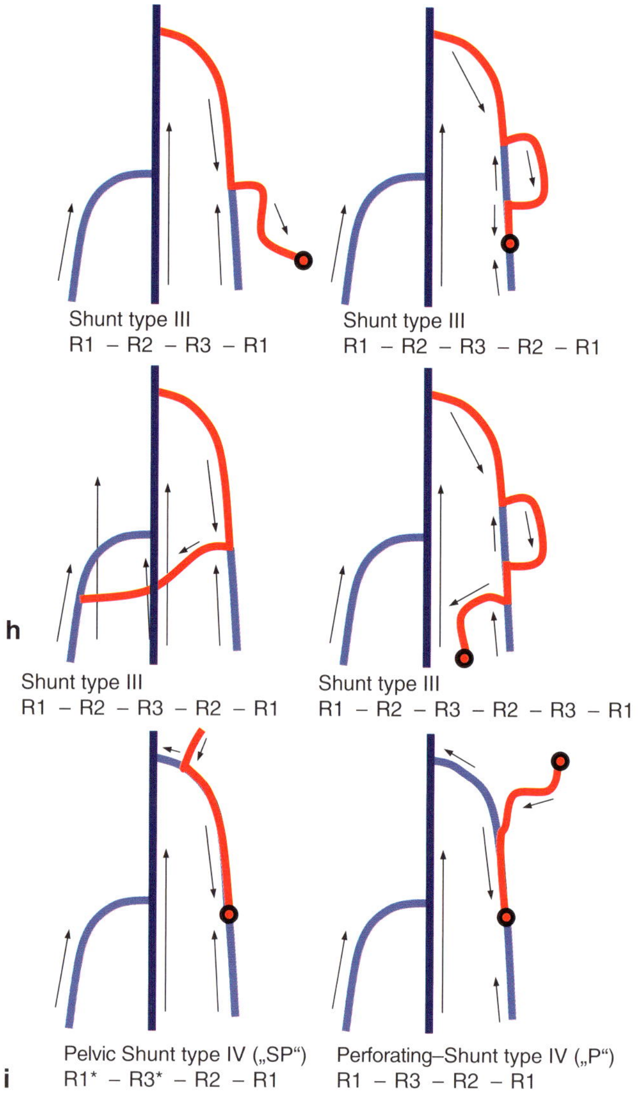

Fig. 4.24 (continued)

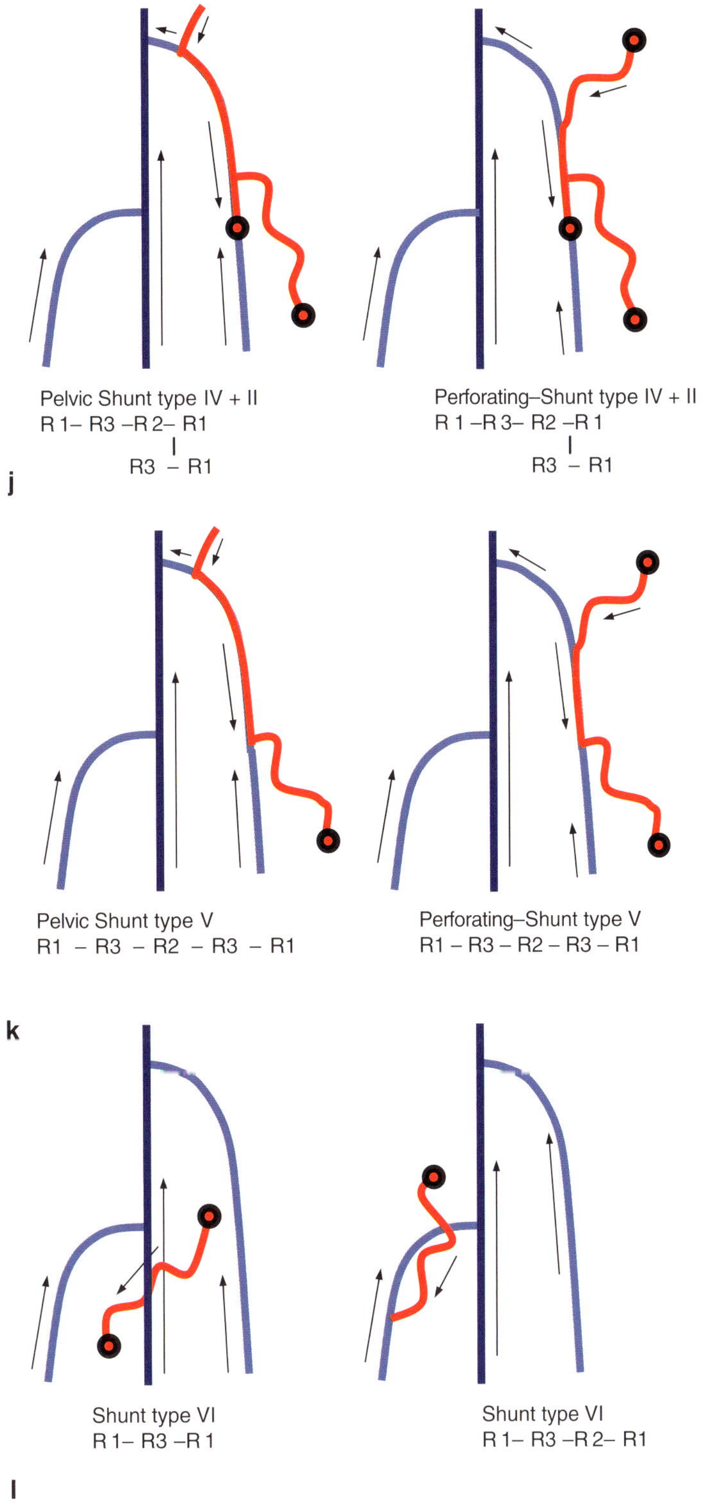

The **date** and **type of examination** should be included in the assessment. Three levels of assessment were defined for diagnosis:

Step 1	History, clinical findings, pocket Doppler
Step 2	Duplex ultrasound, plus optional plethysmography
Step 3	Invasive procedures: phlebography, MRV, spiral CT venography, vein pressure measurement

The current classification is as follows:

Group C: Classification by Clinical Appearance, More Than One Number Can Be Assigned

C_0	No visible varicosities nor venous pathology
C_1	Telangiectasias (<1 mm) and reticular veins (1–3 mm)
C_2	Visible varicosities >3 mm diameter
C_3	Oedema due to venous insufficiency
C_4	Skin changes due to venous insufficiency
C_{4a}	C_{4a} Eczema, hyperpigmentation
C_{4b}	C_{4b} Lipodermatosclerosis, atrophie blanche
C_5	Healed venous ulcer
C_6	Active venous ulcer(s)

Group E: Classification by Cause and Aetiology

E_C	Congenital
E_P	Primary
E_S	Secondary (post-thrombotic)
E_n	No venous cause identified

Group A: Anatomical Classification

The new classification is limited to a general designation of the affected segments:

A_s	Superficial veins
A_d	Deep leg veins
A_p	Perforating veins
A_n	No venous location identified

A patient with a pathological great saphenous vein and refluxive perforating vein would be classified as follows: $A_{s,p}$.

Group P: Classification by Pathophysiology

The original classification into refluxive and obstructive (r, o) was retained and extended by the addition of "n" for no ascertainable venous pathophysiology identified. For use in studies, the pathological veins can be ordered numerically:

Basic CEAP

P_r	Reflux
P_o	Obstruction
$P_{r,o}$	Reflux and obstruction
P_n	No ascertainable venous pathology

Advanced CEAP

Numbers of vein segments:

Superficial vein system	
1	Telangiectasias
2	Great saphenous vein – thigh
3	Great saphenous vein – calf
4	Small saphenous vein
5	Varicose tributary not part of the saphenous vein
Deep vein system	
6	Inferior vena cava
7	Common iliac vein
8	Internal iliac vein
9	External iliac vein
10	Pelvic or gonadal veins, etc.
11	Common femoral vein
12	Deep femoral vein
13	(Superficial) femoral vein
14	Popliteal vein
15	Deep calf veins (anterior and posterior tibial veins, peroneal veins)
16	Gastrocnemius veins, soleus veins and other muscle veins
Perforating veins	
17	Thigh
18	Calf

With this system, the pathology of one or more segments can be defined by numbering the segments involved alongside. The clinical picture with an incompetent perforating vein in the adductor canal (formerly Dodd) and refluxive great saphenous vein to the calf, varicose tributaries and a superficial vein thrombosis in the small saphenous vein would be described as follows:

$$P_{r2,3,5,17,o4}$$

References

Antignani PL, Cornu-Thnard A, Allegra C, Carpentier PH, Partsch H, Uhl JF (2004) Results of a questionnaire regarding improvement of 'C' in the CEAP classification. Eur J Vasc Endovasc Surg 28: 177–181

Cappelli M, Molino Lova R, Ermini S, Turchi A, Bono G, Bahnini A, Franceschi C (2000) Ambulatory conservative hemodynamic management of varicose veins: critical analysis of results at 3 years. Ann Vasc Surg 14:376–384

Eklöf B, Rutherford RB, Bergan JJ, Carpentier PH, Gloviczki P, Kistner RL, Meissner MH, Moneta GL, Myers K, Padberg FT, Perrin M, Ruckley CV, Coleridge-Smith P, Wakefield TW (2004) Revision of CEAP classification for chronic venous disorders (CVD). J Vasc Surg 40:1248–1252

Franceschi C (1993) (Translation of the original, appeared 1988) Theory and practice of the conservative haemodynamic cure of incompetent and varicose veins in ambulatory patients. Armançon, Précy-sous-Thil

Lattimer CR, Kalodiki E, Azzam M, Geroulakos G et al (2012) Varicose veins and severity of chronic venous disorder. Acta Phlebologica 13(2):93–99

Lattimer CR, Kalodiki E, Azzam M, Geroulakos G (2013) An international survey on the interpretation of pigmentation using the C class of the Clinical, Etiological, Anatomical, Pathophysiological Classification. Veins and Lymphatics 2(2):49–54

Mendoza E (2013) Duplexsonographie der oberflächlichen Beinvenen. Springer, Berlin/Heidelberg

Nicolaides AN (2000) Investigation of chronic venous insufficiency – a consensus statement. Circulation 102:126–163

Pittaluga P, Chastanet S, Rea B, Barbe R (2009) Midterm results of the surgical treatment of varices by phlebectomy with conservation of a refluxing saphenous vein. J Vasc Surg 50(1):107–118

Trendelenburg F (1891) Ueber die Unterbindung der Vena saphena magna bei Unterschenkelvaricen. Beitr Klinischen Chir (Tübingen) 7:195–210. English version to be found under www.chiva.info

Zamboni P, Marcellino MG, Cappelli M, Feo CV, Bresadola V, Vasquez G, Liboni A (1998) Saphenous vein sparing surgery: principles, techniques and results. J Cardiovasc Surg 39:151–162

Zamboni P, Gianesini S, Menegatti E, Tacconi G, Palazzo A, Liboni A (2010) Great saphenous varicose vein surgery without saphenofemoral junction disconnection. Br J Surg 97:820–825

Duplex Ultrasound Examination of Superficial Leg Veins

5

Erika Mendoza, Nick Morrison, and Christopher R. Lattimer

Chapter Summary
Certain conditions are indispensible for carrying out duplex ultrasound examinations: the workstation, the general course of the examination, documentation and knowledge of the ultrasound system. These are covered in this chapter.

5.1 The Workstation

Colleagues who regularly carry out duplex ultrasound examination of superficial leg veins should adapt their consulting rooms to the particular requirements of the examination. This will save time, as well as musculoskeletal strain.

E. Mendoza, MD, PhD (✉)
Venenpraxis Wunstorf,
Speckenstraße 10, 31515 Wunstorf, Germany
e-mail: erika.mendoza@t-online.de

N. Morrison, MD
Morrison Vein Institute,
Suite 223, 8575 E. Princess Dr., Scottsdale, AZ, USA

C.R. Lattimer, MD, PhD
Department of Vascular Surgery,
Josef Pflug Vascular Laboratory,
Ealing Hospital and Imperial College, London, UK

5.1.1 Organisational Aspects

The ultrasound room can be the same room to discuss the findings with the patient. The advantage of this is that the doctor can enter the results into the computer or card index while the patient is dressing and may also talk to the patient at the same time. Furthermore, the patient does not need to be accompanied from one room to another. If there is no possibility of printing out the findings during the ultrasound investigation, means must be available for any measurements taken to be noted, without the need stand up, interrupting the examination.

The advantage of separating the ultrasound room from the discussion room is that the new patient can be accompanied into the examination room in advance by an assistant while the doctor is speaking with the previous patient in the discussion room. This saves time lost in dressing and undressing. This may have the disadvantage, however, that patients with walking difficulties take longer to reach the discussion room, even if it is close at hand.

There are no special requirements for the room in which the examination takes place. The only consideration is that it must be possible to darken the room effectively when using older ultrasound machines. This is not necessary with new machines, which offer good picture quality even in a bright light. It is more comfortable if the room is well ventilated, since examinations are sometimes very protracted and most ultrasound machines emit heat. A dimmer control for the

E. Mendoza et al. (eds.), *Duplex Ultrasound of Superficial Leg Veins*,
DOI 10.1007/978-3-642-40731-4_5, © Springer-Verlag Berlin Heidelberg 2014

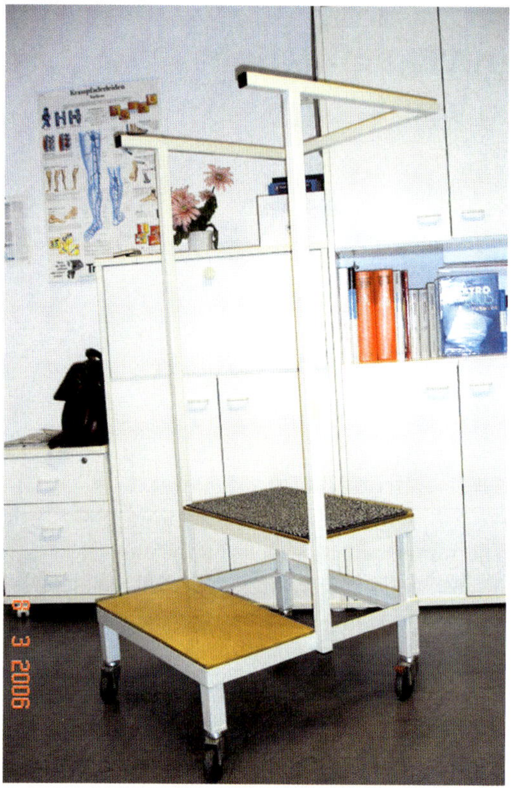

Fig. 5.1 Apparatus for patients to stand on during examination (Dr. Faiez Baghdadi, Neustadt an der Orla; by kind permission) (Copyright: Dr. Faiez Baghdadi, Neustadt an der Orla)

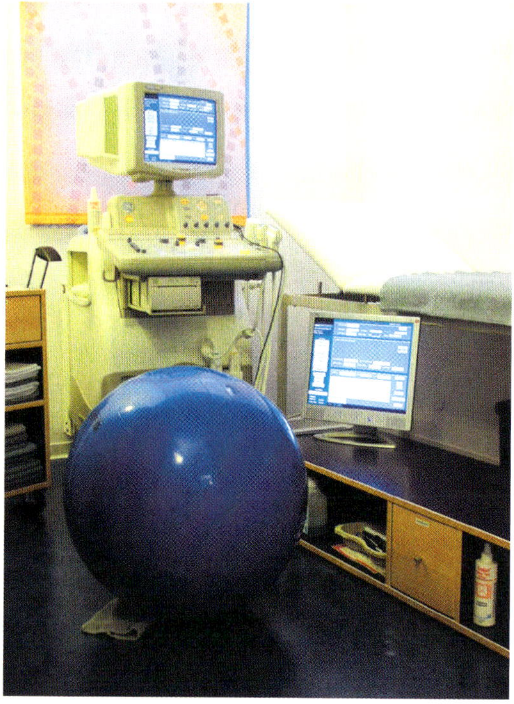

Fig. 5.2 A workstation for superficial leg vein examinations (Copyright: [Author])

room light, located close to the ultrasound machine, eases the task of the examiner, since he does not have to reach for a wall switch every time he needs to adjust the light. A desk lamp placed below the ultrasound machine to light the patient's legs does not generally hinder the view of the B-scan and allows the legs to be inspected even in a darkened room.

5.1.2 Ergonomic Aspects

The patient should be standing for the examination. This produces the difficulty that the patient must be at a certain height for the examiner to probe the calves comfortably. Patients tend to suffer balance problems if they are required to stand for a long period on a relatively small surface (a step is the usual platform). They must also be able to turn round safely.

There are a number of options for raising the patient, ranging from the classic phlebology tilt table to steps and rails which allow the patient to climb and stand safely (Fig. 5.1).

In the author's opinion, the tilt table is unsuitable as the backs of the legs cannot be examined easily because the patient is required to turn around repeatedly on the small step at the end of the table. It would be much easier if they were standing freely.

A raised apparatus with a surrounding railing is more comfortable and stable for the patient (Fig. 5.1). However, the vertical supports may hinder the doctor's work. A further disadvantage is that when patients faint and fall backwards, there is no couch behind to rescue them.

The author therefore prefers a combination of a platform set in front of the examination couch whilst sitting on a low stool or exercise ball (Fig. 5.2).

The ultrasound machine should be placed to the left of the examiner. However, as the monitor is mounted on top of the machine and the patient is standing in front, the examiner must turn his head to the left and upwards to see the monitor.

This position frequently leads to problems in the cervical and thoracic spine. Such can be avoided by installing an additional screen close to the patient's legs to avoid repetitive head turns.

5.2 Examination Modes

5.2.1 Examination of the Patient Standing, Sitting or Lying

The ideal position for the patient is standing for a variety of reasons, the most important being that standing is the position in which patients are most symptomatic and is the position in which identification of reflux is most reliable (DeMuth et al. 2012). Also because the veins become fully distended, even small connecting and perforating veins can be easily identified (Fig. 5.3). Furthermore, reflux due to gravity is accentuated by provocation manoeuvres like manual compression and the Paraná, Wunstorf and orthostatic manoeuvres, which are only possible when standing (Chap. 6). Standing was recommended as the best position in the international consensus document on duplex ultrasound examination of leg veins (Coleridge-Smith et al. 2006).

Patients who are unable to stand or repeatedly feel unwell during the examination can be examined sitting, but the prognostic value of provocation manoeuvres (Chap. 6) is limited under these conditions.

Some colleagues examine veins in the recumbent patient, as this is the usual position for insonating arteries and for detecting deep vein thrombosis. In a lying patient, the common femoral vein in the groin is much smaller than the common femoral artery, whereas in a standing patient, it expands to at least twice the diameter (Fig. 5.3a, b). It is possible to provoke antegrade flow in a lying patient by manual compression or manual activation of the calf muscles by foot movements. However, reflux is sometimes not detected following these manoeuvres because there is insufficient gravitational effect. In a supine patient, reflux can best be provoked by the Valsalva manoeuvre or by applying pressure on the abdomen, even if distal compression may prompt a reflux in proximal portion of the saphenous veins

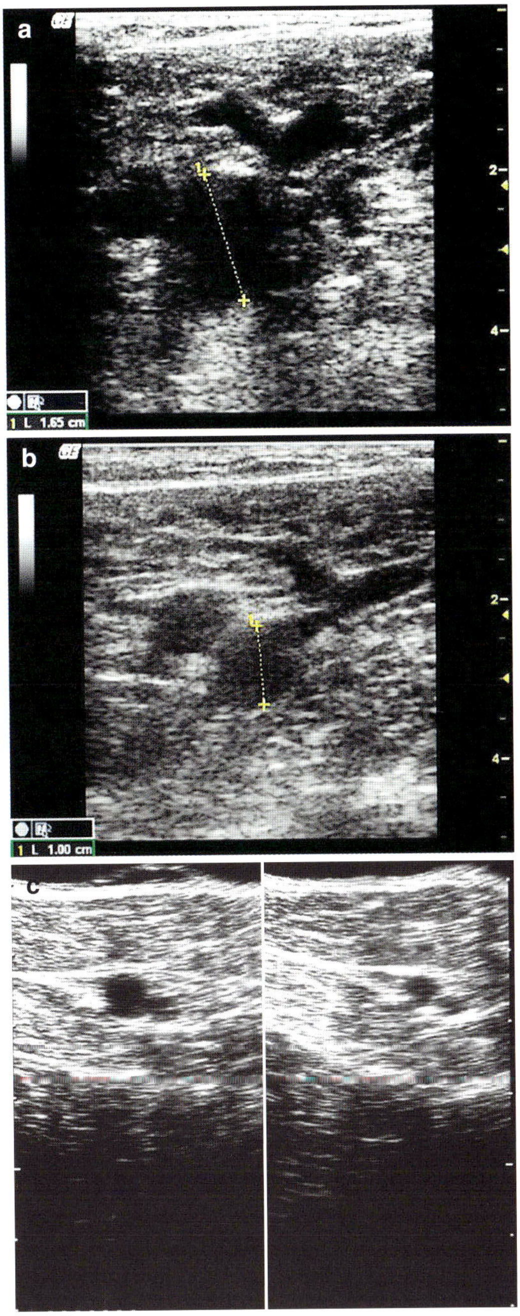

Fig. 5.3 (**a**) Common femoral vein in a standing patient at a diameter of 16.5 mm. Transverse view through the right groin. (**b**) Common femoral vein in the same patient lying down at a reduced diameter of 10 mm. The probe was gently applied so as not to compress the great saphenous vein. (**c**) Transverse view through right thigh great saphenous vein with a perforating vein in the adductor canal (previously Dodd's perforator) in the same patient standing (*left*) and lying (*right*). Note the reduced calibre on lying (Copyright: [Author])

in this position. The examiner will miss many findings by examining underfilled veins. Examination of varices in lying patients should therefore be avoided as far as possible.

5.2.2 Examination in Special Situations

Patients with standing disabilities can be examined sitting down. In this situation, the Wunstorf manoeuvre cannot be used so the patient's calves must be compressed manually. In patients with muscle spasticity, compression manoeuvres should be applied cautiously to avoid triggering muscle cramp which is unpleasant for the patient.

In patients with leg pain and tenderness, the examination should be kept as short as possible and restricted to the central problem. The patient can be re-examined once the leg settles. Manual calf compression should be avoided in so far as possible if it causes pain or performed at a later time. Alternatively, foot compression can be used if the examiner does not wish to apply the Wunstorf manoeuvre or the patient is unable to move his feet or toes.

In patients with pronounced oedema, the veins may be scarcely sonographically visible, especially in the lower leg region. At best, the course of the saphenous trunks can be estimated. Even then, flow may not be demonstrated because the oedema compresses the vessels making them less visible on ultrasound. The correct sequence would be the treatment of the oedema with recall of the patient in order to carry out a fresh examination under improved conditions. Combinations of leg elevation, manual lymphatic drainage and especially compression bandages or stockings are usually successful. If there is a strong suspicion of DVT, it cannot be safely ruled out in this type of patient. Therefore, in such patients, consideration should be given to treatment with anticoagulants until the definitive examination.

Obese patients are more difficult to examine. The veins are deeper, and image resolution becomes poorer with increasing distance from the probe. It is often necessary to switch to a low-frequency probe (Fig. 5.4). The lumen of the vein may be compressed inadvertently in order to get a clearer image. If the examiner tries to get too close by pressing too hard, the vein may disappear altogether.

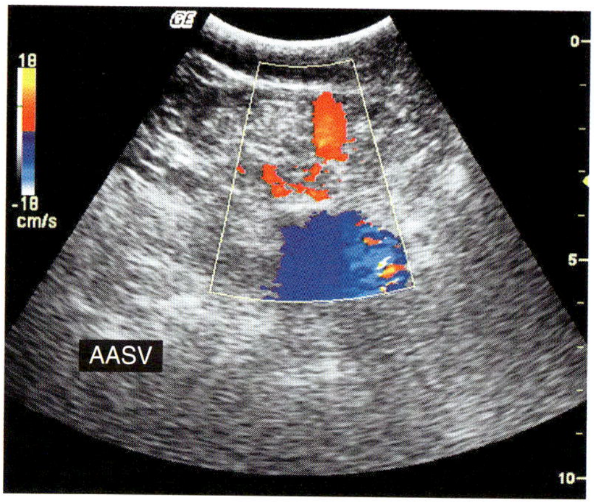

Fig. 5.4 Ultrasound of an obese patient. Transverse view through the left groin with 3.5 MHz curved array probe during muscular systole. The common femoral vein lies at a depth of 5 cm (*blue*); the anterior accessory saphenous vein is refluxive (*red*); the great saphenous vein is not shown (Copyright: [Author])

Patients with venous ulcers must be treated as a priority. Perforating veins may lie beneath and often contribute to the ulceration. General examination of the leg veins can be carried out as described. The author proceeds in patients with inflammatory or suppurating ulcers by first treating the wound and applying compression. As soon as the wound base is clean, the underlying zone can be examined by ultrasound using ultrasound gel. The transducer head should be cleaned before and after the examination with disinfectants recommended by the supplier.

5.3 Course of the Examination

5.3.1 Interview the Patient

It is essential to establish the patient's phlebological case history before the ultrasound examination begins, particularly:

- Type and extent of ailment and when it began
- Prior examinations and results
- Previous interventions like surgery, endothermal ablation or sclerotherapy
- Family and personal history of thrombosis

The answers to these questions may indicate the cause of the condition which may not be venous. The patient should also be asked about underlying conditions and current medication.

5.3.2 Examination

The examination process is a matter of individual preference. The decision has to be made whether the entire superficial vein system, as well as the deep veins in the popliteal region and the groin, should be examined as a matter of routine or only the affected region(s) based on the symptoms. However, important information may be overlooked if only parts of the venous system are examined. It is the author's view that there are certain basic regions which should always be examined before reaching a diagnosis of "superficial venous system free of pathological findings".

In order to avoid overlooking or forgetting any segment, it is recommended that an examination routine should be developed and the same course always followed. Below is a suggested order of examination (minimum requirements are shown in *italics*):

- *Examination of the groin*:
  - *Deep leg veins compressible?*
  - *Flow?*
  - *Saphenofemoral junction refluxive?*
  - *Saphenofemoral junction tributaries refluxive?*
- Course of the great saphenous vein to the knee in the B-scan, with branches and perforating veins, switch on colour and/or PW-mode when sudden changes in calibre are encountered
- *Diameter of great saphenous vein in the thigh if reflux occurs*
- Course of great saphenous vein from knee to ankle in the B-scan, with branches and perforating veins, switch on colour and/or PW-mode when sudden changes in calibre are encountered
- *Examination of posterior tibial perforating veins (Cockett's perforators)*
- *Examination of the popliteal region*:
  - *Deep leg veins compressible?*
  - *Flow?*
  - *Saphenopopliteal junction refluxive?*
  - *Vein of Giacomini present?*
  - *Refluxive?*
- Course of small saphenous vein to the ankle in the B-scan, with branches and perforating veins, switch on colour and/or PW-mode when sudden changes in calibre are encountered
- Examination of back of thigh to exclude refluxive Hach perforating vein
- *Examination of visible side branches to establish origin of reflux*

5.3.3 Transducer Positioning

There is a consensus on probe handling, positioning and use. In longitudinal views, the left of the screen always shows the cranial region of the body, while in transverse views it shows the region which is on the left as seen by the examiner. For legs, this means that when the great saphenous vein in the right leg is examined, the left of the screen shows the ventrolateral region, while in the left leg it shows the dorsomedial region. In examination of the back part of the leg, the left side of the screen will show the lateral zone of the left leg and the medial zone of the right leg. For orientation purposes, it is helpful to mark the probe. The mark should point either upwards or to the left from the examiner's point of view.

When insonating arteries, the probe is placed lengthwise along the vessel revealing a longitudinal view. Longitudinal probe positioning is recommended because these vessels generally run straight so morphological particularities are easier to diagnose. Furthermore, arterial blood flow has to be measured according to strict criteria of angular adjustment, which is only possible with a longitudinal view.

When insonating veins, the absolute flow velocity plays a less important role. More relevant questions are whether there is any flow at all, and the morphology of flow curves measured in PW-mode. As the blood flow is not very rapid and the veins mostly run parallel to the skin, the flow may not always be measured accurately with the probe placed lengthwise. Pressure from tilting the probe may close the vein under examination. It is more effective to measure the flow in varices with a probe held across the course of the vein and slightly tilted. The flow then runs towards or away from the probe, which gives the best results (Figs. 5.5 and 5.6).

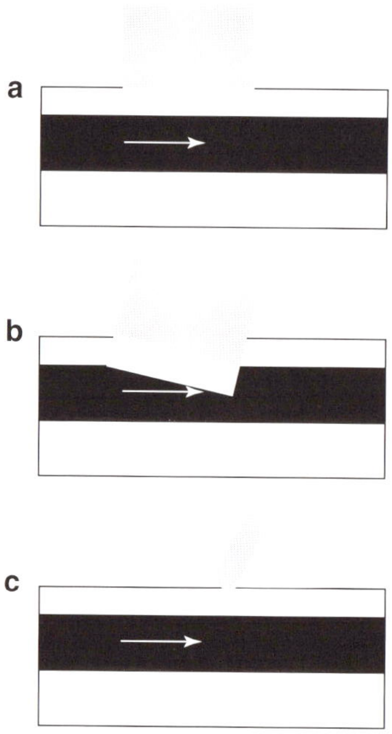

Fig. 5.5 Diagrammatic representation of the possible ways of holding the probe while examining lengthwise along the axis of a vessel: (**a**) The signal is difficult to see, because the blood flow is parallel to the probe. (**b**) If the probe is tilted, this may compress the vein, and the flow may be completely stopped or lost from the image. (**c**) Optimum view with the probe at right angles to the axis of the vessel and slightly tilted (From Mendoza (2002); by kind permission of Arrien GmbH) (Copyright: Arrien, Wunstorf)

Either a frozen B-scan or a moving image can be recorded in PW-mode. The advantage of recording a frozen B-scan is the improved time resolution of the frequency spectrum. Newer equipment has the advantage of simultaneously viewing the B-scan and the PW curve. The advantage of the moving B-scan is that the position of the sample volume can be checked continuously.

In morphological terms, veins, and especially varicose veins, display remarkable variability in their course and network connections. In order to obtain as much data as possible on the region surrounding the vein and not overlook any side branches or perforating veins, optimum examination conditions should be created. It would be ideal to create a three-dimensional image (Figs. 5.7 and 5.8). If the

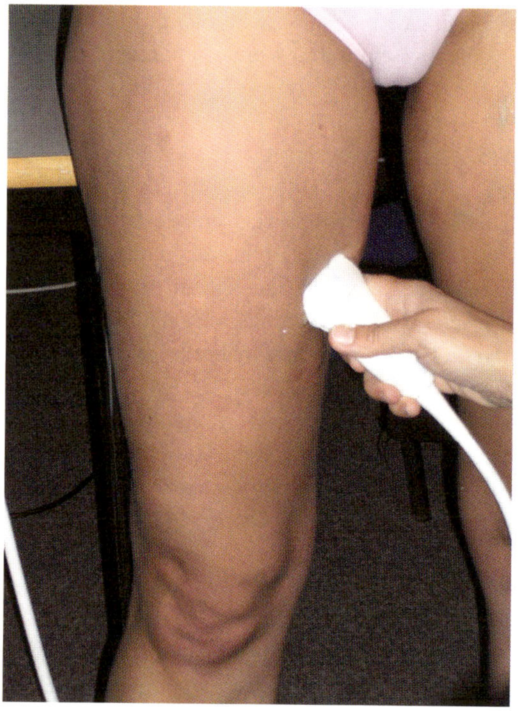

Fig. 5.6 Probe position in examination of great saphenous vein in the thigh in duplex mode (in B-scan the head must not be tilted) (Copyright: [Author])

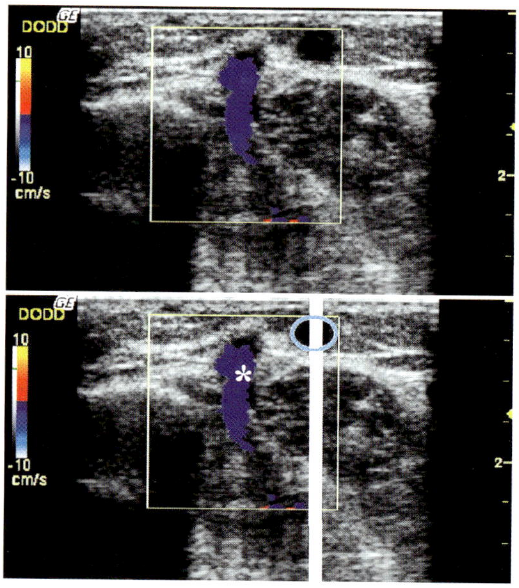

Fig. 5.7 Transverse view of the great saphenous vein in the thigh (*blue circle* in lower image). A perforating vein is seen connecting to the great saphenous vein (marked *). This could easily be overlooked in a longitudinal view of the great saphenous vein (*white line*) (Copyright: [Author])

examiner follows the vein with the probe parallel to its length, the representation remains two-dimensional, and the advantage of duplex ultrasound over phlebography is not exploited. If the vein is viewed transversally, one can build up a mental three-dimensional image of the region surrounding the vein. He is also less likely to miss tributaries.

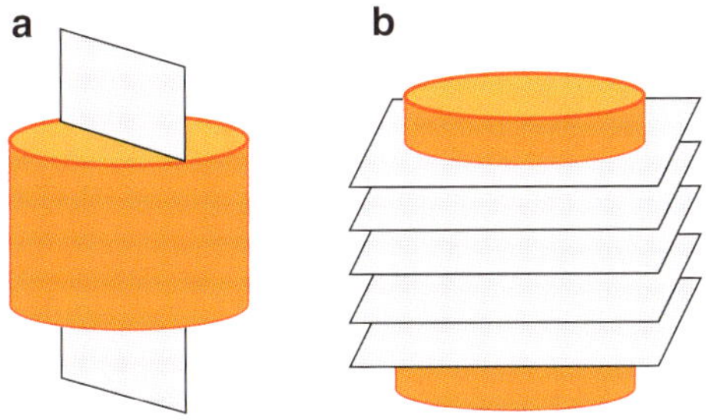

Fig. 5.8 Diagrammatic representation of the leg as an orange cylinder, with the grey planes representing ultrasound images. (**a**) Longitudinal view through the leg. The neighbouring regions cannot be seen. (**b**) Transverse views through the leg. A series of sections build up a three-dimensional image in the examiner's head (Copyright: [Author])

A longitudinal image provides additional information in some regions. These include the saphenofemoral and saphenopopliteal junctions and also for appraising the deep veins and the sources of reflux. It also helps in documenting the extent of a superficial vein thrombosis (phlebitis) in trunk veins.

5.4 Indications for the Examination

There are many more indications for examining the superficial vein system by duplex ultrasound than there are using contrast phlebography.

Table 5.1 lists the indications for examination with additional information on urgency and the need for check-ups.

Table 5.1 Indications for duplex ultrasound examination of leg veins

Indication	Urgency	Check-up	Comments
Telangiectasias	None	As findings progress	Before sclerotherapy, ultrasound exclusion of trunk vein insufficiency
Reticular varices	None	As findings progress	Before sclerotherapy, ultrasound exclusion of trunk vein insufficiency
Visible varices	None	Every 6–12 months	Exclusion of incipient secondary deep vein insufficiency or obstruction
Recent oedema	High	Depending on cause	Examination to exclude thrombosis is important
Long-standing oedema	Medium	Every 6–12 months	Check success of therapy
Skin changes caused by chronic venous insufficiency	Medium	Every 6–12 months	Therapy indication
Venous ulceration	Medium	Every 6–12 months	Check progress, therapy indication
Emergence of new symptoms	Medium to high	Every 6–12 months	Exclusion of thrombosis, therapy indication
Acute pain and swelling in thigh or calf	High	According to findings	Exclusion of deep or saphenous vein thrombosis. Therapeutic or prophylactic anticoagulation
Chronic leg pains	Medium	According to findings	Exclusion of a venous cause
After interventional treatment	Medium	After 6–8 weeks, then every 1–2 years	Screen for DVT, audit and feedback, check progress annually
Superficial vein thrombosis (phlebitis)	High	According to findings	Exclusion of progression into deep veins through perforating veins or at the saphenofemoral junction or synchronous deep venous thrombosis, even in the contralateral extremity (see Chap. 11). Prophylactic anticoagulation

5.5 Clinical Relevance of Findings

Since the introduction of duplex ultrasound, it has become possible to record significantly more pathological findings than previously. Examination is neither painful nor tiresome and can be done at any time. It is being increasingly used as a screening process for oedemas or leg pains. Slight reflux might be defined as a pathological finding. However, not every finding has a clinical correlation, and not every finding must be treated with therapeutic intervention beyond compression.

At the end of the examination, the findings are presented to the patient by the doctor. It should be reported whether the pain, calf cramps or swelling is likely of venous origin. He must also give an opinion as to whether persistent or recurrent pain after an operation results from a recurrence or an untreated varicose vein. The clinical picture is often self-explanatory. Shooting pains of a stabbing nature which radiate often indicate a spinal condition, and dyspnoea suggests heart insufficiency, to give two examples. For this reason, knowledge of the patient history and physical examination in parallel are essential for the diagnosis and to explain the relevance of the findings to the patient.

In the presence of venous insufficiency and concurrent conditions, it may be difficult to decide whether symptoms are mainly venous in origin. In such cases, a therapeutic test with compression stockings is recommended. The patient should wear compression stockings for a month and then come for a further appointment. If the pain has reduced, then relief of symptoms may also be expected from venous intervention.

5.6 Documentation

There is nothing more individual than the progression of varicose veins. Documentation of all the findings after examination is therefore particularly important. To carry out a full examination of the venous system and record nothing more than the fact that the great saphenous vein may be refluxive above or below the knee loses a large amount of information.

5.6.1 Documentation in the Examiner's Records

Recording the haemodynamics of the affected leg is the minimum documentation requirement after a duplex ultrasound examination (Fig. 5.9). The deep leg veins are drawn as straight lines, while the great and small saphenous veins are shown as curved lines which intersect with the deep veins. The direction of flow in these three venous systems is documented with arrows. Arrows also show the direction of flow of reflux in side branches and perforating veins.

If pathologies are discovered, such as aneurysm in the region of the saphenofemoral junction confluence, a hypoplastic segment of great saphenous vein, post-thrombotic changes, etc., these findings can be noted in writing on the drawing. In this way, the findings in the leg, the length of the reflux in the great saphenous vein and the patient's particularities can be seen at a glance.

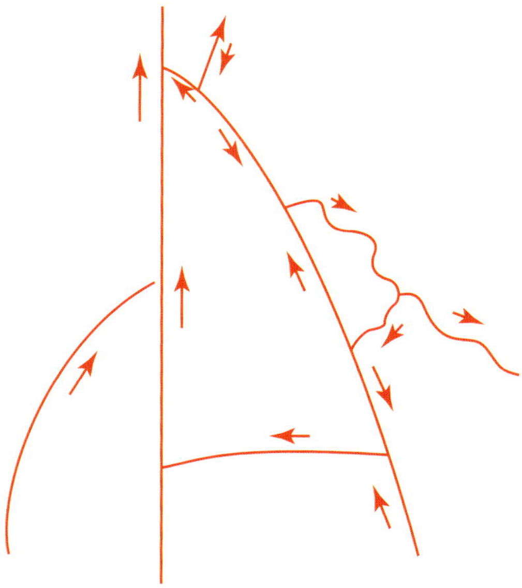

Fig. 5.9 Freehand drawing of findings for documenting haemodynamics (Copyright: [Author])

If electronic records are kept, computer programmes exist for creating these diagrams with comments. However, this is significantly more laborious than a freehand drawing on paper. Alternatively, the findings can be typed in as text; however, these need to be read each time, which is considerably more time consuming than looking at a drawing. Scanning the drawing into the electronic medical record is quite handy and acceptable.

With modern computers, it is possible to archive images in the machine or in an external data storage device. Only those images which are immediately relevant for check-ups, and which cannot be recorded unambiguously as drawings, should additionally be printed out and kept in the patient's records.

It is also advisable to document the following with B-scan images if applicable or available: the saphenofemoral and saphenopopliteal junctions, in transverse and longitudinal views; the course of these two veins, with diameters; the perforating veins; and any particularities such as postthrombotic changes or oedema.

The morphology of the flow curve in PW-mode for reflux in the trunk veins provides information on haemodynamics, so documentation of this is also helpful for later check-ups. The flow curve is a more suitable documentation method than colour presentation because it shows the flow as a function of time, while colour presentation can only show the flow at a given moment and does not provide sufficient information as to whether a vein is competent or refluxive.

Different countries require different levels of documentation for reimbursement purposes. These can range from a compulsory written report to a printout of several images. This is beyond the scope of this book and subject to change. Reimbursement for the doctor or duplex technician can also be determined for an entire session, irrespective of the number of scans that are performed.

The documentation for the finding or exclusion of a thrombosis should be meticulous. This is very important for future check-ups and thrombus evolution, and on occasions a clean copy may be requested for forensic reasons.

The safest way of documenting the presence or absence of an intravascular coagulum is compression ultrasound (Fig. 5.10 and Chap. 14). In the B-scan, it is possible to exclude (Fig. 5.10a) or prove (Fig. 5.10b) the presence of a thrombus.

A further possibility is offered by compression in M-mode (Fig. 5.11). The sample volume is laid against the vein, which is then compressed. The right-hand part of the image documents that the vein can be compressed because the anterior and posterior walls meet in the centre of the lumen. In the popliteal fossa, where vein and artery are superimposed, it can be shown clearly that compression occurred without the probe slipping when the artery maintains a constant calibre and remains in the centre of the image. The M-mode is therefore particularly good for documenting the exclusion of thrombosis at this point.

In B-scan and colour-coded duplex on the other hand, a thrombus permitting partial flow can be very clearly documented (Fig. 5.12).

5.6.2 Reporting Findings to the Primary Physician

The patient's family doctor should gather together all the findings and must be informed of the confirmation or exclusion of ailments.

In the author's experience, colleagues who are not trained in phlebology can learn little from a flow curve (Fig. 5.9). The findings should therefore be clarified in words in a report to the family doctor. As this finding also reports on the condition of the patient's leg, which the family doctor must in turn pass on to other colleagues, all the relevant data must be included, in particular the beginning and end of reflux in the trunk vein, any insufficiencies of perforating veins, the condition of the deep veins and incidental findings like a popliteal cyst or muscular atrophy.

5.6.3 Reporting Findings to the Operating Doctor

Reporting findings to the operating doctor constitutes a special case. If he does not carry out the

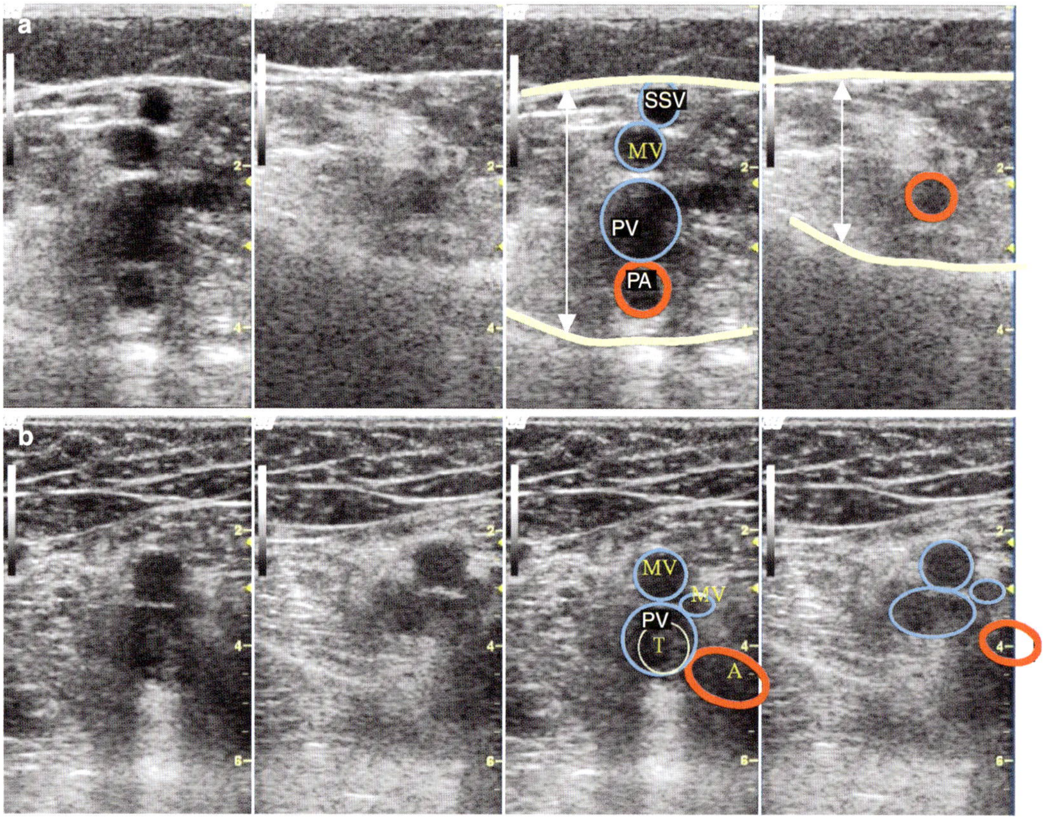

Fig. 5.10 Documentation of confirmation or exclusion of thrombosis. (**a**) Exclusion of thrombosis of the popliteal vein (PV) by compression in B-scan (*left*): normal B-scan with small saphenous vein, muscle vein, popliteal vein and popliteal artery (from *top* to *bottom*). The popliteal fascia (above) and the posterior face of the femur (below) are shown as *pale yellow lines*. The distance between them (*arrow*) is reduced under compression (*right*): compression. The artery (*red*) is still visible under compression, and the veins are not. Therefore, thrombus is not present in these veins (see DVD). (**b**) Compression ultrasound of the popliteal region in the presence of thrombus (*left*): transverse view of popliteal region. The thrombus (*T*) can be seen in the popliteal vein (*PV*). The lumen appears to be clear in both the muscle veins (*MV*) (*right*): With compression, it can be seen that these veins are noncompressible and therefore completely obstructed by thrombus (Copyright: [Author])

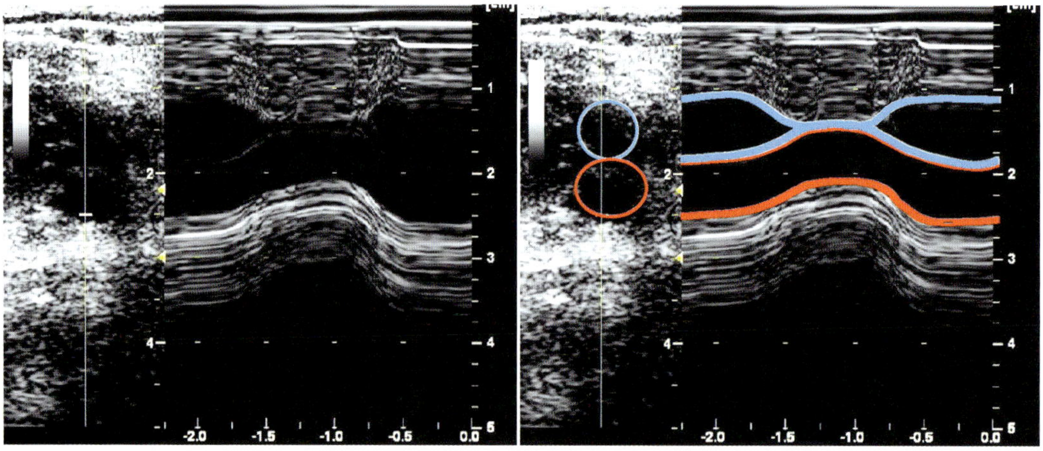

Fig. 5.11 M-mode during compression of the popliteal region. Transverse view through the popliteal fossa with the popliteal vein (*light blue*) and artery (*red*) (Copyright: [Author])

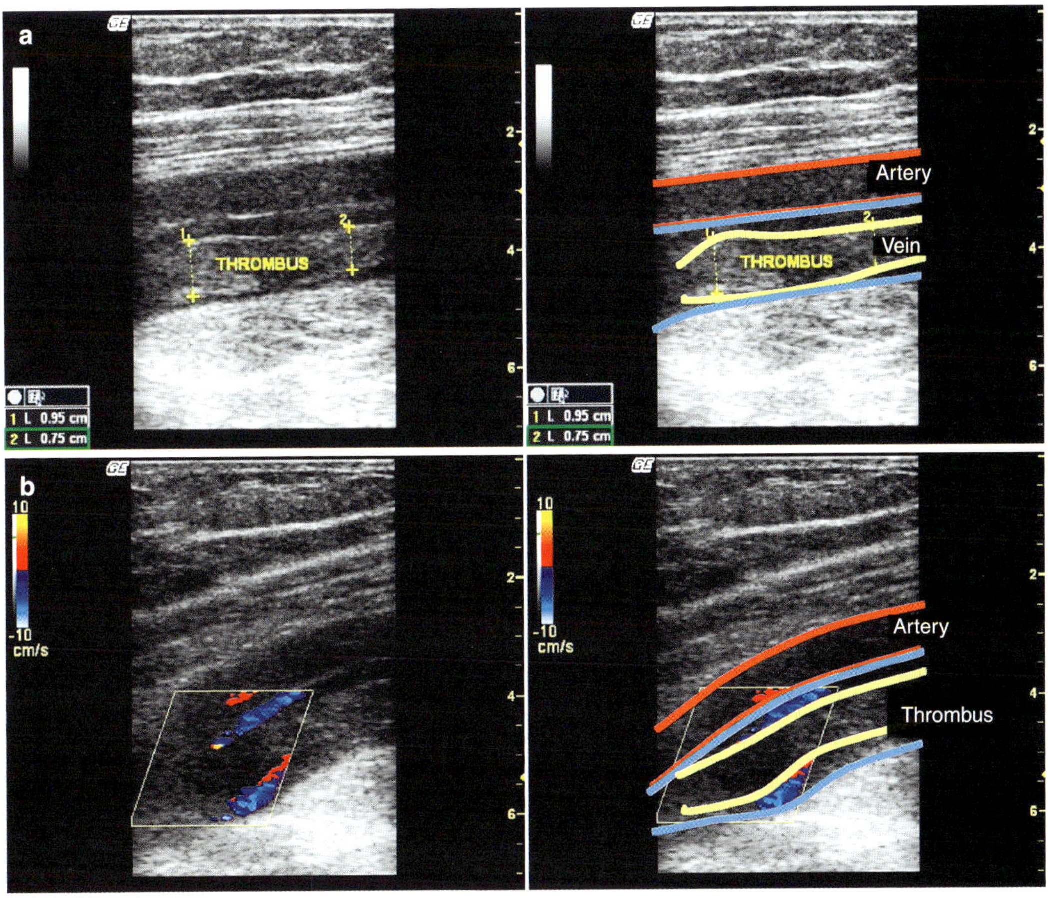

Fig. 5.12 Documentation of thrombosis. (*a*) Longitudinal view of medial side of thigh. The thrombus can be seen in the lumen of the femoral vein; (*b*) colour-coded duplex ultrasound (longitudinal view) of the same patient at the proximal border of the popliteal fossa. There is partial flow around the thrombus (*blue* signal) (Copyright: [Author])

ultrasound examination himself, he must be able to determine information from the findings, such as the location of the pathologically altered perforating veins, the proximal and distal points of insufficiency and if applicable the length of hypoplastic segments [consider adding "status of the deep venous system"]. In the case of surgery on the short ["small"] saphenous vein, details of the height and position (lateral or medial) of its termination into the PV are important.

Ideally, the surgeon should examine the patient himself immediately before the operation and mark all the relevant findings on the skin with a permanent felt-tipped marking pen. If this is not possible, then one of the surgeon's colleagues could carry out the examination immediately before the operation, the day before if necessary, and mark the relevant points on the skin (Mendoza 2002 in Appendix 2). Alternatively, the diagnostic sonographer can also be present and assist during the therapeutic intervention.

These findings must be supplemented by a flow curve with all relevant data. The written report not only is to ensure that the surgeon has the required information if the marks are wiped off but also is essential for legal reasons if complications should arise.

5.6.4 Reporting Findings to the Patient

Some practices have adopted the custom of giving patients a document informing them of the interventions carried out at various stages. This is helpful for subsequent examiners. However, this documentation serves only as a guide for ultrasound examinations on primary varicose veins.

5.7 Knowledge of the Ultrasound System for Phlebology

Ultrasound examination of the leg veins calls for great experience and should ideally be based on well-grounded knowledge of venous anatomy and pathology.

There are many courses on venous duplex examination organised by many societies and colleges. Those who study independently can practise ultrasound examination of the superficial veins on patients. Opportunities arise during scheduled examinations of the leg arteries or deep veins. The trunk veins can be followed in transverse view from top to bottom, and provocation manoeuvres can be practised at the same time.

Another good idea is to shadow competent examiners in practices which regularly carry out superficial leg vein ultrasound examinations. It is also helpful to document findings in one's own patients with a haemodynamic diagram and then ask experienced colleagues to check these results. This will provide the learner with a reliable feedback on his findings and is also a good way of accumulating experience.

References

Coleridge-Smith P, Labropoulos N, Partsch H, Myers K, Nicolaides A, Cavezzi A (2006) Duplex ultrasound investigation of the veins in chronic venous disease of the lower limbs-UIP consensus document, part I. Basic principles. Eur J Vasc Endovasc Surg 31:1–10

DeMuth RP, Caylor K, Walton T, Leonda L, Rosero E, Chung J, Arko F, Clagett GP, Valentine RJ (2012) Clinical significance of standing versus reversed trendelenburg position for the diagnosis of lower-extremity venous reflux in the great saphenous vein. J Vasc Ultrasound 36(1):19–22

Flow Provocation Manoeuvres for the Diagnosis of Venous Disease Using Duplex Ultrasound

6

Erika Mendoza and Christopher R. Lattimer

Chapter Summary
The presence of blood flow is a prerequisite for all duplex ultrasound examinations. Unlike the arterial examination, spontaneous venous blood flow is not sufficient for assessing the superficial and deep veins. In addition to phenomena such as physiological modulation of flow in the deep veins due to respiration, vein compressibility and free movement of the venous valves, it is necessary to apply provocation manoeuvres to augment flow. These increase the diagnostic information by assessing the direction of flow, the patency of the vein and the behaviour of the valves.

6.1 Requirements for Provocation Manoeuvres

The most important factor in the examination is gravity. It is therefore essential to examine the patient in a standing or sitting position when the leg is dependent (Coleridge-Smith et al. 2006).

E. Mendoza, MD, PhD (✉)
Venenpraxis Wunstorf,
Speckenstraße 10, 31515 Wunstorf, Germany
e-mail: erika.mendoza@t-online.de

C.R. Lattimer, MD, PhD
Department of Vascular Surgery,
Josef Pflug Vascular Laboratory,
Ealing Hospital and Imperial College, London, UK

Provocation manoeuvres must satisfy the following criteria:

- Blood flow must be augmented in the vein segment to be examined.
- The manoeuvre must be repeatable and its effect reproducible by different examiners.
- The blood flow must be stimulated repeatedly, in a comparable manner, in the same patient for the duration of the examination.
- The examination result must have a high specificity and sensitivity as a consequence of the manoeuvre.
- The manoeuvre must be easy to carry out. Motion artefacts and shifting of the measurement window can occur easily if the examiner changes position relative to the machine.
- If the manoeuvre requires the active participation of the patient, it must not be too demanding in terms of comprehension and coordination.
- The patient's participation must not be distressing, exhausting or painful.
- Blood flow stimulation should correspond to a physiological process like imitating walking.

6.2 Spontaneous Flow in Veins

6.2.1 Lying Subject

Whilst supine, gravity does not hinder the venous return. The blood flow is **continuous** with 1 or 2 superimposed sine curves depending on the point of examination. The volume flow reflects the

E. Mendoza et al. (eds.), *Duplex Ultrasound of Superficial Leg Veins*,
DOI 10.1007/978-3-642-40731-4_6, © Springer-Verlag Berlin Heidelberg 2014

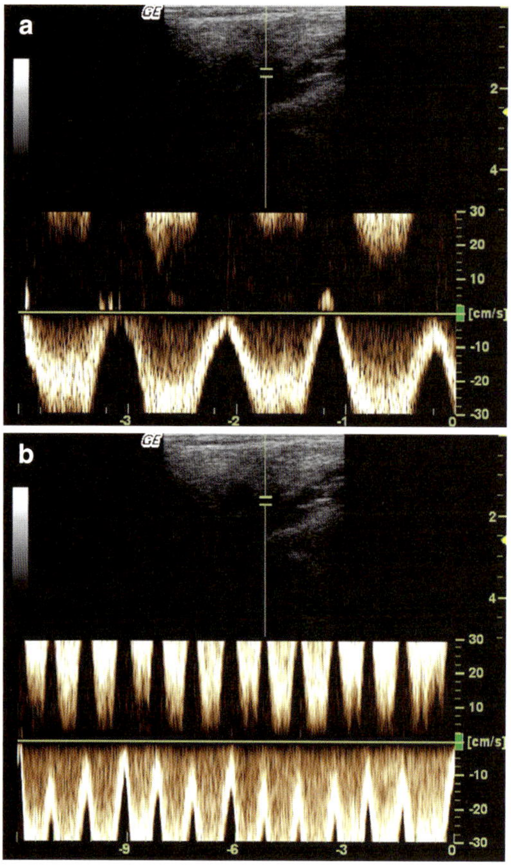

Fig. 6.1 Blood flow (BF) in the right common femoral vein in a lying subject holding his/her breath. The sine curve corresponds to the wave transmitted from the right atrium. It is a composite wave superimposed on the venous return. (**a**) Curve modulation at normal speed (4 s in display). (**b**) Curve modulation at slow speed (12 s in display) Copyright: [Author]

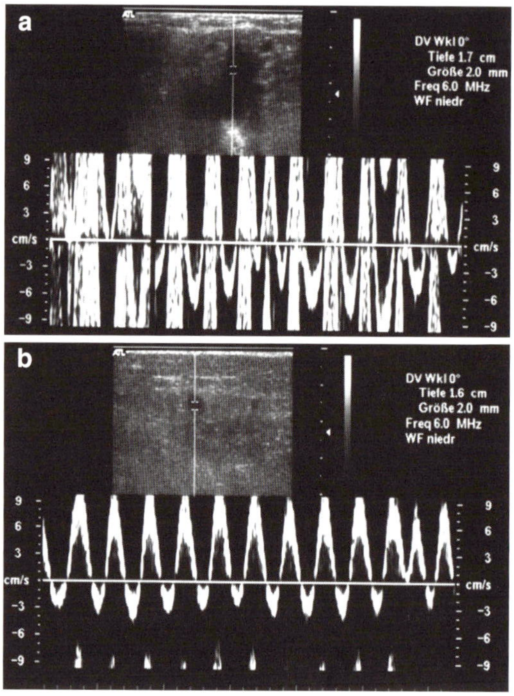

Fig. 6.2 (**a**) Velocity profile of the saphenofemoral region in a patient with an A-V fistula. This fistula resulted from a femoral puncture during a heart catheter examination. (**b**) Velocity profile in the same leg further down the great saphenous vein in the thigh region (12 s in display) Copyright: [Author]

length of time the subject has been lying. Initially, there is a high volume of venous return, but after some time, the spontaneous flow lessens.

In the lying subject, the pressures in the right atrium are transmitted to the large leg veins (Fig. 6.1). This gives rise to the sine curve. In colour duplex mode, these fluctuations in flow are hard to visualise.

This sine curve must be distinguished from the **arterialised flow** in a vein in the case of an arteriovenous fistula. In the immediate vicinity of the fistula, the velocity profile is very similar to arterial (Fig. 6.2a). If the flow is measured directly in the fistula or its immediate vicinity, a greatly increased velocity is found. Further along the course of the vein, the velocity profile becomes weaker with a reduced velocity during cardiac systole. If the sine-shaped velocity profile is found in the great saphenous vein, then an arteriovenous fistula or ventricular septal defect must always be suspected (Fig. 6.2b) (see also Sect. 17.6).

Cyclical flow change in synchrony with the heart rate is not always found and normally has no pathological or diagnostic value. However, in combination with increased velocities, it may indicate an A-V fistula, septal defect or right heart insufficiency (see Sect. 17.5).

This is not the case with **respiration**. The normal venous velocity profile during the respiration cycle in a healthy person is influenced by pressure fluctuations in the abdomen. During inhalation the intra-abdominal pressure increases which increases pressure on the vena cava. This

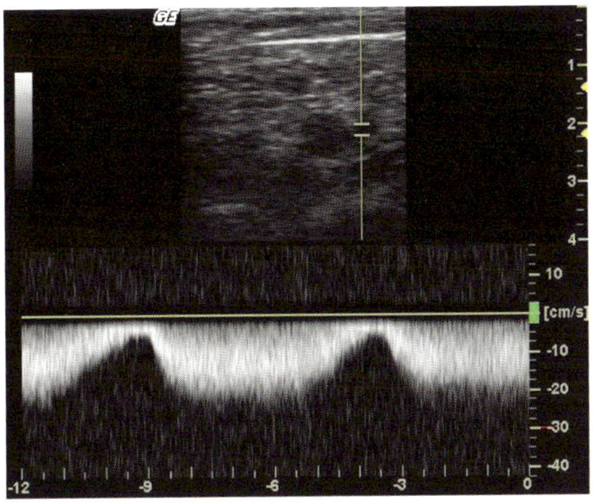

Fig. 6.3 Blood flow (BF) in the right common femoral vein in a supine subject breathing normally, 12 s in display Copyright: [Author]

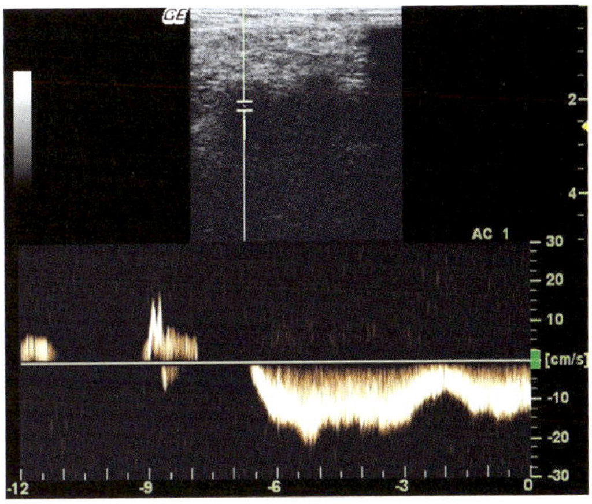

Fig. 6.5 Blood flow (BF) in the right common femoral vein in a supine subject exhaling forcibly. The blood flow stops with two retrograde flow peaks at −12 and −6 s on display. From −6 to 0 s normal respiration resumes Copyright: [Author]

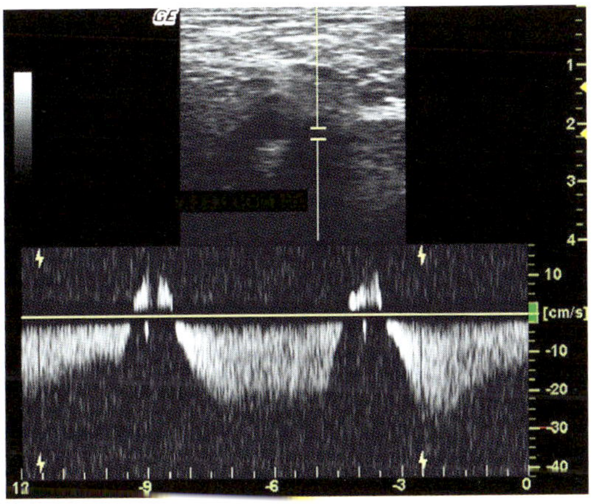

Fig. 6.4 Blood flow (PW) in the right common femoral vein in a supine subject breathing deeply. At the end of inhalation, the blood flow is briefly reversed (peaks), 12 s in display Copyright: [Author]

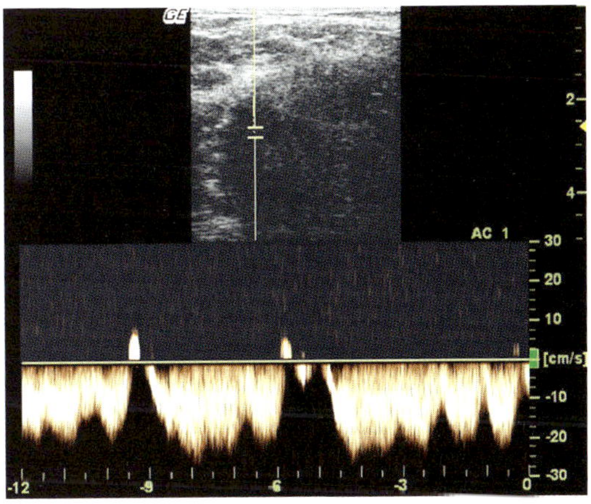

Fig. 6.6 Blood flow (BF) in the right common femoral vein in a supine subject breathing deeply. The transmitted arterial curve is superimposed on the respiration curve to form a composite wave, 12 s in display Copyright: [Author]

hinders the venous return to the right atrium. As a result, towards the end of inhalation, the velocity profile flattens and may disappear almost completely (Fig. 6.3). Occasionally it may become retrograde for an instant (Fig. 6.4). If the subject exhales normally by releasing his/her breath, no pressure occurs in the abdomen and the blood returns freely. If he/she exhales forcibly, it may arrest the venous return, assuming competent valves (Fig. 6.5). If the vein is subject also to the pressure waves transmitted from the right atrium, the two sine curves will be superimposed in the PW curve to form a composite wave. The fast curve synchronised with the pulse and the slow respiration curve (Fig. 6.6). The flow modulations caused by pulse and respiration cannot generally be observed in colour duplex.

The velocity profile changes when there is a **hindrance to flow** above the measurement point. This may be an occlusion caused by thrombosis or external compression of the vein. It may be also an obstruction defined as incomplete closure of the

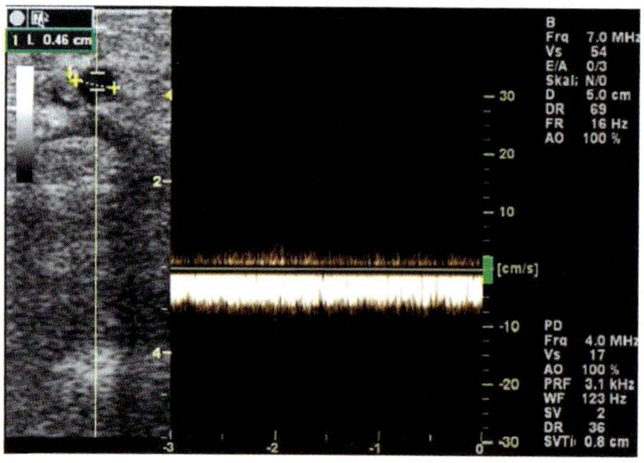

Fig. 6.7 Flow in the cephalic vein when the subclavian vein is nearly occluded. Continuous flow is demonstrated which is not influenced by respiration Copyright: [Author]

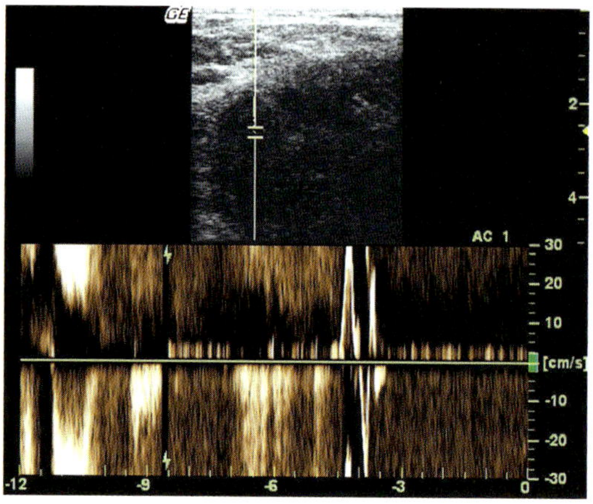

Fig. 6.8 Blood flow (BF) in the right common femoral vein in a healthy test subject who has just laid down after a long period standing; 12 s in display. The blood flows rapidly out of the leg. In the mid-right section of the image, the continuous flow is interrupted at 4 s when the subject coughed briefly Copyright: [Author]

lumen by partial thrombosis or external compression. In the former case, no flow can be measured in the region immediately below the thrombosis. If a diversion route has formed, the flow will behave as an incomplete closure of the vein. This is characterised by a continuous flow pattern without fluctuations in velocity. In the presence of a reduced luminal calibre or a diversion route, the flow will not be influenced by deep inhalation and exhalation (Fig. 6.7).

Immediately after the subject lies down, a continuous flow starts in the deep leg veins, often not modulated by respiration, as the volume of blood collected while standing rapidly drains the leg (Fig. 6.8). A proximal constriction can therefore only be assumed after a period of lying down, which is after approximately 1 min. Raising the leg will accelerate emptying and decrease this time period. If the venous return remains unaffected by respiration, then a proximal obstruction of the iliac veins is a distinct possibility.

6.2.2 Standing Subject

Immediately after standing up, **no flow** is found in healthy leg veins under ultrasound. The venous system has high compliance (Sect. 3.1.2) and can adapt to the increasing volume of blood. It can accommodate a large volume of blood on standing before antegrade flow resumes. On lying down, this reserve empties. When the patient stands up, the venous capillaries and venules are the first ones to fill. When the calf muscle and deep leg veins empty after calf muscle-pump activation, there is no flow initially.

It is only after a time, which varies widely from person to person but has so far not been found to be of pathological relevance, that a slow antegrade flow (towards the heart) is found in the standing subject. This is called "**vis a tergo**" or "force from behind". It arises from the pressure of arterial blood transmitted from the capillaries into the full reservoirs in the calf muscle veins (Fig. 6.9). Respiratory modulation is not observed in the standing person breathing normally, but it becomes apparent when he/she breathes deeply.

6.2.3 Antegrade Flow and Reflux

When walking or when moving the calves and feet, the muscles squeeze the deep veins by segments. They act like a roller pump from the foot upwards pressing the blood up to the heart. In healthy veins return flow is prevented by venous valves. On duplex an antegrade flow towards the heart occurs during the **muscular contraction phase** (systole) (Figs. 6.10 and 6.11. See also Sect. 3.2.2).

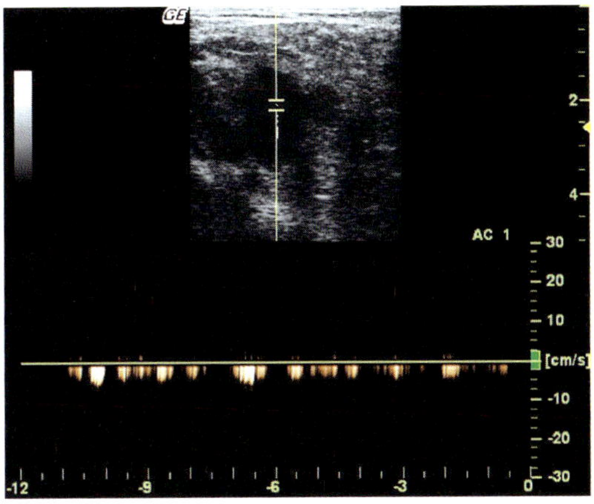

Fig. 6.9 Blood flow (BF) in the right common femoral vein in a motionless standing subject. Continuous slow flow ("vis a tergo") 12 s on display (normal velocity with 4 s on display on online material) Copyright: [Author]

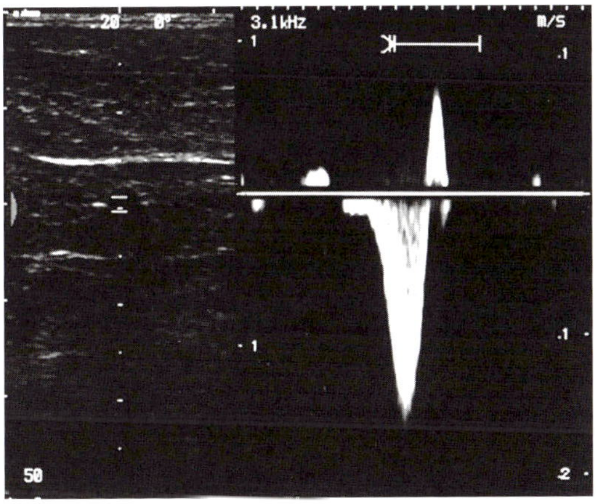

Fig. 6.10 Antegrade flow (downward peak) and a short retrograde flow (upward peak) induced by a manual compression and release manoeuvre of the calf in a competent great saphenous vein. Valve closure limits the duration of retrograde flow Copyright: [Author]

Once the **muscular contraction** is relaxed, the action of pressing the blood towards the heart ceases. If the blood returns down towards the feet under the effects of gravity, a flow towards the probe is recorded. An upwards flow curve or peak is seen on duplex. If the valves close, this flow stops very quickly (Fig. 6.10). If the valves do not close, "reflux" occurs when the blood flows towards the feet for a longer period (Fig. 6.11). This reflux is reported to last 0.5–1 s, depending on the research group (Coleridge-Smith et al. 2006).

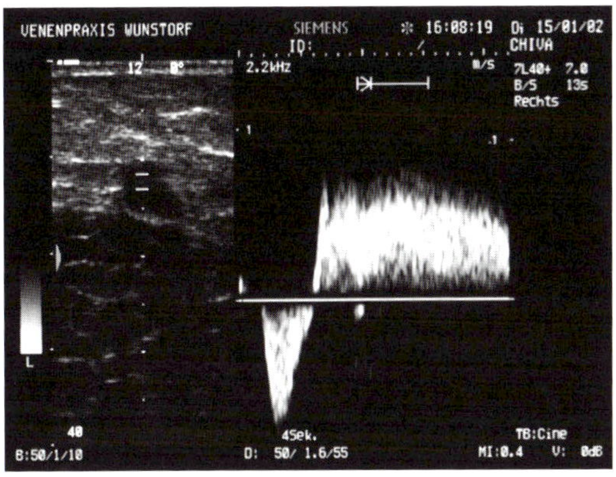

Fig. 6.11 Antegrade flow (downward peak) and retrograde flow (reflux) induced by a manual compression and release manoeuvre of the calf in an incompetent great saphenous vein. Reflux duration is prolonged because the valves are incompetent Copyright: [Author]

A duration of 1 s as a cut-off point between normal and pathological saphenous reflux will avoid a possible grey zone of false-positive findings.

6.3 Valsalva Manoeuvre

In the Valsalva manoeuvre, the patient inhales deeply, holds his/her breath and then creates pressure in the abdomen by contracting the abdominal muscles without exhaling. This **increases the pressure in the inferior vena cava**, which in turn has an effect on hampering the venous return. It is this effect which is measured. The venous system in the legs is a low-pressure system (see also Sect. 3.1.2). If the venous return is challenged by an outflow resistance, like a Valsalva manoeuvre, then antegrade flow ceases. If the venous valves are incompetent, then the blood would run back into the leg veins.

The Valsalva manoeuvre can therefore produce the following results:

- Suspension of blood flow if the valves are competent (Fig. 6.12a).
- Brief reversal of flow due to the blood flowing back out of the abdomen. This reversal of flow causes the valve above of the measurement point to close. By definition, the reverse flow must last longer than 0.5–1 s, to be pathological (Fig. 6.12b).

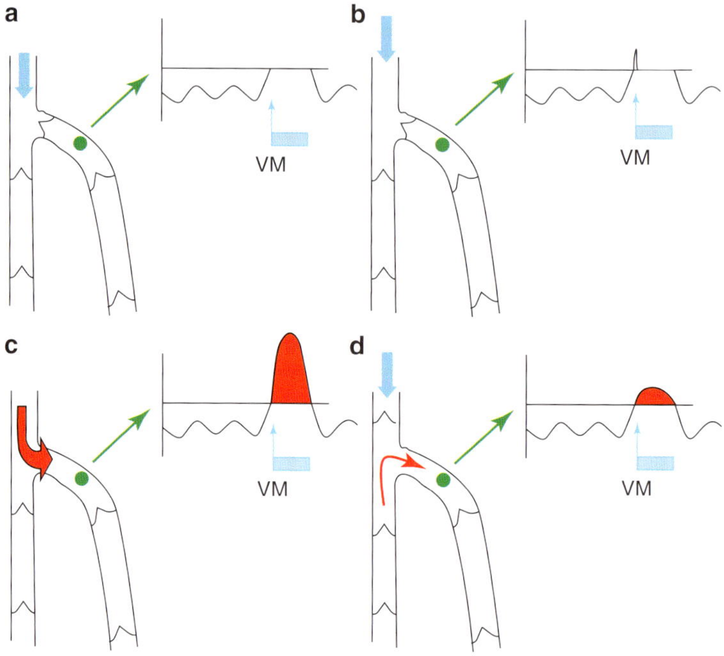

Fig. 6.12 (**a**) *Left*: Diagram of the common femoral vein and its junction with the great saphenous vein. *Right*: Doppler curve of the blood flow in the great saphenous vein measured at the *green point*. The flow curve, modulated by respiration, is interrupted during the Valsalva manoeuvre. The *broad blue arrow* represents the increased intra-abdominal pressure transmitted to the common femoral vein. The *blue rectangle* represents the duration of the Valsalva manoeuvre. (**b**) Flow curve with a competent valve at the saphenofemoral junction. There are no competent valves above the saphenofemoral junction. The *broad blue arrow* represents the pressure in the deep veins. A small amount of blood enters the great saphenous vein causing the valve to close. The measurable reverse flow in the great saphenous vein lasts for less than 1 s. No flow is measured for the remaining time that the patient maintains the pressure. (**c**) Flow curve with an incompetent valve at the junction with the great saphenous vein. There are no incompetent valves above the saphenofemoral junction. The *red arrow* represents the origin and direction of the blood flow, shown in the curve as reverse flow above the zero line (*red area*) (see also Fig. 4.2). (**d**) Flow curve with an incompetent valve at the junction with the great saphenous vein. There is a competent valve above the saphenofemoral junction. The transmitted intra-abdominal pressure causes cessation of flow at the competent iliac valve. There is no retrograde blood flow. The blood flowing up the deep vein from the leg ("vis a tergo") cannot leave the leg. Instead it is diverted into the great saphenous vein, since the valve there is incompetent. The reflux curve in the great saphenous vein is correspondingly weaker. The same situation is found if the small saphenous vein is measured under Valsalva with a competent deep vein system (*VM* Valsalva manoeuvre) Copyright: [Author]

- With incompetent (non-closing) valves, the reverse flow will last as long as the patient exerts pressure (Lattimer et al. 2012) (Fig. 6.12c, d). The flow reversal is clearest if there are no competent valves proximal of the measurement point. In this situation the whole volume of blood from the upper vein segments can reflux back into the segment under examination (Fig. 6.12c). If there is a competent valve proximal of the segment under evaluation, the volume of reverse flow will diminish (Fig. 6.12d). This is frequently the case when the small saphenous vein is assessed using a Valsalva manoeuvre.

Many patients find it difficult to carry out this manoeuvre correctly. Elderly patients often exhale when they exert pressure. However, the Valsalva manoeuvre is only of diagnostic value with deep inhalation and closure of the glottis. Compliance with a Valsalva manoeuvre may be improved by precise instruction like "hold your breath and push your stomach out" or by placing a hand flat on the patient's abdomen and telling him/her to push it away. An apparatus has been developed which can standardise the strength of a Valsalva manoeuvre (Jeanneret et al. 1999). The patient is asked to blow into a tube in order to keep a ball at a certain point. This ensures a constant blowing pressure.

In older ultrasound devices with no simultaneous B scan and PW curve or CW devices (Sect. 1.1.3), the probe may slip from the groin while the patient performs the Valsalva manoeuvre. The absence of a flow signal may mean either that the valve is competent or that the probe has slipped. If antegrade flow is restored when the patient exhales after the Valsalva manoeuvre, then it is likely that the measurement was really taken in the vein. However, the measurement window could also have "slipped back" onto the vein during the relaxation phase. The use of colour duplex or PW with moving B scan is therefore recommended with the Valsalva manoeuvre.

Further research is required to establish whether the Valsalva manoeuvre is a reliable test of the superficial and deep leg veins when the iliac valves in the deep system are healthy and how often it results in a false negative in the popliteal region with competent femoral valves (Basmajian 1952; Moore et al. 2011).

Another limitation of the Valsalva manoeuvre is that it **cannot be repeated indefinitely** without patients suffering symptoms of hyperventilation or syncope.

6.4 Manual Calf Compression and Release

The manual calf compression and release manoeuvre is the commonest induction test used in the evaluation of the leg veins. The calf is compressed with the hand and then relaxed (decompression). The manoeuvre can also be done by compressing the foot or thigh. Calf compression causes antegrade flow in the superficial and deep veins. If venous incompetence is present, there will be reverse flow (retrograde) when the pressure is relaxed (Fig. 6.11).

If the vein segment examined is healthy, there will be no reverse flow on release, or only a very brief reversal. By definition, reflux which lasts for 0.5 or 1 s, depending on the author, is not regarded as pathological. This is because the valve cusps require a retrograde flow to close (Fig. 6.10). Incompetence or reflux is present if a longer duration of retrograde flow occurs.

Certain particularities must be considered when evaluating flow in **perforating veins**.

- Perforating veins connect the superficial and deep veins and pass through a muscle or between two muscles or between the muscle and the tibial border. During muscular contraction the perforating vein is compressed such that generally no flow through it is possible, irrespective of whether or not it is competent.
- In normal gait under physiological conditions during a muscle contraction, the perforators are occluded by the muscle swelling, so that no blood may flow from the deep to the superficial veins via the perforating veins regardless of whether the valves are competent or not. Only dilated perforating veins, which have led to fascial defects, can have an outward flow during muscular contraction.
- During manual compression a relaxed muscle is compressed but remains relaxed. This situation is not physiological. Any flow that arises in the perforating veins may not occur during physiological muscular contraction. This can lead to erroneous conclusions. Under manual compression, a perforating vein which is only dilated to accommodate the increased volume of recirculation re-enters the deep veins (Sect. 3.4) and may have an outward flow. This may never occur under physiological conditions. Consequently, perforating veins in the calf that are dilated secondarily to re-entry flow are frequently diagnosed incorrectly as incompetent (Chap. 9).
- Perforating veins that demonstrate diastolic outward and downward flow into superficial veins are always incompetent, irrespective of a passive or active induction test.
- Isolated perforating vein incompetence without connection to a refluxive superficial vessel does not exist, and assessments should determine the direction of outflow into the superficial and deep veins, for example, out and up or out and down.

The manual compression manoeuvre can be performed any time without the assistance of the patient, and it always causes blood flow in patent veins. In the case of healthy veins, this flow may drain into deep veins and therefore may not reach the thigh or groin. It allows the examiner to evaluate, in a standing patient, whether antegrade flow in deep and superficial veins is followed by reflux.

The **disadvantages** of a manual calf compression and release manoeuvre are:

- The examiner holds the probe in one hand, usually the right, and uses the keyboard of the ultrasound equipment with the left. After setting the measurement programme, he/she must grasp the patient's calf with the left hand whilst the right hand is holding the probe in a steady position. This movement takes a lot of practice and improves with experience or by the assistance of a second person.
- The blood flow that is induced by the compression is not physiological (see above).
- The volume of blood moved is dependent on the size of the examiner's hand, the force applied and the site of compression. If the antegrade flow in the deep veins does not reach the highest incompetent point, reverse flow will never occur in the superficial veins which leads to false-negative results. If digital pressure has obstructed the diseased superficial vein under examination, or the perforating vein that drains it, a particularly long-lasting reverse flow will be found when compression is relaxed. The resulting reflux flow volumes are rather haphazard. The use of a pneumatic calf compression and release device, operated by a foot pedal, can overcome these problems.
- If the measurement point is very close to the foot, it is difficult to apply compression further down, in order to measure an antegrade flow and await the reverse flow.
- If the patient suffers thrombosis or pain in the area to be compressed, manual compression is very distressing.
- Tributaries must often be closed with external digital pressure during the examination in order to simulate the flow conditions expected after therapeutic interruption when applying CHIVA. The examiner then does not have a free hand to perform this additional task.

6.5 Paraná Manoeuvre

In 1997 the Paraná manoeuvre was first published, named after the Argentinean city (Franceschi 1997 in Appendix 2). The examiner shifts the patient's weight slightly forward, e.g. by **pressing on the sacrum** or **pulling on his/her belt**. This causes the patient to tense the soleal muscles involuntarily in order to keep his/her balance. The muscle pump activated in this way causes a powerful antegrade flow in the deep veins.

This manoeuvre is perfectly sufficient to cause a physiological blood flow and can be repeated as often as necessary.

Nevertheless, this manoeuvre has its **disadvantages**:

- The examiner must take his/her left hand off the keyboard.
- The patient also moves which may cause the probe to wander.
- Elderly patients feel insecure because they lose their balance more easily. Patients taking psychotropic drugs may also have difficulties in maintaining their balance. Occasionally, patients may fall over after an enthusiastic manoeuvre.
- Pushing the patient unannounced is not very polite. If the patient is warned he/she tenses in anticipation. This causes erratic flow patterns often making the result inconclusive.
- It is difficult to standardise a push or a pull.

The significant **advantage** of the Paraná manoeuvre is that it corresponds to a physiological process triggering blood flow which simulates walking.

6.6 Wunstorf Manoeuvre

The Wunstorf manoeuvre was proposed in answer to the need for a simple movement, easily executed and not tiring for the patient. Furthermore, it does not require the participation of the examiner. It was inspired by the Paraná manoeuvre. A strong advantage of this manoeuvre is that it does not move the leg whilst remaining a physiological test (Mendoza 2013).

The Wunstorf manoeuvre is performed standing by flexing or extending the forefoot followed

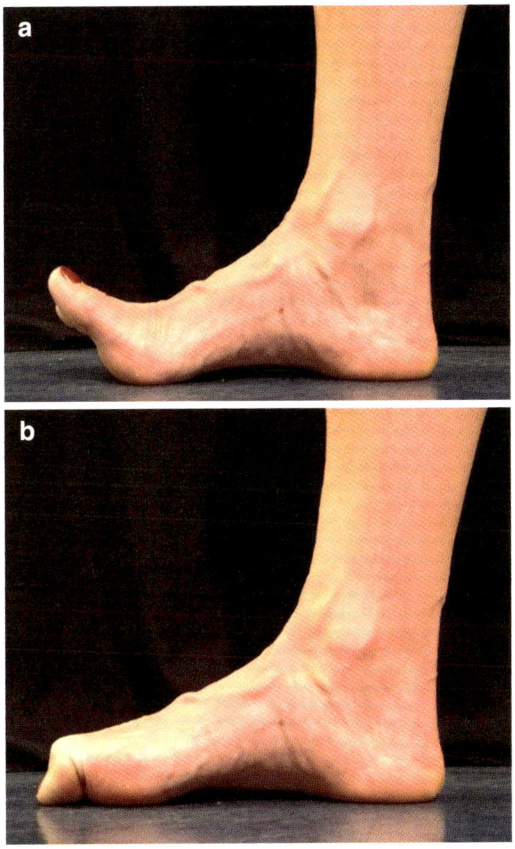

Fig. 6.13 Wunstorf manoeuvre. (**a**) Dorsal flexion of the forefoot. (**b**) Plantar flexion of the forefoot Copyright: [Author]

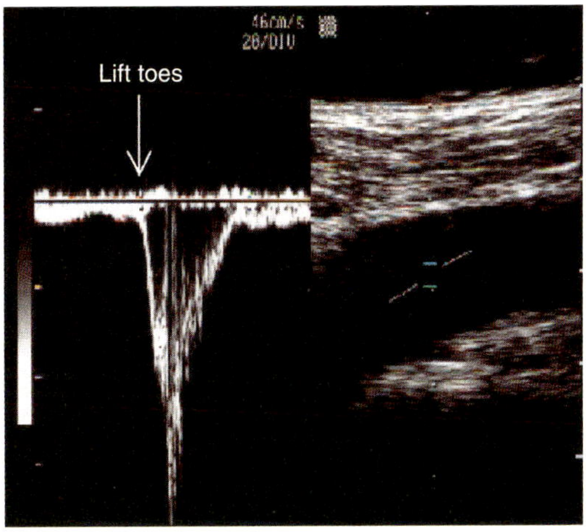

Fig. 6.14 Duplex image of the flow pattern during the contraction and relaxation phase of the Wunstorf manoeuvre. Measured in the common femoral vein of a standing subject. Note the prominent antegrade flow wave but no reflux (Copyright: [Author])

by a relaxation. **Dorsal flexion** involves hyperextension of the toes and raising them off the floor. **Plantar flexion** involves flexing the toes so that they curl under, raising up the metatarsal heads and foot arch. These manoeuvres activate the foot muscle pump (Fig. 6.13).

The effect of dorsal flexion of the foot on venous ejection has been shown by photoplethysmography (Sietzen et al. 1997 in Appendix 2). This study demonstrated that isometric calf muscle contraction by tensing the **Achilles tendon** was more effective at venous emptying than flexing the soleal and gastrocnemius muscles when standing on tiptoe.

In almost all patients, hyperextension of the toes causes an antegrade flow impulse which can be measured up to the common femoral vein (Fig. 6.14). **Antegrade flow** is generally also found in the saphenous trunk veins after the Wunstorf manoeuvre. In patients with deep or superficial vein incompetence, **retrograde flow** (reflux) follows the antegrade flow on relaxation (Fig. 6.15).

The velocity profile induced by the manoeuvre corresponds to the pattern which occurs naturally when walking. It is therefore possible to observe how the venous flow behaves under in vivo conditions.

An interesting aspect of this manoeuvre is that the examiner may determine whether the incompetent re-entry perforating vein is in the calf or higher just from insonating the groin. If the re-entry point is in the calf, reflux will be prevented so long as the patient keeps his/her toes raised. This can be seen from the reflux curve (Figs. 6.15 and 6.16b).

At the beginning of the examination, the patient should be asked to carry out different forms of the Wunstorf manoeuvre while the common femoral vein is observed in PW mode. The patient should be asked to (1) raise the toes, (2) curl the toes and (3) press the soles against the floor and then relax. This allows the examiner to establish which movement is easier for the specific patient and which produces the best augmentation of venous flow.

The Wunstorf manoeuvre is performed by the patient, is painless and does not require assistance

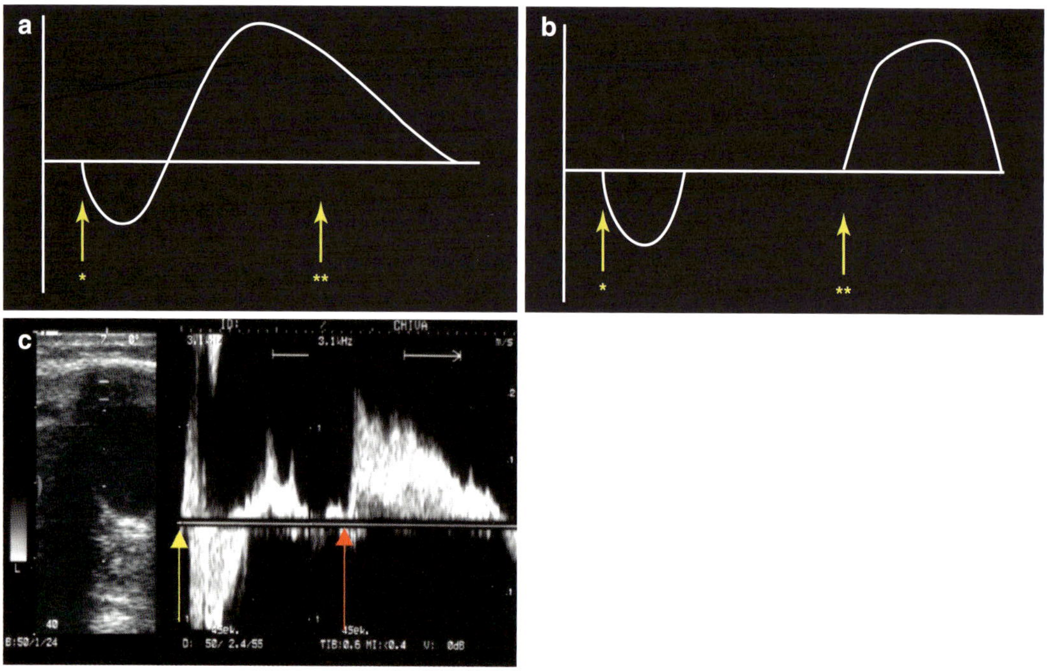

Fig. 6.15 Velocity profile at the saphenofemoral junction (* patient raises toes; ** patient relaxes toes). (**a**) Reflux starts immediately after the antegrade wave and before the relaxation phase. (**b**) If the calf re-entry perforating veins are closed by the manoeuvre, reflux commences only on relaxation. (**c**) Ultrasound image of (b) with flow curve in the great saphenous vein at the saphenofemoral junction (*yellow arrow* toe raising, *red arrow* relaxation) (see also Fig 6.16b) Copyright: [Author]

by the examiner. The movement is not tiring and allows a functional examination of all vein segments.

The Wunstorf manoeuvre failed to cause flow in the groin in only 6 out of 1,230 patients between April 1997 and December 1999 (Mendoza and Berger 2001 in Appendix 2). All six failures occurred in patients suffering from gross leg oedema. The muscle pump may not be functioning adequately in these patients which may have been responsible, in part, for their oedema (see also Sect. 6.8).

6.7 Comparison of Manual Compression and Wunstorf Manoeuvres

These two manoeuvres may induce different patterns of reflux in the same vein with different PW curves. Figure 6.16 shows an example of a standing patient with an incompetent saphenofemoral junction and reflux above and below the knee, examined in the thigh. Evaluation of the two curves shows clearly that the vein is diseased and refluxive but shows different flow and reflux patterns. However, in a healthy great saphenous vein, the Wunstorf manoeuvre may induce little or no antegrade flow since the venous return is usually via the calf perforating veins into the deep veins (Fig. 6.17). The lack of antegrade flow is also true following the manual calf compression and release manoeuvre.

6.8 Elevation-Dependency Manoeuvre

Reflux rate and duration depend on several factors. These include the volume of blood in retrograde flow and the capacity of the venous reservoir and its current level of filling. Venous

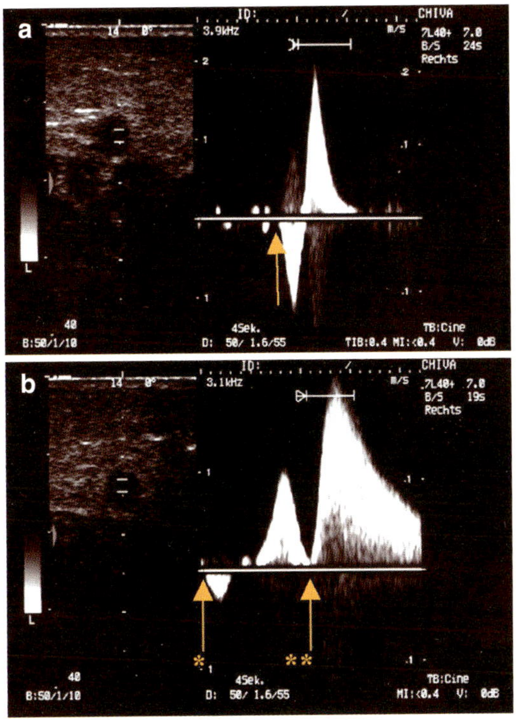

Fig. 6.16 Flow curves with gross incompetence of the great saphenous vein above and below the knee, measured in the mid-thigh: (**a**) manual compression (*arrow*: calf compression). (**b**) Wunstorf manoeuvre (* raise toes, ** relax toes) Copyright: [Author]

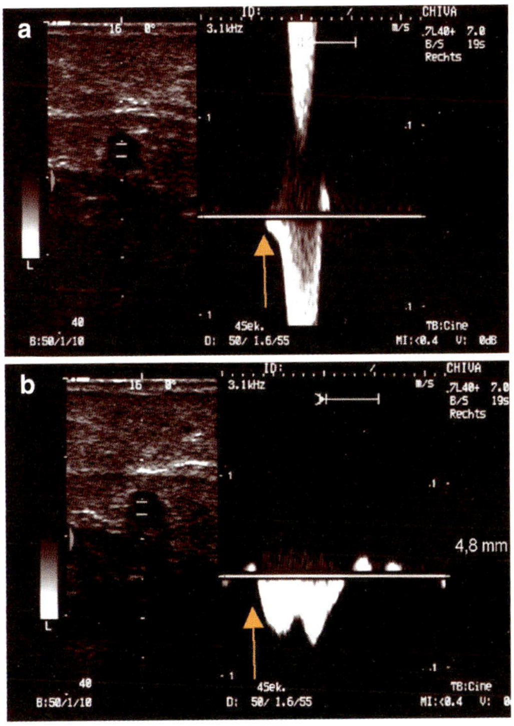

Fig. 6.17 Flow curves with competence of the great saphenous vein, measured in the mid-thigh: (**a**) manual compression (*arrow*: start of compression). (**b**) Wunstorf manoeuvre (*arrow*: raise toes) Copyright: [Author]

compliance and the diameter of the re-entry perforating vein are also significant factors (Sect. 3.2.3). **Poorly drained systems** remain full on standing with no major fluctuations in volume irrespective of walking or other muscle-pump activity. When the patient has been standing for some time, the venous system and the varicose veins are relatively well filled. The calibre of the re-entry perforating veins then has a considerable effect on the flow curve. Small re-entry perforating veins hamper flow into the deep system.

In **well-drained systems**, the diameter of the perforating veins is large. They do not hinder flow. The PW flow curve has a high velocity, and the reflux ends relatively quickly after 2–4 s. However, if the perforating veins are of a smaller calibre than the varicose veins, the flow into them will be slow. In this situation reflux will be small in volume and prolonged on the PW curve (Fig. 6.18). Occasionally, there is no signal visible on colour duplex.

When these patients are standing, a slow, long-lasting retrograde flow is found in the first few minutes of the examination. Subsequently there appears to be no flow in the vein, despite any provocation manoeuvres. This situation sometimes only arises after a few minutes. It is surprising when a vein, which has just been found to be refluxive, has no reflux on a delayed examination with **no measurable flow**. The likely explanation is that the venous reservoir is now full and there is no further capacity for reflux. The veins may appear also to be filled with erythrocytes and can scarcely be distinguished from their surroundings (Fig. 6.19). In this situation it is recommended to get the **patient to lie down** and raise his/her legs for 20–30 s to allow them to drain and then get his/her to stand up again. The veins can then be examined using this elevation-dependency

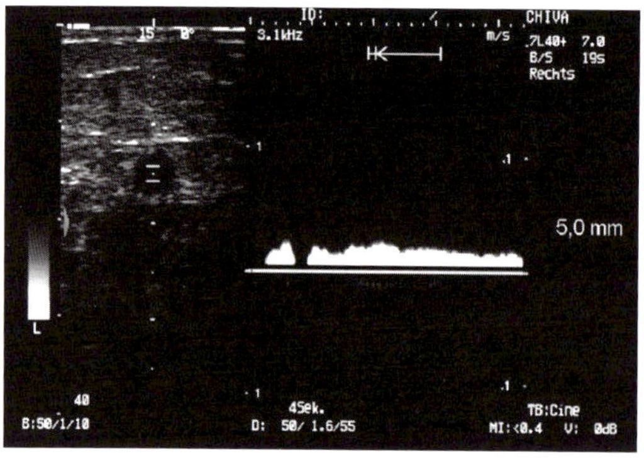

Fig. 6.18 Slow, long-lasting reflux in a poorly drained system Copyright: [Author]

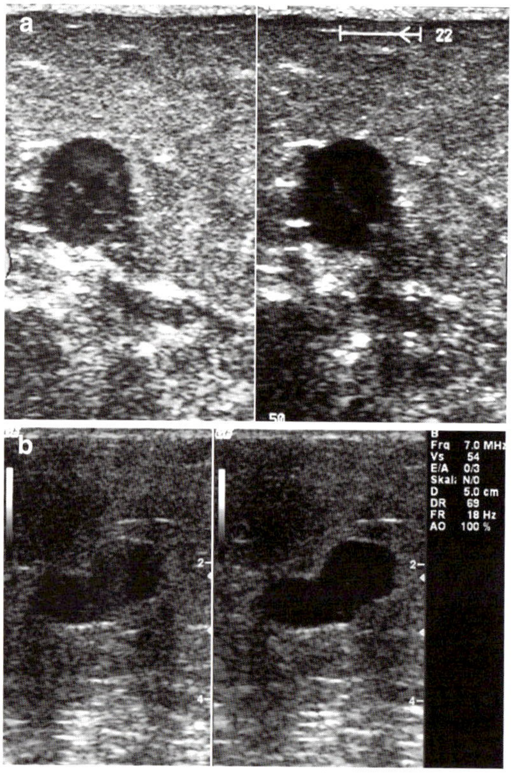

Fig. 6.19 (**a**) Transverse view through the thigh of an obese patient demonstrating a tributary of the great saphenous vein with septa as a consequence of thrombosis, *left* after standing without moving for a long period, *right* after a provocation manoeuvre. In the *left-hand image*, one has the feeling that the erythrocytes are visible and almost stationary. In the *right-hand image*, they have been "flushed away". (**b**) Junction between the great saphenous vein and a tributary; *left* after a long period of standing, *right* after the Wunstorf manoeuvre. Note the improved clarity of the lumen after "flushing" Copyright: [Author]

Table 6.1 Biological aspects of the different provocation manoeuvres

Manoeuvre	Biological advantages	Biological disadvantages
Valsalva	Partly physiological	Only relates to coughing, lifting weight and straining Does not work reliably with competent deep veins
Manual compression	None	Does not correspond to any physiological situation. Misleading in diagnosing perforating veins
Paraná	Physiological	None
Wunstorf	Physiological	None
Elevation dependency	Physiological	Patients may sometimes feel dizzy after standing up

manoeuvre. This procedure can be repeated until all the segments of the vein system have been thoroughly examined. Air-plethysmography may provide additional information on venous filling. Venous reflux time on duplex has been shown to have an excellent and highly significant correlation with venous filling time following an elevation-dependency manoeuvre (Lattimer et al. 2014).

Summary of the different provocation manoeuvres presented above Tables 6.1 and 6.2.

6.9 Tapping Manoeuvre

It is sometimes difficult to determine which vein or perforator is filling a refluxive tributary. In these cases it is helpful to hold the probe in colour mode, or more effectively in PW, over the visible vein, and to tap the leg lightly, further up the leg, in the region in which a perforating vein or incompetent junction is suspected. The finger is then moved over the leg until a signal synchronous with the tapping appears in the vein under examination (Mendoza 2002 in Appendix 2).

It is useful to demonstrate to the patient that the visible veins in the calf are filled from the great saphenous vein in the groin because patients often do not believe that treatment in the groin region is really necessary to treat varicose veins

Table 6.2 Technical aspects of the different provocation manoeuvres

Manoeuvre	Technical advantages	Technical disadvantages
Valsalva	Retrograde flow normally obvious with valve incompetence	Intelligent cooperation by the patient is required. It cannot be repeated indefinitely
Manual compression	Can be repeated indefinitely	Danger of probe drift or a second examiner is needed for the compression. Flow dependent on the examiner's strength and hand size
Paraná	Repeatable	Impolite, danger of probe drift. Elderly patients may lose their balance
Wunstorf	Repeatable, easy to carry out	None
Elevation dependency	Repeatable, sometimes the only way to measure flow in a vein	Very time-consuming

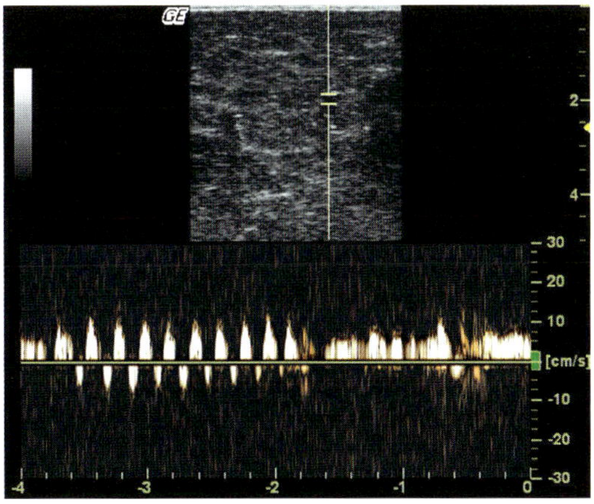

Fig. 6.20 Examination of the refluxive great saphenous vein in the thigh in PW mode demonstrating the tapping manoeuvre. The finger is tapping a tributary in the calf. The manoeuvre is shown in colour duplex in the film (online material) Copyright: [Author]

visible only in the calf. The same procedure can also be performed in reverse by tapping the vein in the calf and holding the probe over the great saphenous vein immediately below the groin (Fig. 6.20). It is more impressive for the patient to see the manoeuvre in PW mode, since he/she can also hear the blood flow.

6.10 Sourcing

A special form of the tapping manoeuvre is called sourcing (Obermayer and Garzon 2010). It is used for examining the sources of reflux in venous ulcers. The refluxive vein(s) in the leg are scanned in colour duplex mode, while the ulcer is continuously compressed and decompressed with one hand (film on online material). This allows the vessel responsible for the ulceration to be determined and treated selectively.

6.11 Practical Procedure

Every examiner will establish his/her own examination procedure; however, it is important to follow a **routine**, which includes all the necessary stages, both for the examination of all vein segments (Sect. 5.3.2) and for the provocation manoeuvres.

A proposal is to start the examination in the **groin** of the standing patient, using PW mode to examine the blood flow in the common femoral vein with the Valsalva manoeuvre, manual compression of the calf and the different forms of the Wunstorf manoeuvre. The manoeuvre which produces the best flow curve will be used in the subsequent examination.

In some patients the saphenofemoral region is competent but reflux may occur after the Valsalva manoeuvre. If reflux is found only under the Valsalva manoeuvre and not under any of the calf stimulation manoeuvres, the patient will only have reflux when there is pressure from the abdominal compartment. This has usually no clinical consequence and does not need treatment; however, it should be observed. If the converse is true, treatment is usually required.

Other vein segments can be examined likewise with whichever manoeuvre produces the best flow curve. In very rare cases, the Wunstorf manoeuvre or manual compression of the calf is not sufficient to generate a flow which can be recorded in the groin (Sects. 6.7 and 6.9) or reflux in all incompetent vein segments. In these patients it is necessary to resort to using the elevation-dependency manoeuvre. Although the examination is considerably lengthened by this provocation test, it may be the only way of achieving a result in such cases.

References

Basmajian JV (1952) The distribution of valves in the femoral, external iliac, and common iliac veins and their relationship to varicose veins. Surg Gynecol Obstet 95(5):537–542

Coleridge-Smith P, Labropoulos N, Partsch H, Myers K, Nicolaides A, Cavezzi A (2006) Duplex ultrasound investigation of the veins in chronic venous disease of the lower limbs-UIP consensus document, part I. Basic principles. Eur J Vasc Endovasc Surg 31:1–10

Jeanneret C, Labs KH, Aschwanden M, Bollinger A et al (1999) Physiological reflux and venous diameter change in the proximal lower limb veins during a standardised Valsalva manoeuvre. Eur J Vasc Endovasc Surg 17:398–403

Lattimer CR, Kalodiki E, Azzam M, Geroulakos G (2012) Volume displacements from an incompetent great saphenous vein during a standardised Valsalva manoeuvre. Acta Phlebologica 13(1):25–30

Lattimer CR, Azzam M, Kalodiki E, Geroulakos G (2014) Venous filling time on air-plethysmography correlates highly with great saphenous vein reflux time on duplex. Phlebology 29(2):90–97

Mendoza E (2013) Provocation manoeuvres fort he duplex ultrasound diagnosis for varicose veins Phlebologie Vol. 42(6):357–362

Moore HM, Gohel M, Davies AH (2011) Number and location of venous valves within the popliteal and femoral veins: a review of the literature. J Anat 219(4):439–443

Obermayer A, Garzon K (2010) Sourcing of superficial Reflux in venous leg ulcers using duplex ultrasound. J Vasc Surg 52:1255–1261

Examination of the Great Saphenous Vein

7

Erika Mendoza, Nick Morrison, and Christopher R. Lattimer

Chapter Summary
The great saphenous vein is by far the most frequently examined and treated vein of all the superficial veins. Furthermore, the majority of venous studies are performed on the great saphenous vein. Duplex ultrasound makes it possible to assess the vein very accurately before and after intervention.

Assessing the great saphenous vein with duplex ultrasound is a relatively new concept with some surgeons still performing surgery without considering the need of a preoperative scan. The first international consensus document appeared in 2006 (Coleridge-Smith et al. 2006) with the object of producing a standard ultrasound protocol which would encourage consistency between treatments, doctors and hospitals. This development was welcomed as it was a first step towards standardisation. Since then there have been several recommendations from various international societies in an attempt to improve the examination of the great saphenous vein and the rest of the superficial venous network.

E. Mendoza, MD, PhD (✉)
Venenpraxis Wunstorf,
Speckenstraße 10, 31515 Wunstorf, Germany
e-mail: erika.mendoza@t-online.de

N. Morrison, MD
Morrison Vein Institute,
Suite 223, 8575 E. Princess Dr., Scottsdale, AZ, USA

C.R. Lattimer, MD, PhD
Department of Vascular Surgery,
Josef Pflug Vascular Laboratory,
Ealing Hospital and Imperial College, London, UK

7.1 Examination Procedure

Every examiner should establish an examination procedure which develops into a well-oiled **routine**. In this way the entire great saphenous vein can be covered including its tributaries and perforating veins so there is less chance of any vein segments being overlooked.

A good place to begin is in the **groin** with the subject standing. Here the anatomy of the saphenofemoral junction and its tributaries can be examined in B scan. The competency of the veins in this region should be tested with the Valsalva manoeuvre and at least one other provocation manoeuvre. Duplex mode should be used for this and it is advisable to use colour duplex.

The whole **course** of the great saphenous vein down the leg should be viewed once in B scan to detect any sudden calibre changes and dilated perforating veins or tributaries. Special attention must be paid to the region of the perforating veins of the adductor canal (formerly Dodd and Hunter) and the paratibial perforating veins (formerly Boyd), as well as the junctions with the anterior and posterior arch veins below the knee. Duplex mode must be switched on repeatedly when running

E. Mendoza et al. (eds.), *Duplex Ultrasound of Superficial Leg Veins*,
DOI 10.1007/978-3-642-40731-4_7, © Springer-Verlag Berlin Heidelberg 2014

over the course of the great saphenous vein. It is more effective to use PW than colour mode for this because changes in the velocity profile are more obvious (Sect. 7.5.2). Tributaries and perforating veins are better assessed in colour on this first pass. However, they must not divert the examination from the saphenous trunk.

7.2 Objectives of the Examination

The following questions should be answered at the conclusion of the examination:

- Is there reflux through the saphenofemoral junction?
- Is the terminal valve competent?
- Is the preterminal valve competent?
- Are the superficial inguinal veins competent?
- Is there any anomaly of the saphenofemoral junction?
- Is an aneurysm present?
- Is the great saphenous vein visible in the fascial compartment throughout its length?
- Is the whole course of the vein interfascial?
- What is its diameter at the standardised point 10 cm below the junction?
- Are there any acute changes in saphenous calibre?
- Is its course typical in relation to topographical anatomy?
- Is its course more lateral than usual at the groin or thigh?
- Is there a duplication present over part of its course?
- Is there an aplastic or hypoplastic segment along its course?
- Is there evidence of thrombosis or post-phlebitic changes?
- Is there reflux in the great saphenous vein?
- Is this reflux well or poorly drained?
- How many saphenous segments are refluxive?
- Where is the proximal reflux source?
- Are any dilated tributaries or perforating veins apparent in the course of the great saphenous vein?
- Are they involved in the recirculation circuit?
- Does the reflux leave the great saphenous vein by a tributary or a perforating vein?
- What is the Hach Class (in the areas it may be used)?
- Which shunt type is present as defined in the CHIVA strategy?
- How does the calibre and course of the great saphenous vein behave distal to the end of the reflux?
- Are there any pathological soft tissue changes surrounding the great saphenous vein?
- Is the flow in the dilated great saphenous vein antegrade, because it is serving as drainage path for obstructed deep veins (secondary varicose veins, Chap. 15)?
- Has all or part of the saphenous vein been treated?

7.3 The Saphenofemoral Junction

In the groin the anterior (formerly medialis) and posterior (formerly lateralis) accessory saphenous veins unite with the great saphenous vein to join the common femoral vein. Since these veins will be mentioned very frequently in this chapter, the former nomenclature will be omitted. Likewise the confluence of the great saphenous vein will be referred to as the saphenofemoral junction (SFJ), as recommended in the consensus document (Coleridge-Smith et al. 2006). The region of the proximal great saphenous vein and the confluence of superficial inguinal veins (sometimes called the "crosse") will be described as the saphenofemoral region.

The saphenofemoral junction is examined with the ultrasound probe lightly pressed against the groin of the standing subject (Fig. 7.1). The anatomy of the saphenofemoral region is examined first in B scan. Next, the effectiveness of the various provocation manoeuvres can be assessed in augmenting antegrade flow and inducing reflux in the superficial and deep veins (Sect. 6.11). Then, the saphenofemoral junction and the anatomy of the confluence of superficial inguinal veins are examined. Flow through the saphenofemoral junction, the superficial tributaries and the great saphenous vein is tested. Particular attention is made in the assessment of valve competence. The terminal valve controls the flow between the common femoral vein and the great saphenous vein and is present in 91 % of cases (Mühlberger et al. 2009). The preterminal valve affects the flow between the saphenofemoral junction, the superficial tributaries and the distal great saphenous vein.

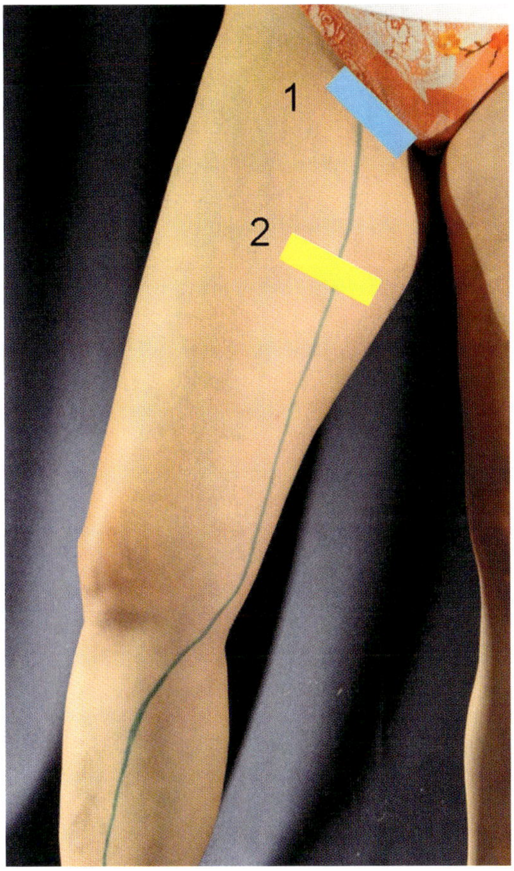

Fig. 7.1 Position of the probe during the examination of the great saphenous vein in a standing subject. *1* Examination of the saphenofemoral junction, *2* measurement of the saphenous vein diameter in the thigh Copyright: [Author]

The superficial tributaries at the saphenofemoral junction (Sect. 2.4) have many anatomical variants which are important to evaluate using duplex ultrasound because this may influence the treatment approach (Fig. 7.2; see also Sect. 7.3.6). It is helpful during surgery if the surgeon knows how many tributaries are expected and how they connect. Occasionally it is difficult to define whether the surgically exposed vein is the junction of the anterior accessory saphenous vein with the great saphenous vein or the true junction of the great saphenous vein with the common femoral vein. This situation is easily avoided if the operator knows exactly how many tributaries join the great saphenous vein at the saphenofemoral junction and their distribution towards lateral and medial. Furthermore, the division of the epigastric and superficial circumflex iliac veins into two or three branches which join the anterior accessory saphenous vein can likewise make this junction look like the saphenofemoral junction, thus adding to the confusion (Fig. 7.2**C**, **D**, **I**, **L**, **M**, **O**, **P** and Sect. 7.3.1).

The veins of the confluence of the superficial inguinal veins are:

- Anterior accessory saphenous vein from distal and lateral (Sects. 7.3.7 and 10.4)
- Superficial circumflex iliac vein from proximal and lateral (Sect. 7.3.5)
- Superficial epigastric vein from proximal, confluence quite variable (Sect. 7.3.5)
- Deep and superficial external pudendal veins from medial (Sect. 7.3.4)
- Posterior accessory saphenous vein from distal and medial (Sect. 10.5)

Some of these veins may not be present. Many of them, especially the proximally arising superficial circumflex iliac and the superficial epigastric veins, have several sub-tributaries which may join to form a single vein at the saphenofemoral junction or enter the confluence of superficial inguinal veins separately. The same is true of the medially arising superficial and deep external pudendal veins which often join the common femoral or the posterior accessory saphenous vein directly. Furthermore, all or any of these veins may join one another before they enter the confluence of the superficial inguinal veins.

Lanz and Wachsmuth have systematised all the **possible anatomical variations of the confluence** (Fig. 7.2). They start with the confluence of all the superficial inguinal veins into the common femoral vein (**A**) and then describe the different variants for the confluence of the individual vessels: **B**–**E** for the anterior accessory saphenous vein; **F**–**G** for the posterior accessory saphenous vein; **H**–**I** for the superficial and deep external pudendal veins, respectively; **J**–**N** for the superficial epigastric vein; and **O**–**R** for the superficial circumflex iliac vein.

7.3.1 Normal Findings

The great saphenous vein joins the common femoral vein from the anteromedial aspect. As a rule a competent great saphenous vein is not very large, but it is always visible in B scan (Fig. 7.3).

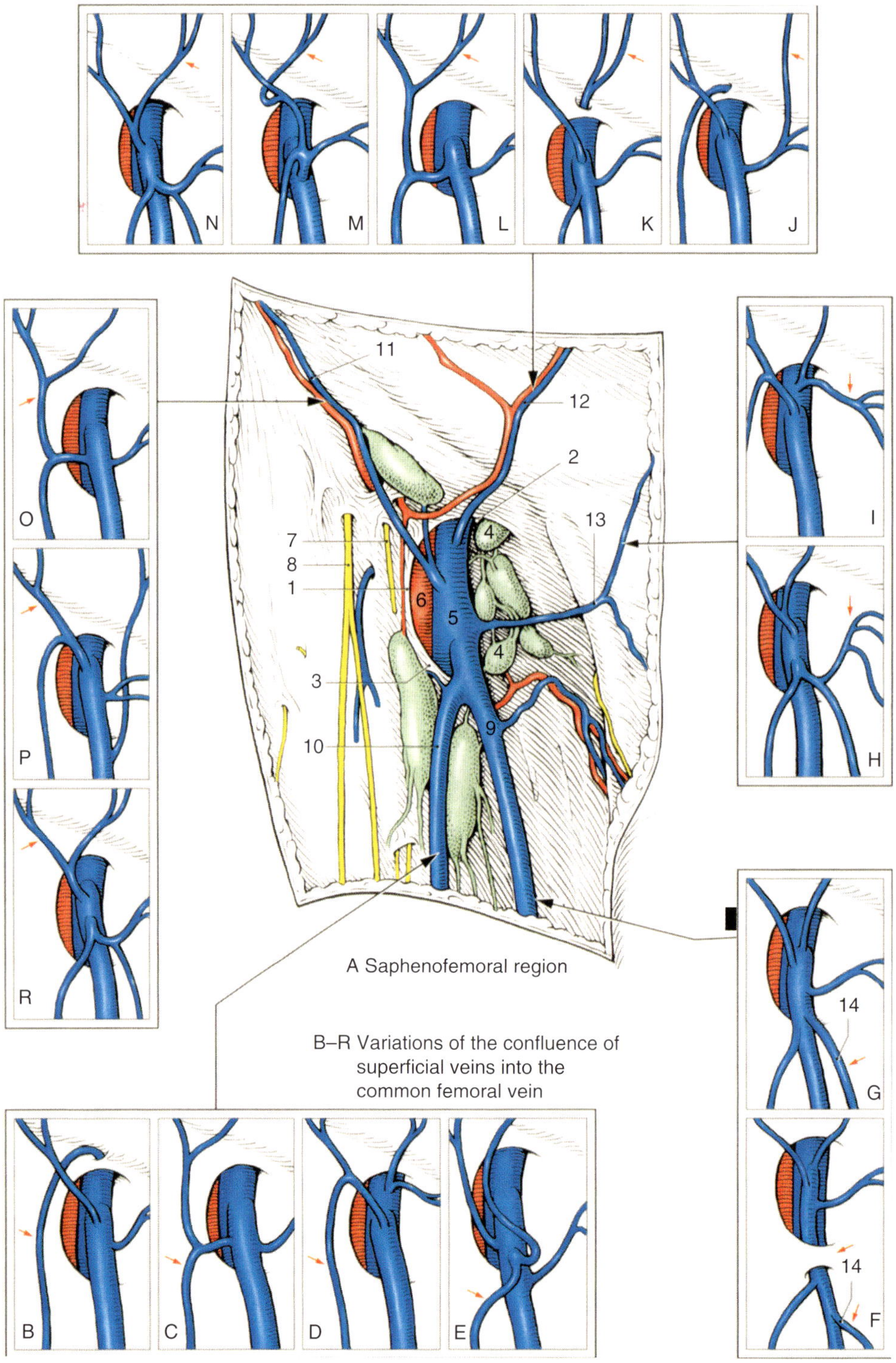

Fig. 7.2 Views of the different confluence variations of the great saphenous vein, its tributaries and the confluence of the superficial inguinal veins with the common femoral vein according to Lanz and Wachsmuth. *1* Falciform margin of the saphenous hiatus with *2* upper cornu and *3* lower cornu. *4* Deep inguinal lymph nodes. *5* Common femoral vein. *6* Common femoral artery. *7* Femoral branch of the genitofemoral nerve, *8* Cutaneous branch of the femoral nerve. *9* Great saphenous vein. *10* Anterior accessory saphenous vein. *11* Superficial circumflex iliac vein. *12* Superficial epigastric vein. *13* Superficial external pudendal vein. *14* Posterior accessory saphenous vein (legends for letters – see text) (From Platzer (2005); by kind permission of Thieme-Verlag) Copyright: Thieme

However, the calibres even of competent veins may differ widely. Some indication of normal vein size may be deduced from the subject's body size and the diameter of the rest of his veins, for example, those visible on the back of the hand. On average, the diameter of the great saphenous vein in the saphenofemoral region in a healthy subject who has been standing for a few minutes is 7.5 mm (±1.8 mm), with a range of 3.5–11.0 mm (Mendoza et al. 2013). Fifteen centimetres below the saphenofemoral junction, it becomes smaller and more uniform in size. The great saphenous vein can be overlooked occasionally in a supine subject.

It is common to see the familiar image of a narrow calibre great saphenous vein terminating in a **broad mouth** at the saphenofemoral junction (Fig. 7.3d). Here the valve leaflets are frequently observed moving with changes in the blood flow (see also Figs. 7.6 and 7.7).

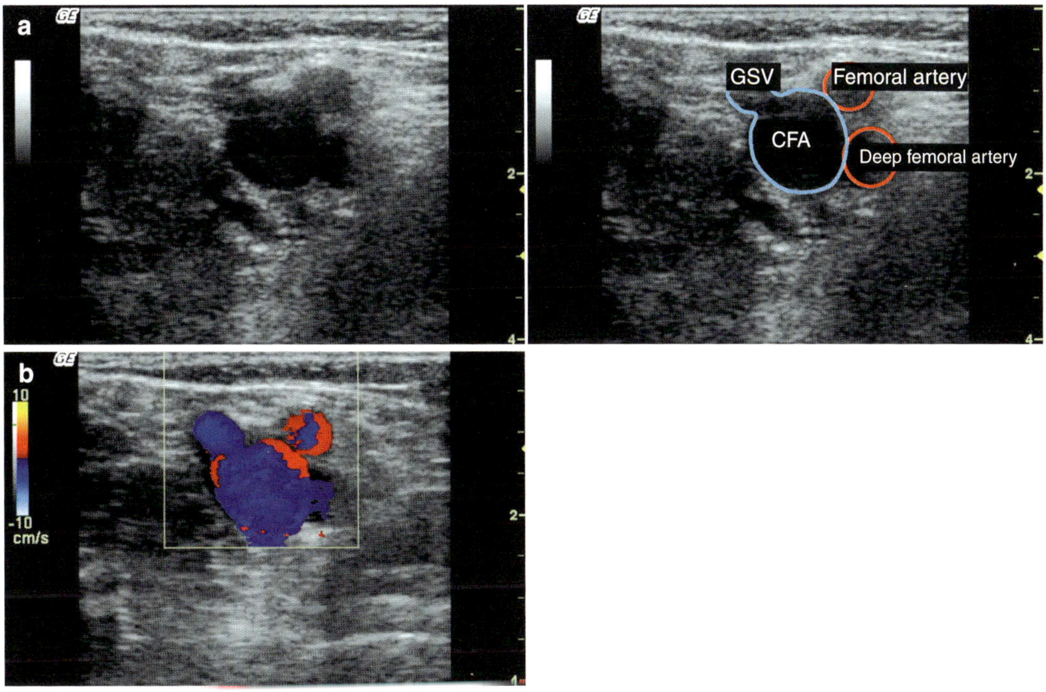

Fig. 7.3 Normal findings of the saphenofemoral junction. (**a**) B scan in transverse view through the left groin of a thin subject standing. Note that the entire venous network, including the common femoral vein is no more than 2 cm below the surface (scale on the right). The saphenofemoral junction is outlined and seen clearer on the moving image (online material). (**b**) Colour duplex ultrasound of the same subject during muscular systole demonstrating antegrade flow in the common femoral vein and saphenofemoral junction. (**c**) B scan of the same subject 1 cm further down where the saphenofemoral junction has separated into a small calibre great saphenous vein and anterior accessory saphenous vein (*AASV*). (**d**) Transverse view through the right groin in a standing subject with small calibre veins. During muscular systole, the blue signal in all the superficial veins represents antegrade flow as they join into the saphenofemoral junction. In this subject the pudendal vein curves anteriorly into the back of the great saphenous vein. For this reason the direction of antegrade flow towards the confluence of superficial inguinal veins is towards the probe and therefore appears *red*. Investigating flow in muscular diastole is important for distinguishing between a normal finding and pathological reflux. If antegrade flow continues in the pudendal vein 1 s after the end of muscular systole, it is pathological. The mouth at the saphenofemoral junction is clearly visible (*yellow arrows*) (*Art.* common femoral artery). (**e**) Transverse view through the right groin with a common drainage of the great saphenous and anterior accessory saphenous veins into the saphenofemoral junction (*SFJ*). There is a separate drainage of the pudendal vein directly into the common femoral vein. The superficial external pudendal artery (*) is visible crossing the saphenofemoral junction. This is a common finding (online material). (**f**) Transverse view through the right groin demonstrating a wide saphenofemoral junction in a big man. Despite its relatively large calibre, the junction was competent (*SFA* superficial femoral artery, *DFA* deep femoral artery, *CFV* common femoral vein). (**g**) Same position as in (f) with colour duplex in muscular systole and antegrade flow (*blue*). In diastole there was no reflux in the saphenous trunk or through the saphenofemoral junction Copyright: [Author]

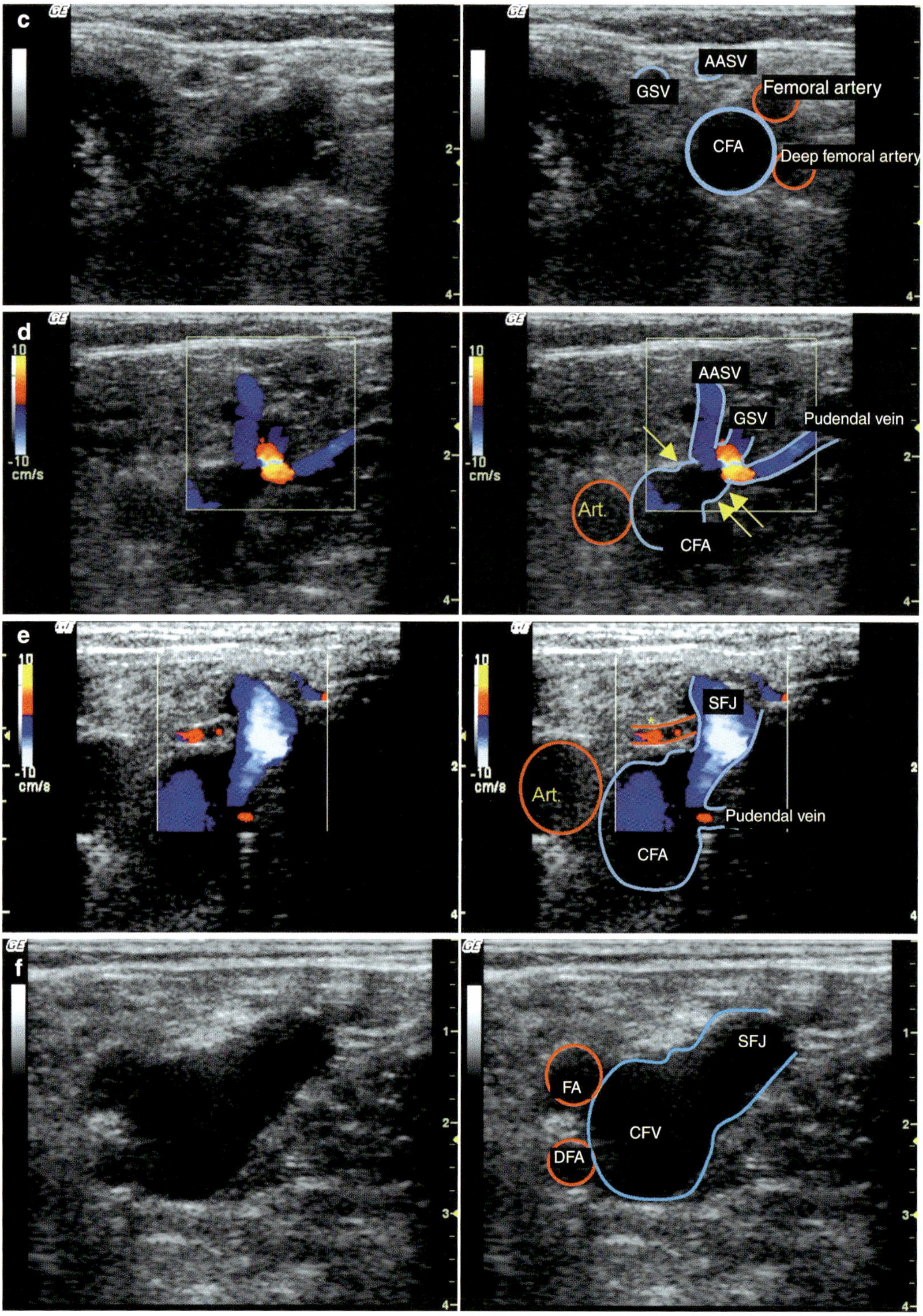

Fig. 7.3 (continued)

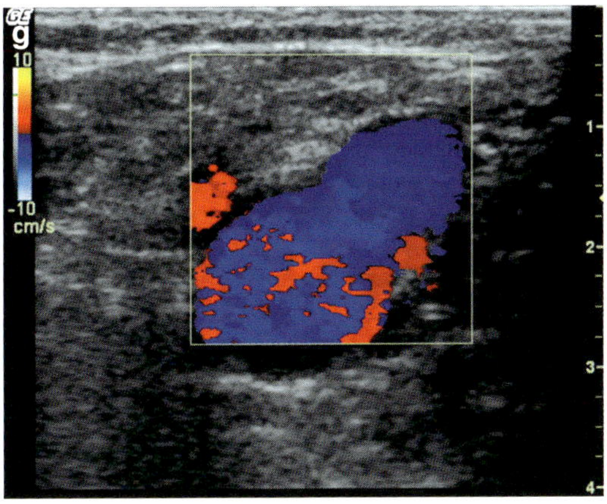

Fig. 7.3 (continued)

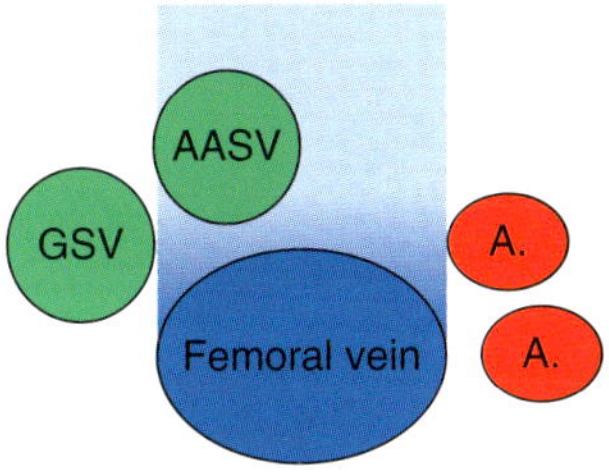

Fig. 7.4 Normal relations of the great saphenous and anterior accessory saphenous veins. This is a transverse view through the left groin of a standing subject slightly below the saphenofemoral junction. The anterior accessory saphenous vein (*AASV*) lies vertically above the femoral vein and the great saphenous vein lies medially ("alignment" sign) Copyright: [Author]

The **anterior accessory saphenous vein** joins the great saphenous vein from the side at an acute angle in the saphenofemoral region. In transverse view it is seen lateral to the great saphenous vein and vertically above the femoral vein (Fig. 7.3c–e). It is not always visible in B scan. A useful rule is if an imaginary line is drawn along a tangent to the medial edge of the common femoral vein, the great saphenous vein lies medial and the anterior accessory saphenous vein lies lateral (Fig. 7.4) (for anatomical variations, see also Sect. 7.3.2; for reflux in the anterior accessory saphenous vein Sect. 7.3.7; and for its anatomical course Sect. 10.4).

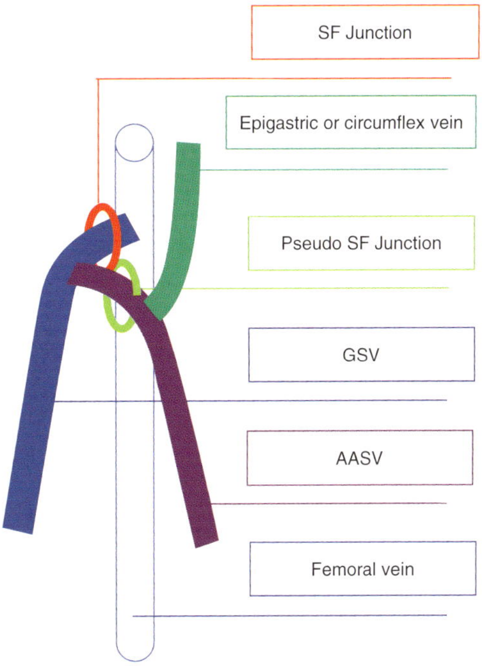

Fig. 7.5 Diagram of a "pseudo" saphenofemoral junction formed by the confluence of a lateral superficial inguinal tributary like the superficial circumflex iliac vein (*SCIV*) or epigastric vein (EV) and the anterior accessory saphenous vein (*AASV*) with the great saphenous vein (*GSV*) (*green circle*). The true saphenofemoral junction lies deeper (*red circle*) Copyright: [Author]

The **superficial circumflex iliac vein** may join either the great saphenous vein or the anterior accessory saphenous vein. It very rarely joins the common femoral vein directly. Using ultrasound it generally appears as a cranial extension of the great saphenous or the anterior accessory saphenous vein. Like the **epigastric vein**, it may consist of several branches which either unite or join the confluence separately. If one of these veins joins the anterior accessory saphenous vein from a cranial direction, then this junction may be mistaken for the saphenofemoral junction (Fig. 7.5). This mistaken identification is a source of error in surgery which may result in an inappropriate ligation (for reflux from these vessels, see also Sect. 7.3.5).

In B scan a **valve** cannot always be seen at the saphenofemoral junction. Although this is said to occur in up to 50 % of subjects, the use of more modern ultrasound machines has increased visualisation of the terminal valve to 91 %. In transverse view the valve leaflets can be seen moving during the various provocation manoeuvres (Fig. 7.6). In longitudinal view the valves can be seen in different positions. The terminal valve lies directly in the saphenofemoral region (Fig. 7.7a–c), and the preterminal valve lies below the confluence of superficial inguinal veins (Fig. 7.8), although the anterior accessory saphenous vein may also join distal to this valve. Valve movement can be detected in B scan. Rigid valve cusps indicate disease; however, flexible cusps do not exclude reflux. PW mode or colour duplex must be used to test for the presence of reflux.

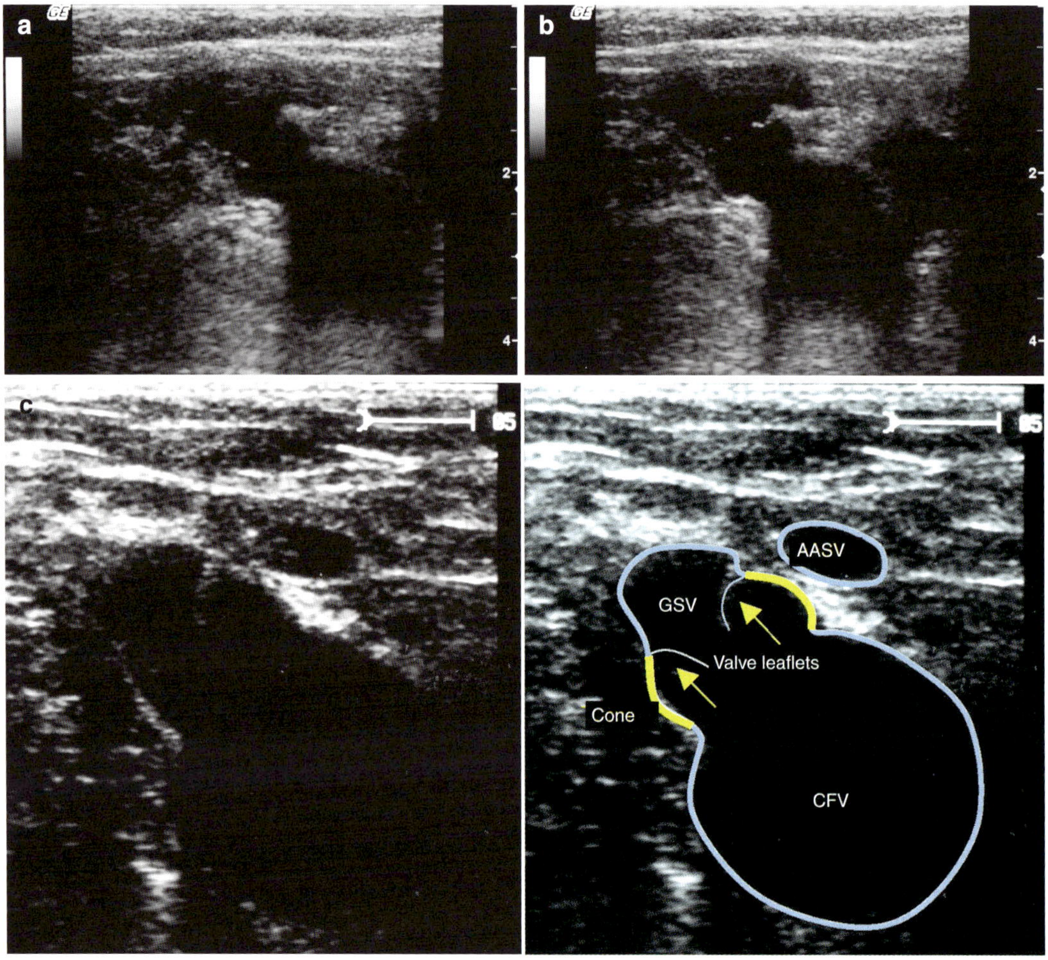

Fig. 7.6 Transverse image of the terminal valve at the saphenofemoral junction. (**a**) During muscular systole the valve leaflets are visible as white lines (*arrow*). (**b**) During muscular diastole the valve curves out towards the great saphenous vein when the junction is competent (muscular systole/diastole cycle on online material). (**c**) The valve (*yellow arrows*) opens during muscular systole causing movements in the mouth of the saphenofemoral junction (*yellow contour*). The anterior accessory saphenous vein (*AASV*) is also seen just before it terminates into the great saphenous vein (*GSV*). (**d**) Same groin in muscular diastole where the returning blood tries to re-enter the great saphenous vein. Here the valve leaflets (*arrowed*) are seen closing back towards the great saphenous vein. (**e**) Transverse view through the right groin this time with complete incompetence of the great saphenous vein. During muscular systole the valve cusps point towards the deep vein. (**f**) During muscular diastole in (e), the valves close back towards the great saphenous vein. It is impossible to establish whether reflux exists from the behaviour of the valves in a static B scan alone. In the film (online material), it is more obvious from the movement of the visualised blood that this valve is incompetent Copyright: [Author]

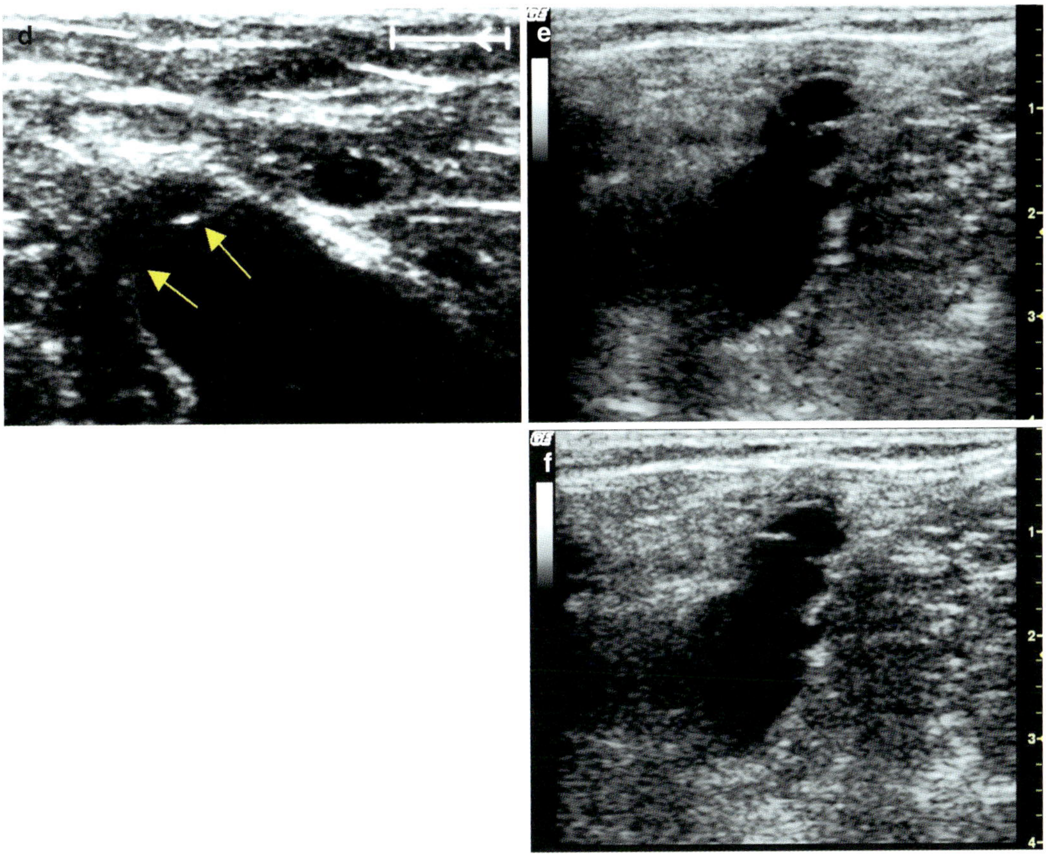

Fig. 7.6 (continued)

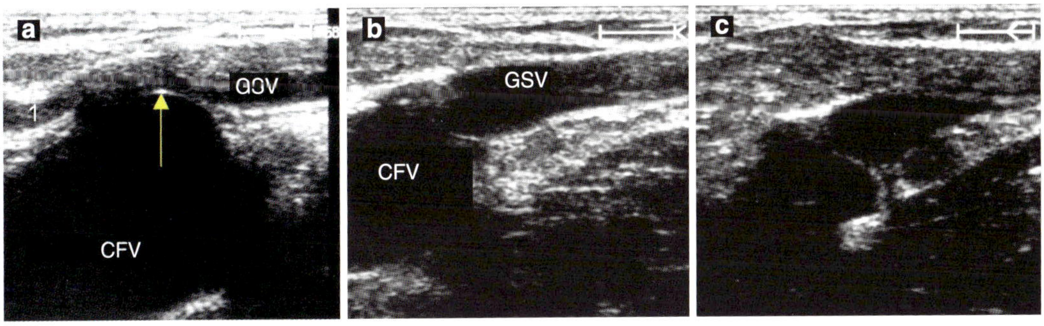

Fig. 7.7 Longitudinal view through the saphenofemoral junction demonstrating a competent terminal valve. (**a**) Longitudinal view during a Valsalva manoeuvre causes the valve (*arrowed*) to curve out into the great saphenous vein (*GSV*). The epigastric vein is seen in the left of the image (1). (**b**) A valve leaflet is seen opening during muscular systole. (**c**) Same subject as in (b) demonstrating a closed valve leaflet curving into the great saphenous vein during a Valsalva manoeuvre (image of a rigid, inflexible valve is seen in Fig. 7.15) Copyright: [Author]

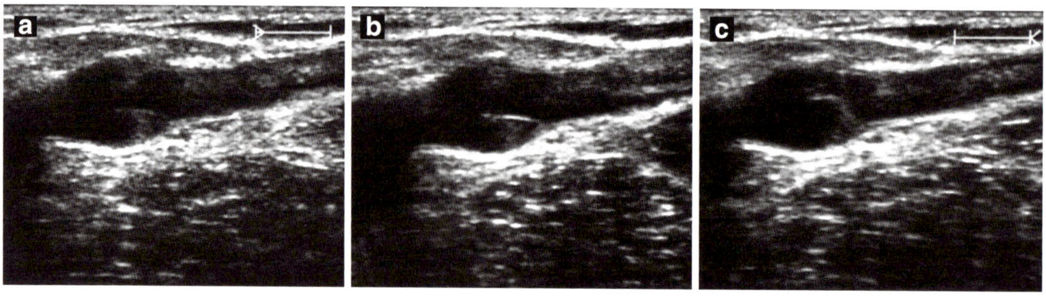

Fig. 7.8 Longitudinal view through the great saphenous vein immediately below the saphenofemoral junction demonstrating the preterminal valve. (**a**) Both valve cusps are visible with the classical "swallow's nest" shape. The valve is seen at rest in the standing subject. (**b**) The leaflet furthest from the surface is very clearly visible at rest. (**c**) The valve closes in muscular diastole Copyright: [Author]

7.3.2 Anatomical Variations of the Saphenofemoral Junction

There are numerous anatomical variations at the saphenofemoral junction. For example, any or all of the superficial inguinal veins may join the common femoral vein directly. Direct drainage occurs frequently with the pudendal vein (Fig. 7.9). If this vein is overlooked during surgery, then it may be the source of a recurrence.

Duplication of the great saphenous vein at the saphenofemoral junction is very rare, even though this is postulated repeatedly as a cause of recurrence. According to Caggiati (personal communication), this variant does not occur. The great saphenous vein may join the common femoral vein directly at the groin or a few centimetres in either direction. Information on the **level of the saphenofemoral junction** is helpful to the surgeon but not as important as determining the level of the sapheno-popliteal junction.

In the majority of cases, the **anterior accessory saphenous vein** terminates in the region of the saphenofemoral junction where it joins the great saphenous vein (Fig. 7.3). Sometimes it may join up to 5 cm further down. It occasionally joins the femoral vein directly immediately adjacent to the great saphenous vein (Fig. 7.10). Very rarely it may join the common femoral vein by passing between the superficial femoral artery and the deep femoral artery (Fig. 7.11). It is equally rare to find a duplication of the anterior accessory saphenous vein in the saphenofemoral region (Fig. 7.12). If these anatomical variations of the anterior accessory saphenous vein are missed preoperatively, they may provide a source of recurrence.

In most cases the **posterior accessory saphenous vein** will not form part of the confluence of superficial inguinal veins but will meet the great saphenous vein in the upper thigh.

The tributaries join medially (pudendal vein and much further distal the posterior accessory saphenous vein) and laterally (epigastric and superficial circumflex iliac from cranial, anterior accessory saphenous vein from caudal). Hildebrandt's diagram provides a simplified classification supplemented by additional information from Mühlberger (Fig. 7.13). Only the pudendal vein drains medially at the saphenofemoral region (Fig. 7.13a). There are laterally joining veins from cranial (epigastric and superficial circumflex iliac veins) and caudal (anterior accessory saphenous vein), which may join above the distal edge of the ostium (dotted line in Fig. 7.13a and fainter in the other images) or below this point. The level at which the anterior accessory saphenous vein joins may be important for positioning the fibre in endoluminal laser treatment. Furthermore, the presence and location of the terminal and preterminal valves should be defined if selective ablation techniques are performed. Some of the anatomical variations are given in Fig. 7.13.

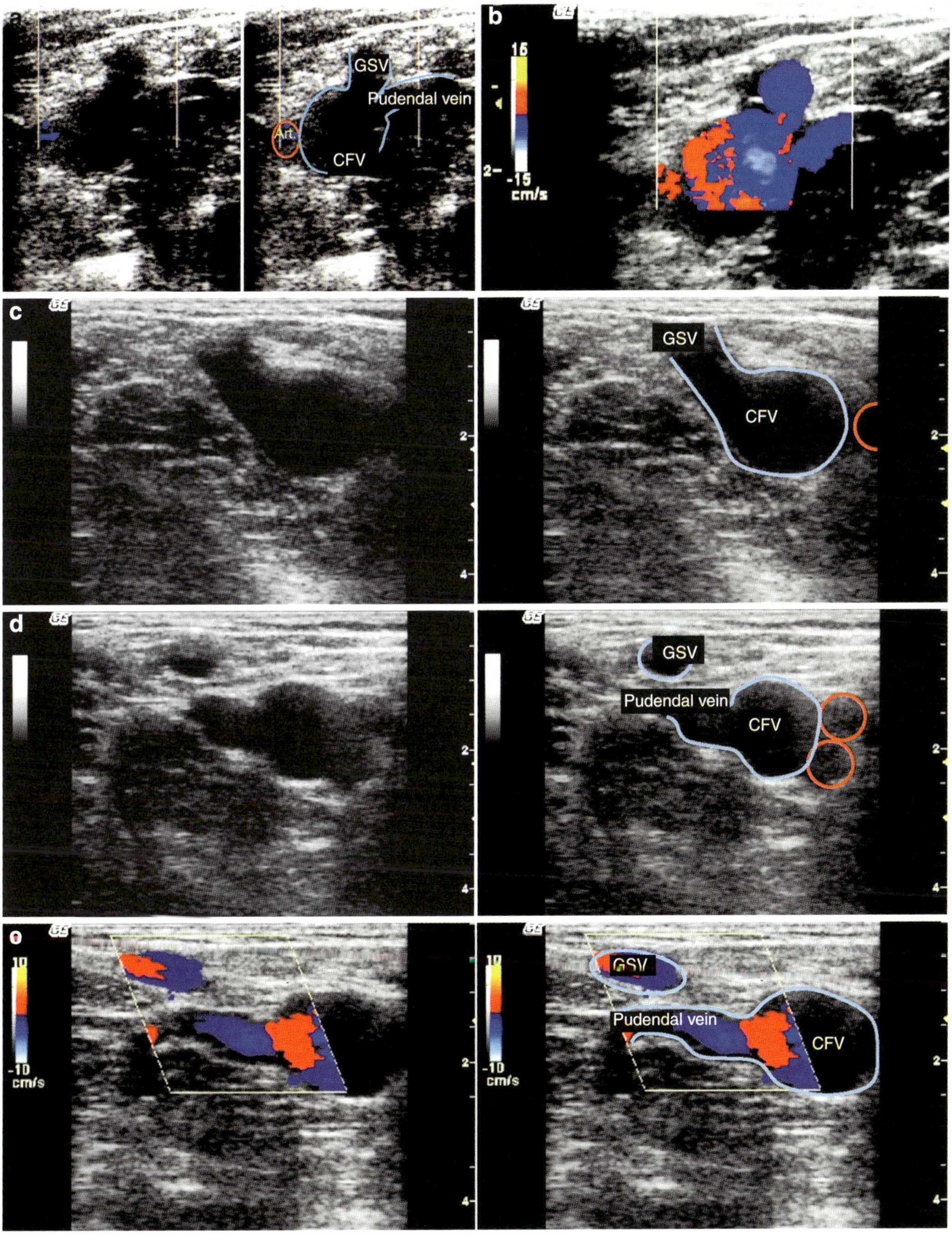

Fig. 7.9 Drainage of the pudendal vein directly into the common femoral vein. (**a**) Transverse view through the right groin. (**b**) Same position showing antegrade flow during muscular systole. (**c**) Transverse view through the left groin. The common femoral artery is circled (*red*). *CFV* common femoral vein, *GSV* great saphenous vein (online material). (**d**) Transverse view approx. 1 cm further distal. The great saphenous vein is visible as an independent vessel. The drainage of a very large pudendal vein is seen entering the common femoral vein directly (online material). (**e**) Same position with colour duplex with the probe tilted slightly so that both veins are visible in one image. At the end of muscular systole, there is a short flow reversal in the great saphenous vein (small red signal) until valve closure. However, long-lasting flow is now apparent in the pudendal vein. It is blue because the blood is refluxing away from the probe and pathological because the flow is prolonged and the pudendal vein is very dilated in comparison to the great saphenous vein (online material) Copyright: [Author]

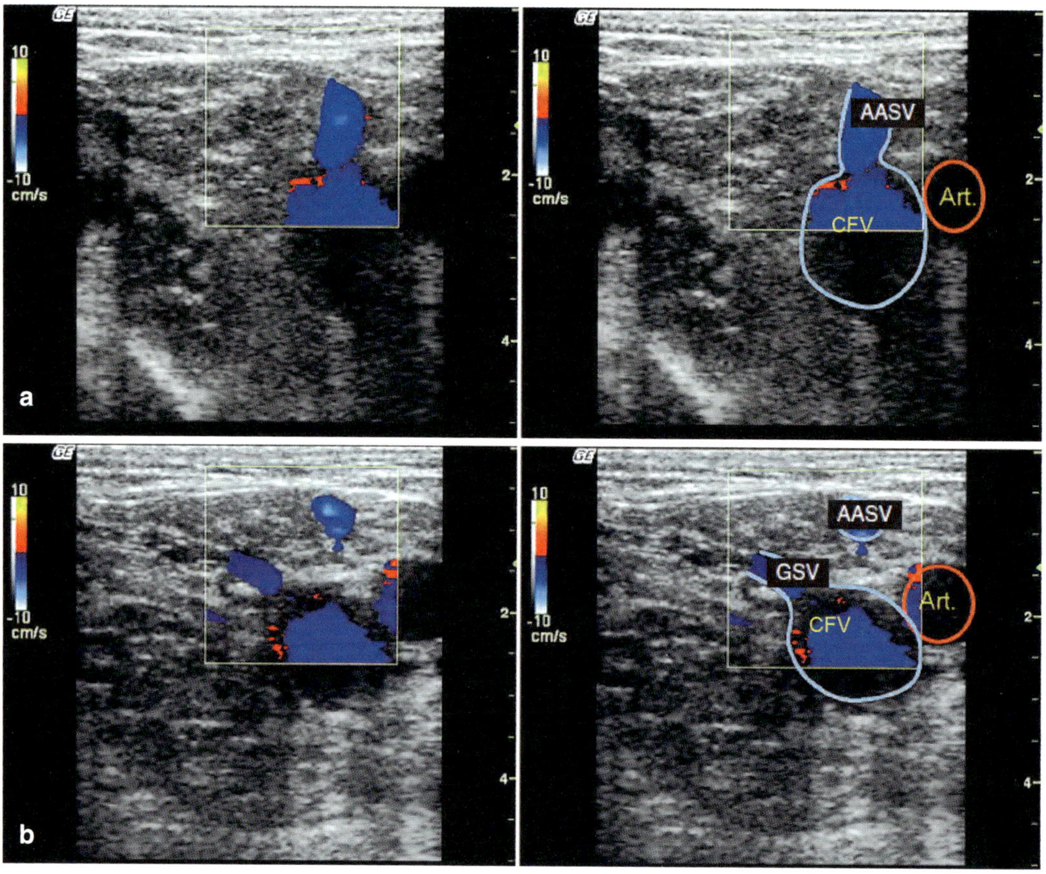

Fig. 7.10 Independent drainage of the anterior accessory saphenous vein (*AASV*) into the common femoral vein (*CFV*) (online material). (**a**) Transverse view through the left groin in a standing subject during muscular systole. There is antegrade flow up the anterior accessory saphenous vein and into the common femoral vein. (**b**) Transverse view 1 cm further distal from (a) demonstrating the great saphenous vein joining the common femoral vein. The anterior accessory saphenous vein is visible as an independent vessel lateral to the saphenofemoral junction Copyright: [Author]

Precise documentation of the saphenofemoral junction should include all the superficial inguinal veins and their relationship and distance from the terminal and preterminal valves. Such information is needed principally for study purposes, but in the context of new treatments which selectively preserve tributaries, pre-procedural documentation may become important.

7.3.3 Reflux from the Common Femoral Vein

The most common source of reflux in the great saphenous vein is the saphenofemoral junction. Here the saphenous trunk is filled refluxively from the common femoral vein. During the Valsalva manoeuvre or muscular diastole, blood flows down from the iliofemoral veins into the great saphenous vein. This can be seen indirectly in B scan from the behaviour of the valves and the dilation of the vein wall during refluxive flow.

The mouth of the **great saphenous vein** generally appears dilated in B scan (Fig. 7.14). The calibre of the great saphenous vein often increases after the subject has been standing for a few minutes. However, reflux may also occur across the saphenofemoral junction even if the vein is not dilated.

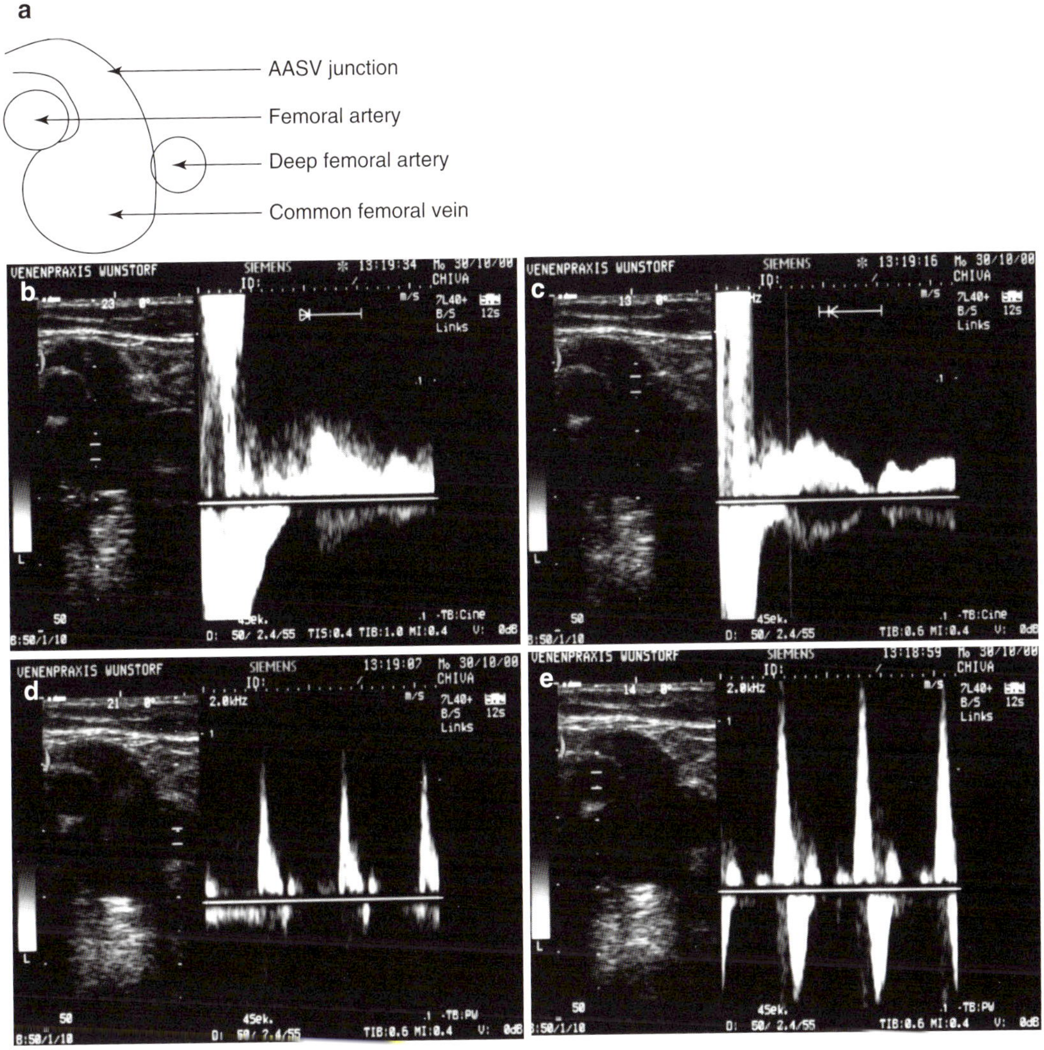

Fig. 7.11 Confluence of the anterior accessory saphenous vein (*AASV*) between the superficial and deep femoral arteries. (**a**) Diagram of the position of the arteries in relation to the confluence. (**b**) Measurement in the common femoral vein which is the reflux source. (**c**) Measurement in the confluence of the anterior accessory saphenous vein which is clearly refluxive. (**d**, **e**) Velocity profiles in the two adjacent arteries Copyright: [Author]

Much information can be gained in B scan:

- The morphology of the saphenofemoral junction and the proximal great saphenous vein
- The morphology of the confluence of superficial inguinal veins
- The presence or absence of thrombus in the common femoral or great saphenous veins (compression manoeuvre, Chaps. 11 and 14)
- Morphology of the valves
- Drainage paths of the insonated veins

7.3.3.1 Morphology of the Saphenofemoral Junction and the Confluence of the Superficial Inguinal Veins

The following questions should be answered:

- Do the superficial inguinal veins join the femoral vein directly or via the great saphenous vein?
- Which superficial inguinal tributaries are present?
- Is the saphenofemoral junction dilated?
- Is there an aneurysm?

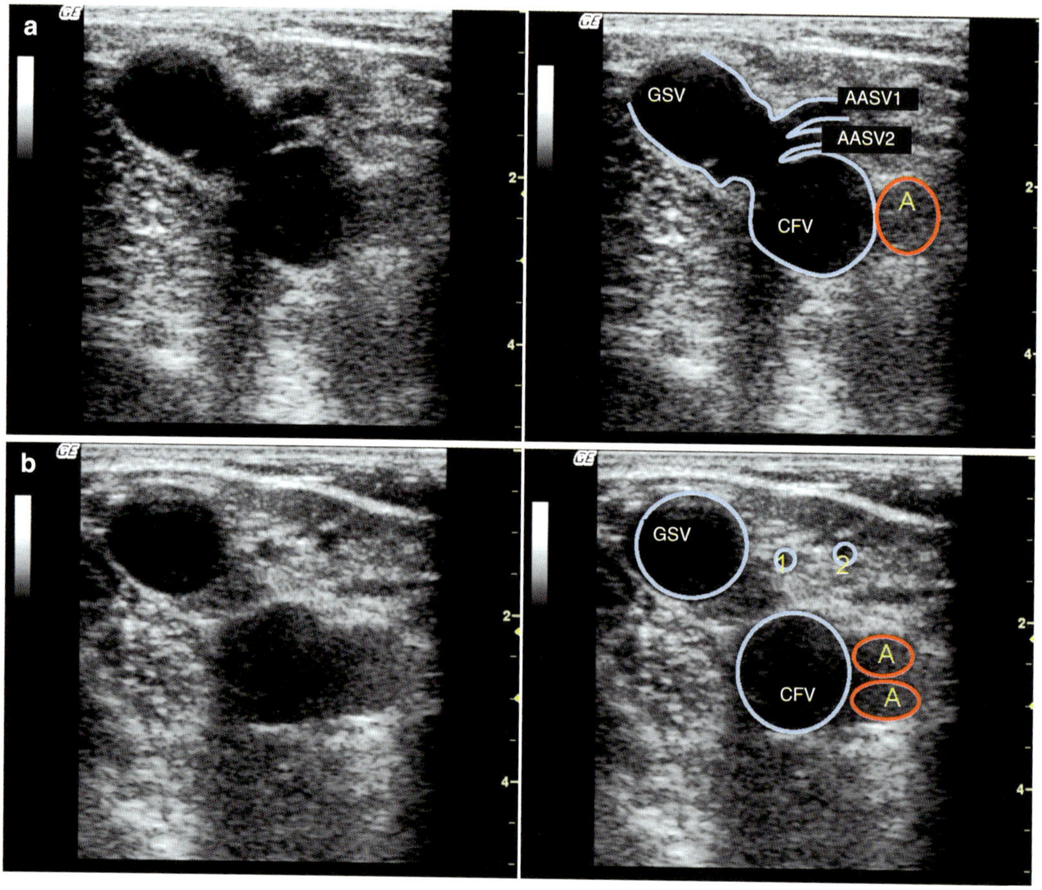

Fig. 7.12 Saphenofemoral junction. Transverse view through the left groin in a standing patient with an incompetent terminal valve and a dilated great saphenous vein (*GSV*) which turns left at the top of the image. Two competent anterior accessory saphenous veins (*AASV*) are seen draining separately into the saphenofemoral junction. (**a**) Region of the drainage points of both anterior accessory saphenous veins. (**b**) 1 cm further distal Copyright: [Author]

Aneurysms of the saphenofemoral region should be identified because of the potential difficulty in surgical treatment. They may be either discrete or fusiform dilatations of the great saphenous vein itself (Fig. 7.15) or dilatations growing out of the vein wall (Fig. 7.16). Surgery on the saphenofemoral junction may be complicated by these thin-walled balloons of blood. They may grow as large as a golf ball and obscure the operating field. Tributaries often flow directly into these aneurysms (Fig. 7.17).

Turbulence is normally observed in aneurysms in B scan during provocation manoeuvres. A thrombus in the lumen of an aneurysm is rare (Pascarella et al. 2005). Surprisingly, in contrast to the arterial circulation, there is no relationship between the presence of an aneurysm and the development of a superficial vein thrombosis (Kalodiki et al. 2012). A combination of a weak vein wall and an overload of refluxive blood volume striking the vein wall may encourage aneurysm formation. The resulting flow characteristics seem to prevent thrombus formation.

Even with incompetence the **terminal valve** is usually seen fluttering. It folds into the great saphenous vein during muscular diastole if reflux is present, or during a Valsalva manoeuvre. If the

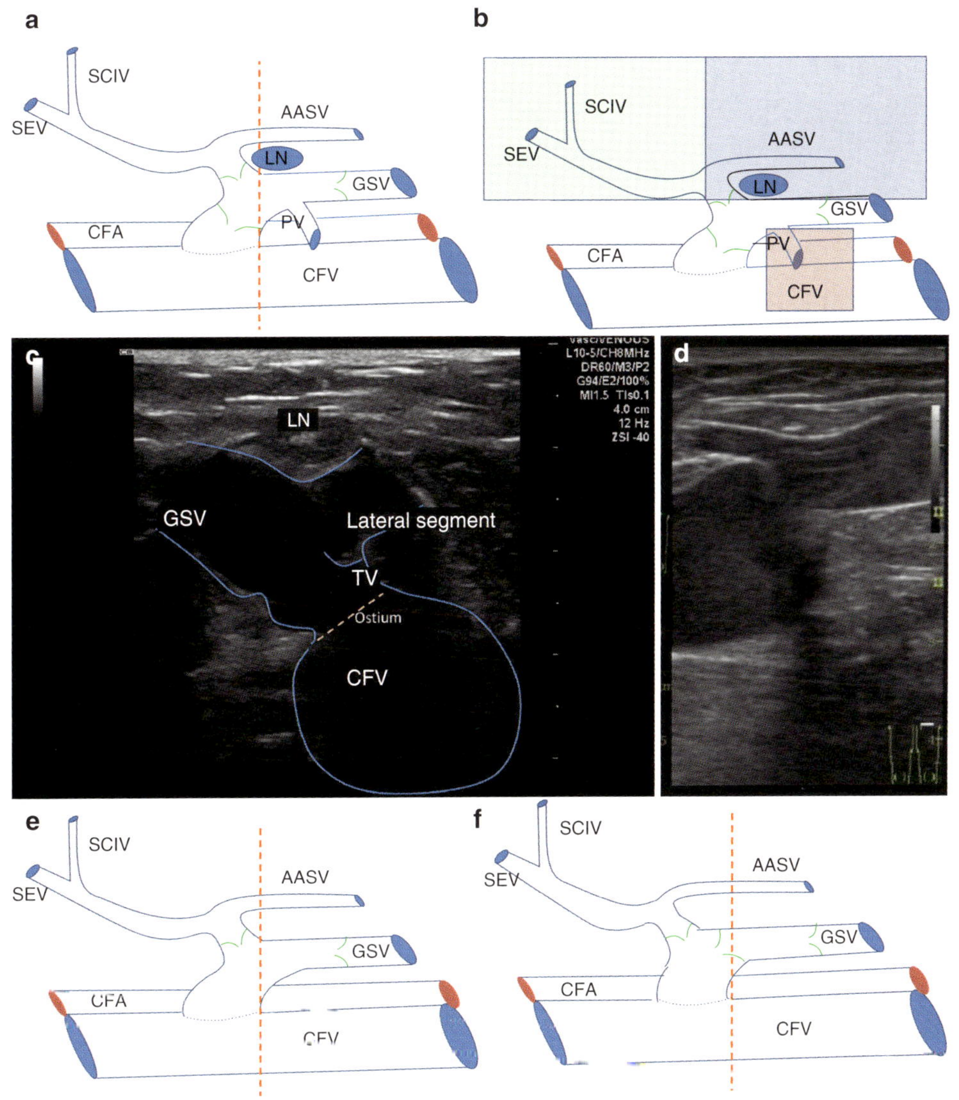

Fig. 7.13 Junctional variations and valves for common or separate inflow from the proximal and lateral tributaries. (**a**) Standard saphenofemoral junction with tributaries. The pudendal vein is the single medial segment which joins between the terminal and preterminal valves. The lateral segment is shown with a common confluence of a cranial and caudal branch and another valve at the level of its junction with the great saphenous vein. The typical position of a lymph node (LN) lateral to the great saphenous vein is shown. The perpendicular *dotted line* marks the caudal edge of the ostium. (**b**) Additional information defining the lateral segment (*light green*/*light purple*) and the medial segment (*light brown*). The lateral segment is divided into cranial (*green*) and caudal (*light purple*) parts. (**c**) Transverse view of the lateral segment distal to the terminal valve (TV). An imaginary dotted line drawn around the front wall of the common femoral vein and passing through the confluence of the great saphenous vein will give the exact point where the great saphenous vein enters the femoral vein. This is known as the *fossa ovalis* or ostium. (**d**) Longitudinal view demonstrating the confluence of the lateral cranial segment also distal to the terminal valve. (**e**) Absent terminal valve. (**f**) Confluence of the lateral segment consisting of the superficial epigastric, circumflex iliac and anterior accessory saphenous veins. Note that here they are proximal to the terminal valve. (**g**) In this image the confluence of the lateral and medial segment are both proximal to the terminal valve. (**h**) All of the superficial inguinal tributaries join between the terminal and the preterminal valves. (**i**) The lateral cranial tributaries may join separately from one another or together as in this illustration between the terminal and preterminal valves. The anterior accessory saphenous vein is not present. (**j**) Isolated entry of the superficial epigastric vein (cranial lateral segment). (**k**) The anterior accessory saphenous vein enters just distal to the preterminal valve (*CFA* common femoral artery, *LN* lymph node, *TV* terminal valve, *CIV* circumflex iliac vein, *SEV* superficial epigastric vein, *PV* pudendal vein, *AASV* anterior accessory saphenous vein, *GSV* great saphenous vein) (Drawings Dr. Andreas Hildebrandt, Berlin; by kind permission) Copyright: Dr. A. Hildebrandt, Berlin

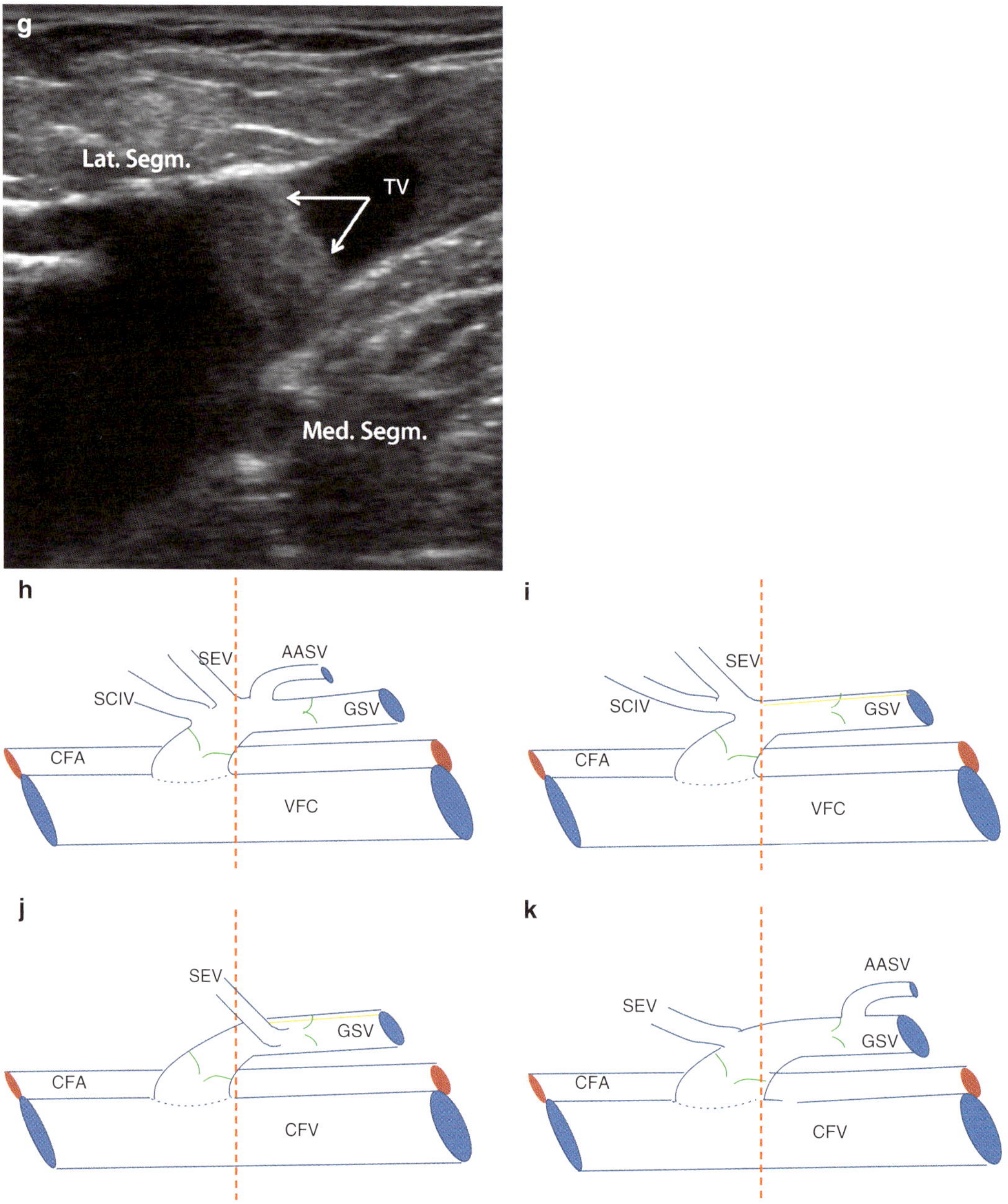

Fig. 7.13 (continued)

valve is rigid and immobile, this may suggest a primary valve defect or post-thrombotic scarring (Fig. 7.15).

If the system is poorly drained (Sect. 3.2.3), echoes appear in B scan inside the great saphenous vein immediately after a provocation manoeuvre. These may make the vein appear homogeneous with a similar echogenicity as the surrounding tissue. This depends on the accumulation of erythrocytes and the formation of so-called erythrocyte sludge. If the vein appears heterogeneous, this may indicate turbulence and varying flow velocities (Fig. 7.15). Patients presenting with this turbulence may go on to develop an aneurysm at the saphenofemoral region.

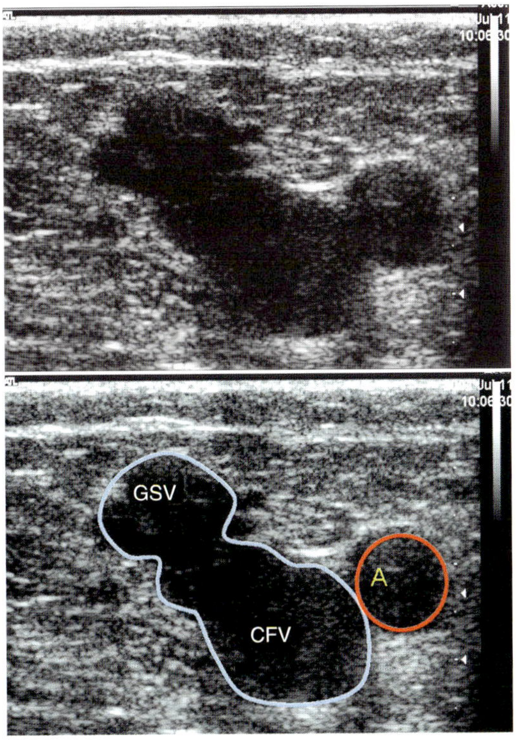

Fig. 7.14 Incompetent saphenofemoral junction of the left leg in B scan. The diameter of the great saphenous vein (*GSV*) is grossly dilated (c.f. Fig. 7.3) (*A* common femoral artery, *VFC* common femoral vein) Copyright: [Author]

The direction of blood flow can be seen in B scan from the erythrocyte sludge. However, reflux can be seen much more clearly using colour duplex ultrasound. This allows us to answer the following questions:

- Does the reflux flow from the common femoral vein through the saphenofemoral junction into the superficial veins?
- Does it fill the great saphenous vein, anterior accessory saphenous vein or both refluxively?
- Is any other superficial inguinal tributary also refluxive?
- Is isolated reflux present in a named superficial inguinal tributary?

Reflux from the common femoral vein through the saphenofemoral junction via an incompetent terminal valve is measurable at the saphenofemoral region (Fig. 7.18). This is termed **complete incompetence** of the great saphenous vein. This finding must be distinguished from the tributary type **incomplete incompetence**. In this situation the reflux arises from the deep leg veins via an incompetent superficial inguinal tributary. The terminal valve remains competent (Sects. 7.3.4 and 7.3.5).

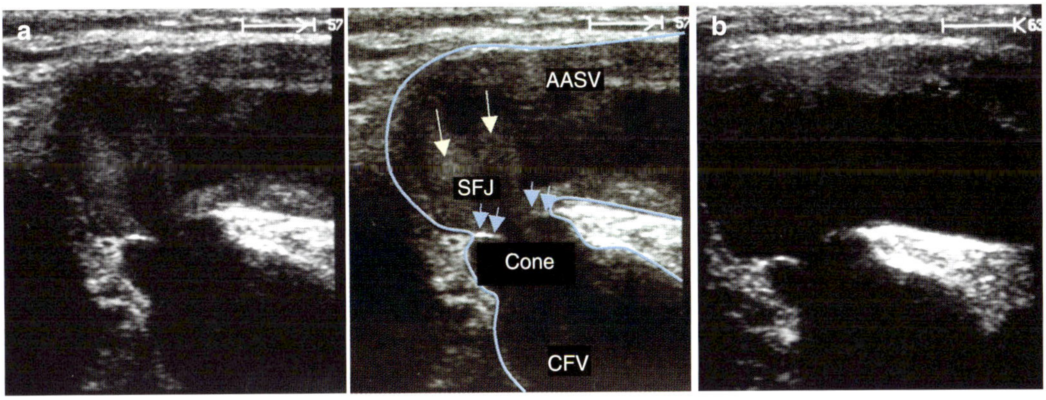

Fig. 7.15 Aneurysm at the confluence of the great saphenous vein and the anterior accessory saphenous vein (*AAVS*) with incompetence of the terminal valve and a competent preterminal valve (complete, Hach Class I). (**a**) Transverse view through the left groin demonstrating the saphenofemoral junction (*SFJ*) during muscular diastole. Blood refluxes from the common femoral vein through the incompetent terminal valve into the great saphenous vein and directly into the laterally positioned anterior accessory saphenous vein. Turbulence can be observed in the aneurysm (*white arrows*). Although this is during diastole and there is reflux, the valve cusp point towards each other They are not curved back into the great saphenous vein as would be expected with reflux but are rigid (*blue arrows*) (*CFV* common femoral vein). (**b**) Same position after the end of diastole. The erythrocyte sludge has gone, and the valve cusps remain rigid in the same position as during diastole. The narrow lumen between the rigid valve cusps caused a jet-effect which may have led to the development of the aneurysm (online material) Copyright: [Author]

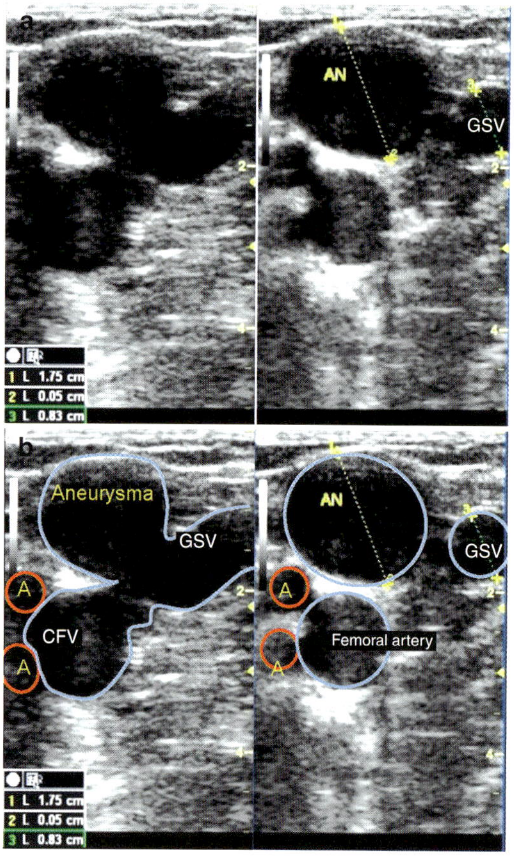

Fig. 7.16 Aneurysm formed by a bulge in the side wall of the vein. (**a**) Transverse view through the right groin with an incompetent saphenofemoral junction. The aneurysm looks like a mushroom growing out of the great saphenous vein (*GSV*). (**b**) 1 cm further distal the aneurysm (*AN*) and the great saphenous vein look like two different vessels Copyright: [Author]

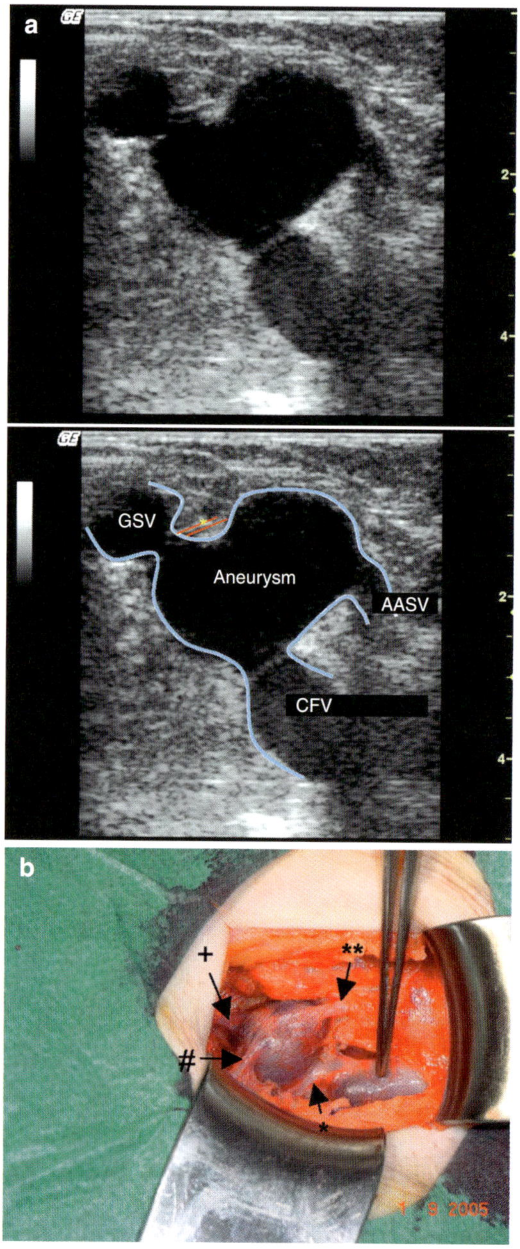

Fig. 7.17 Side aneurysm of the great saphenous vein (*GSV*) at the saphenofemoral junction. (**a**) Transverse view through the left groin in B scan. The anterior accessory saphenous vein (*AASV*) is seen draining into the aneurysm. The superficial external pudendal artery (*) crosses between the aneurysm and the great saphenous vein (online material). (**b**) Intraoperative photograph of the aneurysm exposed showing its connections with the pudendal (#) and epigastric (+) veins. The forceps are pointing to the normal calibre great saphenous vein just below the band-like superficial external pudendal artery (*) (** anterior accessory saphenous vein) Copyright: [Author]

In addition to the reflux from the common femoral vein, it is not uncommon to find a **tributary** (usually the pudendal vein) which is also **refluxive** or at least dilated (Fig. 7.19). Antegrade flow will be found in both these veins during muscular systole. The course of the pudendal vein to its termination in the saphenofemoral region may show red representing flow towards the probe. In diastole it is important to clarify whether flow can be observed from the deep vein into the great saphenous vein (*red*) and whether the pudendal vein presents a long-lasting flow. The colour red or blue depends on the course of the pudendal vein towards the probe. However, it

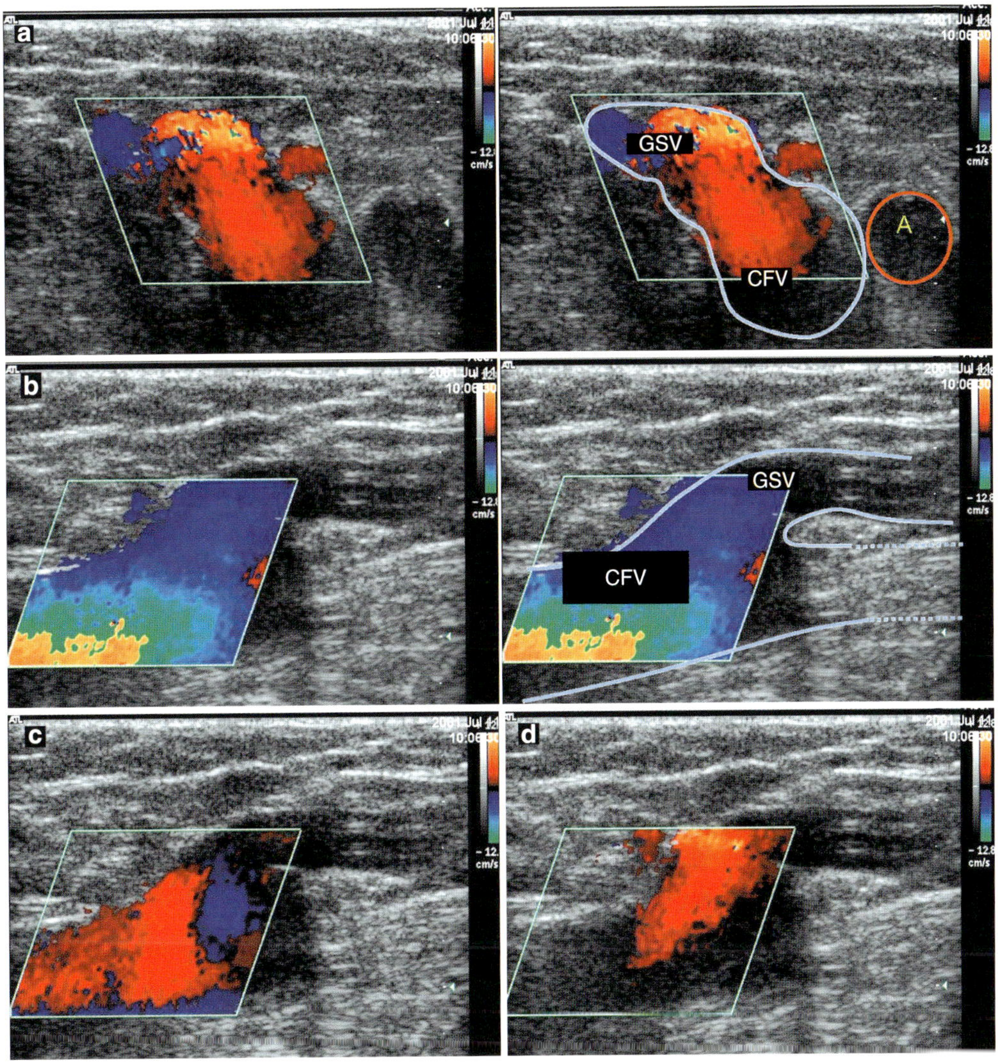

Fig. 7.18 Incompetent saphenofemoral junction in colour duplex in the patient from Fig. 7.13a). (**a**) Transverse view through the groin during muscular diastole demonstrating reflux from the common femoral vein (*CFV*). The blood flows from the deep vein towards the probe (*red*). Note that the common femoral vein and saphenofemoral junction are both coloured *red*. (**b**) Longitudinal view through the junction in the same patient during muscular systole. The blood flow is antegrade in both the deep and superficial veins. (**c**) Same longitudinal position at the very beginning of muscular diastole. The blood starts to change direction and flows out of the common femoral vein. (**d**) During muscular diastole the blood flows out of the common femoral vein and into the great saphenous vein. Only with this unequivocal finding is it correct to speak of incompetence of the saphenofemoral junction Copyright: [Author]

is pathological if this flow is prolonged in diastole. Here it may fill the great saphenous vein refluxively or drain into the common femoral vein through the saphenofemoral junction (Sect. 7.3.6).

Sometimes the findings at the saphenofemoral junction are **contradictory**. It may be competent during the Valsalva manoeuvre and incompetent with another provocation manoeuvre, or vice versa. Occasionally it is incompetent and then competent consecutively using the same manoeuvre twice. When this happens the veins are not usually very dilated. The contradiction may result from the different intensities of the manoeuvres. The calf compression applied or the effort in raising the toes may not have been the same both

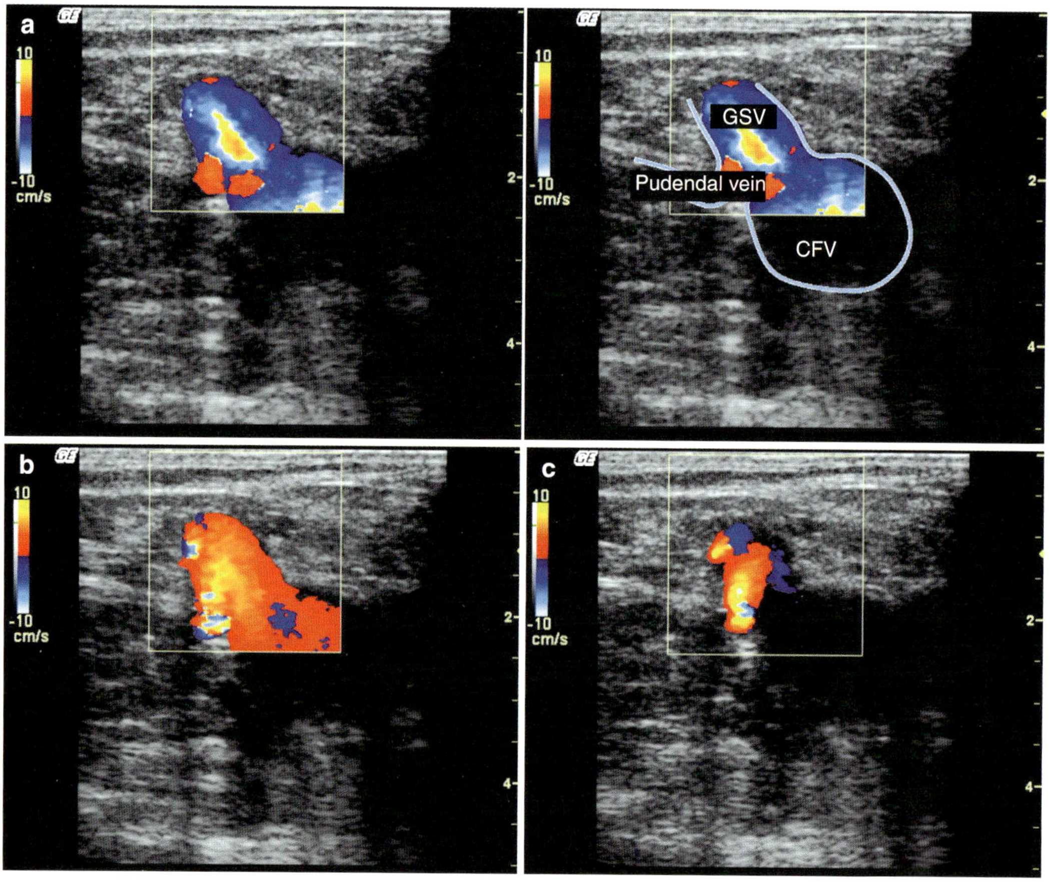

Fig. 7.19 Incompetent saphenofemoral junction with a refluxive pudendal vein (online material). (**a**) Transverse view through the left groin during muscular systole demonstrating antegrade flow in both veins (great saphenous and pudendal). In the pudendal vein antegrade flow towards the probe (*red*), flow is only visible at the confluence with the great saphenous vein (*GSV*). (**b**) At the beginning of muscular diastole, there is clear reflux from the common femoral vein through the saphenofemoral junction. The reflux from the pudendal vein cannot be evaluated at this early timepoint. (**c**) Towards the end of muscular diastole, it becomes clear that in addition to reflux from the common femoral vein (*CFV*), the great saphenous vein is also filled refluxively by the pudendal vein Copyright: [Author]

times. The frequency of the challenge test is also important because this affects the volume of blood which collects in the leg prior to the subsequent manoeuvre. Poorly drained systems may likewise give contradictory results (Sect. 3.2.3). In the latter case, an elevation-dependency manoeuvre may clarify what is happening (Sect. 6.9). As the patient stands up from a period of leg elevation, a long-lasting reflux will be observed in the vein if it is pathological (Lattimer et al. 2013). Competent valves may be found in the common femoral vein which may result in a negative Valsalva reflux but a positive reflux following a calf compression or contraction manoeuvre (Lattimer et al. 2012b). If the contradiction cannot be resolved, then the subject must be called in again for more testing. However, this problem only arises in borderline cases of pathology and in the early stages of incompetence where treatment is rarely required.

The **deep femoral vein** joins the femoral vein from posterior in the proximal thigh to form the common femoral vein. Normally this confluence cannot be seen during the examination of the saphenofemoral junction. The deep femoral vein may join at an acute angle in which case it will be the same colour (blue) on duplex as the femoral vein. Sometimes a red jet can be seen entering the common femoral vein from posterior (Fig. 7.20a, b). This means that the deep femoral vein joins at right angles. This finding is not pathological.

A special situation occurs when there is **reflux** arising from the **deep femoral vein** which flows directly into the **great saphenous vein** (Fig. 7.20c, d). In rare cases the deep femoral vein joins immediately opposite the saphenofemoral junction. It meets the femoral vein from behind and its blood flows anteriorly to enter directly into the great saphenous vein. Simple interruption of the saphenofemoral junction in patients with this configuration leads to an improvement in their varicose veins. A cause may be postulated that a systolic jet from the deep femoral vein during activity strikes the valve of the great saphenous vein with enough force to cause damage. After endoluminal procedures that close the great saphenous vein without ligation of the tributaries, recurrence may occur in this unusual configuration because of the relentless jet from the deep femoral vein.

With constant reflux from the common femoral vein into a very dilated pudendal vein, this may result in cross-pelvic communications and shunting (**Spontaneous Palma shunt**, Chap. 15).

7.3.4 Reflux from the Pudendal Vein

The pudendal vein joins the saphenofemoral junction from the medial side. It may join the great saphenous vein, the saphenofemoral junction or directly into the femoral vein (Fig. 7.9). Occasionally it joins the great saphenous vein from a posterior direction. These variants are helpful to the surgeon. Reflux arising from the pudendal vein when it joins the saphenofemoral junction and takes it to the great saphenous vein can easily be confused with reflux arising from the common femoral vein directly (Fig. 7.21). Colour duplex is better than PW mode for distinguishing these conditions. The pudendal vein may also be described as the medial segment.

7.3.5 Reflux from the Epigastric and Superficial Circumflex Iliac Veins

The epigastric and superficial circumflex iliac veins may also account for incompetence of the great saphenous vein. This is possible in addition to reflux from the saphenofemoral junction (incompetent terminal valve) or independent of it (with competent terminal valve). The two together are also known as the cranial section of the lateral segment (Fig. 7.13).

Both the epigastric and the superficial circumflex iliac veins may also join the anterior accessory saphenous vein first and deliver their reflux either only distally into this vein or through the anterior accessory saphenous vein into the great saphenous vein from the lateral side. Here, as with the pudendal vein, only precise examination can shed light on these different reflux sources (Figs. 7.22 and 7.23).

The epigastric vein unlike all the situations described so far (see also Fig. 7.2) is never the last vein to join the junction segment of the great saphenous vein before the saphenofemoral junction. In research in surgical preparations (Mühlberger et al. 2009), the average distance between the confluence of the epigastric vein with the saphenous vein and the confluence of the great saphenous vein with the common femoral vein was found to be 1.2 cm. In only 30 % of epigastric veins was this distance reduced to 0–0.7 cm.

Reflux in the cranial part of the lateral segment must not only be sought in the confluence region. The whole proximal great saphenous vein must be examined systematically for inflows. The groin region proximal of the saphenofemoral junction must be examined for refluxive vessels. They must then be followed to their confluence with the deep veins or refluxive leg veins.

7.3.6 Physiological and Pathological Flow in Groin Tributaries

It is often difficult to determine whether a tributary is refluxive. In these vessels the physiological flow is into the great saphenous vein and towards the foot. Therefore, no conclusion can be drawn from the **flow direction** alone.

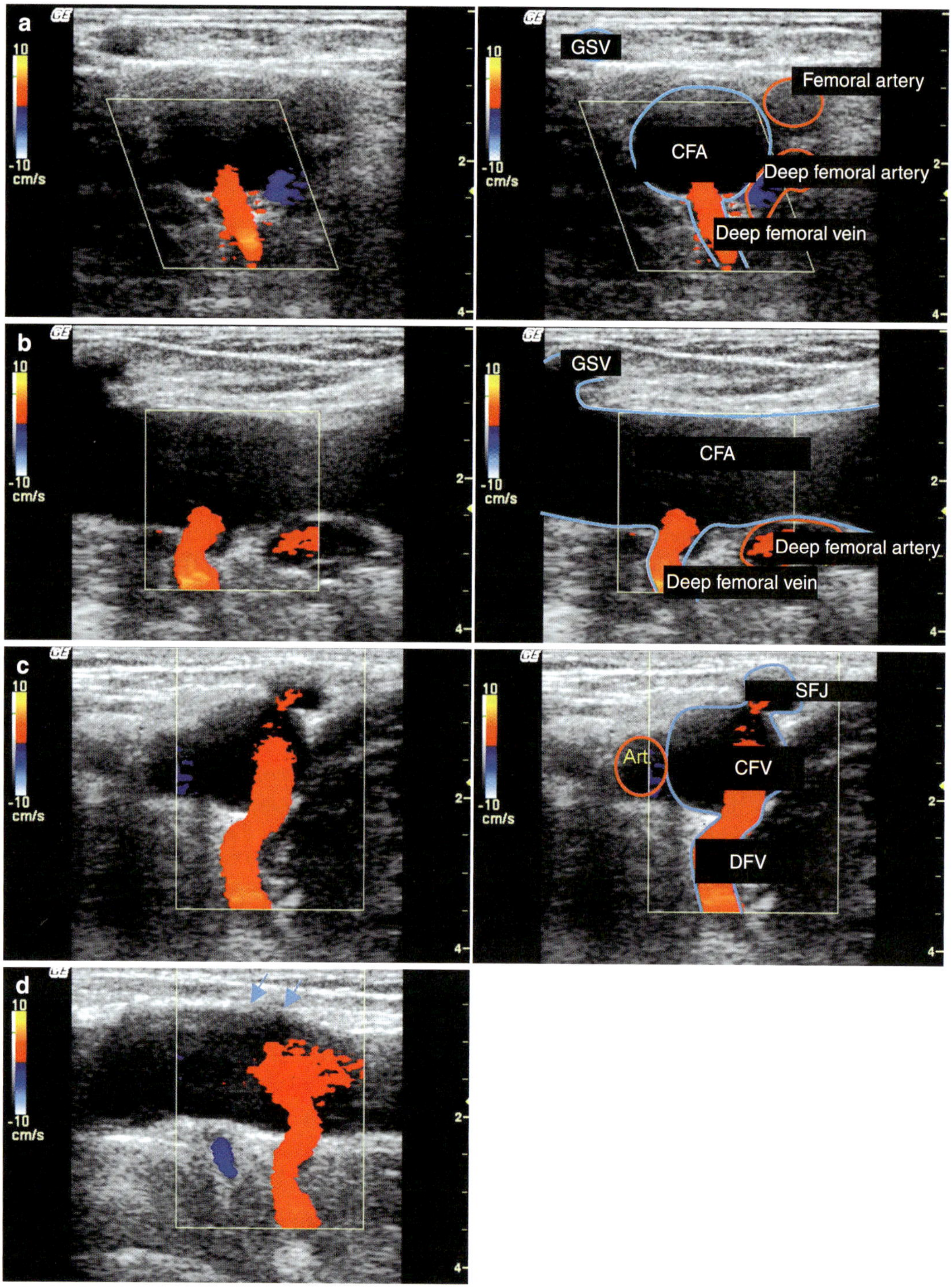

Fig. 7.20 Confluence of the deep femoral vein in the groin. (**a**) Transverse view of the left groin showing the common femoral (*CFV*), deep femoral (*DFV*) and great saphenous veins (*GSV*). The deep femoral vein joins below the saphenofemoral junction. Therefore, the great saphenous vein appears separate from the common femoral vein (online material). (**b**) Longitudinal view in the same subject. (**c**) Transverse view of the right groin showing the common femoral, deep femoral and great saphenous veins. The deep femoral vein joins immediately opposite the great saphenous vein. It looks as if the deep femoral vein fills the great saphenous vein refluxively (red) because the flow is towards the probe. (**d**) Longitudinal view in the same subject. The saphenofemoral junction is indicated opposite the confluence of the deep femoral vein (*blue arrows*) Copyright: [Author]

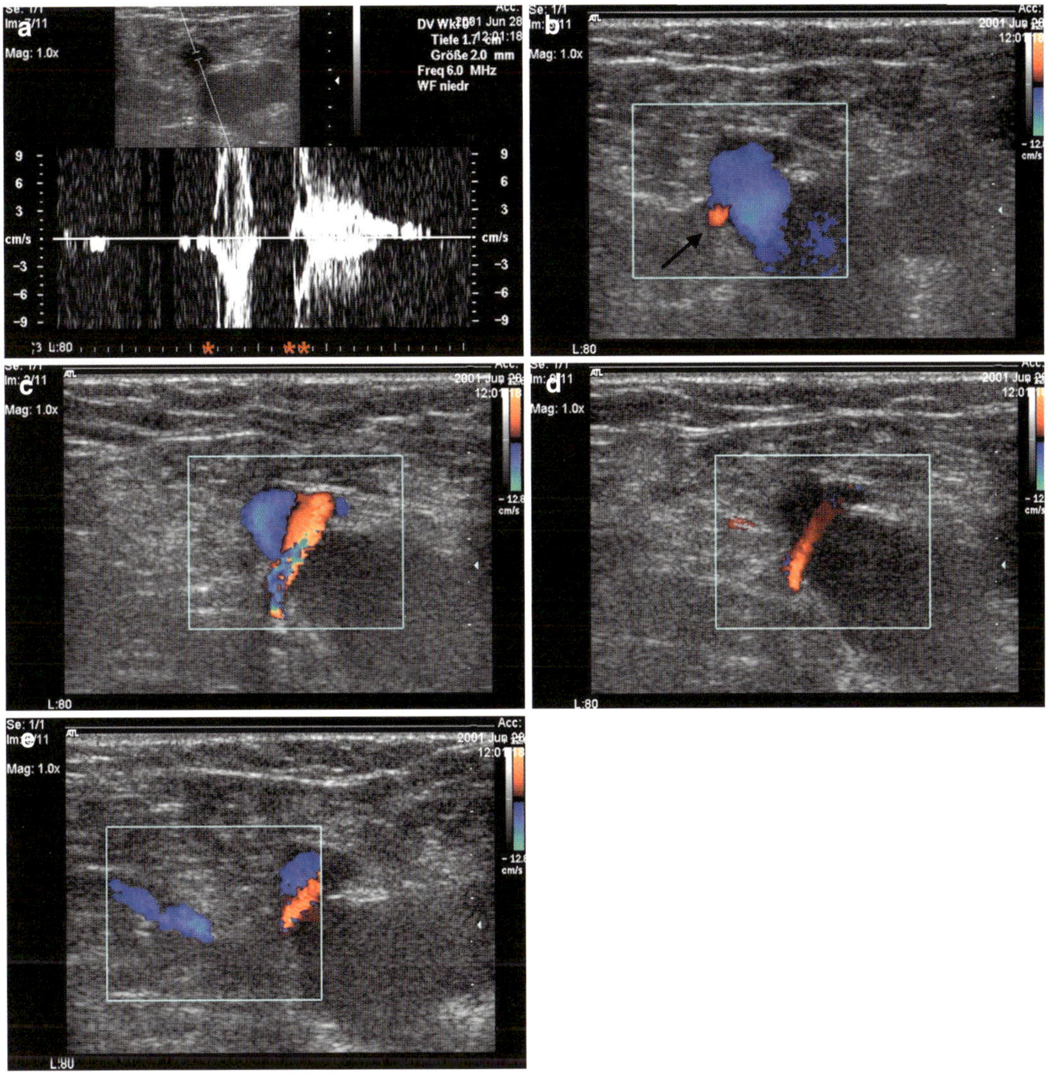

Fig. 7.21 Transverse view through the left groin. (**a**) Velocity profiles in the great saphenous vein just below the saphenofemoral junction demonstrating antegrade flow during systole (*) and retrograde flow after relaxation of the toes (**). (**b**) During muscular systole antegrade flow is seen in the great saphenous vein with inflow from the pudendal vein (*arrowed*). (**c**) During muscular diastole there is no reflux from the common femoral vein. The only reflux present is from the pudendal vein into the great saphenous vein. (**d**) Flow from the confluence of superficial inguinal veins "at rest". The subject is standing without moving. Note the constant flow from the pudendal vein. (**e**) Another image showing a permanent flow (reflux) from the pudendal vein at rest (reflux from the pudendal and epigastric veins on online material) Copyright: [Author]

Analysis of the velocity profile is decisive. After manual compression of the calf, the Wunstorf manoeuvre or during the Valsalva manoeuvre, a short, not very rapid, flow in these tributaries is normal. The description "short" in this context needs to be defined. In venous assessment the backflow should last no more than 0.5 or 1 s, depending on the author, if it is physiological. The short backflow in a healthy vein lasts between 0.1 and 0.2 s and represents the time taken for the valve to close. Regarding superficial inguinal tributaries, a precise time cut-off point is less meaningful because these veins drain physiologically into the deep veins during muscular diastole. A variety of components interact in these cases adding further difficulties to a time definition, as

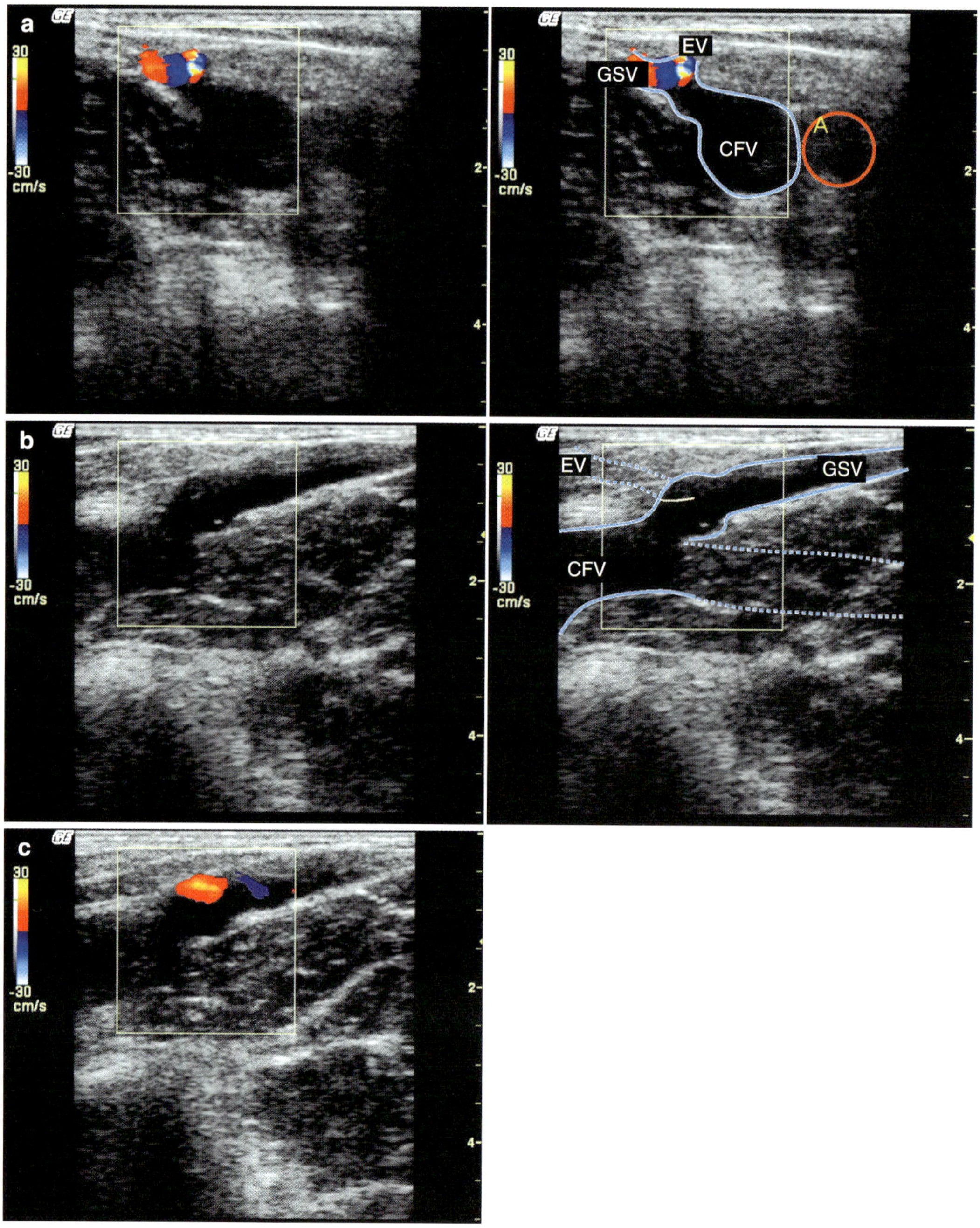

Fig. 7.22 Reflux with competent terminal valve of the great saphenous vein. (**a**) Transverse view through the left groin. Reflux from the epigastric vein (*EV*) into the great saphenous vein (*GSV*) without incompetence of the saphenofemoral junction. The reflux from the epigastric vein flows away from the probe into the great saphenous vein and is therefore shown in blue (online material) (*CFV* common femoral vein). (**b**) Longitudinal view through the same groin. The epigastric vein does not run on this plane and therefore indicated with a *dotted line* in the upper left of the second image. One valve leaflet is shown in *yellow*. (**c**) Longitudinal view in muscular diastole. Reflux from the epigastric vein is seen flowing into the great saphenous vein Copyright: [Author]

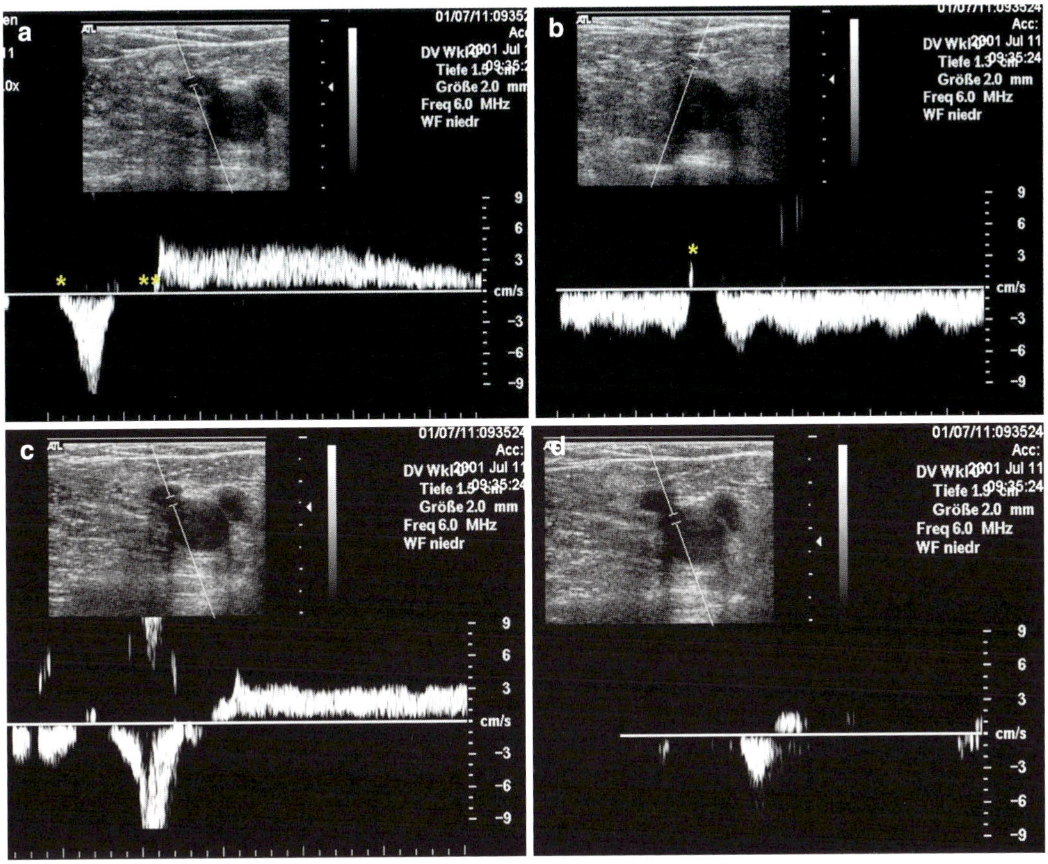

Fig. 7.23 (**a**) PW measurement in the great saphenous vein immediately below the saphenofemoral junction, * muscular systole giving rise to antegrade flow, ** muscular diastole evidencing reflux. (**b**) Measurement in the epigastric vein of the same subject demonstrating a long-lasting flow towards the feet and into the saphenofemoral junction. The flow is continuous and prolonged with only a short interruption during muscular systole (*). (**c**) Measurements taken at the saphenofemoral junction in the same patient. Here it might be supposed that the reflux comes from the common femoral vein because it was recorded in the immediate vicinity. (**d**) Measurement in the common femoral vein at the saphenofemoral junction. No reflux is recorded. Flow from the epigastric vein fills the great saphenous vein. The reflux profile from the epigastric vein in (b) coincides with the great saphenous vein in (a). This is an additional support for the conclusion that the blood volume in the great saphenous vein comes from the epigastric vein Copyright: [Author]

can be seen in Figs. 7.24 and 7.25. The concept of “flow volumes” in the diagram should be regarded as a semi-quantitative measure and refers to the area under the velocity profile.

Healthy tributaries can be seen in B scan as small calibre vessels usually only when they are being specifically targeted. In colour duplex they are easier to find during muscular diastole. A tributary which is obvious during a B scan examination is usually pathological and requires further assessment. If the flow in the tributary is longer than 1 s, its velocity profile must be compared with that of the great saphenous vein.

In poorly drained systems (Sect. 3.2.3), there is often reflux from one of the superficial inguinal tributaries. The identification of a refluxive tributary is important for the **prognosis** after treatment. The highest reflux source in these patients may be from a pelvic origin. Therefore, whatever endovenous leg procedure is selected, this source is unlikely to be included in the treatment. This

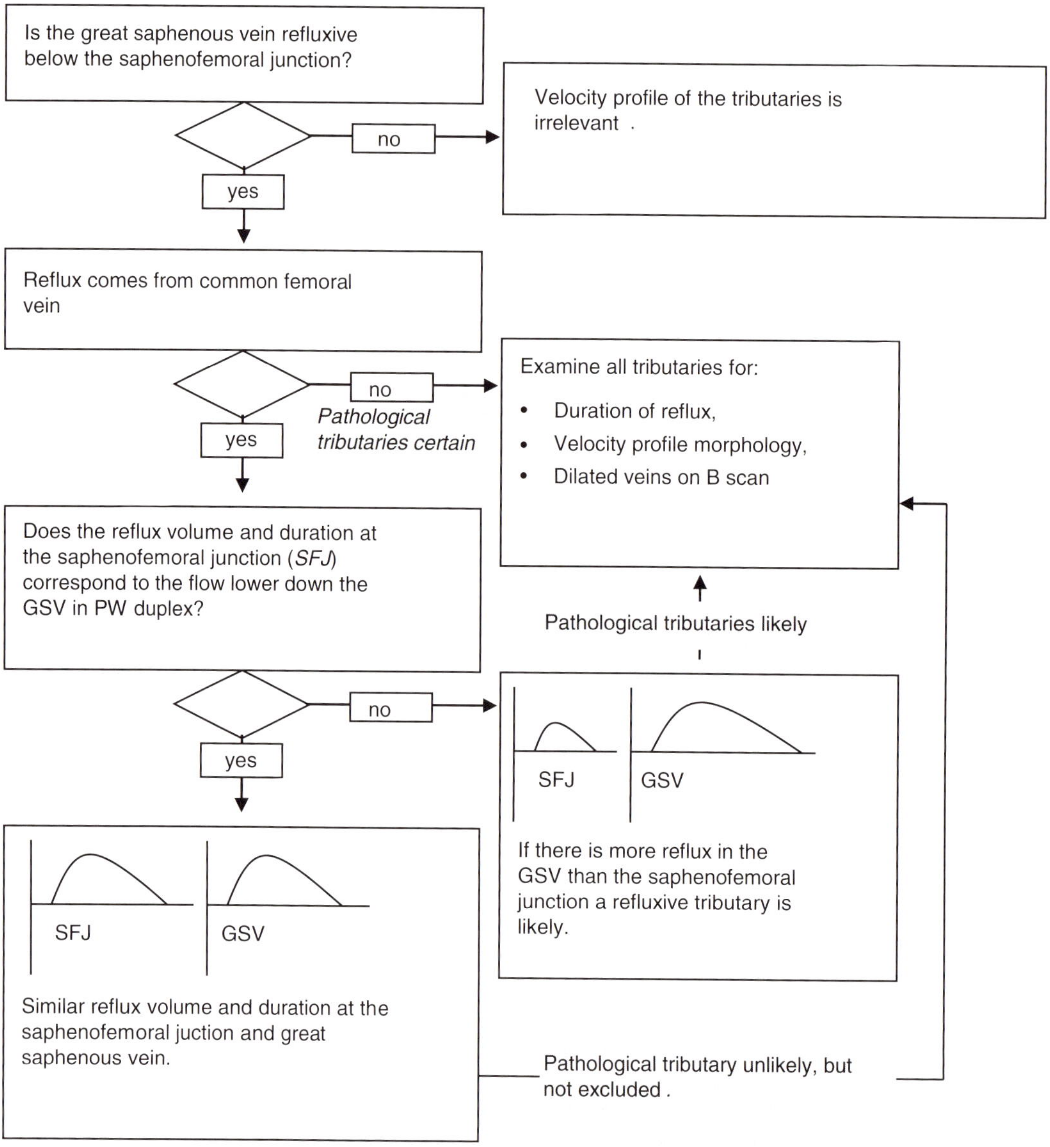

Fig. 7.24 Algorithm for assessing reflux in the saphenofemoral region to determine whether the incompetence of the great saphenous vein (*GSV*) is complete or incomplete Copyright: [Author]

It has been shown that female patients with reflux from the superficial inguinal tributaries have high oestradiol levels in the blood of the varicose veins themselves. More surprising was that there were also increased levels of testosterone in comparison to male patients (Oswald 2005). This discovery must be examined with further research for its clinical implications and prognostic significance. Nevertheless, it confirms that gonadal venous blood is present in leg veins which may have originated from a proximal reflux source.

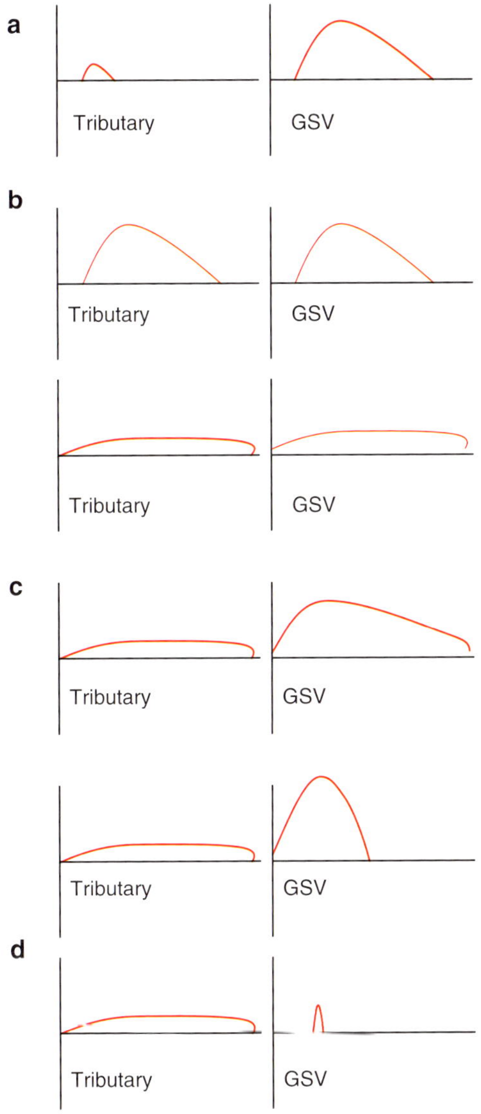

Fig. 7.25 Comparison of the velocity profiles between a tributary and the great saphenous vein. (**a**) Short backflow with small volume in a healthy superficial inguinal tributary. (**b**) The backflow in this tributary has an identical profile to the great saphenous vein, making it clearly responsible for the reflux into the great saphenous vein. This is regardless of whether the profiles are steep or relatively flat. (**c**) Reflux volumes in this great saphenous vein are greater than in the tributary, but just as prolonged. Here, the tributary is partly responsible for the reflux and therefore pathological, but it is obvious that the great saphenous vein is filled from several sources. (**d**) Reflux in this great saphenous vein is shorter than in the tributary (*upper*) or absent (*lower*). The tributary in both these cases has a clear pathological flow and must be considered refluxive. It is likely that they are draining through the saphenofemoral junction into the deep veins or the flow is too small to be recognised if it drains down into the increased calibre great saphenous vein Copyright: [Author]

may lead to early recurrences in the patient (Sect. 13.3).

7.3.7 Reflux in the Anterior Accessory Saphenous Vein

The anterior accessory saphenous vein joins the great saphenous vein in the groin. Rarely it joins the common femoral vein directly. Occasionally there is duplication in the region of its termination (Figs. 7.2, 7.3, 7.4, 7.5, 7.6, 7.10, 7.11, and 7.12). An anterior accessory saphenous vein is found in only 50 % of cases (Mühlberger et al. 2009). The average distance between the confluence of the anterior accessory saphenous vein with the great saphenous vein and the saphenofemoral junction is 2 cm. In 90 % of legs, the anterior accessory saphenous vein is joined by one or more tributaries (epigastric or superficial circumflex iliac vein) before it terminates into the great saphenous vein.

Normally the anterior accessory saphenous vein is distinguished from the great saphenous vein because of its lateral position in relation to the great saphenous vein and common femoral vein (Fig. 7.4). However, this anatomy is sometimes not so easy to detect if its **course** is followed carefully. Occasionally, the vein which appears in the groin from a lateral position may prove to be the great saphenous vein (Sect. 7.4). Aplasia of the proximal section of the great saphenous vein may lead to a mistaken identity.

If there is reflux in the anterior accessory saphenous vein in the groin, there are three possible findings:

- Reflux from the common femoral vein through the saphenofemoral junction:
  - With a healthy great saphenous vein in its downward course. The proximal great saphenous vein is only incompetent down to the confluence of the anterior accessory saphenous vein, Hach Class I (Figs. 7.26 and 7.28a)
  - With an incompetent great saphenous vein where the anterior accessory saphenous vein is a refluxive tributary of the refluxive great saphenous vein (Figs. 7.27 and 7.28b).

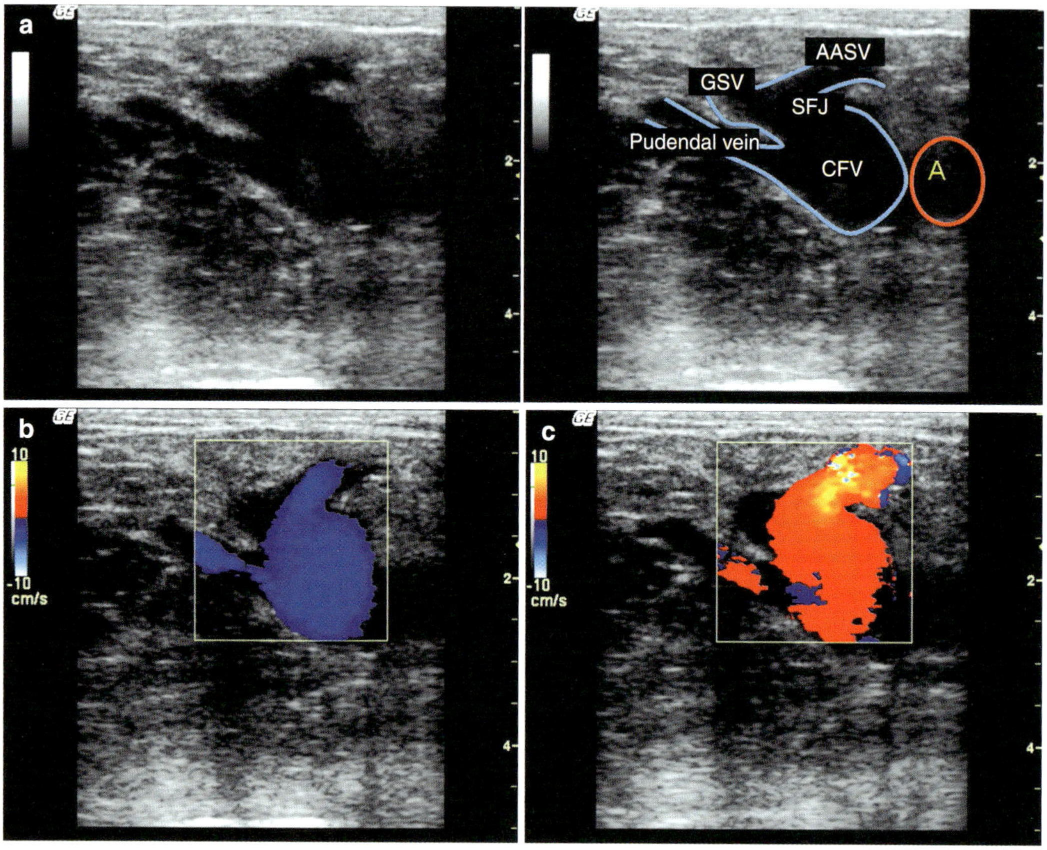

Fig. 7.26 Transverse view through the groin with an incompetent terminal valve and reflux escaping through the accessory anterior saphenous vein. This is complete incompetence of the great saphenous vein, Hach Class I. (**a**) The saphenofemoral junction (*SFJ*) is dilated to accommodate the drainage of the great saphenous vein (*GSV*) and anterior accessory saphenous vein (AAS*V*). There is an incidental finding of independent drainage of the pudendal vein (*PV*). (**b**) During muscular systole there is antegrade flow (*blue*) in the common femoral vein (*CFV*), the anterior accessory saphenous vein and pudendal vein, but no flow in the great saphenous vein. (**c**) During muscular diastole there is reflux through the saphenofemoral junction into the anterior accessory saphenous vein. There is no reflux in the lower part of the great saphenous vein (online material) Copyright: [Author]

- Reflux from the confluence of superficial inguinal veins into the anterior accessory saphenous vein without reflux of the great saphenous vein or the saphenofemoral junction (Fig. 7.28c).
- Reflux from the antegrade flow in the great saphenous vein into the anterior accessory saphenous vein. The deep veins are not involved in this type of recirculation (Fig. 7.28d).

It is important to distinguish these findings for the purposes of deciding on a treatment strategy and in making a prognosis. The prognosis is less good with reflux arising from the confluence of the superficial inguinal veins.

7.3.8 Pelvic Venous Reflux Through Franceschi's P and I Points

When there is reflux arising from within the pelvis, the blood flow escaping into the subcutaneous compartment can be observed at two points (see also Sect. 3.3.6).

The **I point** is located in a standing subject approximately 1–3 cm above and lateral to the

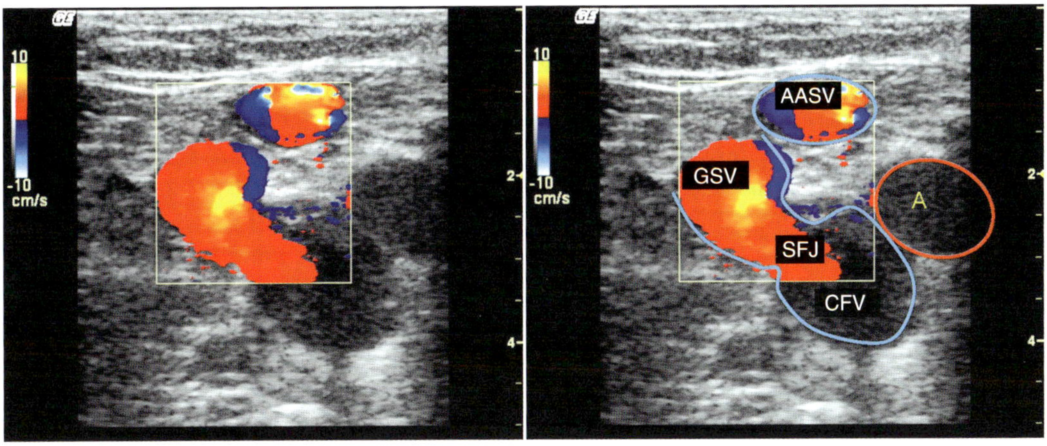

Fig. 7.27 A tortuous and dilated anterior accessory saphenous vein (*AASV*) in the groin. The saphenofemoral junction (*SFJ*) is refluxive with the reflux flowing into both the great saphenous vein (*GSV*) and the anterior accessory saphenous vein. The anterior accessory saphenous vein is so tortuous that it is already visible as an independent vessel in the image of the saphenofemoral junction. It lies lateral to the tangential line through the medial circumference of the common femoral vein (*CFV*) (see also Fig. 7.4) Copyright: [Author]

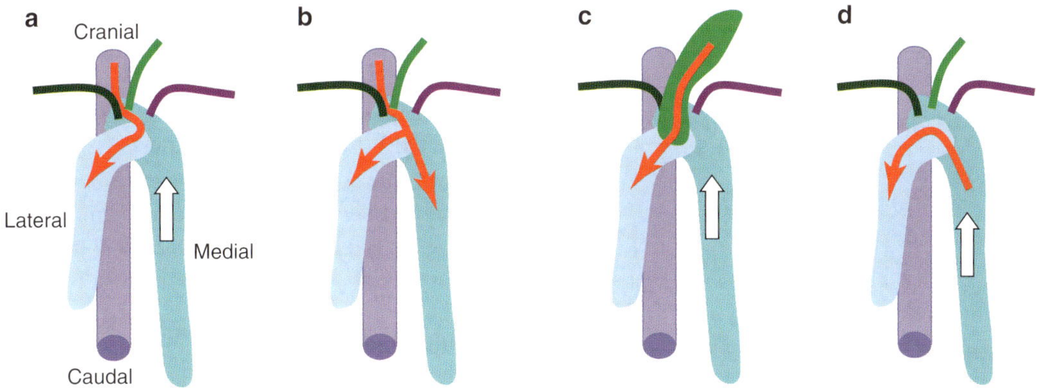

Fig. 7.28 Possible forms of reflux in the confluence of the anterior accessory saphenous vein using the right groin as an example. (**a**) Reflux (*red arrow*) from the common femoral vein through the saphenofemoral junction into the anterior accessory saphenous vein. The great saphenous vein is healthy in its further course with antegrade flow (*white arrow*). (**b**) Reflux (*red arrow*) from the common femoral vein through the saphenofemoral junction which is directed into both the anterior accessory saphenous vein and the lower part of the great saphenous vein. (**c**) Reflux (*red arrow*) from the epigastric vein which joins the anterior accessory saphenous vein directly. The great saphenous vein is healthy in its further course downwards with antegrade flow (*white arrow*). (**d**) Reflux (*red arrow*) from the great saphenous vein flowing into the anterior accessory saphenous vein. The saphenofemoral junction and great saphenous vein are competent Copyright: [Author]

saphenofemoral junction. It is medial to the epigastric veins. If the I point is incompetent, a refluxive round ligament vein will be found above the inguinal ligament in transverse view. Reflux is best observed here during the Valsalva manoeuvre. It is also present, but less obvious, using other provocation manoeuvres.

The **P point** is located in the lithotomy position with the probe applied at right angles or slightly skewed near the labia. If the P point is incompetent, it is best demonstrated during the Valsalva manoeuvre. There will be a strong reflux signal between the vaginal cavity and the ischiopubic bone (Fig. 7.29).

7.3.9 Reporting the Superficial Inguinal Veins

Examination findings can be documented on a line diagram or template during the examination and described in writing. However, recording the findings in a table is fast and easy to review. A suggested table is shown (Table 7.1).

7.3.10 Clinical Implications of Different Reflux Sources in the Groin

In the pre-ultrasound era, treatment of varicose veins was restricted to stripping of the great saphenous vein including ligation of all superficial inguinal tributaries in a crossectomy. Neovascularisation was considered to be the only cause of recurrence assuming a well-performed initial operation. The introduction of ultrasound allowed new treatment procedures to be developed.

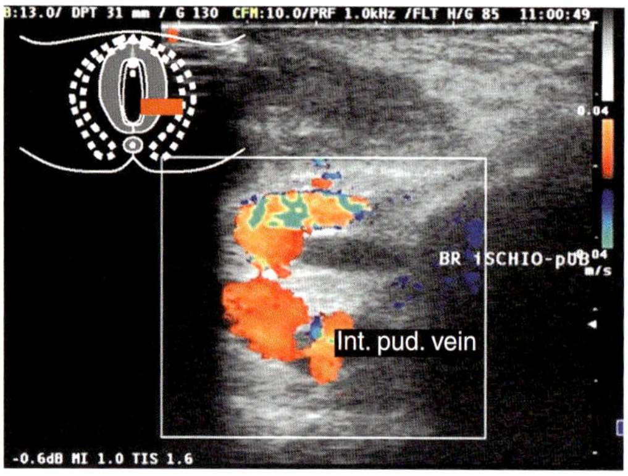

Fig. 7.29 Image showing reflux at the P point near the left labium. The probe is applied at right angles as shown in the diagram. Reflux is seen passing from the internal pudendal vein to the external pudendal vein Copyright: [Author]

In the early days of endoluminal laser ablation, the confluence of superficial inguinal veins was intentionally left unclosed. Current practice in most units is to leave with a gap of about 2 cm between the lower margin of the ostium and the tip of the laser. However, controversy remains as to the ideal placement of the laser tip with some advocates pursuing a "flush" ablation and others a more "selective" ablation. These different techniques continue because there remains a lack of an agreed definitive solution.

A post-operative ultrasound examination is able to determine the nature of recurrent veins in the groin. For example, an inflow from the epigastric veins without reflux can be distinguished from a neovascularisation wherein newly formed veins develop and connect to the common femoral vein. The former recurrence may arise when reflux from the epigastric veins existed prior to the operation and the crossectomy deprived them of a drainage route (Sects. 13.3.1 and 13.4.1). A similar situation may be seen after ligation of the confluence of superficial inguinal veins when reflux from the pelvis existed prior to the operation. These veins quickly enlarge and develop to find a connection to the distal great saphenous vein which was not initially removed. A recurrence often results (Sect. 13.3.2).

Duplex ultrasound plays an important part in the preoperative diagnosis, accurate documentation and follow-up of the groin regardless of whatever treatment was used. If the source of preoperative reflux is detected precisely in advance, then the optimum treatment for the saphenofemoral region can be selected in accordance with the drainage routes. Options may include closure of the pelvic reflux path or closure

Table 7.1 Reporting findings at the confluence of superficial inguinal veins

Vein	Number	Dilated	Refluxive	Remarks
Anterior accessory saphenous vein		Yes/no	Yes/no	
Superficial circumflex iliac vein		Yes/no	Yes/no	
Epigastric vein		Yes/no	Yes/no	
Pudendal vein		Yes/no	Yes/no	
Posterior accessory saphenous vein		Yes/no	Yes/no	

of the great saphenous vein distal to the entry point of the pudendal vein to allow drainage.

Stücker summarised the different possibilities of reflux in the groin into three types (Stücker et al. 2013):

Type 1: Incompetence of the terminal but sufficiency of the preterminal valve with reflux escaping through anterior accessory saphenous vein

Type 2: Sufficiency of the terminal but incompetent preterminal valve with reflux originating in tributaries and not in deep vein

Type 3: Incompetence of the terminal and the preterminal valve with reflux emerging from deep vein and descending along the great saphenous vein

7.4 B Scan Examination Along the Great Saphenous Vein

The anatomy of the great saphenous vein has already been described (Sects. 2.4.1, 2.4.2, 2.4.3, 2.4.4, and 2.4.5). The great saphenous vein is generally examined starting at the groin and going down to the foot.

The subject should be standing with the majority of their weight on the contralateral leg whilst holding onto a frame for light support. The test leg should be dependent, slightly externally rotated with the foot lightly resting on the floor and pointing laterally (Fig. 7.1). As a matter of routine, once the superficial inguinal tributaries have been identified and assessed (Sect. 7.3), a **compression manoeuvre** should be carried out on the saphenofemoral junction and the deep veins to exclude thrombosis (Fig. 7.30).

The diameter of the great saphenous vein is often measured to check if the vein is incompetent and for study purposes. The UIP (Union Internationale de Phlebologie) consensus document suggests measuring the vein at the saphenofemoral junction or within the first 3 cm of the great saphenous vein and in the middle of the thigh (Coleridge-Smith et al. 2006). However, these recommendations have not been validated by studies.

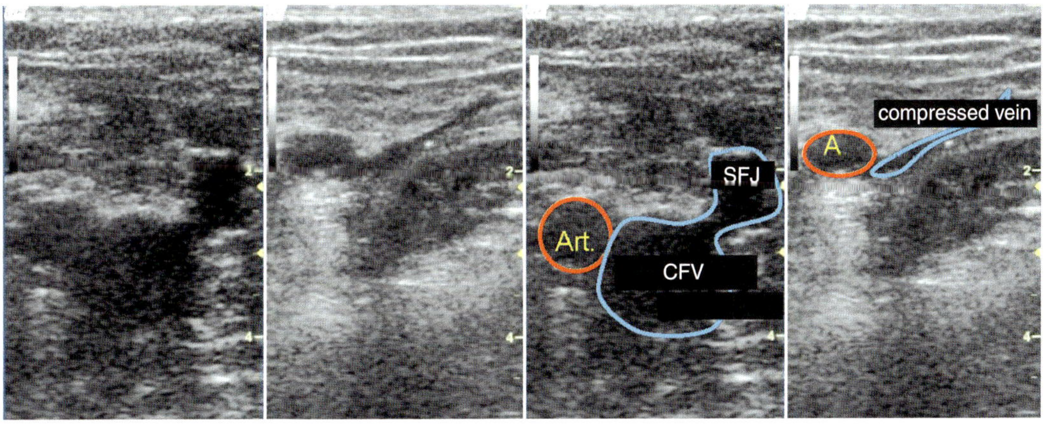

Fig. 7.30 Compression manoeuvre in the groin. Transverse view of the right groin in a standing subject. The *first* image shows the normal state of the saphenofemoral junction (*SFJ*) and the *second* image the appearances during compression with the probe. The artery is slightly squashed (*A*) during compression, but the common femoral vein (*CFV*) and saphenofemoral junction (*SFJ*) become a narrow slit Copyright: [Author]

Optimum Point for Measuring the Diameter of the Great Saphenous Vein

Current data suggest a second measurement point in the proximal thigh 10–15 cm from the groin (Fig. 7.31, see also Fig. 7.1). In a population of 182 legs, the diameter of the great saphenous vein was measured in the standing subject 2–3 cm and also 10–15 cm below the saphenofemoral junction. Sixty legs had a healthy great saphenous vein, and 122 presented with reflux beginning in the groin. Fifty-one of these were refluxive above the knee only (Hach Class II), and 71 were refluxive above and below the knee (Hach Class III and IV). The diameter did not correlate with age or sex at either measurement point. Correlations were found with weight, moderate correlations between the diameter and the clinical class of CEAP, as well as the refilling time. Although a high correlation was found between the diameters at the groin and in the thigh, the predictive value of the diameter in the proximal thigh was better for the presence of reflux and the clinical class. The great saphenous vein at the proximal thigh was more uniform, easier to measure and more representative as a single measurement point.

The average diameter in subjects with healthy veins was 7.5 mm (±1.8) at the saphenofemoral junction and 3.7 mm (±0.9) in the proximal thigh. In subjects with reflux, the average diameter was 10.9 mm (±3.9) at the saphenofemoral junction and 6.3 mm (±1.9) in the proximal thigh. The diameter did not correlate with the Hach Class (Mendoza et al. 2013).

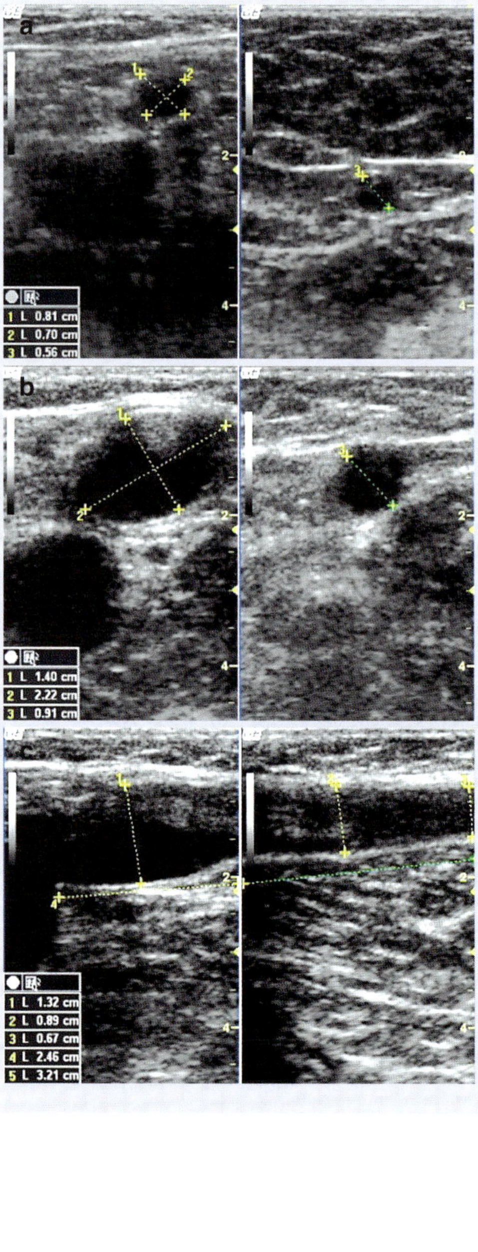

Fig. 7.31 Diameter measurements in the great saphenous vein. (**a**) Transverse views through the right groin (*left half of image*) and the thigh 10–15 cm below the groin (*right half of image*) in a normal subject. The great saphenous vein was measured at both points. The diameter in the groin was 0.81 or 0.7 cm depending on which axis was taken. In the thigh it was smaller at 0.56 cm. **b**: Transverse view through the right groin in a patient with venous insufficiency. The great saphenous vein is elliptical in shape. Gross differences in the measurements were obtained depending on the axis taken (1.4–2.2 cm). The diameter at the thigh was significantly smaller at 0.9 cm. **c**: Longitudinal view through the course of the proximal great saphenous vein. The left and right halves of the image show the great saphenous vein in continuity. A uniform and reliable measurement point is difficult to obtain because of the progressive reduction in the calibre of the great saphenous vein Copyright: [Author]

Diameter measurements should be taken in a transverse image. It remains controversial whether the probe should be at right angles to the skin or diagonal in position. As shown in Fig. 7.31, the variability demonstrated at the saphenofemoral junction measurement point, the preferred point chosen by most phlebologists, is so great that this is unlikely to provide meaningful information. For studies it is important always to use the same method of measurement and to describe this method exactly.

For the reasons mentioned above, it is preferable to measure the diameter in the thigh, 10–15 cm from the groin, in a segment where the walls of the great saphenous vein run parallel and there are neither inflows nor outflows. The ideal probe position is at about the height of the yellow line in Fig. 7.1.

Interval compression manoeuvres in B scan should be performed to exclude a thrombosis along the course of the great saphenous vein (see also Chap. 11). Furthermore, the **course of the vein** within its fascia (Sect. 7.4.1) and any **aplastic/hypoplastic** (Sect. 7.4.2) or **duplications** (Sect. 7.4.3) should be identified at this stage of the examination.

The great saphenous vein should be examined over its entire course in transverse view so that tributaries and perforating veins are not overlooked. **Variations in calibre** must always be examined with care. In such cases it is important to check for reflux in the distal segment after the separation of a refluxive tributary. The smaller calibre great saphenous vein below a refluxive tributary is frequently competent; however, this is not necessarily always the case.

7.4.1 Saphenous Eye

Bailly proposed the term "saphenous eye" for the typical appearance of the great saphenous vein in the thigh and calf in transverse view (Bailly 1992 in Appendix 2). The eye consists of the muscle fascia (lower lid), saphenous fascia (upper lid) and the great saphenous vein itself, representing the iris and pupil (Figs. 7.32 and 7.33). The saphenous fascia lies directly on or just above the great saphenous vein. Occasionally a thin additional fascia can be seen in the subcutaneous fatty tissue (Figs. 7.34a and 7.36). This fascia if present separates the subcutaneous tissue into two layers and runs parallel to the muscle fascia.

If the upper and lower lid of the saphenous eye cannot be identified in association with a vein in transverse view, it is not the great saphenous vein. Any tortuous structure visible from the exterior is a tributary. The great saphenous vein is straight and cannot become tortuous within its fascial compartment because it is anchored by the saphenous ligament and surrounding connective tissue. Tortuous and dilated veins are always tributaries. This difference is very important for establishing the **Hach Class** (Sect. 4.1).

To the novice examiner, refluxive **tributaries** may be taken for the great saphenous vein if they appear to be straight downward continuations (Fig. 7.34).

7.4.2 Aplasia/Hypoplasia of the Great Saphenous Vein

An aplastic or hypoplastic segment of the great saphenous vein is found in 12 % of subjects with healthy veins and 24 % of those with refluxive great saphenous veins (Sect. 2.4.4). A straight or tortuous tributary runs parallel to this aplastic segment in the subcutaneous tissue carrying the blood from distal to enter the patent proximal part of great saphenous vein (or vice versa if there is reflux). In aplastic segments the saphenous eye appears "empty" (Fig. 7.35). However, if the empty saphenous eye is studied histologically, a rudimentary saphenous vein is always found. In case of very thin saphenous vein, many phlebologists use the term hypoplastic (Sect. 2.6.3).

7.4.3 Duplication of the Great Saphenous Vein

As described above (Sect. 2.4.3), only those veins which course through the saphenous compartment can be defined as saphenous veins. Thus,

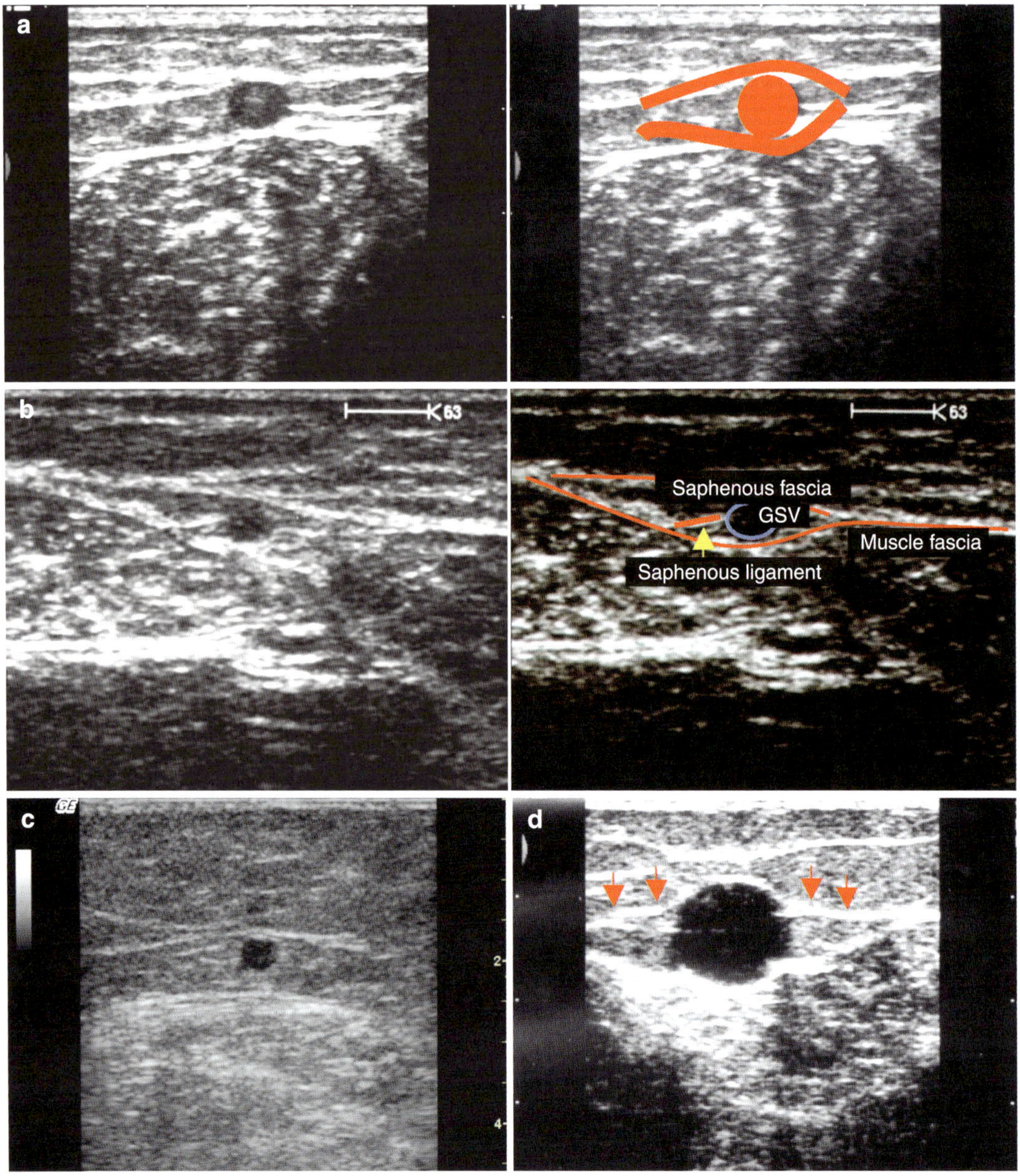

Fig. 7.32 Variations of the saphenous eye in the thigh. (**a**) Transverse view through the inner thigh with normal appearance of the saphenous eye. (**b**) The appearance may be asymmetrical depending on the level of the section and the fat content of the leg. (**c**) When the fat content is high, there may be a space between the lower lid and the iris. If the saphenous compartment is filled with fat, the great saphenous vein (*GSV*) does not lie directly on the muscle fascia. (**d**) If the great saphenous vein is refluxive, the iris will appear very big. In this image the connective tissue anchoring the great saphenous vein, the saphenous ligament (*arrowed*), is very clear Copyright: [Author]

there is only a duplication when both the branches run parallel inside this compartment. **True duplication** is found in 1 % of subjects (Fig. 7.36). A tributary running through the subcutaneous fatty tissue parallel to the great saphenous vein is found in the thigh of 26 % of legs. This is a pseudo duplication, Fig. 7.37. In subjects with healthy veins, the lumen of this accompanying vein is often larger than that of the great saphenous vein itself. In phlebography there was no way of distinguishing whether the course of a vein is intrafascial or extrafascial. Consequently,

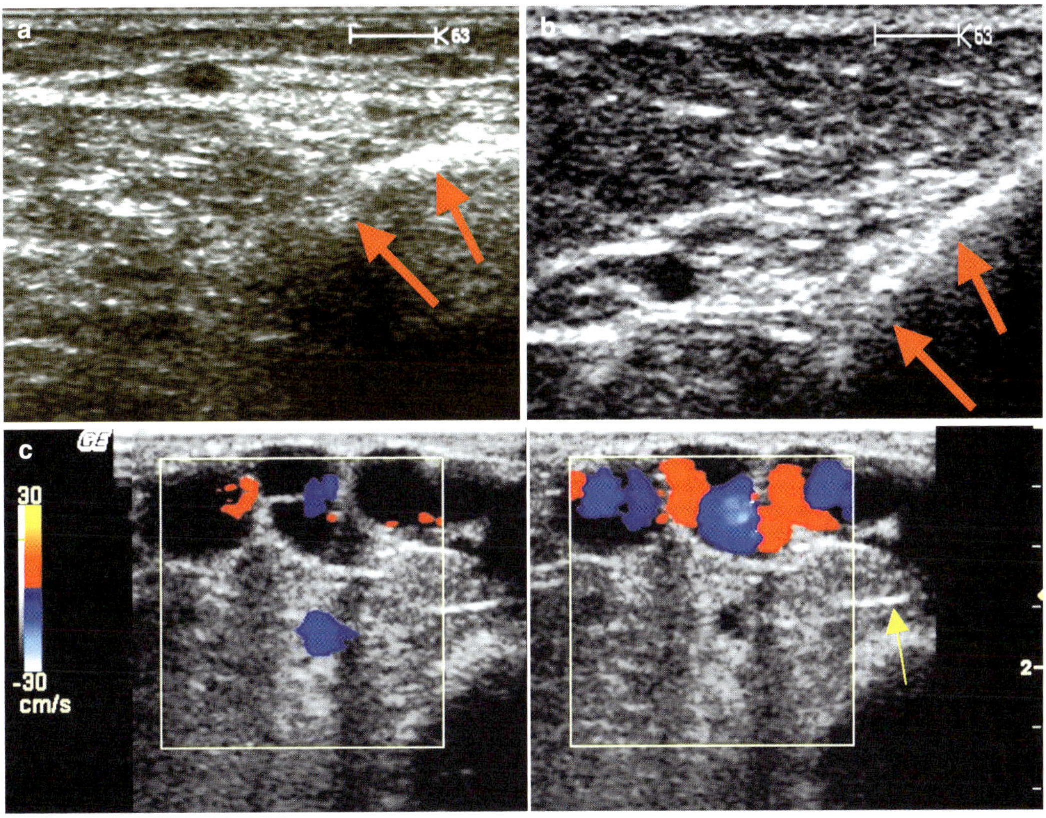

Fig. 7.33 The saphenous eye in the lower leg. (**a**) Transverse view through the left calf, approximately10 cm below the posterior skin crease of the knee. The saphenous eye is harder to identify in the calf, because there is much less fat in this region. The edge of the tibia is on the *right* of the image (*arrows*). (**b**) It is difficult to distinguish the eye clearly from the surrounding tissue in the calf as demonstrated in the left leg of an obese subject. The tibial edge is *arrowed*. (**c**) In the calf the fascial compartment helps in differentiating between the saphenous vein and the tributaries. The *left* image shows a refluxive tributary and great saphenous vein in muscular systole. There is antegrade flow in the great saphenous vein (*blue*). The *right* image is during muscular diastole. There is no flow in the great saphenous vein, but the tributaries are filled refluxively. The fascia is just discernible in the lateral part of the compartment to the right of the colour window immediately above the tibial edge (*arrowed*) Copyright: [Author]

pseudo and true duplications were classified together which increased the frequency of a duplicate system to 27 % (Sect. 2.4.3).

If the great saphenous vein is refluxive, this does not necessarily mean that both limbs of a duplication are refluxive (Fig. 7.38).

7.4.4 Course of the Great Saphenous Vein

The great saphenous vein appears on ultrasound medial to the confluence of the superficial inguinal veins. In disease it is a large vessel coming up from the thigh (Fig. 7.39). The greatest volume of antegrade flow will be observed during provocation manoeuvres. Occasionally the great saphenous vein in the groin can be situated in a medial or lateral position which may cause confusion with the anterior or posterior accessory saphenous veins (Fig. 7.40; see also Sects. 10.4 and 10.5).

There are several ways of confirming the identity of the great saphenous vein:

- If the probe is passed to and fro along the **inner thigh** in transverse view, the saphenous eye will always be found whether “filled” or “empty” Figs. 7.32 and 7.35). In the distal thigh, there

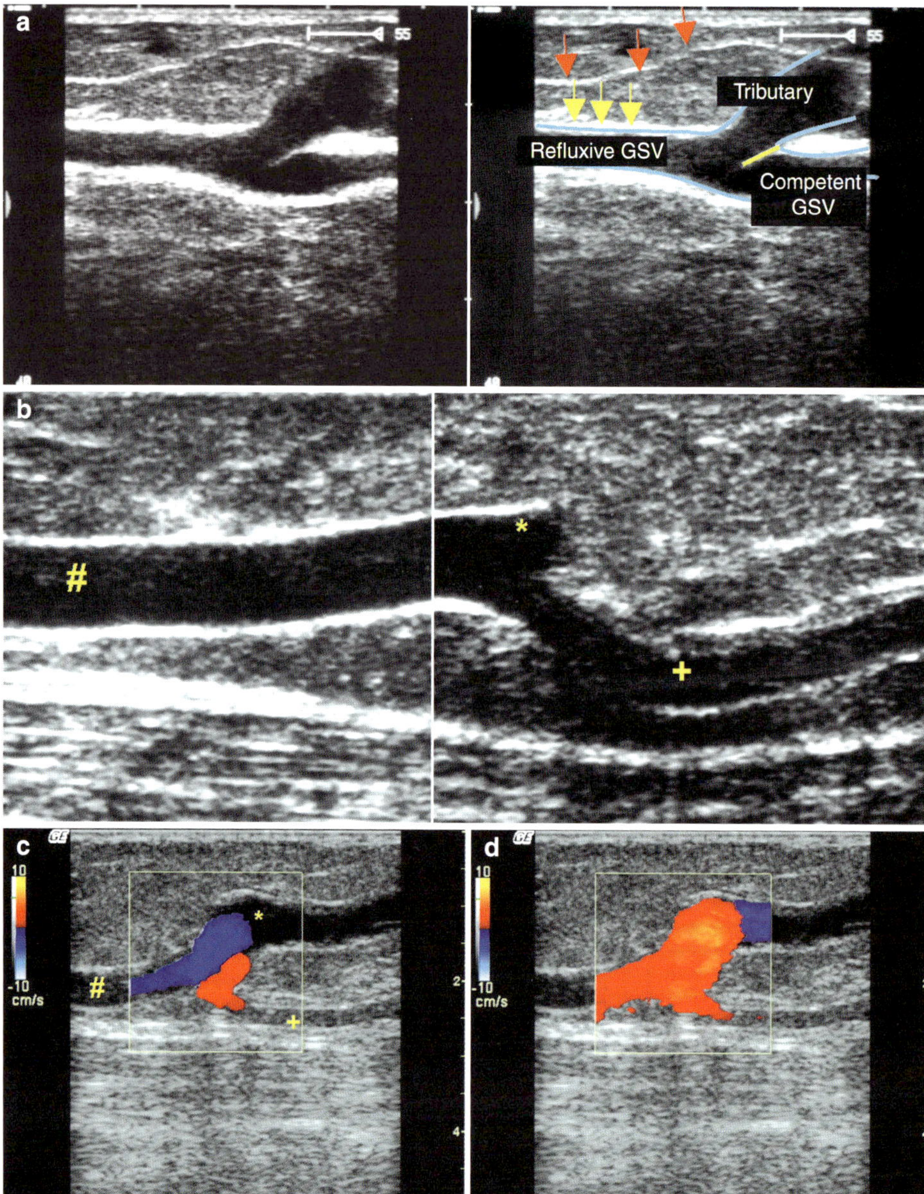

Fig. 7.34 Junction of the great saphenous vein in continuity with a tributary. (**a**) Longitudinal view through the inner thigh. The axes of the proximal (refluxive) and distal (competent) great saphenous vein (*GSV*) usually run in a straight line as shown. The tributary comes off at an angle of varying degrees. A valve leaflet is visible at the junction of the tributary with the great saphenous vein (marked in *yellow*). The sharp white contour of the great saphenous vein is prominent because it represents a thick vein wall. The tributary in contrast has a thin wall which is much less apparent (saphenous fascia *yellow arrows*, subcutaneous fascia *red arrows*). (**b**) Longitudinal view through the inner thigh demonstrating a refluxive great saphenous vein (#) in continuity with a refluxive tributary (*). Its further course disappears from the right of the image because it becomes tortuous. The great saphenous vein itself is competent (+) more distal. The large calibre of the great saphenous vein and associated tributary gives the false impression that the distal great saphenous vein is a tributary because it forms an angle with the axis. (**c**) Another patient demonstrating the junction of the great saphenous vein with a straight continuation of a tributary. During muscular systole there is antegrade flow in all veins. The great saphenous vein is tented up towards the skin, making the antegrade flow in the distal section of the vein appear red because the flow here is towards the probe. The tributary is dilated. (**d**) During muscular diastole there is gross reflux into the dilated tributary and antegrade flow in the distal great saphenous vein (online material) Copyright: [Author]

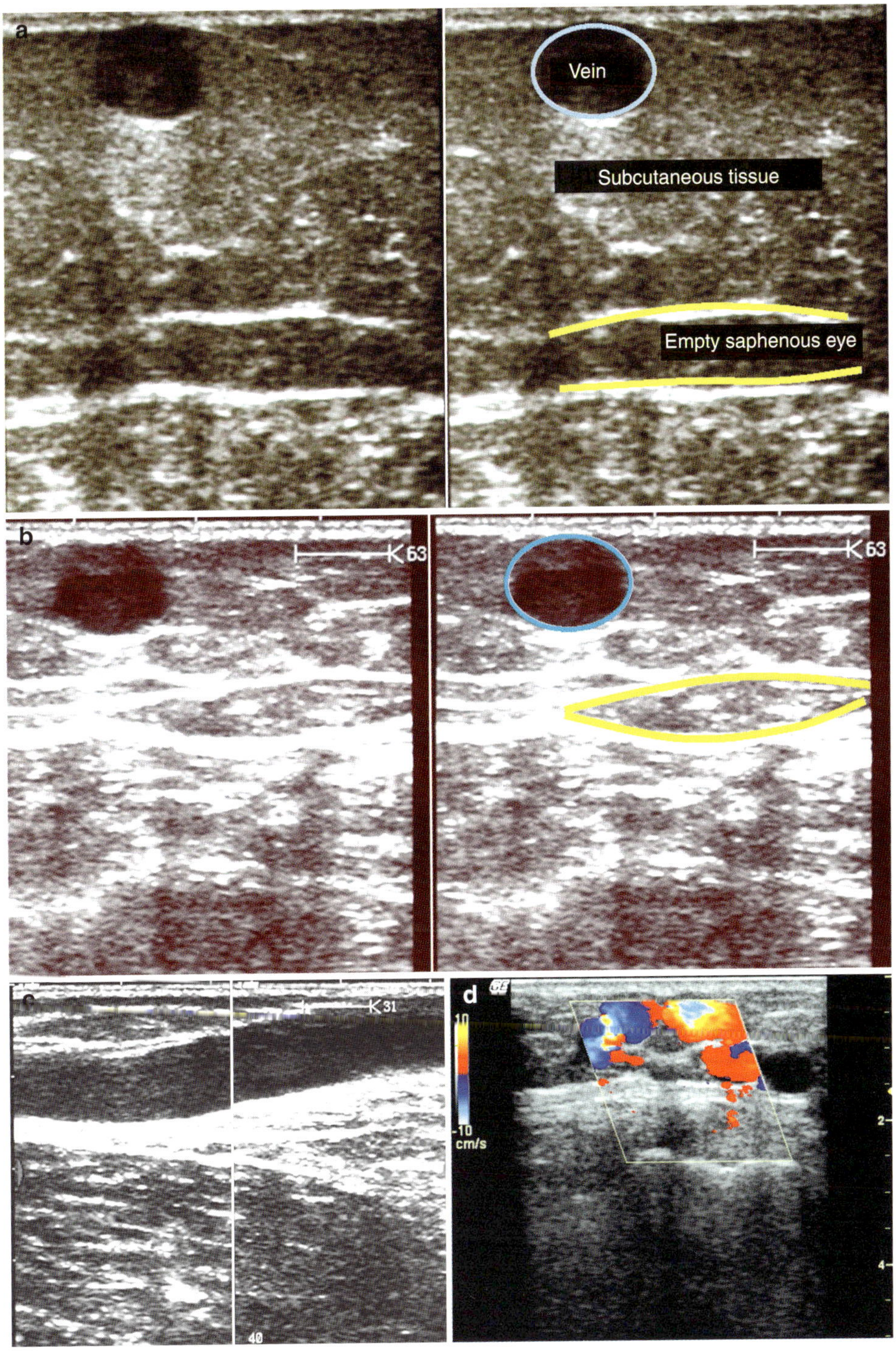

Fig. 7.35 Aplastic segment of the great saphenous vein. (**a**) An "empty" saphenous eye in the thigh with a dilated tributary directly under the skin. (**b**) With less fatty tissue the "eye" is smaller. Transverse view above the aplastic segment demonstrating the junction of the great saphenous vein with the extrafascial tributary is seen on the online material. (**c**) Longitudinal view in the same leg at the point where the tributary leaves the saphenous compartment. No visible vein remains within this saphenous compartment. (**d**) Longitudinal view though the distal thigh in colour duplex demonstrating a very short aplastic segment. The reflux bypasses the aplastic segment of the refluxive great saphenous vein (*arrowed*) by running above the vein in a tributary for a short distance. It then rejoins the great saphenous vein further down. A competent great saphenous vein with an aplastic segment is shown on the online material Copyright: [Author]

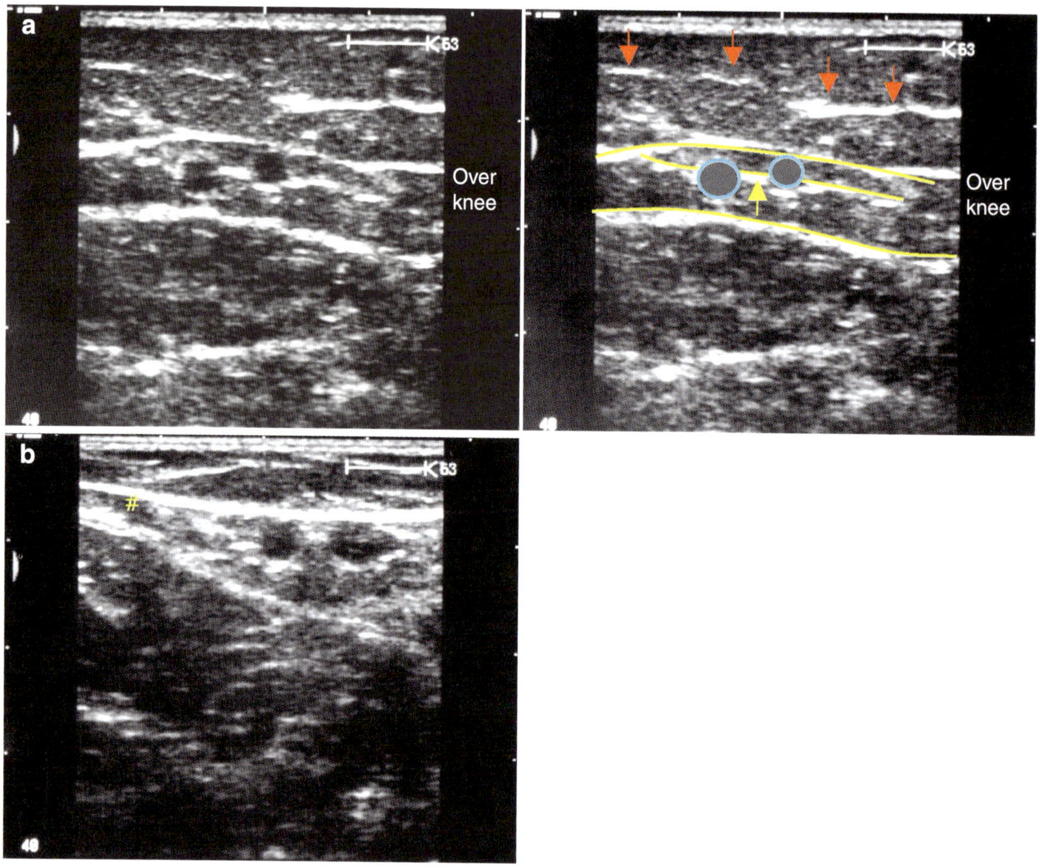

Fig. 7.36 Subject with a true duplication of the great saphenous vein in the right leg starting 3 cm below the saphenofemoral junction down to the posterior knee crease. (**a**) Transverse view just above the knee with both great saphenous veins in close proximity. The saphenous ligament (*yellow arrow*) connects the two veins. An additional layer of connective tissue is visible within the subcutaneous fat (*red arrows*) online material. (**b**) Transverse view approximately 10 cm below the groin in the same subject. The saphenous compartment contains both great saphenous veins. Further lateral an anterior accessory saphenous vein is apparent (#). The online material contains two more images of the same subject at the mid and distal thigh. The two veins are slightly further apart at these points but are still within the same compartment and connected together by the saphenous ligament Copyright: [Author]

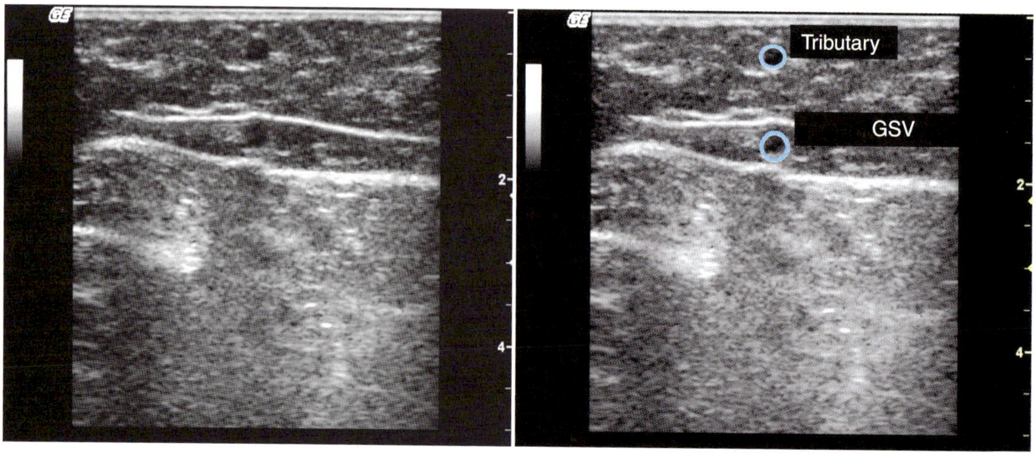

Fig. 7.37 Pseudo duplication of the great saphenous vein. Transverse view through the thigh. A second vein is seen running parallel to the great saphenous vein within the subcutaneous fat. This is a straight tributary accompanying the great saphenous vein (online material) Copyright: [Author]

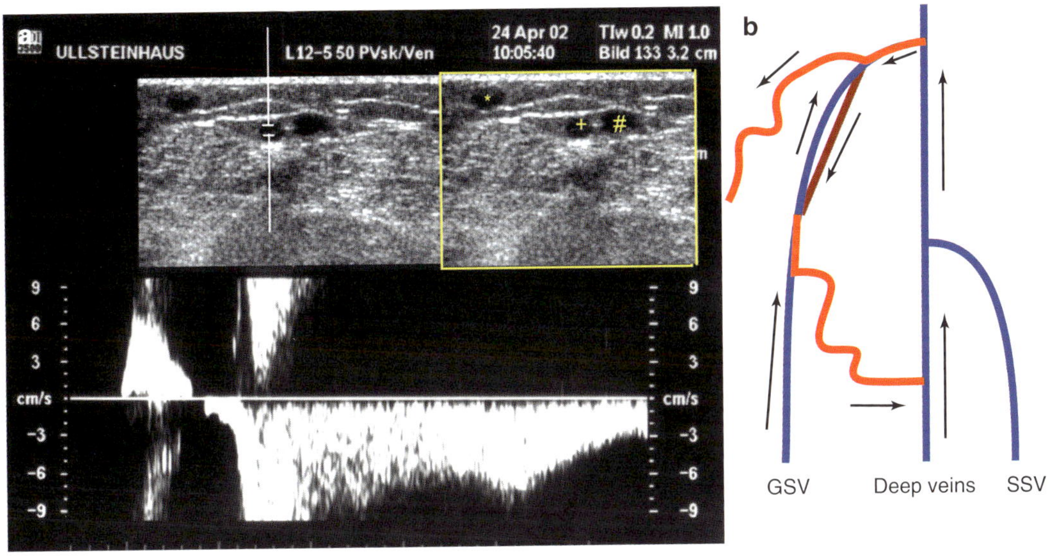

Fig. 7.38 (**a**) Transverse view through the inner thigh demonstrating a duplication of the great saphenous vein (*GSV*) in the saphenous compartment with an accompanying tributary (*). The right vessel of the duplication (#) and the tributary are refluxive (online material). The left vessel (+) is competent (▶ velocity profile at bottom). As the refluxive vessel joins the competent vessel further down, it delivers its reflux into the competent vessel provoking a permanent antegrade flow. That means that blood flow is antegrade in the competent vessel during muscular diastole (*right* B scan unmarked, *left* B scan marked). (**b**) Diagram of the recirculation circuit. The refluxive vessel of the duplication is shown dark *red* (*SSV* small saphenous vein) Copyright: [Author]

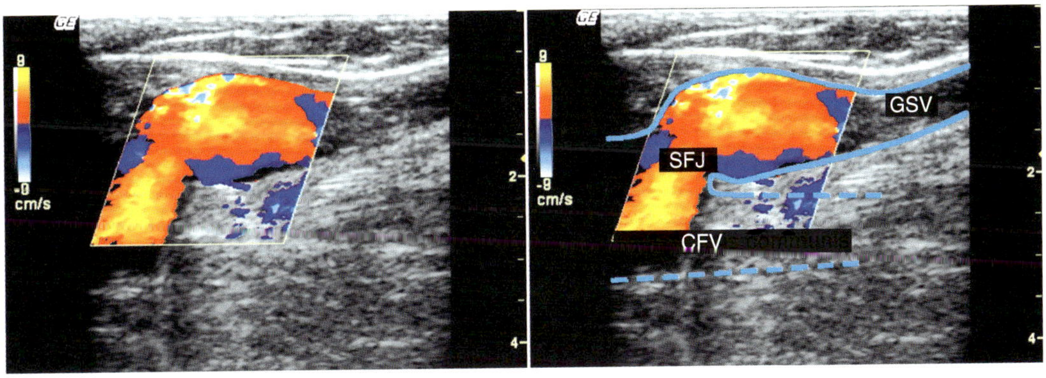

Fig. 7.39 Longitudinal view of the normal course of the great saphenous vein (*GSV*) in the groin in a patient with an incompetent terminal valve. During muscular diastole turbulent flow from the common femoral vein (*CFV*) is seen entering the great saphenous vein via the saphenofemoral junction (*SFJ*). The common femoral vein is marked with *blue dotted lines* because it leaves the plane of this image Copyright: [Author]

may be a palpable fascial defect which can be felt as a "hole" in the tissue. This is often assumed to be the point where a perforating vein passes through the musculature. However, in B scan it can be seen that this is incorrect. The vein at this point is usually either uniformly dilated (Fig. 7.41a) or demonstrates a focal dilatation along one side of the wall (Fig. 7.41b, c).

- The great saphenous vein is always posterior to the medial condyle of the knee (Fig. 7.48a).
- One to two hand's breadths below the knee, the great saphenous vein is always found between the **tibial edge** and the extensor hallucis longus muscle (Fig. 7.33a–c).
- At the ankle the great saphenous vein lies on or is slightly anterior to the medial malleolus

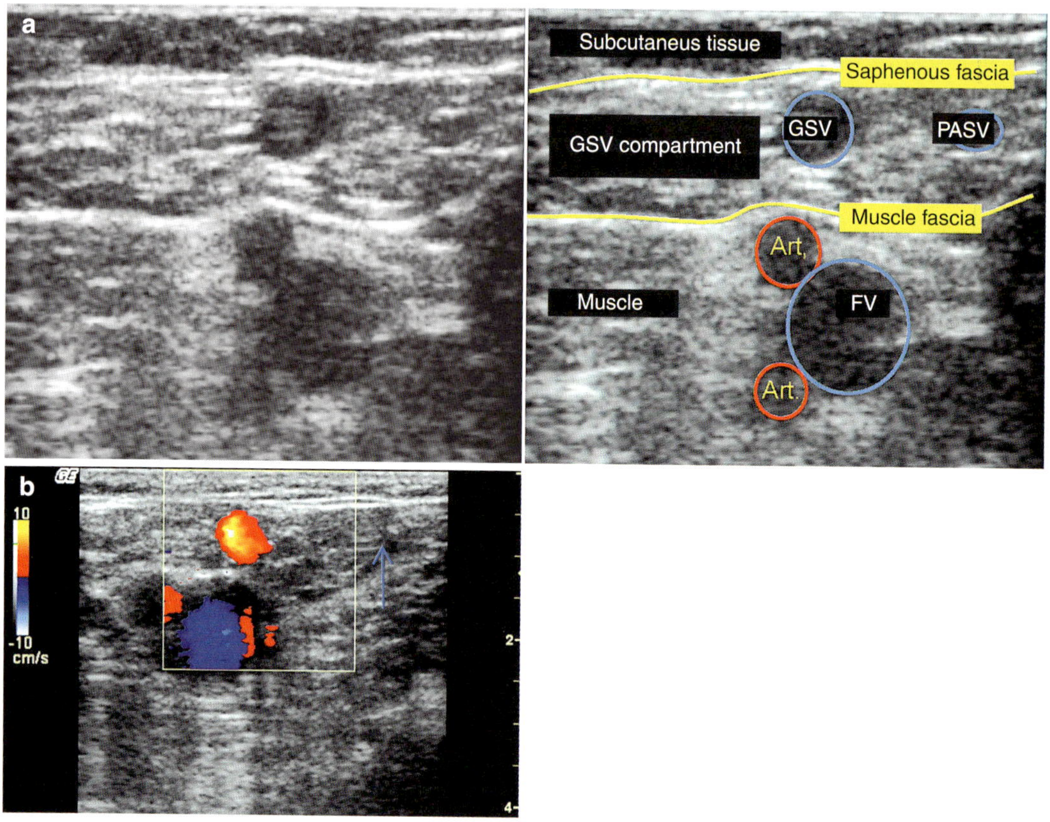

Fig. 7.40 (**a**) Transverse view through the right groin just below the saphenofemoral junction. A large vein is observed in a lateral position with a smaller less defined vein further medial. The classic assumption would be that the anterior accessory saphenous vein is incompetent (see also Fig. 7.10b) and the great saphenous vein is healthy. With further assessment of the course of the veins, it becomes apparent (online material) that the refluxive vein running laterally in the groin is the great saphenous vein (*GSV*) and the medial competent vein is the posterior accessory saphenous vein (*VSAP*). (**b**) Transverse view through the same leg further proximal in colour duplex. The lateral vein is refluxive (*red*), the much smaller medial vein (*arrow*) is not (*no signal on colour duplex*) Copyright: [Author]

(Fig. 2.5). This is difficult to demonstrate using ultrasound because the contact area of the probe is minimal. If this area is followed up the leg, the great saphenous should be found a few centimetres above the ankle.

Despite a systematic examination, a great saphenous vein along its typical course may not be identified in some subjects. This happens occasionally after the subject has been standing for some time (Fig. 7.42). In these subjects erythrocyte sludge may settle in the vein filling it with a homogeneous grey colour instead of a black void. This is difficult to differentiate from the surrounding tissue. There are various ways of "clearing" the vein to return it to its echo-free state. These include vein compression with the probe, manual calf compression or the Wunstorf manoeuvre. The main objective is to create flow in the vein to "flush out" the erythrocytes.

7.5 Measuring Blood Flow Along the Great Saphenous Vein

Duplex ultrasound offers two ways of measuring blood flow in the great saphenous vein. These are PW (velocity profile analysis) and colour-coded duplex. In contrast to the arteries veins are collapsible tubes without a regular pump from behind. This makes consistent velocity measurements difficult to obtain. Therefore, a **semi-quantitative evaluation** of the velocity

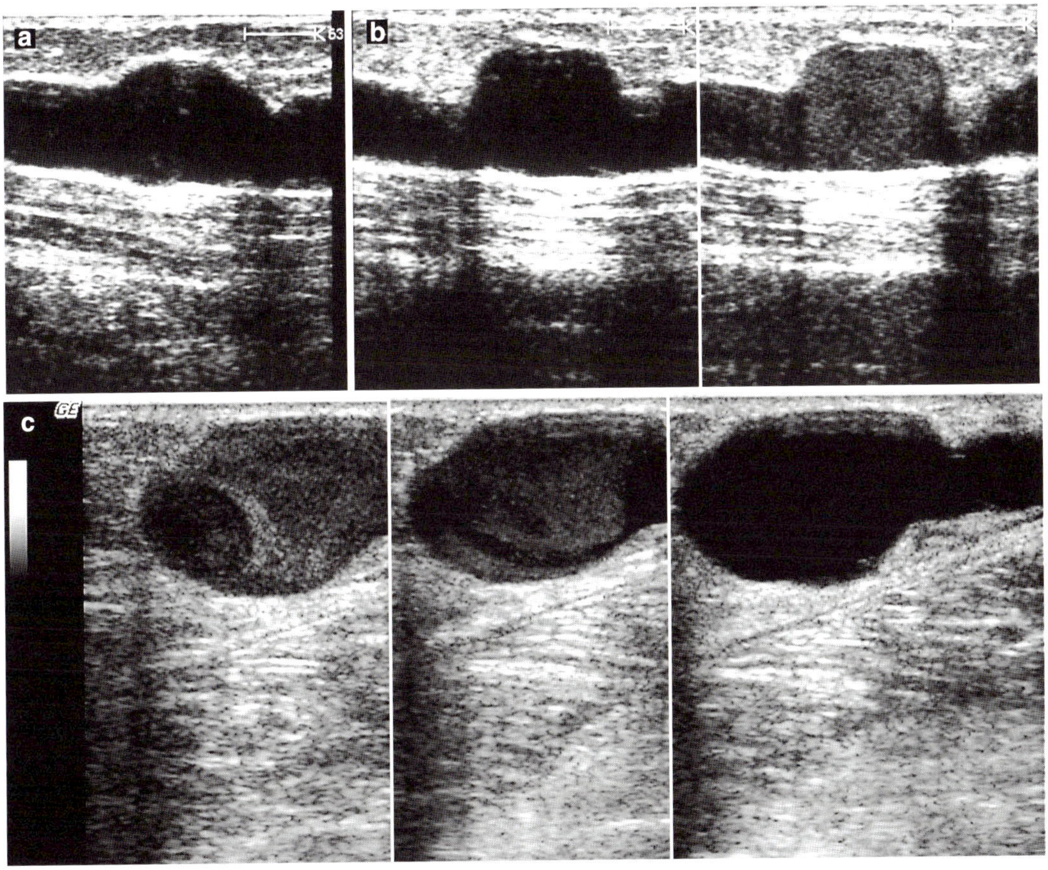

Fig. 7.41 Image of a dilated section of the great saphenous vein in the distal thigh. (**a**) Longitudinal view through the inner thigh just above the knee demonstrating a dilation of the great saphenous vein. A perforating vein in this region cannot be identified. (**b**) Longitudinal view in the distal thigh showing the great saphenous vein and a very marked bulge (*left*) which fills with erythrocyte sludge if the subject stands still for a few seconds (*right*). Note the increasing prominence of the acoustic shadow (objects in B scan, Chap. 1). (**c**) Longitudinal view through the distal thigh in a different subject with erythrocyte sludge in an aneurysmally dilated region of the great saphenous vein. *Left* after the subject has been standing still, *middle* with extension of the toes, *right* after muscular diastole Copyright: [Author]

profile is all that is usually possible (Fig. 1.20). The angle of insonation in relation to the course of the vein is not as important as it is with arteries.

7.5.1 Normal Findings

In a standing subject, the great saphenous vein has a poor, hardly measurable, upward flow. Therefore, a **provocation manoeuvre** will be required to assess flow in this vein (Fig. 7.43a, b; see also Chap. 6).

Muscle contraction of the calf (Wunstorf manoeuvre) or a manual calf compression is sometimes insufficient to provoke adequate flow

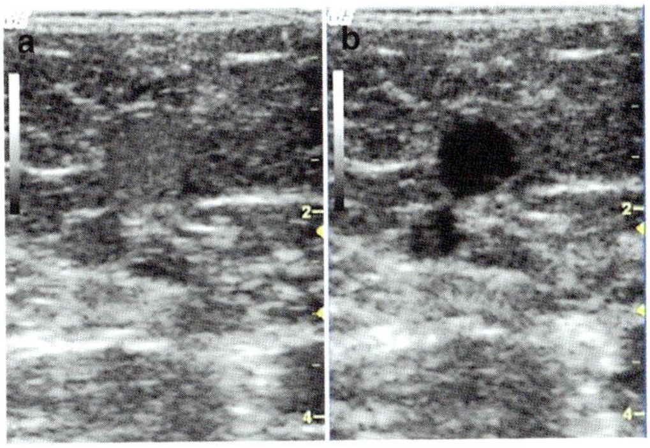

Fig. 7.42 (**a**) Transverse view through the inner thigh demonstrating an almost invisible great saphenous vein. The erythrocyte sludge has eliminated the contrast between the vein and the surrounding tissue. The accompanying tributary could be easily overlooked. (**b**) After the Wunstorf manoeuvre, both the great saphenous vein and a refluxive tributary are clearly visible Copyright: [Author]

in a healthy great saphenous vein. This is because the blood leaves the great saphenous vein partially or completely through perforating veins before it reaches the probe (Fig. 7.43b). To measure flow in the proximal thigh, both methods (muscle contraction and manual compression) should therefore be used (Fig. 7.43a, b). Manual compression of the thigh immediately distal of the probe is a useful complement. In healthy veins **antegrade flow** is observed. The velocity profile is down and away from the probe in PW (Fig. 7.43a, b) On colour duplex the vein is coloured blue (Fig. 7.43c). This antegrade flow may be followed by a short backflow. This is represented in PW as a short upward curve (Fig. 7.43a, b). On colour duplex there is a flicker of red (Fig. 7.43c).

This short backflow is caused by gravity. The blood flows back under the force of gravity until the **valve closes**. Additionally, as has been reported by Lurie and Kistner, B mode has demonstrated a vortex effect in the sinus of the valve that actually initiates closure of the valve during antegrade flow. Then, retrograde flow of a small volume is necessary to approximate and push the valve cusps back into the lumen thereby closing the valve (Lurie et al. 2003).

Measuring the **diameter** alone is not enough to judge whether a vein is competent or incompetent.

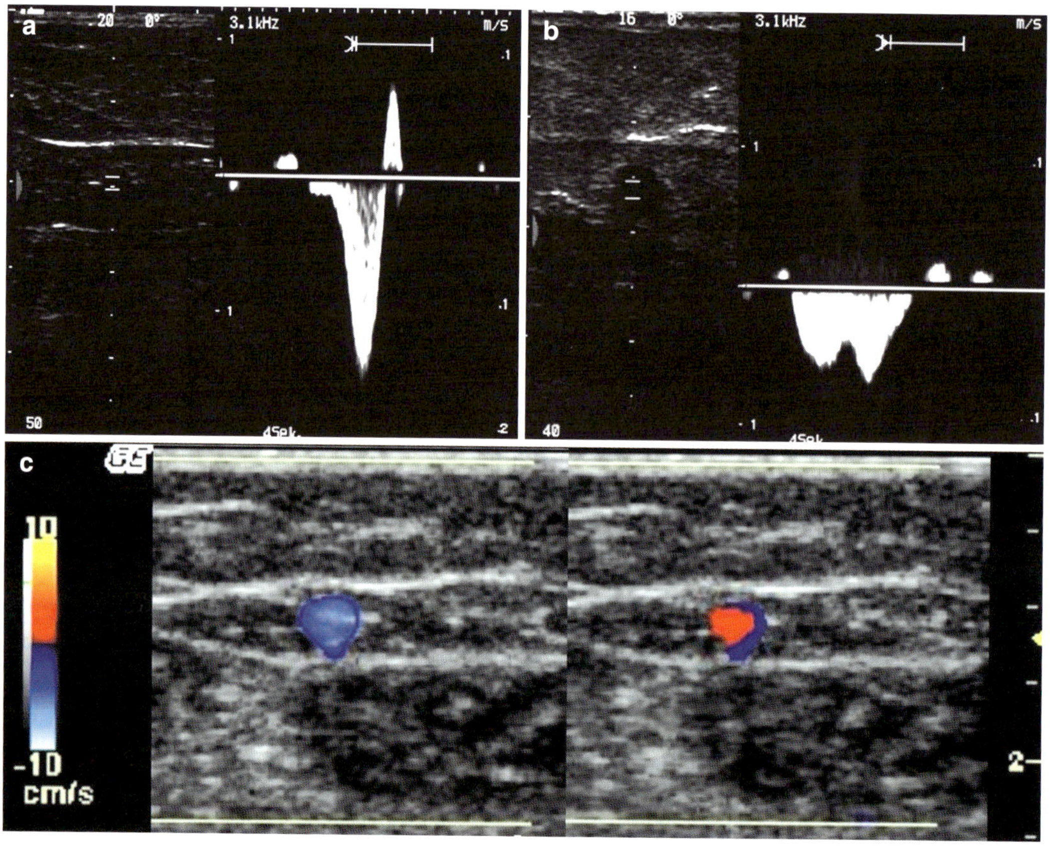

Fig. 7.43 The antegrade volume flow generated by a provocation manoeuvre varies in every subject. (**a**) PW measurement in the great saphenous vein 10 cm below the groin during a manual calf compression and release manoeuvre. (**b**) The same measurement during a Wunstorf manoeuvre. The flow in this case is more prolonged. (**c**) Colour duplex image in the great saphenous vein 10 cm below the groin; *left* under a Wunstorf manoeuvre, the flow is antegrade (*blue*). After the toes are relaxed, there is a short change of colour to red (*right*), corresponding to the short backflow until the valve closes. (**d**) A large 6.1 mm diameter competent great saphenous vein in the thigh shown with colour duplex. (**e**) Measurement of the same vein in PW mode demonstrating antegrade flow with a short backflow. (**f**) Reflux in the great saphenous vein in the thigh in a vein of only 3.5 mm in diameter Copyright: [Author]

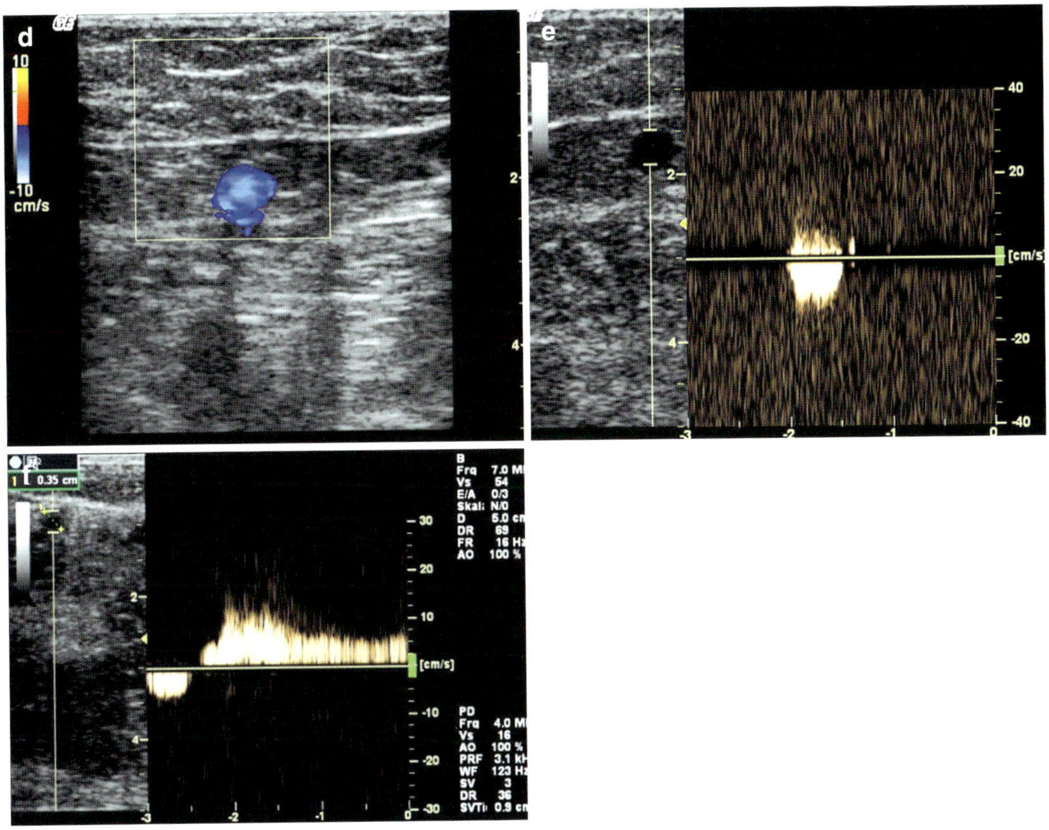

Fig. 7.43 (continued)

It is not unusual for large calibre veins to be competent (Fig. 7.43d, e) and very small calibre veins to be refluxive (Fig. 7.43f). Special attention must be paid to large calibre veins with exclusively or predominantly antegrade flow, especially during muscular diastole. This may indicate a secondary dilation due to deep venous obstruction (Chap. 15).

In the absence of visible varices, a competent saphenofemoral junction may give a false reassurance of normality with the temptation not to examine the rest of the veins. Even in the absence of significant perforating veins or tributaries in B scan, the flow patterns should still be examined at various points. As a **minimum requirement**, the great saphenous vein should be assessed at the following points:

- The point at which the diameter was measured (10–15 cm below the groin)
- The distal thigh at the level of the perforating veins of the adductor canal (formerly Dodd and Hunter)
- Below the knee at the height of the paratibial perforating veins (formerly Boyd)
- Just above the ankle

Occasionally the great saphenous vein forms part of a recirculation circuit without being filled itself in retrograde flow. In this situation it may be filled with refluxive blood from a perforating vein or tributary where it carries this blood in antegrade flow to a refluxive tributary further up the leg. In B scan an increase in diameter is observed with the velocity profile showing antegrade flow during both systole and diastole, usually with a much larger volume flow in diastole (Fig. 9.10). This condition is called **antegrade incompetence**.

7.5.2 Reflux in the Great Saphenous Vein

When a subject with an incompetent great saphenous vein is standing, antegrade flow during a provocation manoeuvre will be followed by **reflux**. Usually there is a greater volume of refluxive blood than that observed in antegrade flow. The reflux may be short and rapid (Fig. 7.44a) or slow and long-lasting (Fig. 7.44b), or a combination of these two extremes (Fig. 7.44c). In colour duplex the reflux appears as a red colour in the lumen (Fig. 7.44c, d). If the curve in PW duplex disappears after the short, necessary backflow for valve closure, it is easy to stop observing and overlook a low-volume reflux which continues for much longer (Fig. 7.45).

The reflux volume is the blood volume which first flows upwards during a provocation manoeuvre and then flows down again during the relaxation phase of the manoeuvre (Chap. 3). By the definition from the international consensus document (Coleridge-Smith et al. 2006), the retrograde flow must last at least between 0.5 and 1 s before it can be regarded as reflux. The clinical importance of reflux between 0.5 and 1 s has never been fully assessed in a study. It may be sensible to use the 1 s cut-off point to define pathology because shorter flows often correlate with reflux volumes which are very small with questionable clinical significance.

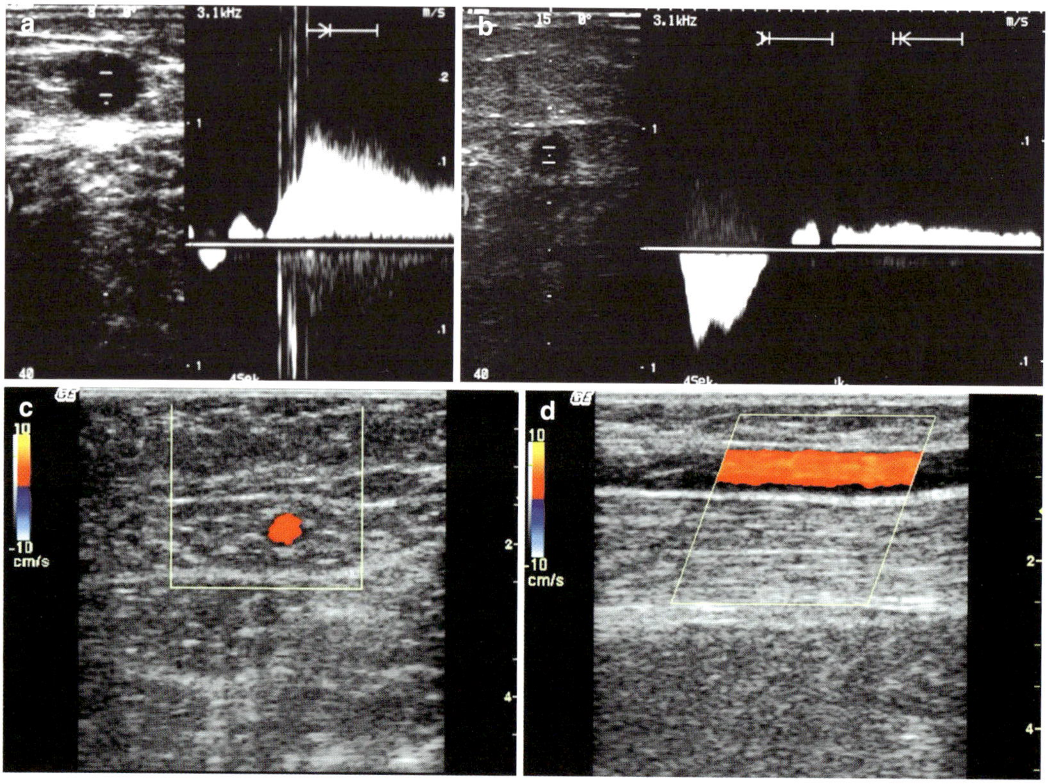

Fig. 7.44 (**a**) Transverse view through the inner thigh with a refluxive great saphenous vein. In PW a short antegrade flow is observed (*downward curve*) followed by a large volume of reflux (*upward curve*). (**b**) Transverse view through the inner thigh with a refluxive but poorly drained great saphenous vein. The reflux is slow and long-lasting. This is easily overlooked using colour duplex. (**c**) Transverse view through the inner thigh in colour duplex. The great saphenous vein maintains a *red* colour in its lumen for a long time (online material). (**d**) Longitudinal view through the great saphenous vein with reflux in colour duplex. This image is obtained by angling the measurement window along the great saphenous vein as it runs parallel to the skin Copyright: [Author]

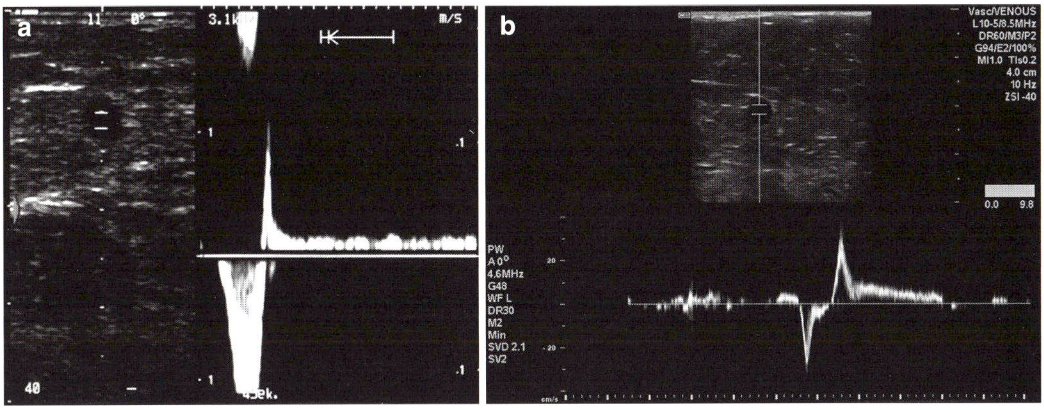

Fig. 7.45 (**a**) Transverse view through the thigh using PW mode. After a provocation manoeuvre causing antegrade flow, there is a short, rapid reflux causing valve closure followed by slower, longer-lasting reflux. The first part of the curve is the backflow signalling terminal valve closure in the groin. The second part is much slower and represents the reflux carried from the posterior accessory saphenous vein flowing into the great saphenous vein. This finding would be overlooked if the examination concluded prematurely after recording the short backflow curve. (**b**) Transverse view through the thigh with backflow causing saphenofemoral junction closure (*steep upward curve*) followed by prolonged low-volume reflux arising from the epigastric vein (*flat upward curve*) Copyright: [Author]

The curve is never unequivocal. Reflux phenomena may occur at volumes similar to the volumes observed in antegrade flow (Fig. 7.46a). Clarification can be obtained by using different provocation manoeuvres (Fig. 7.46b). The examiner must pay special attention in cases where the examination may be painful. In the presence of oedema from chronic venous insufficiency, the great saphenous vein may be only moderately dilated with very little flow observed during provocation. The antegrade and retrograde flow curves in PW mode may be too diminished to be clinically useful. In this situation an elevation-dependency manoeuvre (Sect. 6.9) may be very helpful in clarifying pathology.

When the great saphenous vein is dilated, the **valves** can be seen "open" in muscular systole and "closed" in diastole. Even if the valve appears closed, the vein may still be incompetent (Fig. 7.47).

7.5.2.1 Identifying the Reflux Source of the Great Saphenous Vein

In the vast majority of cases, the great saphenous vein is filled refluxively at a single point like the saphenofemoral junction. However, when looking for proximal reflux sources, there may be other pathological inflows. These include an additional refluxive inguinal tributary, a perforating vein or refluxive flow from the anterior accessory saphenous vein.

Interesting

Most dilated perforating veins in the course of a refluxive great saphenous vein are well drained and not refluxive (Chaps. 3 and 9).

Once the **junction** of the great saphenous vein with the common femoral vein has been examined (Sect. 7.3), it may be competent or refluxive. If the saphenofemoral junction or a superficial inguinal tributary is incompetent and fills the great saphenous vein, then this will identify the proximal reflux source (Fig. 7.39a).

However, if the saphenofemoral junction is competent, then the vein should be examined from proximal to distal. The probe should be held in transverse view to determine possible reflux sources. These include sites where dilated perforating veins or tributaries join the vein. Usually these inflows are associated with alterations in calibre. The vein is usually smaller in calibre proximal to the inflow compared to further down (Fig. 7.48a).

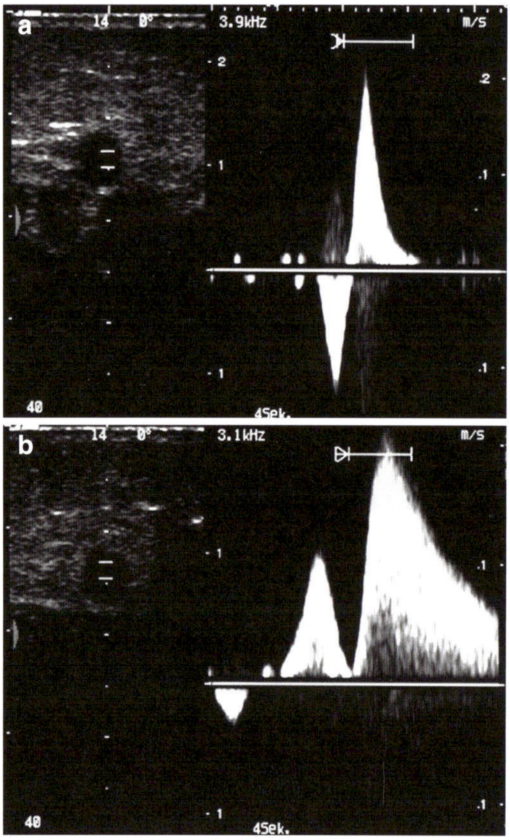

Fig. 7.46 Incomplete incompetence of the great saphenous vein filled by reflux from a paratibial perforating vein (formerly Boyd). (**a**) Examination of the great saphenous vein in the calf below the reflux source from the incompetent perforating vein using manual compression. In B scan note that the reflux duration is relatively short. (**b**) Examination of the same great saphenous vein using the Wunstorf manoeuvre. The antegrade flow is smaller but the reflux is of much greater volume. There are two peaks. The first reflux curve appears while the forefoot is still elevated. After relaxation more reflux is allowed to flow out from the perforating vein. The Wunstorf manoeuvre appears to be more reliable than manual compression when assessing incompetence in perforating veins Copyright: [Author]

Common reflux sources into the great saphenous vein:

- Posterior accessory saphenous vein. The reflux originates from the small saphenous vein (Fig. 4.9a), the pelvis through the labial veins (Fig. 4.7b) or from the perforating vein at the back of the thigh (Fig. 4.8b).

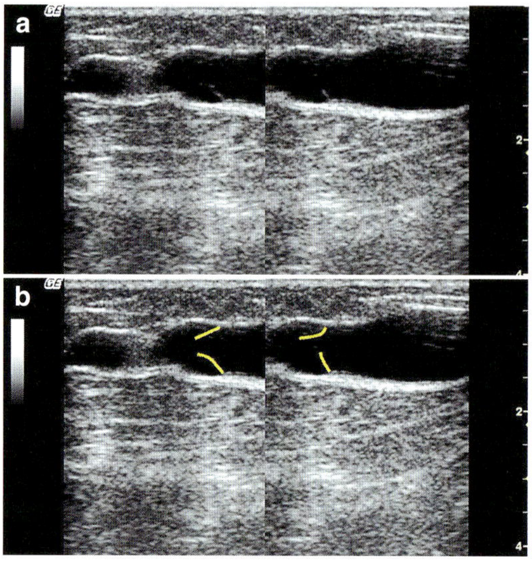

Fig. 7.47 Valves in a refluxive great saphenous vein. Longitudinal view through the inner thigh in the same subject as seen in Fig 7.44d but further proximal. (**a**) Observed during muscular systole (*left*) and muscular diastole (*right*). The upper valve leaflet in the image appears to be rigid because it does not seem to close across the lumen (online material). (**b**) Valve wings marked (*yellow*) Copyright: [Author]

- Perforating vein of the adductor canal (formerly Dodd; Fig. 4.8a).
- Connecting vein between the anterior accessory vein and great saphenous vein in the mid thigh (Fig. 4.7c).
- Paratibial perforating veins (especially formerly Boyd; Fig. 7.48b).
- Intersaphenous vein between the small and great saphenous veins in the calf (Fig. 4.9b).
- Connecting vein between the posterior arch vein and the great saphenous vein in the distal calf (Fig. 4.8c).

Uncommon reflux sources into the great saphenous vein:

- Perforating vein from the deep femoral vein approx. 5–10 cm below the groin
- Distal perforating vein of the adductor canal (formerly Hunter)
- Paratibial perforating vein after thrombosis
- Perforating vein directly from the tibia after a tibia fracture; Sect. 9.10)

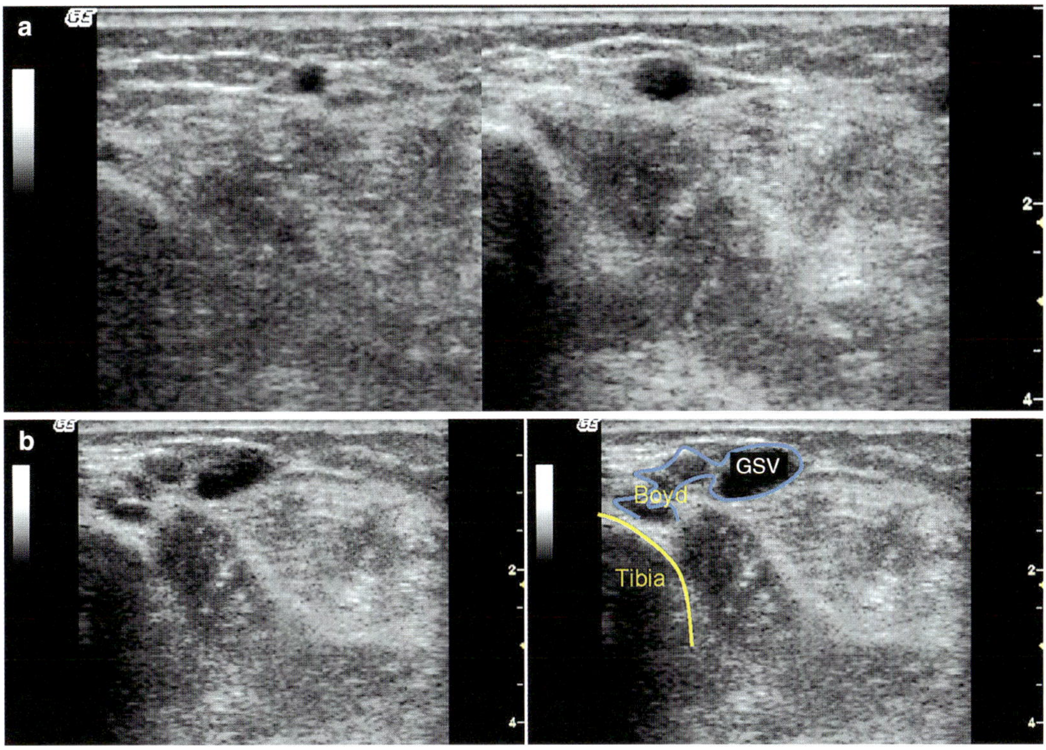

Fig. 7.48 Reflux source from the proximal paratibial perforating vein (formerly Boyd). (**a**) Great saphenous vein below the knee proximal of the perforating vein (*left*) and distal (*right*). The enveloping saphenous fascia can be seen at both points. There is a clear change in calibre with reflux below the entry of the perforating vein and competency above (additional material online). (**b**) Transverse view through the calf at the level of the paratibial perforating vein. The junction of the refluxive perforating vein with the great saphenous vein is shown (additional material online) Copyright: [Author]

Special attention must be paid to these sites when examining the great saphenous vein from proximal to distal. They may be the main proximal reflux source or an additional source of proximal pathological flow. If this second variant is overlooked prior to a saphenofemoral ligation, then **recurrence** is inevitable because the refluxive inflow into the great saphenous vein has not been completely eradicated. This commonly occurs with a refluxive perforating vein of the adductor canal (formerly Dodd) or with reflux into the great saphenous vein through the posterior accessory saphenous vein.

A situation may occur called **reflux without source** (Mendoza 2002 in Appendix 2). This is where the saphenofemoral junction is competent, but many healthy tributaries drain retrograde along the downward course of the great saphenous. This causes an increasing volume of reflux to build up without a definite source. The reflux in this situation does not come from the deep system but only from the tributaries. The diameter of the great saphenous vein and the reflux volume remain small (Fig. 7.49 and Sect. 3.3.4).

7.5.2.2 Identifying the Reflux Drainage from the Great Saphenous Vein

Reflux may leave the great saphenous vein in several places. Tributaries and perforating veins are usually involved.

Almost all the visible, dilated **perforating veins** down the course of the great saphenous

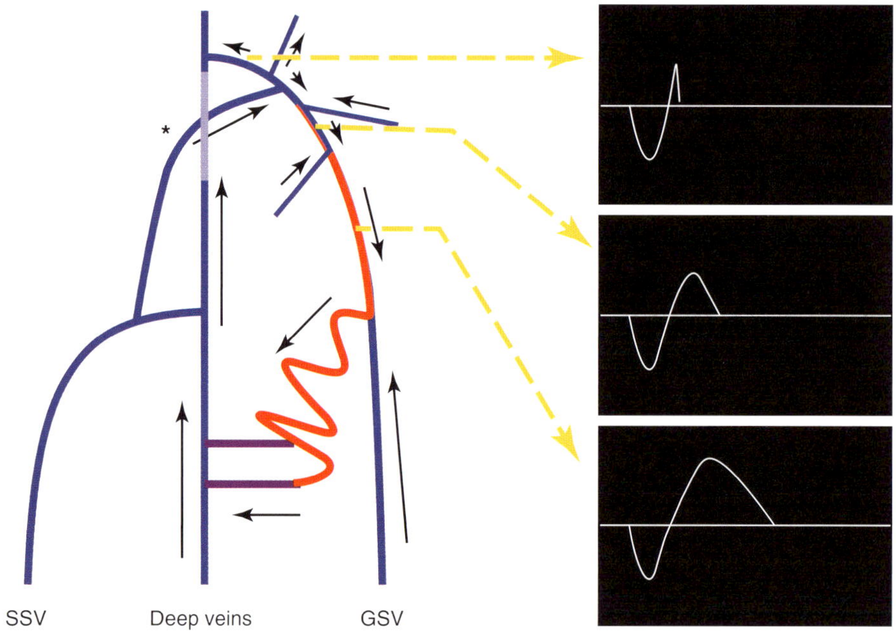

Fig. 7.49 Reflux without source according to Cappelli and Franceschi. The terminal valve of the great saphenous vein (*GSV*) remains competent. Blood from healthy tributaries, including the posterior (*) and anterior accessory saphenous veins, drain progressively into the great saphenous vein in a retrograde fashion. There is no pathological connection with the deep system. The reflux curves are of small volume but progressively increase down the great saphenous vein (shown on the right at three different stages, *SSV* small saphenous vein) (online material) Copyright: [Author]

vein may serve as re-entry points for reflux (Sects. 3.4 and 9.3). If the refluxive section of the great saphenous vein ends at one of these perforating veins, then this can be established as the distal reflux drainage point (Fig. 7.50).

Multiple drainage points are not usually visible on phlebography. For this reason Hach always stated that the varicose tributary was the lowest reflux drainage point when using his classification. A draining perforating vein on the great saphenous vein is present in 47 % of legs with incompetence. Additional refluxive tributaries are usually, but not necessarily, associated with this recirculation circuit.

Reflux is drained exclusively through **tributaries** in 53 % of recirculations involving the great saphenous vein. These then carry their reflux back through perforating veins or the small saphenous vein and into the deep veins. These tributaries are usually clinically visible on the surface of the leg as varicose veins.

In an unpublished study where 82 consecutive legs with great saphenous reflux were examined with duplex (Table 7.2), 48 (59 %) were found to have only one refluxive tributary which drained all the reflux from the great saphenous vein (Fig 7.51a). In 32 % of the legs, there were two refluxive tributaries, in 8 % the vein was drained by 3 tributaries and in 1 % by 4. The most distal tributary in each case was the **distal reflux drainage point**. The great saphenous veins were all competent below this point, by definition, down to the ankle. An alteration in the calibre of the great saphenous vein is usually found at the distal reflux drainage point (Fig. 7.51c).

7.5.2.3 Identifying the Number of Refluxive Segments of the Great Saphenous Vein

A refluxive tributary may refill the great saphenous vein lower down where the flow is antegrade causing it to reflux once more (Sect. 4.1.3). Thus, all parts of the great saphenous vein below the first competent segment must be examined. In 16 % of incompetence in the great saphenous vein, there is a competent section between the proximal reflux source and the distal re-entry point. This is where a refluxive tributary takes the

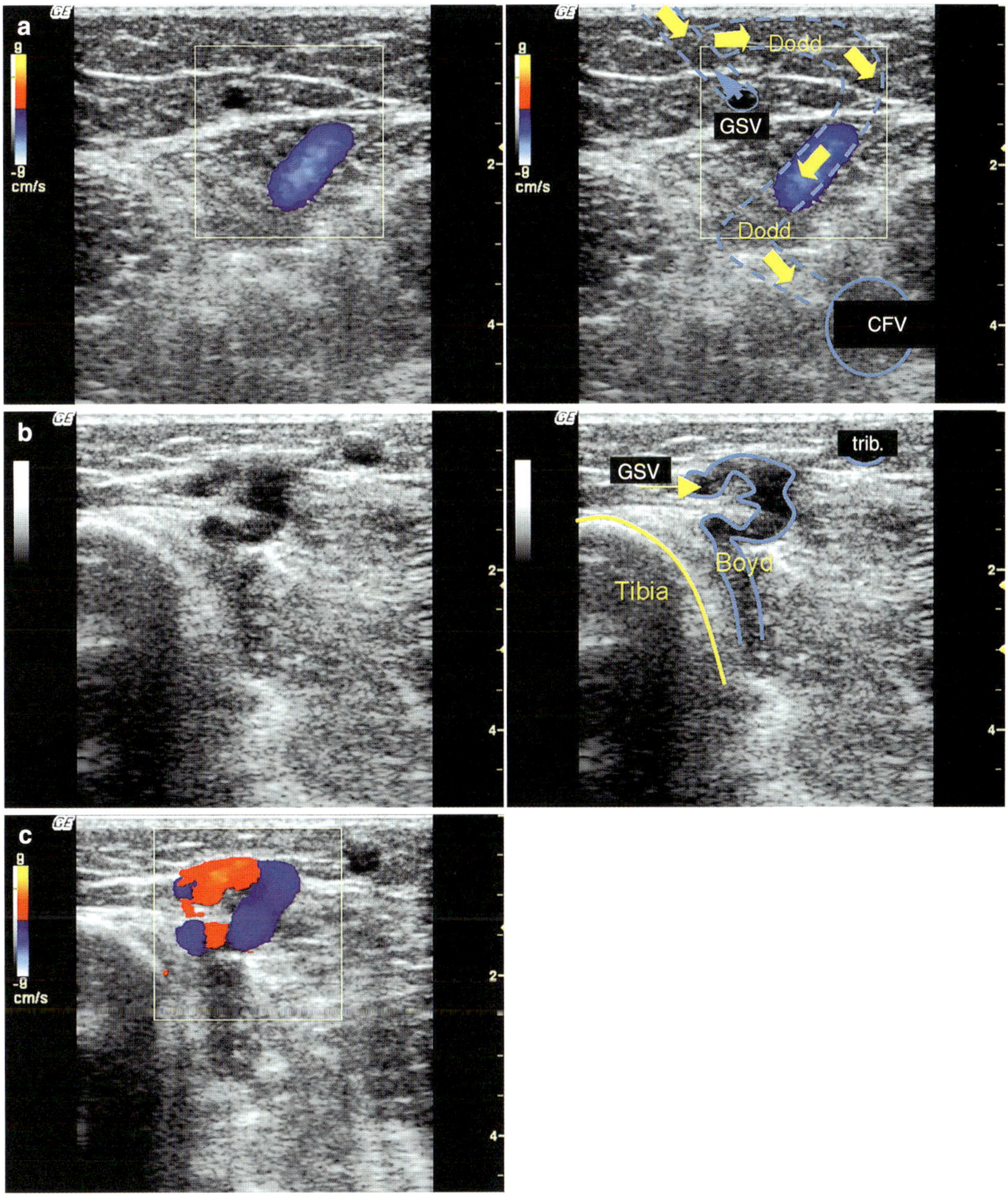

Fig. 7.50 (**a**) Transverse view through the inner thigh at the height of the perforating vein of the adductor canal (formerly Dodd). The terminal and preterminal valves are incompetent with a refluxive great saphenous vein from the groin. This is draining through the perforating vein back into the deep vein. There are no refluxive tributaries present. This is classified as a complete incompetence of the great saphenous vein (*GSV*), Hach Class II. This was a concurrent finding during the examination of the leg of a subject with post-traumatic varicose veins in the calf (Fig. 9.14). The groin reflux was not apparent clinically because this recirculation did not include any varicose tributaries. The perforating vein of the adductor canal runs slightly distal. For this reason the image shows the competent great saphenous vein as well as the dilated perforating vein which carries the reflux to the deep vein. The connection between the two is shown with a dotted line as it is not in the plane of this image. The reflux is indicated by yellow arrows. (**b**) Transverse view through the upper third of the calf. The tibial edge is shown on the *left*. The great saphenous vein is incompetent above and below the knee with a refluxive tributary (*trib*) leaving the great saphenous vein just above the proximal paratibial perforating vein (formerly Boyd). This is classified as a complete incompetence of the great saphenous vein, Hach Class III (additional material online). The reflux in the great saphenous vein ends in the perforating vein which carries the majority of the reflux volume back into the deep system. (**c**) Same position as (b) shown in colour duplex Copyright: [Author]

reflux away from the great saphenous vein and carries it back into the great saphenous vein further down the leg (Fig. 4.11a).

Table 7.2 Refluxive tributaries of the great saphenous vein

Number of refluxive tributaries	Number of legs examined	Percent [%]
1	48	58.6
2	26	31.7
3	7	8.5
4	1	1.2
Total	*82*	*100*

7.5.2.4 Identifying a Draining Perforating Vein Along the Refluxive Course

For those who use the **CHIVA** method of treatment, it is important to differentiate the shunt types. If there is a perforating vein draining the refluxive segment of the great saphenous vein (shunt type I), the proximal reflux source should be interrupted. The saphenous vein will then drain via this perforating vein. If there is no perforating vein (shunt type III), manual tributary occlusion will arrest the retrograde flow in the saphenous trunk. This is a shunt type 3 where the proposed treatment is to ablate or ligate only

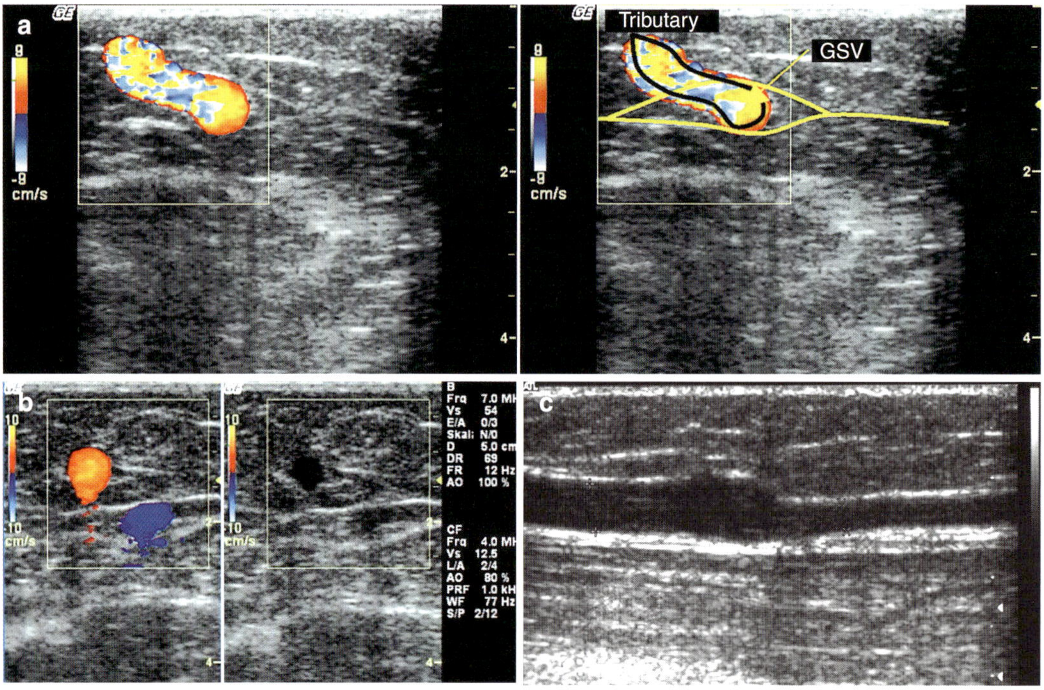

Fig. 7.51 Junction of a single tributary draining the great saphenous vein (*GSV*). (**a**) Transverse view through the inner thigh demonstrating the refluxive tributary in colour duplex. The refluxive great saphenous vein is visible in the saphenous eye where it fills a tributary. Below this point the great saphenous vein is competent. This is a complete incompetence of the great saphenous vein, Hach Class II. The colour "overloads" the image causing the vein to appear much larger than the one in B scan (*black outline*) (additional material online). (**b**) Transverse view below the refluxive tributary. The great saphenous vein is competent and the tributary is refluxive. At the end of muscular systole, the flow in the great saphenous vein is still antegrade (*blue*) while it is already refluxive (*red*) in the tributary (*Left*). When the patient stands still, there is no flow in both these veins (*Right*) (additional material online). (**c**) Calibre reduction below the branch point of the refluxive tributary in a patient with complete incompetence of the great saphenous vein in the thigh, Hach Class II. On the *left* the diameter of the great saphenous vein is 4.8 mm, on the *right* it is 2.9 mm Copyright: [Author]

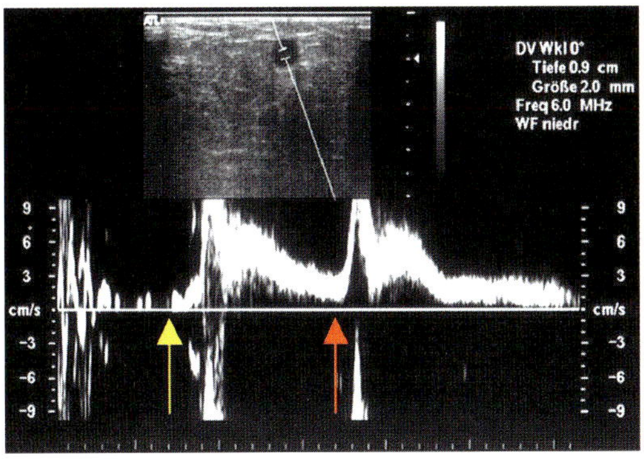

Fig. 7.52 Transverse view through the thigh with PW recordings of the velocity profile of the great saphenous vein. The great saphenous vein is refluxive with two draining tributaries which were compressed digitally by the examiner. Starting from the *left*, movement artefacts occurred only as the subject raised and lowered his toes with the provocation manoeuvre. Tributary occlusion seems to control the saphenous reflux. At the *yellow arrow* and the *red arrow*, digital compression of the proximal and distal tributaries were released, respectively. Both resulted in gross saphenous reflux. It may be concluded that there are no draining perforating veins on the great saphenous vein because, if there were, tributary compression would not have controlled the reflux Copyright: [Author]

the tributary and leave the saphenofemoral junction intact. Apart from an examination in B scan, a simple test can clarify this situation (Figs. 7.52 and 4.23). A velocity profile is first taken in the proximal region of the refluxive great saphenous vein in PW mode during a Wunstorf manoeuvre. The refluxive tributary close to its junction with the great saphenous vein is then compressed with a finger without compressing the great saphenous vein at the same time (Fig. 4.23). Then, the Wunstorf manoeuvre is repeated. If antegrade flow is present in the proximal great saphenous vein, this confirms that the vein itself is not compressed by the finger. If there are **no draining perforating veins** between the probe and the compressed tributary, no reflux will be recorded, after the brief antegrade curve. Directly after the digital compression of the tributary is released, reflux will resume (Mendoza 2002 in Appendix 2; Zamboni et al. 2010). In Fig. 7.52, there were two refluxive tributaries which were

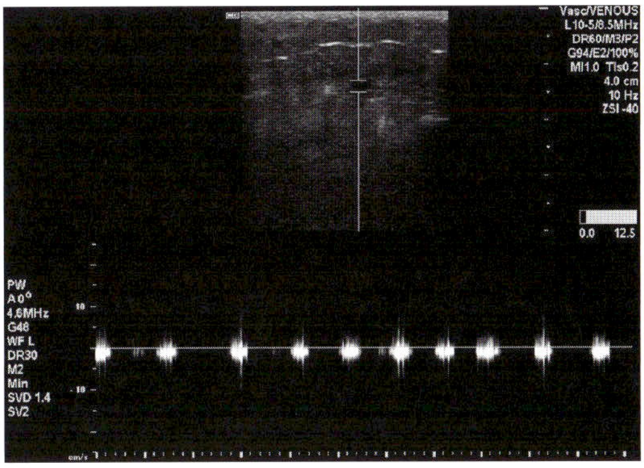

Fig. 7.53 Spontaneous saphenous pulsation, neither dependent on respiration nor synchronous with the cardiac cycle, is a marker for advanced chronic venous insufficiency. Pulsation is detected in the great saphenous vein of a dependent leg in a patient with chronic venous insufficiency after about 1–2 min Copyright: [Author]

compressed with two fingers and released one at a time.

7.5.3 Pulsatility Within the Great Saphenous Vein

If the subject sits on the edge of a couch with the legs in a dependent position, antegrade flow will soon commence within an incompetent great saphenous vein. Closer inspection will reveal that this flow is pulsatile (Lattimer et al. 2012a). It was suggested that the more marked the pulsation, the more pathological the chronic venous insufficiency of the leg (Fig. 7.53).

Two out of 44 legs with healthy veins (4.5 %) presented spontaneous pulsation in the great saphenous vein. In contrast 75 % of legs with refluxive great saphenous vein presented pulsation. Pulsation also correlates with clinical findings. In the absence of visible veins or skin alterations, pulsation is found in the great saphenous vein in 4.5 % of cases and in 94.1 % of cases with vein-related skin alterations. The presence of pulsation also correlates with the diameter in the middle third of the thigh. With no pulsation the average diameter of the great saphenous vein was 3.5 mm. With pulsation the average diameter was 7 mm.

References

Coleridge-Smith P, Labropoulos N, Partsch H, Myers K, Nicolaides A, Cavezzi A (2006) Duplex ultrasound investigation of the veins in chronic venous disease of the lower limbs-UIP consensus document, part I. Basic principles. Eur J Vasc Endovasc Surg 31:1–10

Kalodiki E, Stvrtinova V, Allegra C et al (2012) Superficial vein thrombosis: a consensus statement. Int Angiol 31:203–216

Lattimer CR, Azzam M, Kalodiki E, Makris G, Geroulakos G (2012a) Saphenous pulsation on duplex may be a marker of severe chronic superficial venous insufficiency. J Vasc Surg 56(5):1338–1343

Lattimer CR, Kalodiki E, Azzam M et al (2012b) Volume displacements from an incompetent great saphenous vein during a standardised Valsalva manoeuvre. Acta Phlebologica 13(1):25–30

Lattimer CR, Kalodiki E, Azzam M, Geroulakos G (2013) Reflux time estimation on air-plethysmography may stratify patients with early superficial venous insufficiency. Phlebology 28(2):101–108

Lurie F, Kistner RL, Eklof B, Kessler D (2003) Mechanism of venous valve closure and role of the valve in circulation: a new concept. J Vasc Surg 38:955–961

Mendoza E, Blättler W, Amsler F (2013) Great saphenous vein diameter at the saphenofemoral junction and proximal thigh as parameters of venous disease class. Eur J Vasc Endovasc Surg 45(1):76–83

Mühlberger D, Morandini L, Brenner E (2009) Venous valves and major superficial tributary veins near the saphenofemoral junction. J Vasc Surg 49:1562–1569

Oswald M (2005) Our blue wonder. To be read at: www.ourbluewonder.com

Pascarella L, Al-Tuwaijri M, Bergan JJ, Mekenas LM (2005) Lower extremity superficial venous aneurysms. Ann Vasc Surg 19(1):69–73

Platzer W (2005) Taschenatlas der Anatomie. Stuttgart, Thieme

Stücker M, Moritz R, Altmeyer P, Reich-Schupke S (2013) New concept: different types of insufficiency of the saphenofemoral junction identified by duplex as a chance for a more differentiated therapy of the great saphenous vein. Phlebology 28(5):268–274

Zamboni P, Gianesini S, Menegatti E, Tacconi G, Palazzo A, Liboni A (2010) Great saphenous varicose vein surgery without saphenofemoral junction disconnection. Br J Surg 97:820–825

8 Examination of the Small Saphenous Vein

Erika Mendoza and Christopher R. Lattimer

Chapter Summary

The small saphenous vein is less often refluxive than the great saphenous vein. Nevertheless, it should be included always in any duplex ultrasound examination. This chapter will only cover aspects in which the small saphenous vein differs from the great saphenous vein. Basic items which apply equally for the small saphenous vein, like flow measurement and the changes in reflux volumes from joining tributaries or perforating veins, are explained in detail in Chap. 7.

8.1 Examination Procedure

It is important to develop a routine so as not to overlook any vein segments. The whole length of the vein must be examined, including the tributaries and perforating veins.

A good place to begin is in the **popliteal fossa** with the subject standing. First, the popliteal vein and its flow should be assessed (Chap. 14). Next, the junction of the small saphenous vein with the deep venous system should be identified and examined, and the anatomy of the muscular veins as well as the presence of a vein of Giacomini. Finally, the venous flow is measured under provocation manoeuvres. In contrast to the great saphenous vein, the Valsalva manoeuvre is less appropriate for the small saphenous vein. The colour duplex mode is the best starting point to assess venous flow. Ultrasound of the back of the thigh is an essential part of the examination to look for a possible refluxive proximal extension of the small saphenous vein or Giacomini anastomosis.

The course of the small saphenous vein should be scanned in B mode, keeping an eye out for any sudden calibre changes and dilated perforating veins or tributaries. The diameter can be measured in B mode 5 cm below its junction. Duplex mode must be switched on repeatedly when running over the course of the small saphenous vein to record flow velocity and direction. PW mode is more effective than colour mode for this purpose, since changes in the velocity profile are more apparent (Sect. 7.5.2). Tributaries and perforating veins are better assessed using colour-coded duplex in the preliminary assessment. However, this must not divert the examination away from the saphenous trunk.

E. Mendoza, MD, PhD (✉)
Venenpraxis Wunstorf,
Speckenstraße 10, 31515 Wunstorf, Germany
e-mail: erika.mendoza@t-online.de

C.R. Lattimer, MD, PhD
Department of Vascular Surgery,
Josef Pflug Vascular Laboratory,
Ealing Hospital and Imperial College, London, UK

E. Mendoza et al. (eds.), *Duplex Ultrasound of Superficial Leg Veins*,
DOI 10.1007/978-3-642-40731-4_8, © Springer-Verlag Berlin Heidelberg 2014

8.2 Examination Objectives

The examination must provide answers to the following questions:

- Does the small saphenous vein join the popliteal vein?
- At what level is the saphenopopliteal junction in relation to the posterior knee crease?
- Is the small saphenous vein connected to muscle veins in the region of the junction?
- Does a thigh extension of the small saphenous vein exist?
- Does it build a Giacomini vein?
- Is the thigh extension or the vein of Giacomini competent?
- Are the muscle veins competent?
- Is there any anomaly in the junction of the small saphenous vein?
- Is the junction of the small saphenous vein refluxive, dilated or even aneurysmal?
- Is the whole course of the small saphenous vein interfascial?
- What is its diameter at a standardised point, 5 cm below its junction?
- Are there any sudden changes in calibre?
- Is its course typical or does it deviate or duplicate?
- Does any segment have superficial vein thrombosis or post-thrombotic alteration?
- Is there reflux?
- Is this reflux well or poorly drained assessed by the profile of the reflux curve in PW mode?
- How many segments are refluxive?
- Where is the proximal reflux source?
- Are there any dilated tributaries or perforating veins along the small saphenous vein's course?
- Are they involved in a recirculation loop?
- Does the reflux leave the small saphenous vein by a tributary or a perforating vein?
- How long is the refluxive segment?
- Which shunt type is found?
- How does the calibre and course of the small saphenous vein behave below the end of the reflux?
- Are there any remarkable findings in the tissues surrounding the small saphenous vein?
- Is the flow in the dilated small saphenous vein antegrade because it is serving as drainage for the deep system? Secondary varicose veins are discussed in Chap. 15.

8.3 The Saphenopopliteal Junction

The junction of the small saphenous vein with the popliteal vein is quite **variable** (Sect. 2.5.1 and Fig. 2.31). The first task in duplex ultrasound is to locate this junction. This is far less easy than with the great saphenous vein. The probe should be positioned transversally over the popliteal region and moved proximal and distal in B scan. Once the popliteal vein is located, the small saphenous vein should be seen some centimetres further down where it can almost always be found. If this is not the case, the small saphenous vein must be followed from the mid calf upwards.

8.3.1 Anatomy and Flow

The small saphenous vein courses from the calf to the popliteal fossa within its own fascial compartment. At first, the compartment lies in the groove between the bellies of gastrocnemius. It then widens as it extends up into the popliteal fossa. As with the great saphenous vein, the small saphenous vein at its junction is not enclosed in a narrow compartment. It curves inwards towards its termination where it joins the popliteal vein (Fig. 8.1). In healthy veins, the saphenopopliteal junction is usually situated above the posterior skin crease of the knee (Sect. 2.5.1).

In 65 % of legs, the small saphenous vein has a cranial extension. If this vein joins the great saphenous vein, it is called either the Giacomini anastomosis or the femoropopliteal vein. The physiological flow in the cranial extension of the small saphenous vein is towards the small saphenous vein, which is downwards (Fig. 8.2 and Sect. 2.5.3). Alternatively, the proximal extension of the small saphenous vein may terminate directly into a perforating vein on the back of the thigh.

Superficial veins along their course are best seen in transverse view. Junctions are demonstrated better in longitudinal view.

8.3.2 Refluxive Anatomy and Flow

If the small saphenous vein is incompetent, it may divert to a greater or lesser degree from the

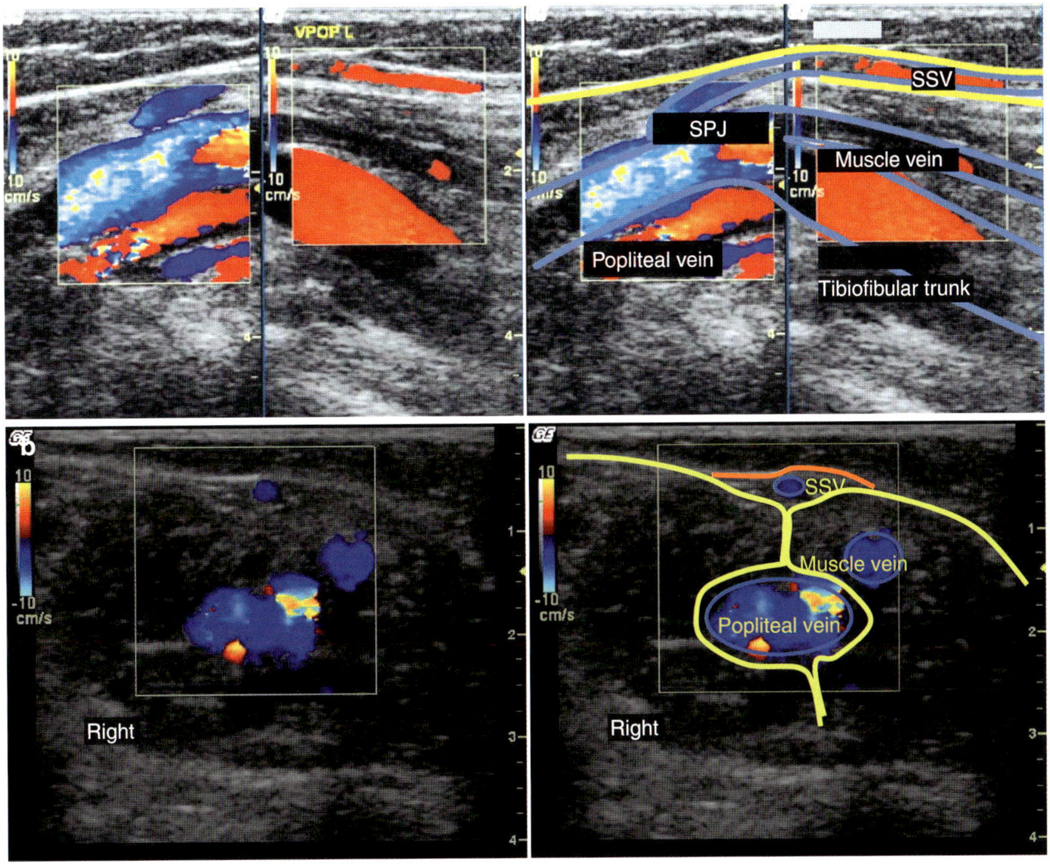

Fig. 8.1 Junction of the small saphenous vein (*SSV*) in the popliteal fossa with no reflux. (**a**) Longitudinal view through the popliteal fossa demonstrating the small saphenous vein curving inwards into the popliteal vein, which is also curved. The probe is tilted showing flow away from the probe (*left*, *blue*) and towards the probe (*right*, *red*). On the right, a muscular vein is seen draining into the tibiofibular trunk. Fasciae are shown in *yellow*: The muscle fascia follows the gastrocnemius heads (*yellow lines*) to form the base of the popliteal depression which is completely overarched by the saphenous fascia (*orange line*) (online material). (**b**) Transverse view through the popliteal fossa during muscular systole demonstrating antegrade flow in healthy veins (*blue*) Copyright: [Author]

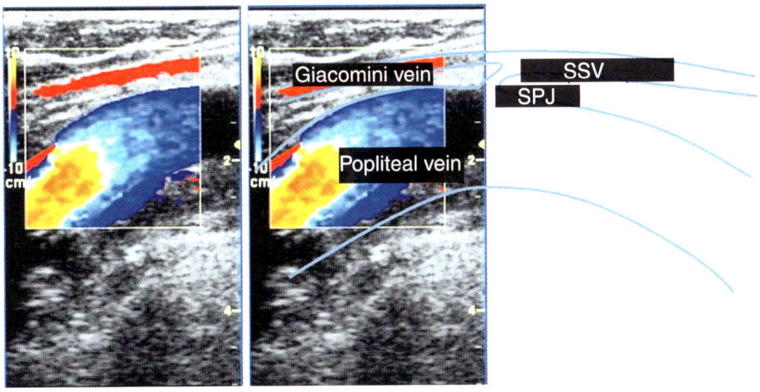

Fig. 8.2 Longitudinal view through the upper part of the popliteal fossa demonstrating the proximal extension of the small saphenous vein or Giacomini vein (online material). Note the physiological downward flow (*red*) in the Giacomini vein which drains into the small saphenous vein. High-velocity aliasing artefacts are seen in the popliteal vein (*yellow and orange*) Copyright: [Author]

normal locations described. This usually depends upon the lateral spaces which are devoid of investing saphenous fascia and the reflux volume (Fig. 8.3a, b). In cases where the reflux has existed for a long time, it is no longer possible to show the vein in a single image. This is because

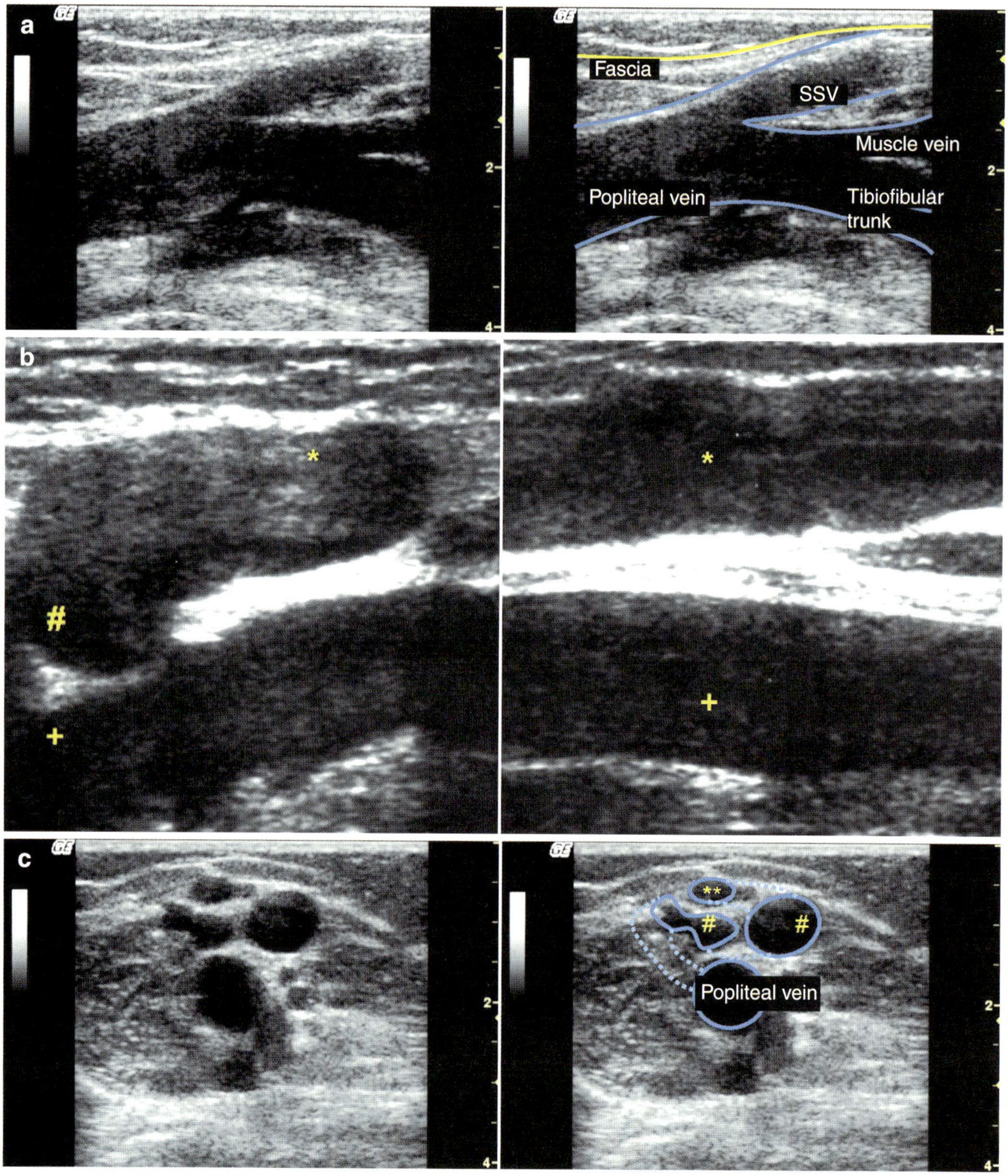

Fig. 8.3 Refluxive small saphenous vein (*SSV*) at a typical junction with the popliteal vein. (**a**) With early incompetence, the calibre of the small saphenous vein appears large. The anatomy is almost like a normal finding without reflux (online material). (**b**) Longitudinal view through the popliteal fossa and proximal calf demonstrating a grossly dilated small saphenous vein (*) at its junction (#) with the popliteal vein (+) (online material). (**c**) Transverse view through the popliteal fossa with long-standing incompetence of the small saphenous vein. The junction is hard to visualise and the termination is very tortuous occupying several layers (online material). Just below the fascia is the non-refluxive vein of Giacomini (**) immediately before its junction with the small saphenous vein (not shown). The tortuous termination (#) is cut twice in this image. The dotted line reconstructs the terminal course of the vein. (**d**) Longitudinal view through the same popliteal fossa. The termination of the small saphenous vein appears in the image as a lengthwise vein (#) rather than an inward curve. This can be distinguished from a muscular vein because it cannot be traced further down (@) due to its tortuosity. It eventually meets the straight part of the small saphenous vein (*) Copyright: [Author]

Fig. 8.3 (continued)

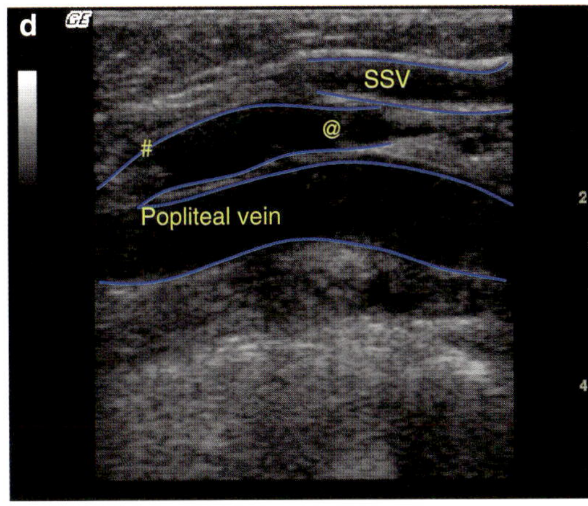

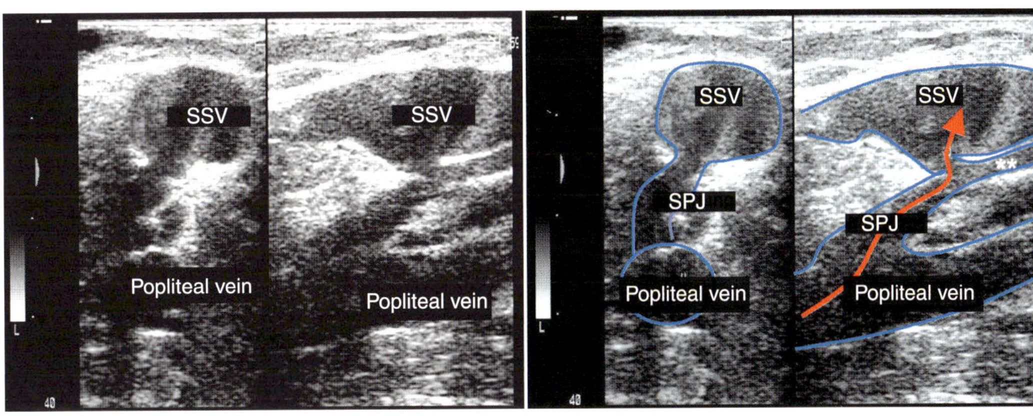

Fig. 8.4 Left transverse, right longitudinal view through the popliteal fossa demonstrating a venous aneurysm at the termination of the small saphenous vein (*SSV*). This joins the popliteal vein together with a competent muscle vein (**). The aneurysm has partially thrombosed (Fig. 11.5b). The *arrow* indicates the direction of flow of the refluxive blood Copyright: [Author]

it becomes very tortuous (Fig. 8.3c, d). This pathological feature is not typical of the great saphenous vein. The explanation may be the fact that the small saphenous vein in the popliteal fossa is not held in a straight course by its fascia. The distance between the popliteal vein and the beginning of the fascial sheath of the small saphenous vein is significantly greater than the corresponding distance in the great saphenous vein. This may be the reason why the great saphenous vein never becomes tortuous at its termination. However, a very dilated termination may still occur.

On rare occasions, an aneurysm may form at the termination of the small saphenous vein which may contain a thrombus (Figs. 8.4 and 8.5).

8.3.3 Level of Termination of the Small Saphenous Vein

If the small saphenous vein is followed up from the middle of the calf, in very rare cases (<1 %; Sect. 2.5.1), a junction is found with muscle veins or a communicating vein to the great saphenous vein (Fig. 8.6). In this case, the small saphenous vein is no longer visible within its fascia at the proximal calf and the saphenopopliteal junction is absent.

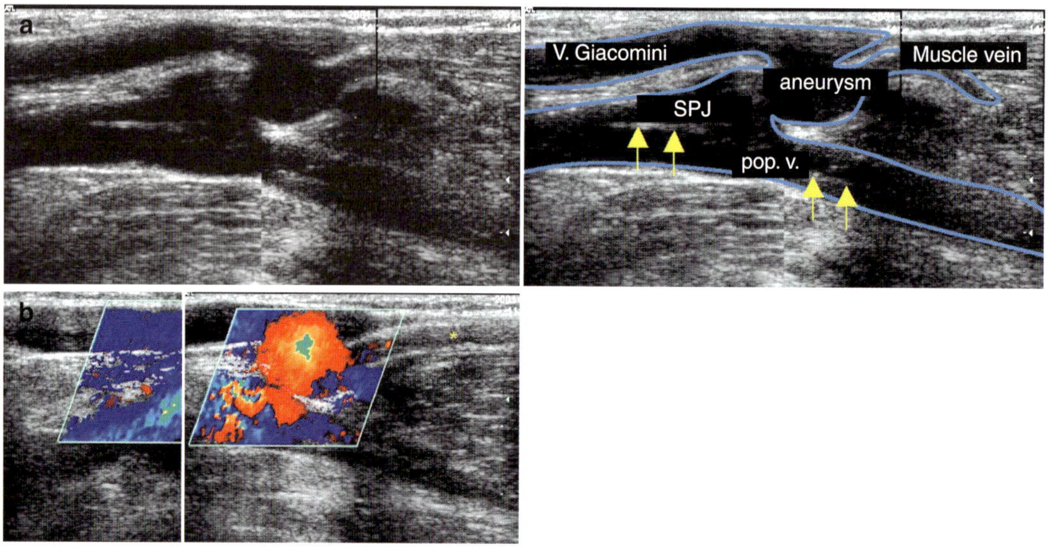

Fig. 8.5 (**a**) Longitudinal view through the popliteal fossa demonstrating the aftermath of a femoropopliteal vein thrombosis. Septal formation is apparent in the deep veins (*arrowed*) which is refluxive (**b**). The Giacomini vein is dilated and refluxive at its junction with the small saphenous vein. The muscular vein is competent (online material). (**b**) The same leg as in **a** with colour duplex ultrasound during muscular diastole. There is an antegrade upward flow (*blue*, away from probe) in the vein of Giacomini (reflux), which is filled through the incompetent saphenopopliteal junction (*red*, towards probe). In the *right half* of the image, the probe was positioned further lateral to demonstrate the small saphenous vein (*) Copyright: [Author]

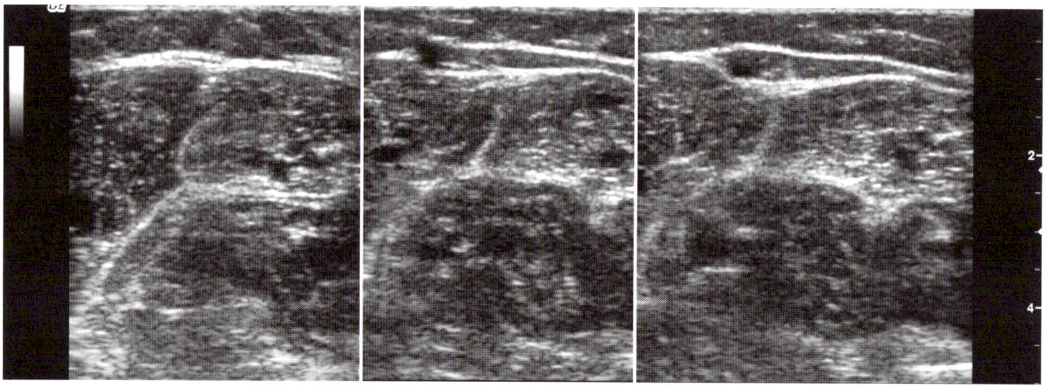

Fig. 8.6 Transverse view through the back of the calf demonstrating agenesis of the small saphenous vein junction. In the upper third of the calf, flow from the small saphenous vein passes through a communicating vein to the great saphenous vein. *Left* (upper calf) shows the empty fascial compartment. *Middle* (lower part of upper calf) shows the vein piercing the fascia. *Right* (mid calf) shows the typical small saphenous vein enclosed in its fascial layers (online material) Copyright: [Author]

According to Caggiati, 54 % of small saphenous veins join the popliteal vein above the posterior skin crease, and 38 % are higher still at or above the apex of the popliteal fossa (Sect. 2.5.1). It is important to identify preoperatively those cases in which the **junction lies under the distal thigh musculature**, since dissection with local anaesthesia is much more difficult (Figs. 8.7 and 2.31d). The small saphenous vein does not pierce the muscle. Instead it runs upwards under the musculature for a variable distance. The small saphenous vein seldom

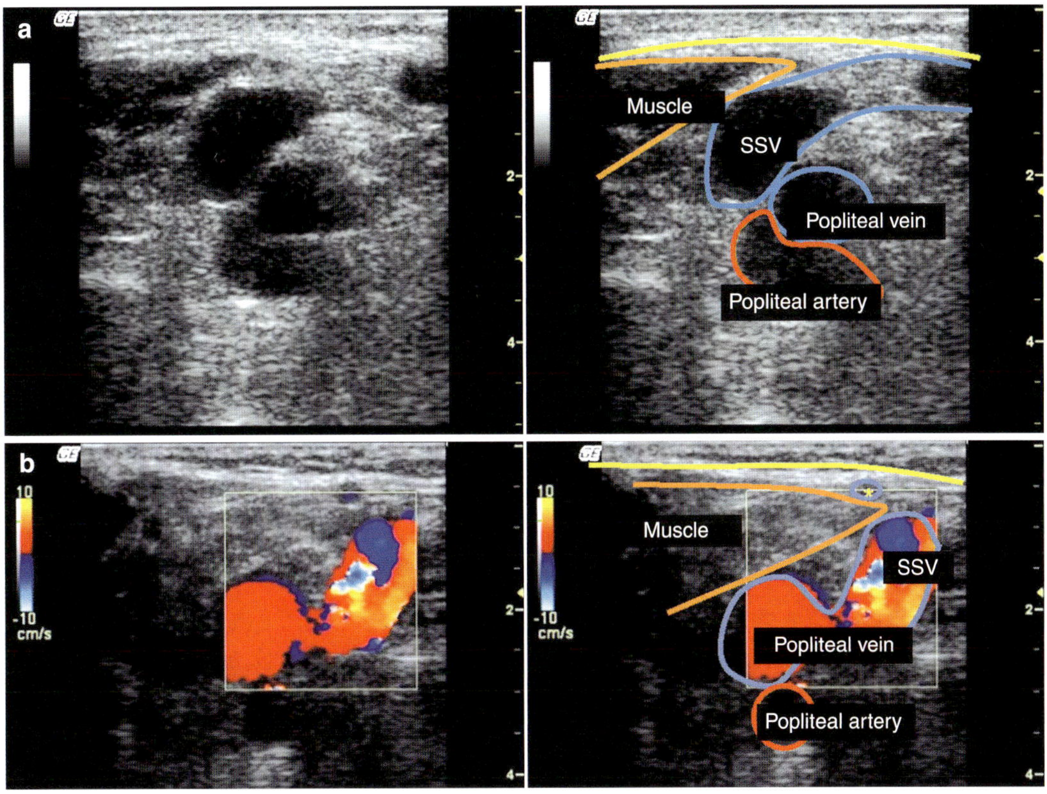

Fig. 8.7 (**a**) Transverse view 7 cm above the left popliteal skin crease demonstrating a high junction of the small saphenous vein (*SSV*). This is at the apex of the popliteal fossa where the vein is seen running underneath the thigh musculature to join the popliteal vein from a lateral approach (online material). (**b**) Transverse view through the distal thigh of the left leg with the small saphenous vein joining the popliteal vein from the medial side (* vein of Giacomini) Copyright: [Author]

joins the popliteal vein directly from a posterior route (Fig. 8.3a). More often it joins the deep vein from lateral or medial (Fig. 8.7a, b). When there is a high junction, the tibial and peroneal nerves run close to the veins (Sect. 17.6). It is essential to scan the patient just prior to surgery in order to assess the expected anatomy. This information can make the vein easier to find and identify during dissection.

When the **junction is above the apex of the popliteal fossa**, a large incision is required to expose the deep leg vein prior to ligation. The importance of a preoperative ultrasound scan cannot be overestimated for planning the surgical strategy. This should complement the ultrasound scan report performed at the time of diagnosis. In these cases, the junction lies very deep under the thigh musculature (Fig. 8.8).

8.3.4 Reflux in the Small Saphenous Vein from the Femoropopliteal Vein

If the great and posterior accessory saphenous veins are incompetent, reflux from the groin can reach the junction of the small saphenous vein through the vein of Giacomini and fill it refluxively (Fig. 4.13a). If the great saphenous vein alone is treated when there is reflux from the femoropopliteal vein, recurrence is certain. Obtaining an image with the probe against the back of the thigh when examining the small saphenous vein is therefore obligatory.

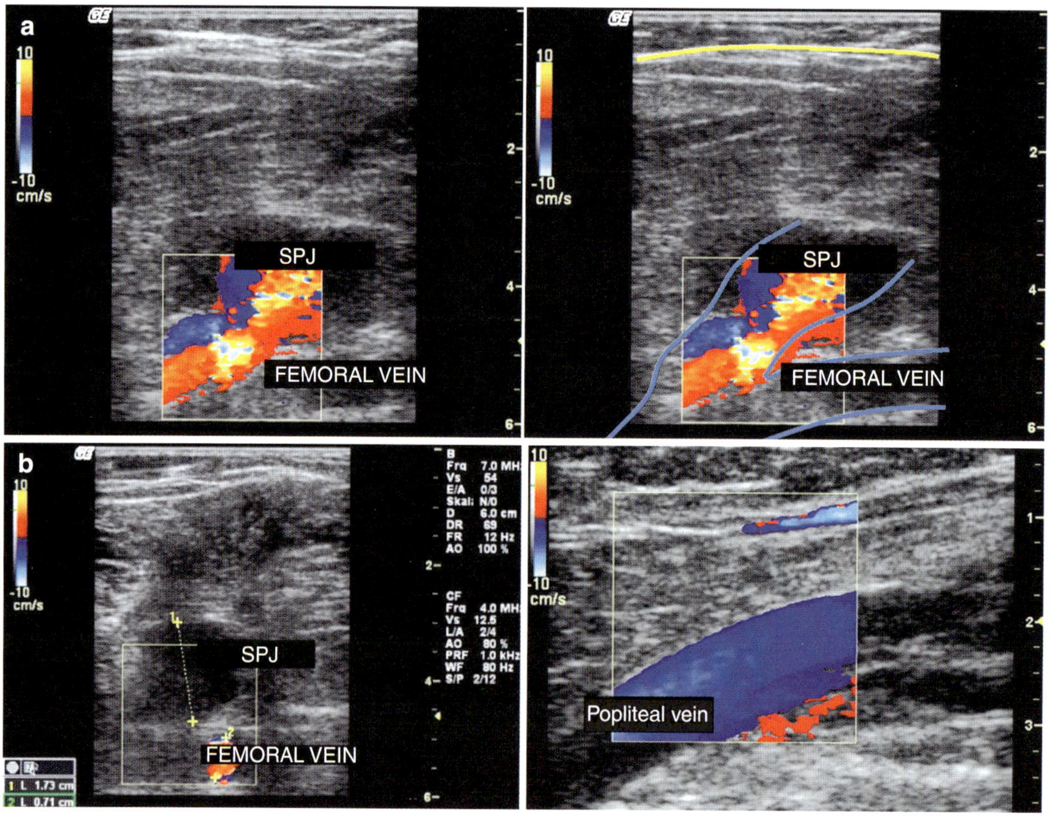

Fig. 8.8 Junction of the small saphenous vein at the back of the thigh. (**a**) Longitudinal section showing the junction of the small saphenous vein (*SSV*) with the superficial femoral vein below the musculature at a depth of 6 cm (online material). (**b**) Transverse view 2 cm below the junction of the small saphenous vein in the same subject as in (a): The diameter of the small saphenous vein (17.3 mm) is clearly bigger than the femoral vein (7.1 mm). (**c**) Longitudinal view through the popliteal fossa demonstrating that the small saphenous vein passes through without joining the popliteal vein (online material) Copyright: [Author]

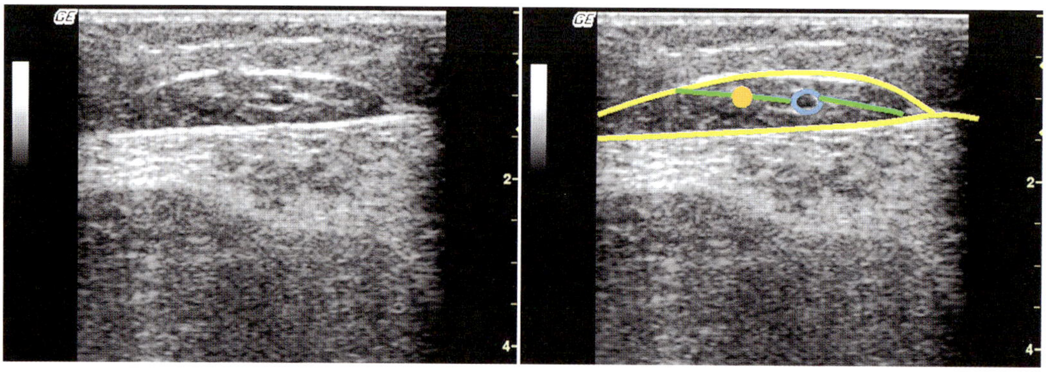

Fig. 8.9 Transverse view through the back of the calf showing the normal small saphenous vein (*blue*) in the fascial compartment (*yellow*) and its attachment by the saphenous ligament (*green*). Occasionally the accompanying sural nerve can also be seen (*yellow dot*) (online material) Copyright: [Author]

8.4 Course of the Small Saphenous Vein

8.4.1 Normal Findings

The small saphenous vein has a very constant course within its fascial compartment in the back of the calf. The fascial compartment contains a variable amount of fatty tissue depending on the constitution of the subject (Figs. 8.9, 2.33 and 2.34). Apart from rare aplasias in the junction area (Fig. 8.6), aplastic segments have not been described in the course of the vein.

A good place to measure the diameter of the small saphenous vein is a point 5 cm below the junction. The diameter is measured in transverse view with the subject standing (Fig. 8.10).

In 4 % of cases, there is duplication of the small saphenous vein (Sect. 2.5.2). Both lumina may be competent, both refluxive (Fig. 8.11a) or only one refluxive (Fig. 8.11b). Duplication must be distinguished from a refluxive vasa vasorum. This is found occasionally and seen as a smaller vein winding around the small saphenous vein (Fig. 8.12).

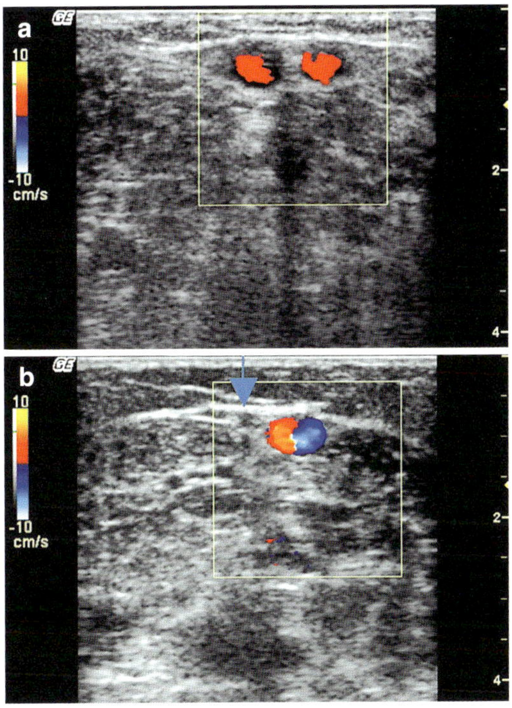

Fig. 8.11 Duplication of the small saphenous vein. (**a**) Transverse view through the back of the calf with reflux in both lumens of the small saphenous vein (online material). (**b**) Another case where only the lateral lumen is refluxive (*blue and red from aliasing*). The medial lumen is competent and very small (*blue arrow*) (online material) Copyright: [Author]

8.4.2 Findings with Reflux

The small saphenous vein is most often filled refluxively in the popliteal region. The reflux

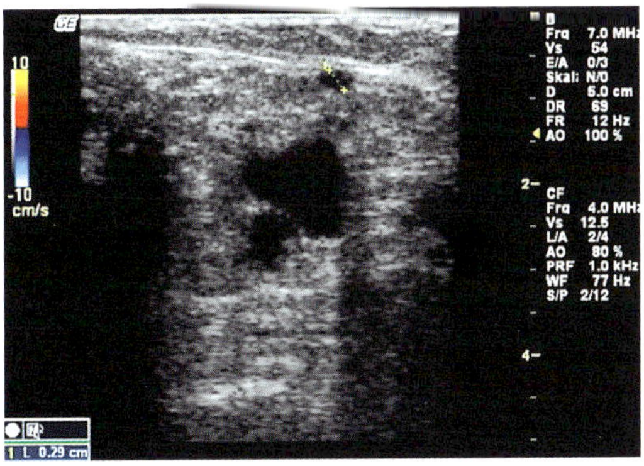

Fig. 8.10 Small saphenous vein 5 cm below the junction in transverse view through the back of the upper calf. Although the vein has a diameter of only 2.9 mm, it is refluxive (online material) Copyright: [Author]

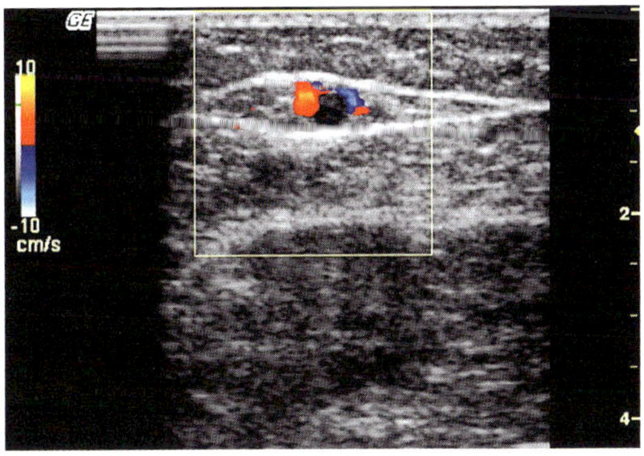

Fig. 8.12 Refluxive vasa vasorum of the small saphenous vein. Duplication must be distinguished from the very occasional occurrence of a refluxive vasa vasorum. Transverse view through the back of the calf in muscular diastole. The small saphenous vein is competent with a lumen that remains black. The vasa vasorum are refluxive (online material). Copyright: [Author]

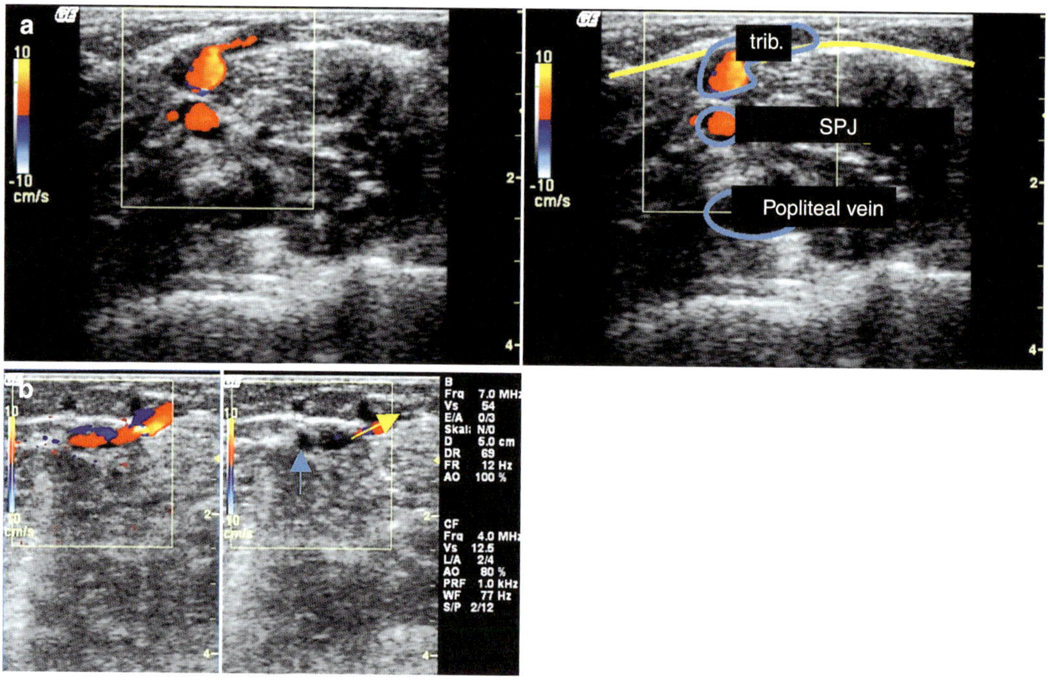

Fig. 8.13 Tributaries of the small saphenous vein (*SSV*). (**a**) Transverse view through the popliteal fossa demonstrating a direct refluxive tributary. The saphenopopliteal junction is incompetent. As soon as the reflux from the small saphenous vein reaches the fascia, it enters a tributary (*SA*). The small saphenous vein remains competent for the rest of its downward course. (**b**) Refluxive tributary of the small saphenous vein in the mid calf. The small saphenous vein is seen in the middle of the fascial compartment (*blue arrow*). The reflux is carried laterally by the tributary which pierces the fascia to enter the epifascial region (*yellow arrow*). Perforating veins often leave these tributaries to drain the reflux into the deep veins (online material) Copyright: [Author]

source is either through its junction or more seldom from the vein of Giacomini. Like the great saphenous vein, it is held and fixed within the fascial compartment and therefore courses in a straight line to the lateral malleolus. The calibre of the vein depends on the reflux volume (Figs. 8.3b and 8.4). Reflux may occur in small calibre veins. A small diameter cannot be a reliable indicator of normality (Fig. 8.10).

After a **thrombosis**, the small saphenous vein presents a typical image with a double contour (Fig. 11.6).

8.4.2.1 Reflux Exit Points

Reflux can leave the small saphenous vein at any point along its course. Tributaries are imaged with ultrasound in the same way as the great saphenous vein (Sects. 7.5.2 and 10.6.3).

In the popliteal fossa, reflux may leave the small saphenous vein by the vein of Giacomini or through separate knee tributaries (Figs. 8.13a, 4.6a and 4.16a). Reflux arising from the small saphenous vein through the vein of Giacomini as a source of reflux for the great saphenous vein is easily overlooked. Clinically this appears as a prominent great saphenous vein with varicosities along its course. Early "recurrence" after treatment of the great saphenous vein is expected if the true reflux source was not identified or treated.

Various branches may leave the refluxive small saphenous vein over its course. In the middle of the calf, these refluxive tributaries are very often connected to perforating veins. The soleus perforating vein (formerly May) is the most well known. They can connect also to muscle veins. These usually all serve as re-entry points carrying their reflux into the deep veins (Fig. 8.13b).

In the distal third of the calf, an interfascial branch may connect the small saphenous vein with the posterior arch vein. This is not easily seen on ultrasound because the leg at this site has a very small contact area with the probe. However, it is usually obvious clinically. This vein can carry the reflux from the small saphenous vein to the medial malleolus.

If the small saphenous vein is refluxive along its entire length, it may be devoid of any refluxive tributaries over its course. In this case the reflux enters the deep veins at the ankle or through the foot veins.

8.4.2.2 Reflux in the Presence of a Competent Saphenopopliteal Junction

If the junction of the small saphenous vein is competent, the vein may become refluxive along its downward course. Reflux sources may arise from the vein of Giacomini (see above and Figs. 4.11a, 4.12b and 4.13a), tributaries of the great saphenous vein, perforating veins or muscle veins. The most frequent source of reflux for the small saphenous vein is the great saphenous vein through the communicating vein on the inside of the calf (Sect. 10.6.4 and Fig. 4.13b).

The small saphenous vein may also be filled refluxively by tributaries of a refluxive **anterior accessory saphenous vein** communicating from the lateral side (Fig. 4.11b).

The **soleus perforating vein** (formerly May) is very seldom an independent proximal reflux source. In such cases, a trauma to the back of the calf has usually occurred. This can be detected in the patient's history (Fig. 4.12a). Very often the reflux has arisen after a thrombosis (Fig. 15.5).

A reflux source unique to the small saphenous vein is from the **muscle veins**. These may carry reflux from the deep system through the calf muscle compartment to the small saphenous vein. The epifascial veins can also receive this reflux. Occasionally in hyperextension of the knee, the popliteal vein may be compressed provoking a retrograde flow in the small saphenous vein in case of muscle contraction (standing) or in prone position.

8.5 Muscle Veins

In the popliteal fossa there are muscle veins in varying numbers and with variable courses that join the small saphenous vein (Figs. 8.14, 8.15, 8.16 and 8.17; see also Figs. 8.4 and 8.5) or the popliteal vein (Figs. 8.1a and 8.3a). They represent the drainage from the upper part of the calf muscle venous reservoir (Sect. 3.1). As shown in Fig. 8.14a, b, these veins can run parallel to the small saphenous vein causing confusion in identification. This can be a problem after surgery because, even after an expert examination, a muscle vein may be confused with the now absent small saphenous vein (Fig. 8.14d). In rare cases a refluxive muscle vein may fill the small saphenous vein refluxively further down its course (Fig. 8.15).

The **key to differentiating** between a muscle vein and the small saphenous vein is their relationship to the musculature and the saphenous fascia. The small saphenous vein always lies on the musculature between the saphenous fascia and the muscle fascia. Its course is parallel to the skin and does not vary. The muscle veins may start running parallel to the small saphenous vein, but then they turn into the musculature and away from the skin (Fig. 8.14d).

A preoperative assessment with precise documentation of the anatomy and flow within muscle veins and their relation to the small saphenous and popliteal vein is helpful. The following combinations are all possible:

- Refluxive small saphenous vein and refluxive muscle veins in the popliteal fossa which have no further contact in their downward course.
- Refluxive small saphenous vein and refluxive muscle veins in the popliteal fossa which communicate during their downward course (Fig. 8.15c). After a proximal ligation of the small saphenous vein, these muscle veins, if not eliminated, may result in continued reflux further down the small saphenous vein.
- Refluxive small saphenous vein and competent muscle veins (Fig. 8.16).
- Both veins are competent, but the muscle veins may appear dilated, depending on how long the subject has been standing (Fig. 8.14c).
- Competent small saphenous vein and refluxive muscle vein. The latter delivers reflux into the lower part of the small saphenous vein (Fig. 8.15a, b) or directly into epifascial tributaries (Fig. 8.17)

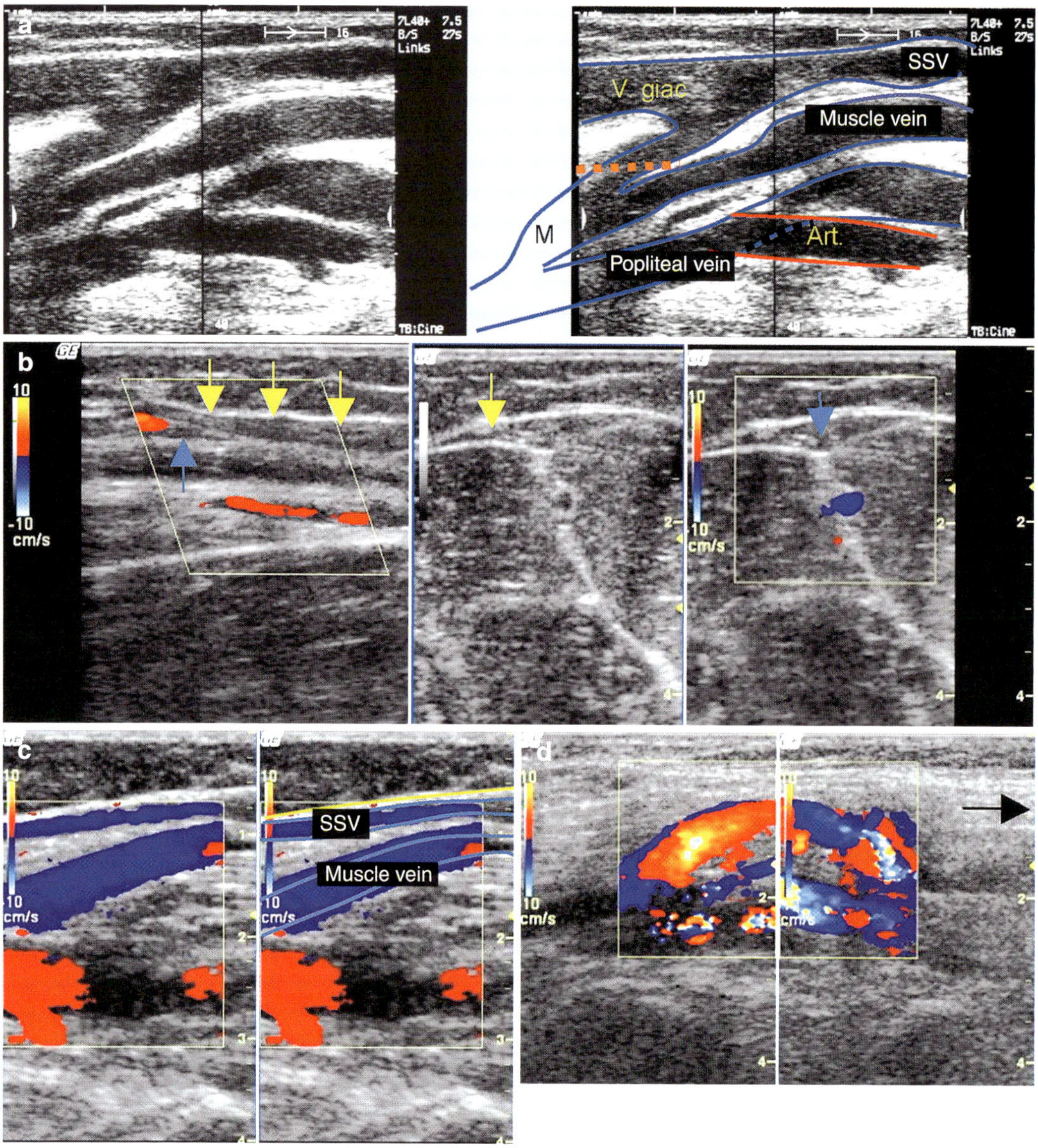

Fig. 8.14 (**a**) Longitudinal section through the popliteal fossa demonstrating a refluxive small saphenous vein (*SSV*) and an accompanying healthy but large muscle vein. Both join together to enter the popliteal vein (*M*). Intra-operatively, the confluence of the small saphenous vein with the muscle vein may easily be mistaken as the saphenopopliteal junction. The site of a proposed ligation and section to disconnect this vein has been marked (*dotted orange line*). It is easy to imagine how after the elimination of the small saphenous vein in this case, the muscle vein might be mistaken for an intact small saphenous vein (see d) (online material). (**b**) Downward course of a competent small saphenous vein and an accompanying muscle vein during calf muscle systole. *Left* Longitudinal section, *middle* and *right* transverse section with and without flow. The muscle vein (*blue* flow signal in image on *right*, extended *red* flow signal in image on *left*) runs in the septum between the two gastrocnemius muscles. The small saphenous vein is very small (*blue arrow*), and the saphenous fascia is seen in very close proximity (*yellow arrows*). (**c**) Competent small saphenous vein and accompanying competent muscle vein in the upper calf curving inwards to the junction (not shown). The muscle vein appears as the dominant vein. However, they can be clearly distinguished because the true small saphenous vein runs directly on the muscle beneath the fascia (*yellow*) (online material). (**d**) Longitudinal view through the popliteal fossa after stripping of the small saphenous vein. The popliteal vein has thrombosed. A large refluxive muscle vein is seen as it runs first towards the skin (*left half* of the image). It later becomes deeper where it re-enters the muscle tissue (*right half* of the image). It is clearly not on the level of the saphenous compartment (*arrow*). It can thus be safely distinguished from the small saphenous vein Copyright: [Author]

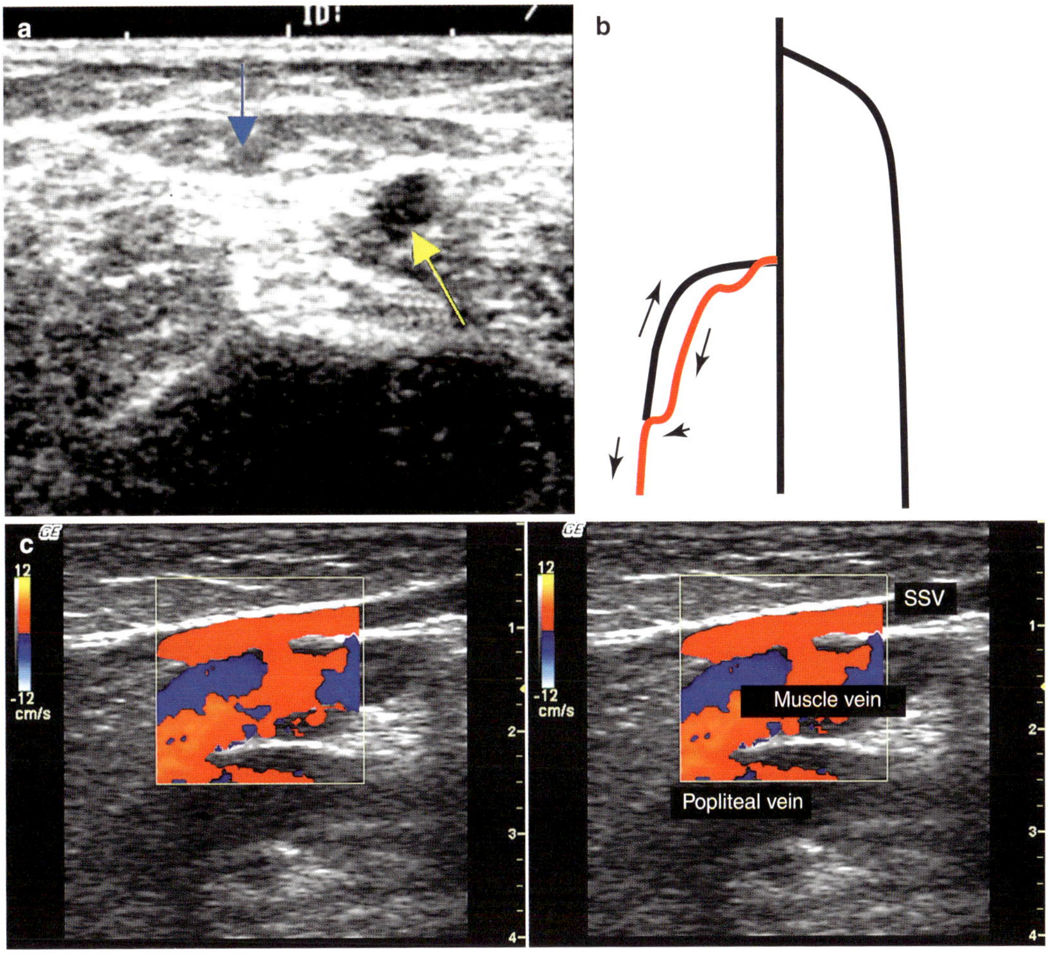

Fig. 8.15 (**a**) Transverse view through the back of the calf showing a competent small saphenous vein (*blue arrow*) and a refluxive muscle vein (*yellow arrow*). (**b**) Diagram of the recirculation circuit with incompetence of a muscle vein arising from the popliteal fossa. This fills the lower part of the small saphenous vein which is also refluxive (online material). (**c**) Longitudinal view through the lower part of the popliteal fossa similar to (a). However, the small saphenous vein (*SSV*) is also refluxive at the junction. The junction of the small saphenous vein lies in the lower thigh. There is quite often a connection with the muscle vein in this region. If only the junction of the small saphenous vein is interrupted, because the connection was not discovered in preoperative scan, reflux may persist (online material) Copyright: [Author]

8.6 Systolic Flow in the Small Saphenous Vein

The general indications for examining flow direction in the small saphenous vein are given in Sect. 7.5. In contrast to the great saphenous vein, the small saphenous vein has a unique feature. In the great saphenous vein, there is antegrade flow during all muscular provocation manoeuvres. These include the Wunstorf manoeuvre or manual calf compression. Antegrade flow occurs irrespective of whether the vein is competent or not. However, in the small saphenous vein during muscular systole, there may be flow in the direction of the feet (Fig. 8.18). As depicted, systolic reflux occurs with muscle contraction (Fig. 8.18a) but not with manual calf compression (Fig. 8.18b). This suggests a functional hindrance in the thigh veins precipitated by calf contraction which compresses the proximal popliteal or distal femoral vein. The precise cause

Fig. 8.16 Longitudinal view through the back of the calf with a refluxive, grossly dilated small saphenous vein (*) and a competent muscle vein (#). The muscle vein runs directly on the muscles, immediately underneath the muscle fascia Copyright: [Author]

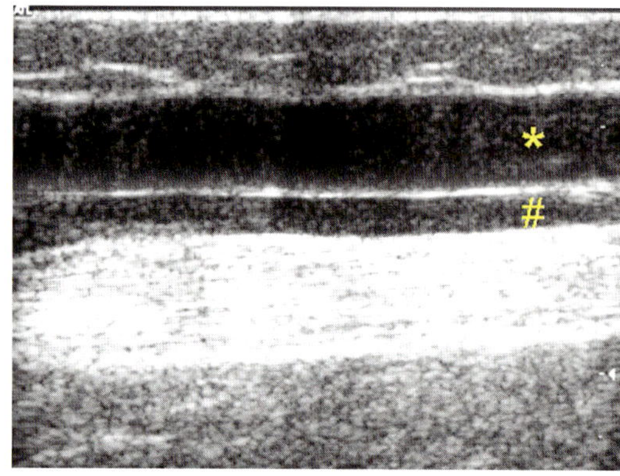

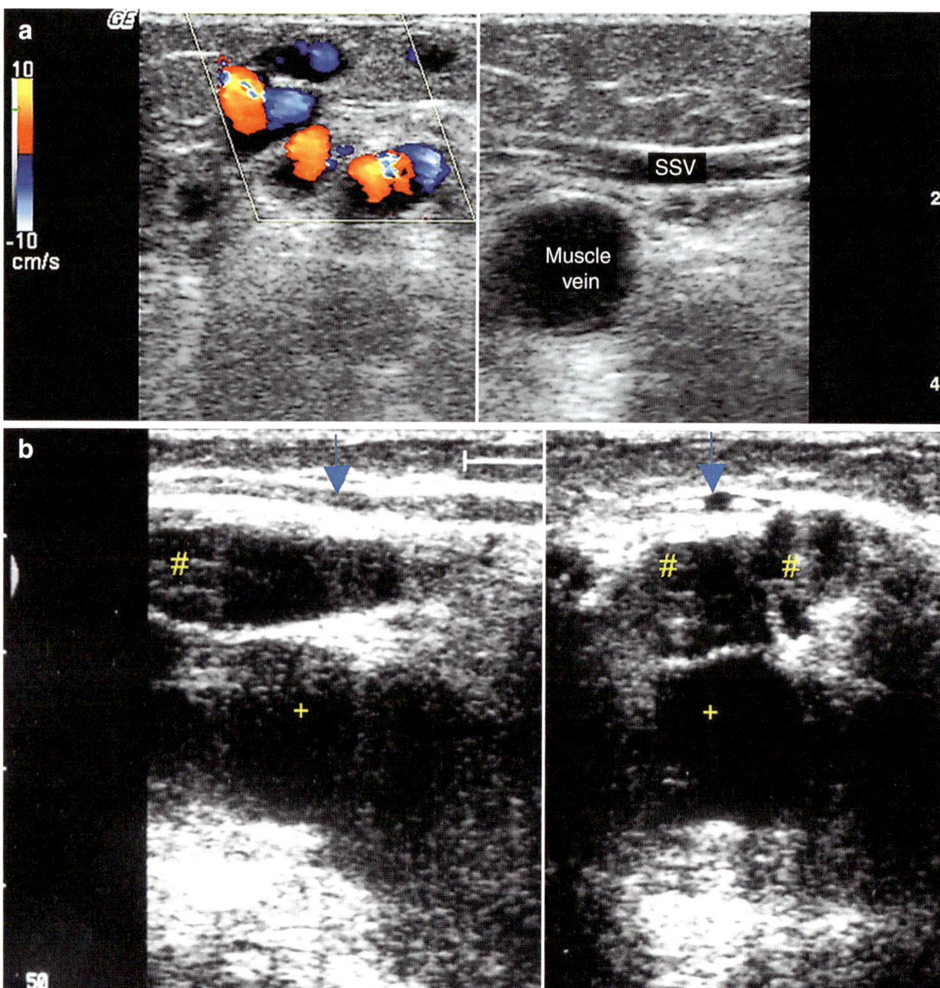

Fig. 8.17 (**a**) Refluxive muscle vein and competent small saphenous vein. Left is a transverse view of where the reflux leaves the muscle vein to enter the epifascial veins. Right is a longitudinal view with a section of the competent small saphenous vein (*SSV*) and the grossly dilated muscle vein (*MV*). (online material). (**b**) A longitudinal (*left*) and transverse (*right*) view through the upper calf. A refluxive muscle vein (#) could easily be mistaken for the small saphenous vein. The latter is small and runs in its own fascial compartment (*blue arrow*) Copyright: [Author]

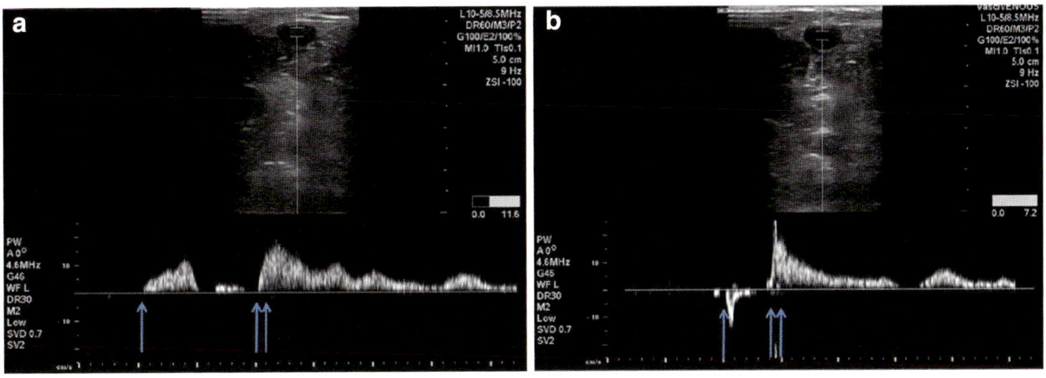

Fig. 8.18 Transverse view of the popliteal fossa with PW measurement in a refluxive small saphenous vein immediately below the saphenopopliteal junction. (**a**) Velocity profile induced by a Wunstorf manoeuvre (muscle contraction/systole *1 arrow*; relaxation/diastole *2 arrows*). Reflux is present in both systole and diastole. (**b**) Velocity profile in the same place induced by a manual calf compression (*1 arrow*) and release (*2 arrows*) manoeuvre. Note the antegrade flow on manual compression Copyright: [Author]

and mechanism are not clear. In post-thrombotic occlusion of the deep veins, reflux can be observed in the refluxive small saphenous vein even during the first phase of manual compression.

There are several studies of systolic reflux in the small saphenous vein by M. Cappelli and A. Obermayer (not yet published). They explain this phenomenon by a functional or physical obstruction of the femoral vein proximal of the junction of the small saphenous vein, so that during muscular systole, flow emerges from the deep leg veins into the small saphenous vein.

9 Perforating Veins

Erika Mendoza and Christopher R. Lattimer

Chapter Summary

Perforating veins form the connection between the superficial and deep veins. Physiologically, they serve to drain the superficial veins into the deep veins. In case of venous insufficiency with recirculation of blood in superficial leg veins, they may reflux or act as a drainage pathway. These are termed "re-entry" points.

Perforating veins very seldom run a straight horizontal course from the superficial to the deep veins. Instead, they curve and wind through the musculature. This means that during muscular contraction, the perforating vein is compressed and thus closed by the shear forces and pressure exerted by the muscle movement.

Although hundreds of perforating veins are present in the leg (see also Sects. 2.4.7 and 2.5.5), only those which are pathologically dilated are relevant for the examination of a recirculation. If a perforating vein is barely recognisable in B scan, it generally plays no part in the recirculation.

Perforating veins which drain saphenous veins very seldom do so directly. The blood is usually routed via a tributary. Only the paratibial perforating vein below the knee (formerly Boyd) joins the back of the great saphenous vein directly. The perforating veins of the adductor canal (formerly Dodd and Hunter) are more or less equally likely to leave the great saphenous vein directly or via a small saphenous tributary.

It must not be forgotten that the saphenofemoral junction and saphenopopliteal junction are the most common perforating veins; however, they are usually described separately.

E. Mendoza, MD, PhD (✉)
Venenpraxis Wunstorf,
Speckenstraße 10, 31515 Wunstorf, Germany
e-mail: erika.mendoza@t-online.de

C.R. Lattimer, MD, PhD
Department of Vascular Surgery,
Josef Pflug Vascular Laboratory,
Ealing Hospital and Imperial College, London, UK

9.1 Examination Procedure

Most perforating veins of clinical importance lie along the course of the saphenous veins and their major tributaries. They are usually included in the examination of the saphenous vein. However, remote perforating veins must be examined separately with the probe. These include the perforating veins in the back and the lateral side of the thigh. **Varicose tributaries** must be checked for perforating veins, especially on the inside of the calf.

In B scan, perforating veins appear as echo-free structures running inwards from the surface towards the deep veins. The site of a perforating vein is identified as an interruption of the muscle

E. Mendoza et al. (eds.), *Duplex Ultrasound of Superficial Leg Veins*,
DOI 10.1007/978-3-642-40731-4_9, © Springer-Verlag Berlin Heidelberg 2014

fascia. This can be observed as the probe is moved along the leg. The fact that a perforating vein is dilated is no guarantee that it is refluxive. It may be a re-entry point, dilated by volume overload (Sect. 3.4).

Perforating veins can be visualised in colour duplex and during provocation manoeuvres, since the flow is either towards or away from the probe. The colour does not permit any conclusions on flow direction because this flow is often turbulent. In this case, PW mode is the only way of establishing whether the perforating vein is refluxive.

Perforating veins are best examined with the subject standing. Dependency results in well-filled veins and assists in the diagnosis. The physiological flow in a perforating vein is from superficial to deep. After the subject has been standing without moving for a long time, the pressures in the superficial and deep veins equalise resulting in stasis within perforating veins.

During muscle contraction, the blood is first expelled from the deep system with upward and outward forces. Initial flow towards the superficial veins occurs until the point at which the valves close or the calf muscles close the perforating veins. This arrests further outward flow and encourages upward flow. Thus, an initial outward flow in a perforating vein does not necessarily indicate incompetence, any more than a short duration of retrograde flow (<0.5 s) necessary for valve closure in a saphenous vein after a provocation manoeuvre (Sect. 9.3).

9.2 Examination Objectives

The following questions should be answered in the examination of perforating veins:

- Are there any dilated perforating veins in the courses of the great and small saphenous veins?
- Are there any visible perforating veins in other typical locations like the posterior arch vein and the back or lateral side of the thigh or calf?
- If so, is it a muscle perforating vein (connection between deep vein, muscle vein via perforator to a superficial vein), and is there a post-traumatic cause in case of dilation?
- Have the perforating veins suffered post-thrombotic damage?
- What is their diameter?

The following should be clarified in perforating veins of large diameter (>3 mm):

- Does the perforating vein form the upper end of a recirculation (reflux source)?
- Does the perforating vein form the lower end of a recirculation (re-entry point)?
- Does the perforating vein present a blowout?
- Is the perforating vein located under an ulcer?

9.3 Blood Flow in a Perforating Vein

Physiologically, blood in leg veins is supposed to flow from superficial to deep, which means that the blood will show an inward flow in normal perforating veins. However, with manual compression, it has been shown that competent perforating veins have an outward flow in 21.7 % during manual compression lasting less than 0.5 s and in 70 % after release (Delis et al. 2001). It is not known whether these percentages of outflow are the same following physiological provocation manoeuvres (Paraná, Wunstorf, see Chap. 5).

If a recirculation is present (see Sect. 3.2), only those perforating veins which are dilated (>3 mm) in B scan need to be examined using duplex ultrasound. Perforating veins which are not visible in B scan are generally not involved in a recirculation. The volume and direction of blood flow in a large-calibre perforating vein must be measured to decide whether it is a reflux source or a re-entry point.

The following criteria are important for the examination of dilated perforating veins:

Position relative to the superficial veins (Sects. 9.4, 9.5, 9.6, 9.7, 9.8, 9.9 and 9.10):

- In the course of a saphenous vein
- In the course of a tributary

Direction of flow, to clarify:

- The reflux source (Sect. 9.3.1)
- The re-entry point (Sect. 9.3.2)
- Combinations (Sect. 9.3.2)

To examine the blood flow in a perforating vein, it must first be augmented. Muscular provocation manoeuvres like the Wunstorf manoeuvre (Sect. 6.7) close the perforating veins in their course during calf muscle systole, irrespective of whether the valves are functioning. In exceptional cases, grossly dilated perforating veins may not close.

The pressure in the deep veins is increased by muscular contraction and manual calf compression. As a result, blood tries to flow upwards but also outwards into the perforating veins. If these are dilated because they are refluxive or suffer volume overload from a recirculation, the flow direction during muscular systole or manual compression will be outwards (Fig. 9.1).

The flow after muscle relaxation is essential for diagnosis (Fig. 9.1). All perforating veins should be assessed during **muscular diastole**. If there is outward flow during diastole, the perforating vein is incompetent (Fig. 9.1e). However, it is more common to find a higher pressure in the incompetent superficial vein than in the deep vein after muscular contraction. In this case, the blood flows inwards through the dilated perforating vein during diastole (Fig. 9.1b–d). Further studies have to enlighten the direction taken by the blood before and after flow through a perforating vein. For example, these interactions could be out and up, out and down, up and in and down and in, depending on the situation. This may help also to identify whether the perforating vein acts as a source of reflux or a re-entry point. Outward and upward flow, for example, may be less detrimental than outward and downward flow. The extent this has on therapeutic decisions needs further investigation.

The practice of applying a tourniquet above the perforating vein in order to measure its flow under manual compression and decompression may give a false pathological result. If the incompetent vein is occluded above the perforating vein by the tourniquet, the refluxive recirculation downwards will not occur in diastole. However, a perforating vein which is dilated by recirculation is often in contact with an incompetent vein further down. After decompression, the blood will flow out of the deep veins, through the dilated perforating vein and into the incompetent distal segment of the superficial vein. A vein thus appears incompetent which under physiological conditions (without the tourniquet) serves as a re-entry point.

9.3.1 Perforating Veins as Sources of Recirculation

Diastolic **reflux** or outward flow during muscular diastole is a sine qua non for describing a perforating vein as a reflux source.

The further down the leg, the less likely a perforating vein is to serve as the reflux source for a recirculation. The only exception is secondary varices after trauma to the calf which may occur with periosteal injuries to the tibia (Sect. 9.10). It is not unusual to find a single refluxive muscle vein after trauma, for example, in footballers. These fill varicose tributaries and form a proximal source of reflux. The proximal reflux source is often the proximal perforating veins of the adductor canal (formerly Dodd) (Fig. 9.2), less often the distal perforating vein of the adductor canal (formerly Hunter; Fig. 9.1e) and very rarely the proximal paratibial perforating veins (formerly Boyd; Figs. 9.3 and 7.48). The latter are more often refluxive with secondary varices arising from reflux in the deep axis above the posterior tibial vein.

Incompetent muscle veins may be the source for subcutaneous reticular varices on the **back and lateral or medial aspect of the calf** (Fig. 9.4 and Sect. 9.9). These frequently develop after trauma. A perforating vein in the back of the thigh may be incompetent, refluxing into the Giacomini anastomosis or a varicose tributary (Fig. 9.5). Occasionally, a perforating vein arising directly from the popliteal vein may be found near the saphenopopliteal junction or slightly further proximal (Fig. 9.6).

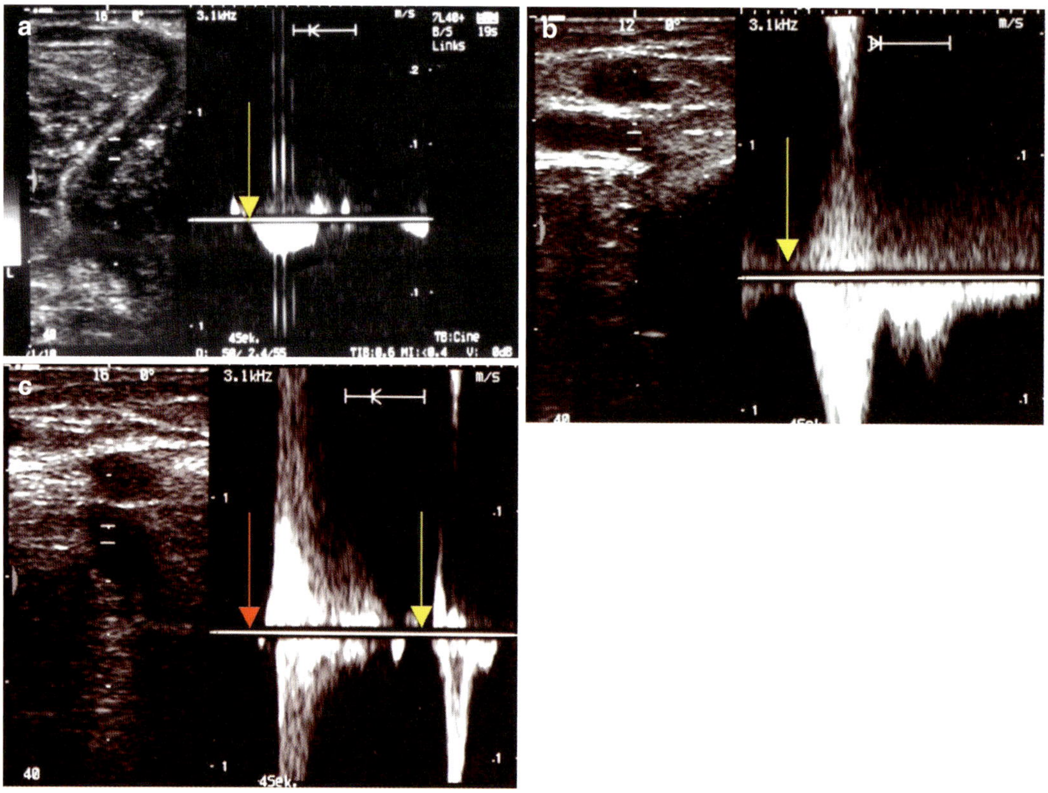

Fig. 9.1 Blood flow in perforating veins under provocation manoeuvres; *red arrow*, start of muscular systole; *yellow arrow*, start of muscular diastole; *above baseline*, outward reflux; and *below baseline*, antegrade inward flow. (**a**) Flow in a grossly dilated paratibial perforating vein with an incompetent great saphenous vein. The blood flows through this perforating vein to the deep vein. This results from secondary dilation, not primary incompetence. (**b**) Flow in a grossly dilated paratibial perforating vein to the deep vein with an incompetent great saphenous vein. The inward flow results from secondary dilatation, not primary incompetence. (**c**) Flow in the posterior tibial perforating vein (formerly Cockett 2). The volume which flows outwards during muscular systole appears to be greater than the inward re-entry volume. This subject had severe varicose veins with secondary deep vein incompetence. However, since the diastolic blood flow is still inwards, drainage must be initially through a perforating vein dilated by the reflux volume, which is not in itself incompetent. In procedures which eliminate the reflux source, it is possible to wait before treating this vein. Once the recirculation has been eliminated, it will become apparent whether the perforating vein recovers its normal calibre or must be interrupted. (**d**) A muscle vein in the calf at the end of a varicose tributary. The blood flows inwards towards the deep veins during both muscular systole and diastole. This perforating vein has bidirectional flow from secondary dilatation; it is not primarily a refluxive vein. (**e**) Distal perforating vein of the adductor canal (formerly Hunter) as a proximal reflux source of a recirculation. Outward flow occurs during both muscular systole and diastole. This is a clear diagnosis of an incompetent perforating vein. (**f**) Transverse view through the inner thigh showing the perforating vein of the adductor canal (formerly Dodd) joining the side of the great saphenous vein. The perforating vein appears refluxive in calf muscle systole with outward flow (*red* in colour duplex). Manual compression of the calf causes an increase in pressure in the deep veins driving blood through the perforating vein in the relaxed musculature of the thigh and then into the superficial veins (online material). (**g**) Relaxation phase in the same subject as in (f) demonstrating flow reversal. Inward flow from the refluxive great saphenous vein via the perforating vein into the deep vein. The perforating vein is not a reflux source for recirculation, but a re-entry drainage point. (**h**) Transverse view through the inside of the calf demonstrating a dilated paratibial perforating vein (formerly Boyd) with incompetence of the great saphenous vein (*GSV*), above and below the knee. There is distal drainage through the perforating veins of the posterior tibial veins (formerly Cockett group). The Wunstorf manoeuvre is demonstrated by the film sequences on the online material which show inward flow during muscular diastole. Colour artefacts are observed during muscular contraction which are unavoidable as the musculature is moving in the image. The flow after prolonged standing can also be seen with small volumes of blood flowing from the deep to the superficial system. This indicates that there is a re-entry perforating vein Copyright: [Author]

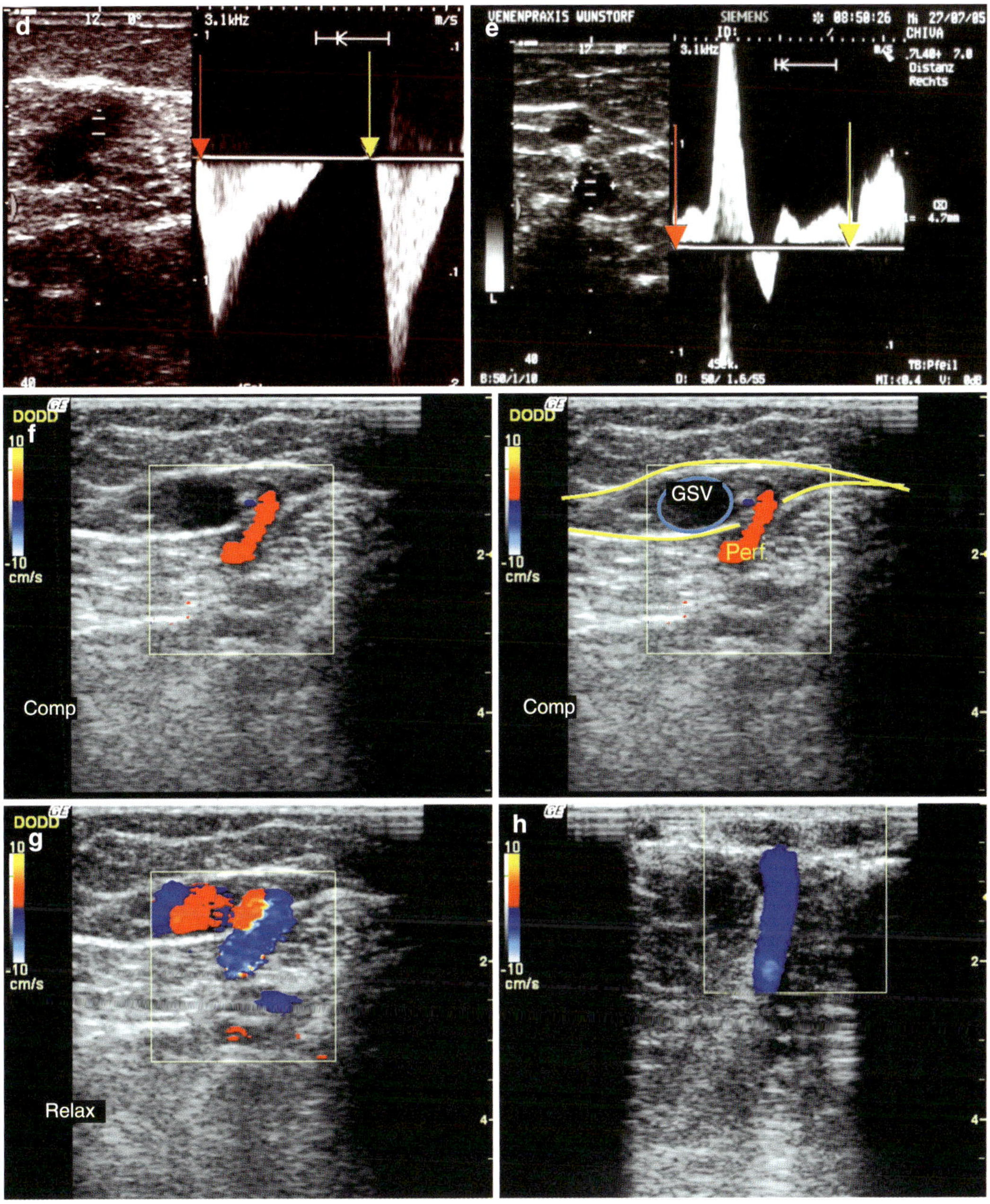

Fig. 9.1 (continued)

It is also rare for a dilated perforating vein to fill an already refluxive vein with more reflux from the deep vein. However, this can occur when secondary varices appear after a deep vein thrombosis. If the saphenous vein is already refluxive above the perforating vein, the velocity profiles in each must be compared before diagnosing the latter as incompetent. Firstly, their velocity profiles must show a predominantly outward flow. Secondly, the velocity profile in the distal section

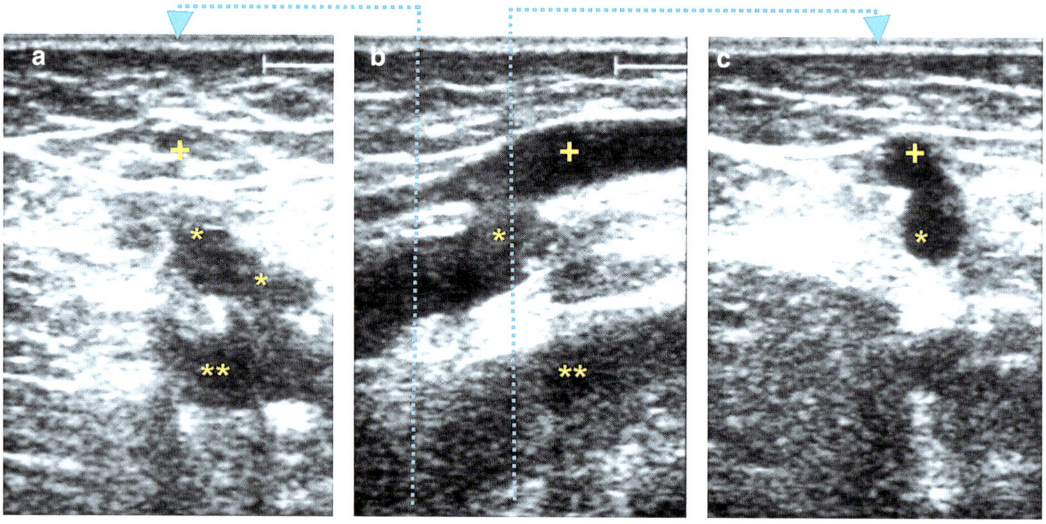

Fig. 9.2 (**a**) Transverse view through a competent great saphenous vein (+) in the mid thigh. Beneath it, an incompetent perforating vein of the adductor canal (formerly Dodd) (*) is seen connecting to the femoral vein (**). (**b**) Longitudinal view at the junction of the perforating vein with the great saphenous vein which becomes refluxive and dilated. The perforating vein typically arises from the deep system and courses downwards. (**c**) Junction of the perforating vein and the great saphenous vein in transverse view (*dotted line* in **b**: section levels for **a** and **c**) Copyright: [Author]

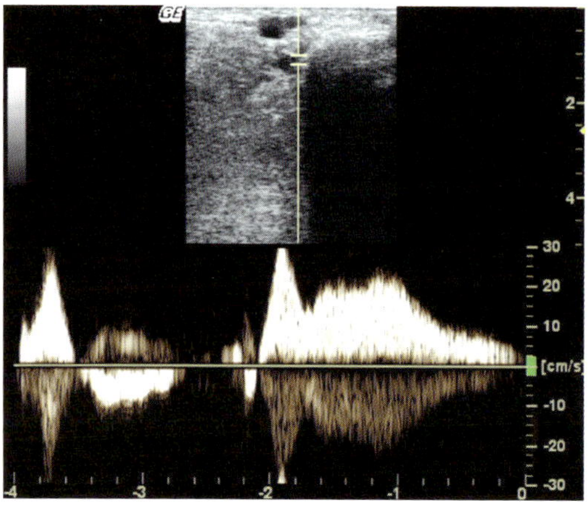

Fig. 9.3 Transverse view through the upper third of the left calf demonstrating an incompetent proximal paratibial perforating vein (formerly Boyd). The perforating vein is dilated and acts as a reflux source for the great saphenous vein. Note the outward flow during calf diastole Copyright: [Author]

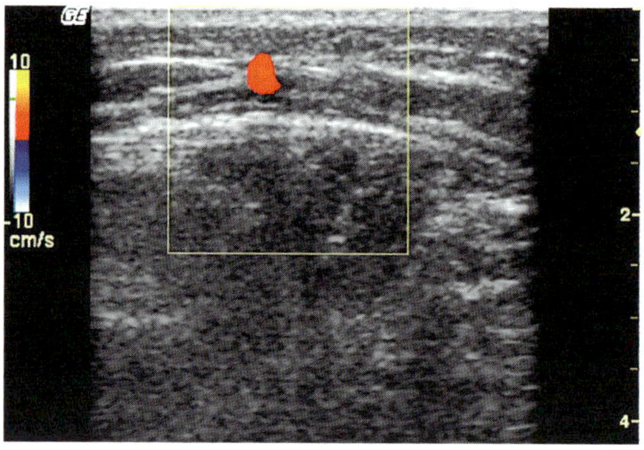

Fig. 9.4 Transverse view through the back of the left thigh. A small-calibre, refluxive perforating vein is seen emerging from the muscle fascia to fill a subcutaneous reticular network. Subcutaneous treatments of reticular veins are less likely to succeed in the presence of a feeding perforating vein unless this is also treated Copyright: [Author]

of the great saphenous vein must carry a larger reflux volume than the proximal great saphenous vein. This means that the perforating vein is adding to the reflux volume and should be treated. This distinction can only be made in PW mode.

9.3.2 Perforating Veins as Re-entry Points for a Recirculation

Dilated perforating veins usually act as re-entry points and are not primarily incompetent vessels:

- They provide the drainage for a large-calibre vessel, and consequently, they must also have a large calibre to drain the increased volume.

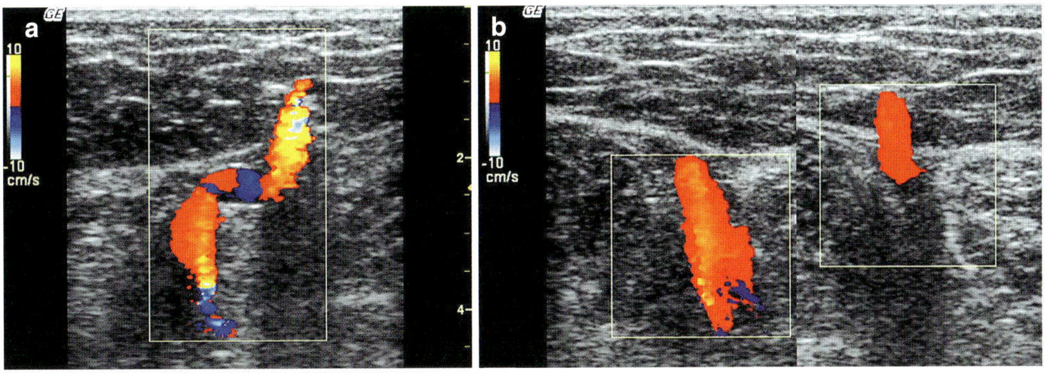

Fig. 9.5 (**a**) Longitudinal view through the back of the thigh in a patient with a visible varicose tributary above the knee. A large, refluxive perforating vein is seen with duplex running distally for a short distance under the muscle fascia and then piercing the fascia and filling the tributary (online material). (**b**) Transverse view of the same perforating vein; *left* (further proximal) where it is still deep, *right* (further distal) where it pierces the fascia to become superficial Copyright: [Author]

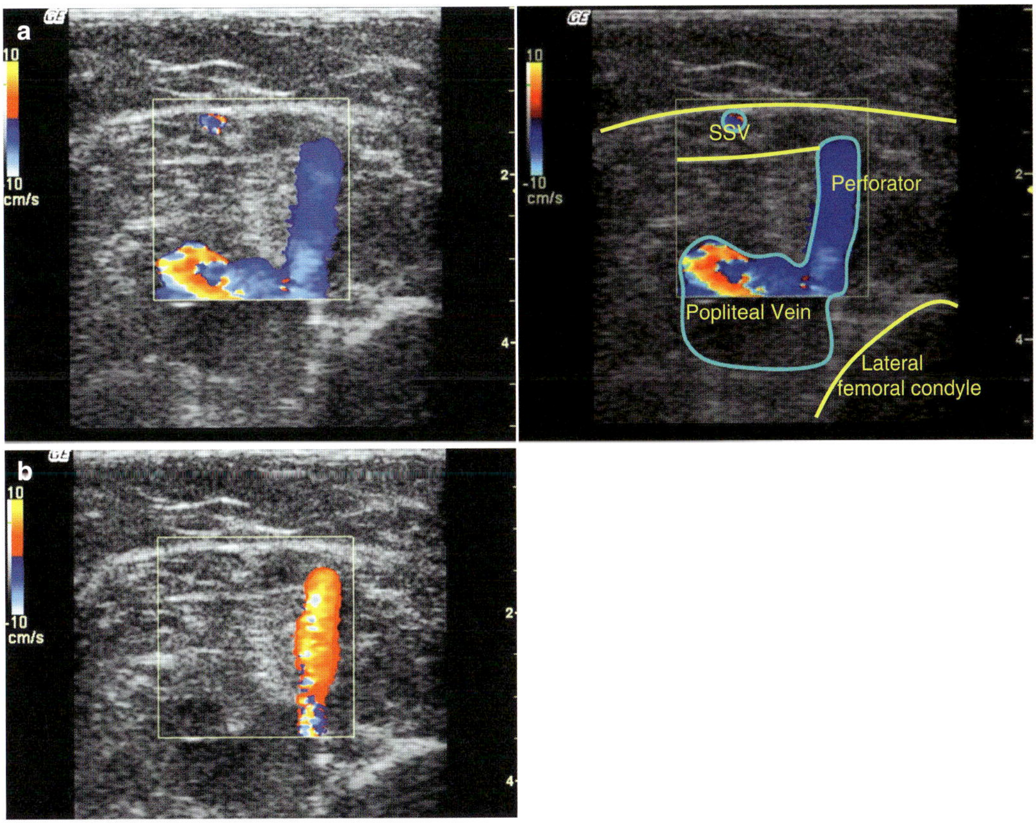

Fig. 9.6 Transverse view through the right popliteal region. The saphenopopliteal junction is 10 cm higher up. A large perforating vein is seen arising from the popliteal vein and refluxing into a (not shown) subcutaneous varicosity. (**a**) During muscular systole, there is antegrade flow in small saphenous vein and inward flow in the perforating vein. (**b**) During muscular diastole, there is reflux arising from the popliteal vein with outward flow in the perforating vein. The film sequences on the online material show first the B scan with the probe travelling from distal to proximal and then the colour duplex scan. The Wunstorf manoeuvre causes a long-lasting reflux in diastole Copyright: [Author]

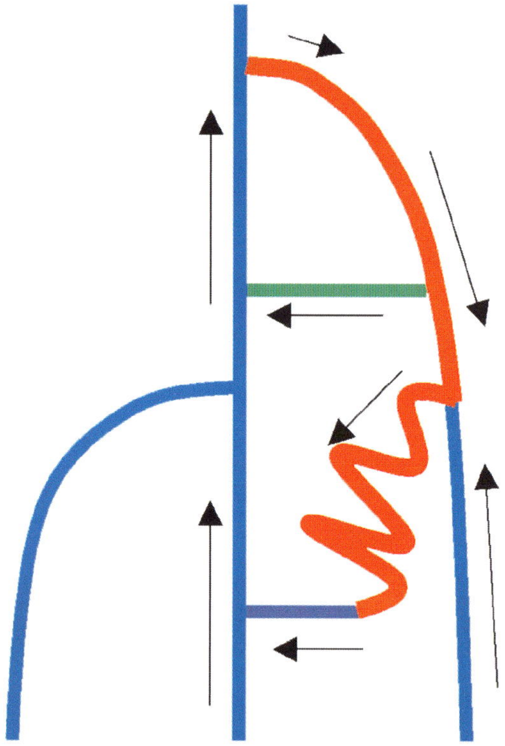

Fig. 9.7 Reflux in great saphenous vein (GSV) above and below the knee. Drainage is via the perforator in the adductor canal in the thigh (formerly Dodd; green connection between great saphenous vein and deep vein, see Fig. 9.1f, g) and through the perforating veins of the posterior tibial veins (formerly Cockett group; *blue connection* from the tributary to the deep leg vein) (SSV small saphenous vein) Copyright: [Author]

- During muscular diastole, the blood flows inwards through these veins to the deep veins (Fig. 9.1a–h).
- If the recirculation is interrupted by crossectomy, stripping, endovenous means or saphenous conservation surgery, the calibre of these re-entry perforating veins will be reduced (Mendoza 2013).

The further distal the perforating vein, the greater the probability that it serves as a drainage pathway (see also Sect. 3.4). It may lie on the course of a refluxive vein and therefore only deliver a part of its recirculation volume to the deep veins (Fig. 9.7). The perforating vein of the adductor canal (formerly Dodd or Hunter) is such an example. Alternatively, it may be at the end of the refluxive section (Fig. 9.7). This is typical of the posterior tibial group of perforating veins (formerly Cockett). Perforating veins at the end of a refluxive section are also called **terminal perforating veins** (Franceschi and Zamboni 2009).

All perforating veins can serve as a drainage pathway in a recirculation. The most frequent ones are the calf veins, especially the **posterior tibial group** (formerly Cockett group), and the **paratibial perforating veins**. The veins in the dorsal part of the foot can also play a part in the drainage of superficial reflux above the ankle. They are connected with the deep vein system on the medial and lateral aspect of the foot.

Blowout veins are terminal perforating veins which represent the re-entry points at the lowest point of superficial reflux. They become grossly dilated because, whenever the calf muscle contracts, blood is pushed out of the perforating vein. It cannot drain distally and it is met with a hydrostatic column proximally. Hence, the pressure changes are great. Thus, blood in this segment continues to oscillate between muscular systole and diastole, and the resulting turbulence and pressures lead to a dilatation of the vein wall (see also Sect. 3.1).

9.3.3 Re-entry Perforators of the Saphenous Veins

In the classification of shunts according to Franceschi (1993), it is important to differentiate if the reflux enters the deep venous system directly through a perforator connected to the saphenous vein (Shunt I or IV) or via a tributary which bridges between the saphenous vein and the re-entry perforator (Shunt III or V). This can be achieved with the reflux elimination test (Zamboni et al. 2010), described in Fig. 4.23.

9.4 Perforating Veins in the Thigh Along the Great Saphenous Vein

There is a perforating vein in the upper thigh which is seldom clinically relevant. It connects the deep femoral vein to the great saphenous vein

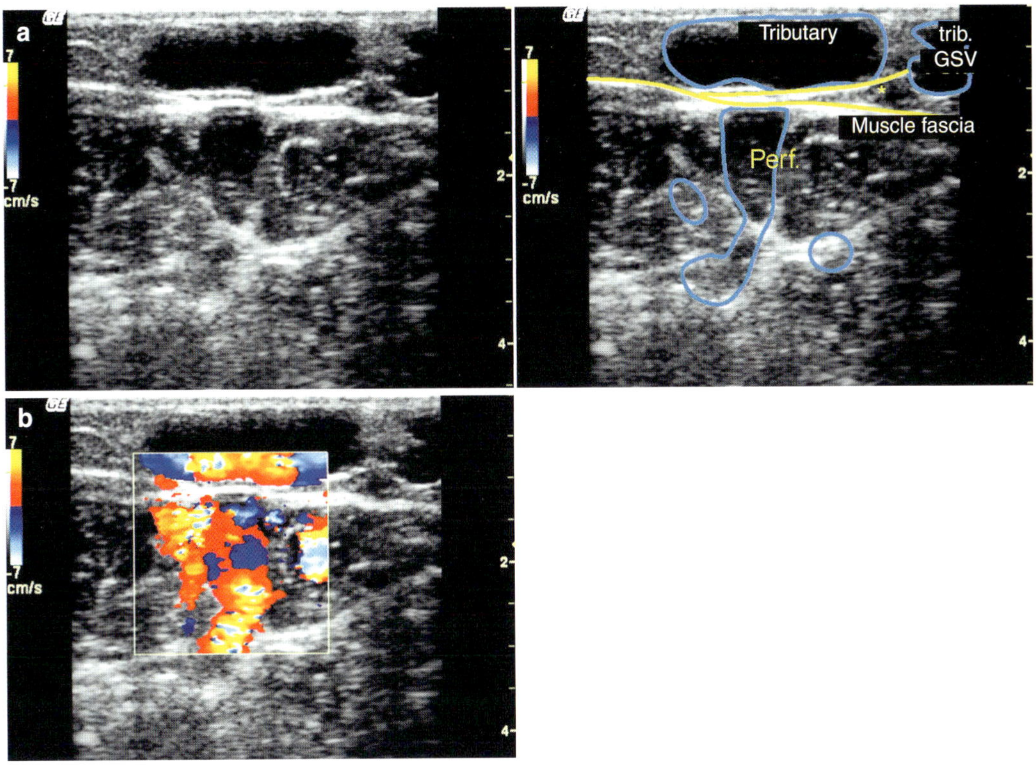

Fig. 9.8 (**a**) Transverse view through the inner thigh showing a dilated perforating vein of the adductor canal (formerly Dodd), which fills a tributary of a competent great saphenous vein (*GSV*). The perforating vein winds markedly making it impossible to see where it pierces the fascia. * indicates the saphenous fascia which merges into the muscle fascia in the left-hand third of the image. (**b**) Same configuration as in (a) during muscular diastole demonstrating turbulent flow in the tributary and the dilated perforating vein Copyright: [Author]

approximately 5 cm below the saphenofemoral junction.

According to new nomenclature, the perforating veins in the thigh along the course of the great saphenous vein are now known generally as the **perforating veins of the adductor canal**. They include the former Dodd perforating veins in the middle third of the thigh and the less important Hunter perforating veins in the lower third.

The most important perforating vein in the thigh is the one found at the border between its middle and lower third. It runs an oblique course from the femoral vein down to the great saphenous vein. In very rare cases, it is almost vertical forming a plane in-line with the great saphenous vein. The more proximal of the two middle third perforating veins is at the border between the upper and middle thirds of the thigh or at the mid thigh.

A refluxive perforating vein of the adductor canal may join a tributary of the great saphenous vein (Fig. 9.8). This tributary will then either carry the reflux further as a varicose vein or fill the great saphenous vein refluxively. The perforating vein may also join the great saphenous vein directly (Fig. 9.9, see also Fig. 9.2). A further tributary is often filled refluxively in the immediate vicinity of the incompetent perforating vein directly from the refluxively filled saphenous trunk. Thus, only a small segment of the great saphenous vein serves as a conduit for reflux, making its participation in recirculation minimal. On rare occasions when there is a refluxive tributary above the perforating vein, reflux can ascend up the great saphenous vein (Fig. 9.10). This is called ascending pathological reflux or **antegrade incompetence** (Sect. 7.5.1). Trauma can also result in dilatation of the perforating veins (Fig. 9.11).

The most distal perforating vein of the adductor canal (formerly Hunter) runs on the inside of

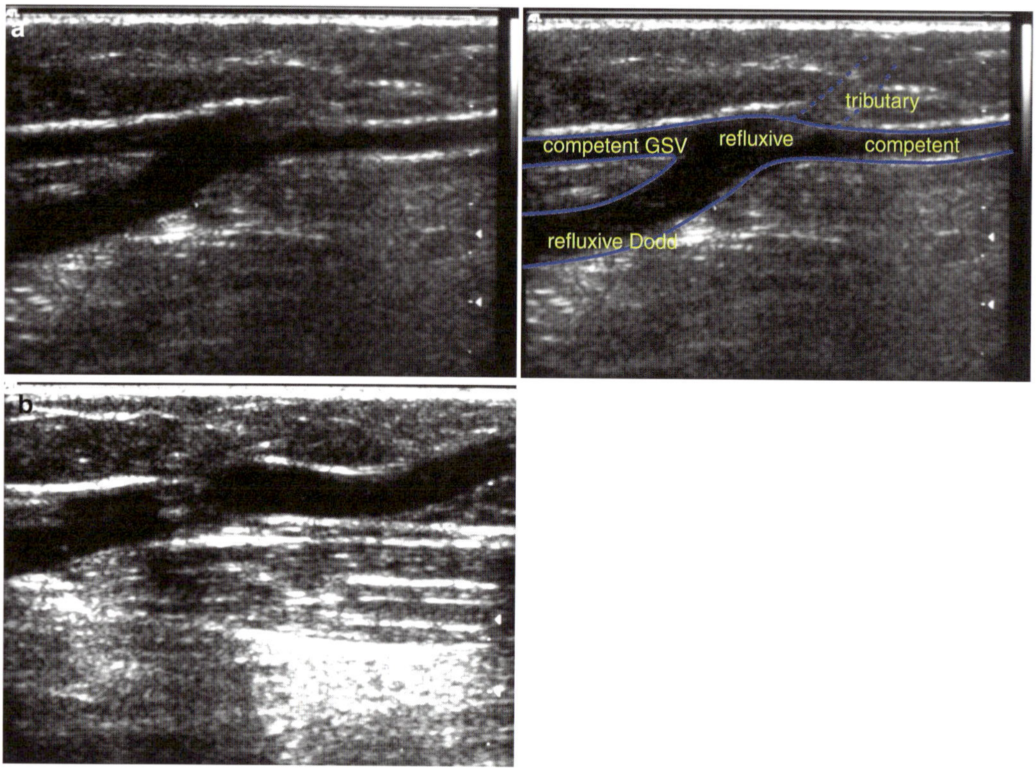

Fig. 9.9 (**a**) Longitudinal view through the inner thigh. A refluxive perforating vein of the adductor canal is seen as a reflux source for the great saphenous vein. The perforating vein comes from above which is typical for this vein. The great saphenous vein remains competent above and below because it is only filled refluxively across a very short segment where the reflux stream exits into a refluxive tributary. (**b**) Same leg as in (a) with the probe axis tilted laterally to demonstrate the course of the refluxive tributary. This is represented by the dotted contour in (a) (*right*) Copyright: [Author]

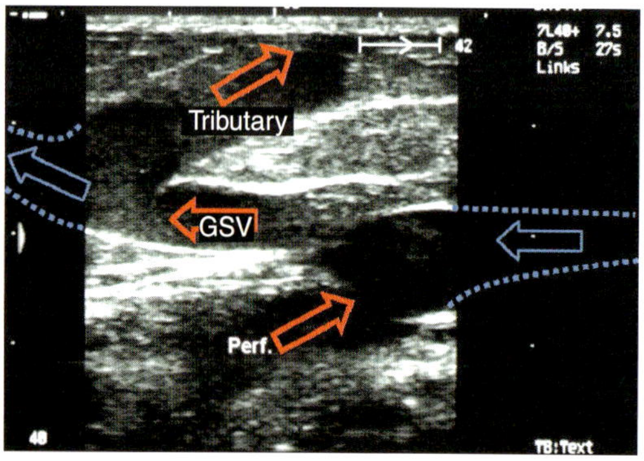

Fig. 9.10 Longitudinal view through the inner thigh, left upper, right lower. A refluxive perforating vein of the adductor canal (*red arrow*) is seen joining a competent great saphenous vein (*GSV*), *blue arrow*. The refluxive blood flows up in the great saphenous vein for 2 cm until it fills a refluxive tributary. The great saphenous vein is volume overloaded with antegrade flow for 2 cm of its course. Although it forms part of the reflux path, the flow remains antegrade. This is called antegrade incompetence Copyright: [Author]

the leg above the knee and is seldom significantly dilated or incompetent. Its course is fairly straight (Fig. 9.1e).

9.5 Proximal Paratibial Perforating Vein

The posterior and anterior arch veins join the great saphenous vein below the knee. At this level, the proximal paratibial perforating vein (formerly Boyd) joins the great saphenous vein. It runs close to the medial edge of the tibia and is not always visible. When the great saphenous vein is incompetent above and below the knee, it often drains into this vein together with a refluxive tributary which also joins at this point (Fig. 9.1h). Occasionally, it forms the proximal reflux source especially with reflux in the deep veins after thrombosis (Fig. 9.3).

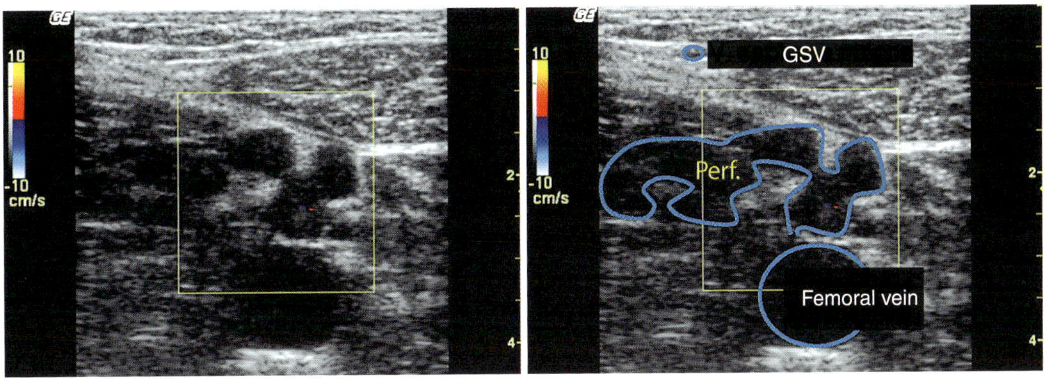

Fig. 9.11 Transverse view through the inner thigh at the level of the perforating vein of the adductor canal with a large intramuscular and subfascial tortuous vein without flow to demonstrate the anatomy. Flow images to be found online: antegrade flow is seen in the great saphenous vein. The patient presented with calf varicose veins. During the examination of the great saphenous vein, an incidental intramuscular varicose tributary was discovered (see accompanying online material). A large reflux volume was observed arising from the common femoral vein and flowing directly into this varicose subfascial tributary. Although the patient was asymptomatic, on closer questioning he remembered a severe bicycle accident with a direct blow against the handlebars Copyright: [Author]

9.6 Other Paratibial Perforating Veins

The course of the paratibial perforating veins is S-shaped. They run anterolaterally from the great saphenous vein to the tibia and then pass between the tibia and the musculature to the posterior tibial vein (Fig. 9.1a). When the great saphenous vein is refluxive, they often provide a drainage pathway. Occasionally an epifascial varicose tributary may drain into the deep veins via this perforating vein if it is very dilated (Fig. 9.1b).

9.7 Posterior Tibial Perforating Veins

The posterior tibial perforating veins (formerly Cockett group) are classified according to their height above the floor into Types I–III. They drain the medial calf. In varicose subjects, blood drains into them from the posterior arch veins, the great saphenous vein and sometimes the small saphenous vein. The posterior arch vein runs along the Linton line (Sect. 2.10 and Fig. 2.19). As explained in Sect. 10.7, a refluxive posterior arch vein runs a winding course. This vein is connected to the great and small saphenous veins and various posterior tibial perforating veins by numerous tributaries and connecting veins in a complex venous network. It is therefore recommended to examine the whole inside of the calf systematically from top to bottom with the probe in the transverse position, so as not to miss any dilated perforating veins.

Dilated posterior tibial perforating veins are often designated as incompetent and surgically interrupted. Cockett himself (Cockett and Jones 1953) only recommended surgical interruption when the deep veins were incompetent. Interestingly, incompetence of the deep veins is one of the few circumstances in which refluxive perforating veins are found on the Linton line. Duplex ultrasound and venous preservation approaches have led to a change in thinking about the treatment of this group of perforating veins. Accurate examination of the direction and volume of flow (Sect. 9.3) is the only way of distinguishing between a draining vein and one that is primarily incompetent.

9.8 Perforating Veins of the Small Saphenous Vein

Connections with the gastrocnemius muscle veins are often found in the region of the saphenopopliteal junction. These may be of no primary pathological importance, or they may form the reflux source (Fig. 8.14).

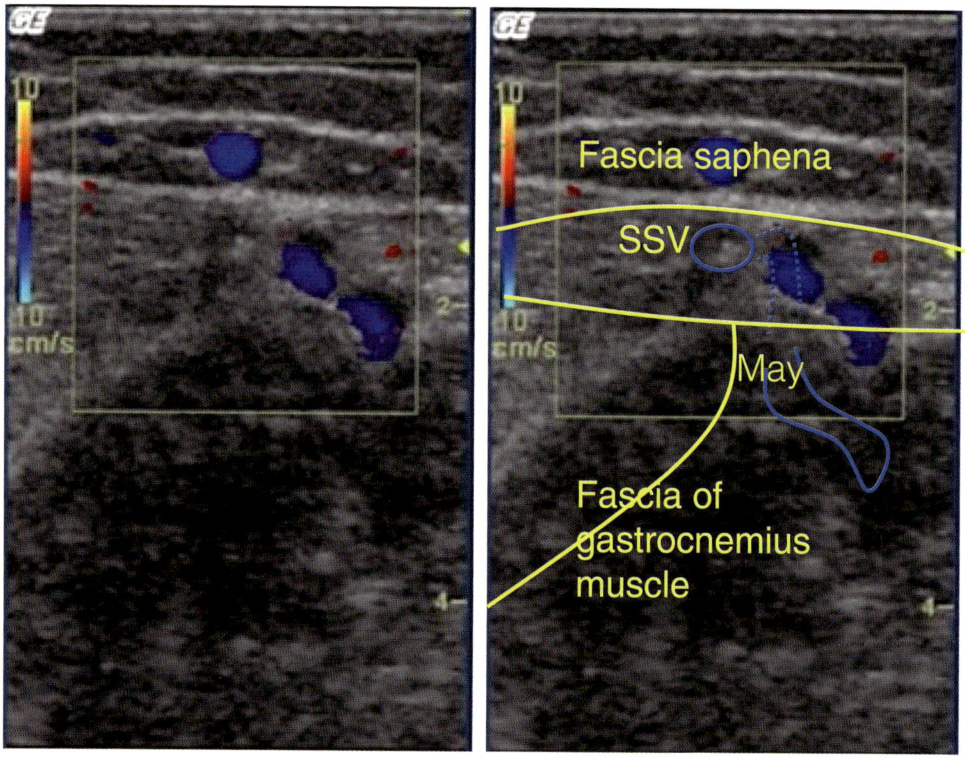

Fig. 9.12 Transverse view through the back of the calf, middle third, showing the soleus perforating vein (formerly May). It is seen joining the small saphenous vein (*SSV*) from medial just proximal of the section level (*dotted line*) Copyright: [Author]

On ultrasound, the soleal perforating vein (formerly May) is most often visible where it may drain a refluxing small saphenous vein (Fig. 9.12). Occasionally, a proximally competent small saphenous vein may be filled distally and reflux by retrograde flow through this perforating vein or other refluxing muscle veins (Fig. 8.15).

At the ankle is the para-Achillean perforating vein (formerly Bassi). It often serves as an inward drainage path for reflux.

9.9 Perforating Veins on the Back of the Leg

There are numerous possible sites in the back of the thigh which may be reflux sources for varices. Connections with **muscle veins** may exist as far up as the gluteal fold. This is also a common site after trauma. The reflux volume in these cases is small because the reticular vein network is not well drained. The diameter of these perforating veins is less than 5 mm.

A special part is played by the perforating vein in the **back of the thigh** (formerly Hach). It is a well-defined perforating vein, which may be connected to the femoropopliteal vein or the Giacomini anastomoses. Alternatively, it may fill large varicose tributaries. On ultrasound, it is very deep and may be hard to trace into the back of the thigh (Fig. 9.5).

In the **popliteal region** and higher perforating veins may form a connection between the popliteal vein and the epifascial vein system without the participation of the small saphenous vein (see above and Fig. 9.6).

Muscle veins are often found in the calf which serves as an inward drainage path for recirculation (Fig. 9.13), especially on the inside of the calf for draining an incompetent great saphenous vein. In very rare cases, these can become refluxive, usually after a trauma or a deep vein thrombosis (Sect. 9.3.1).

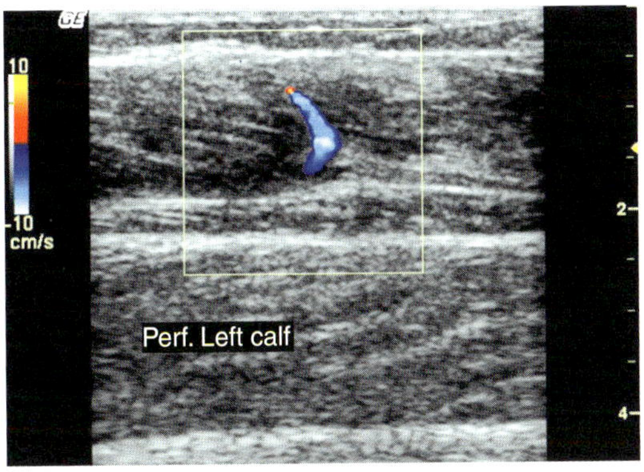

Fig. 9.13 Longitudinal view through the left calf mediodorsal to the great saphenous vein. On duplex, a muscle vein is seen coloured blue. It is draining a varicose vein in muscle diastole. It is blue because the direction of flow is into the leg and away from the probe Copyright: [Author]

9.10 Transtibial Perforating Vein

In very rare cases, varicose veins may develop after a severe contusion of the tibia. Typically, there is no fracture, but the cortex is breached. This is visible on ultrasound. The saphenous veins are competent and there is an absence of a perforating vein to bring the reflux from the deep veins. An interruption of the otherwise echogenic line of the periosteum can be observed which is crossed by a perforating vein arising directly from the bone marrow (Fig. 9.14). The blood flows exclusively outwards without flow during muscular systole. Alfred Obermayer demonstrated pathological flow from the tibiofibular veins into the marrow using MRI. Further

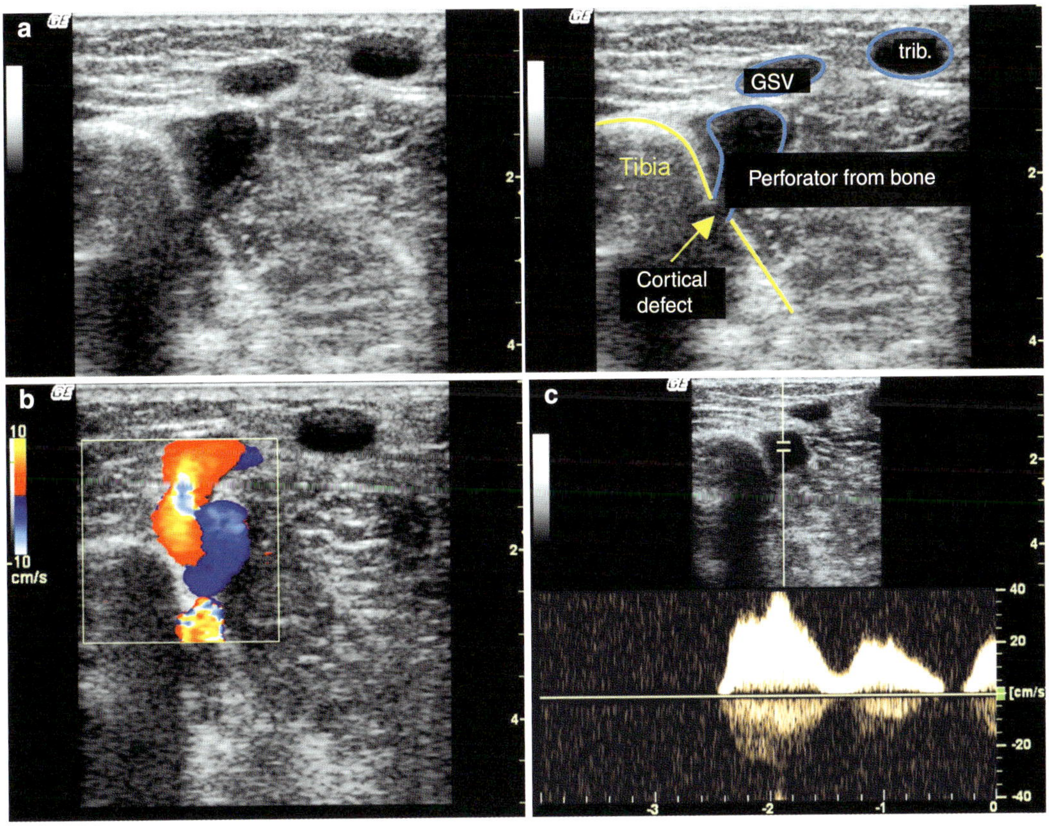

Fig. 9.14 (**a**) Transverse view through the inside of the calf, top third. There is a hole in the cortex of the medial tibia edge. An echo-free structure originates from this hole which connects with the great saphenous vein (*GSV*) and the epifascial tributaries (*trib.*). This is a vein (online material). (**b**) Same view as in (a) with colour duplex demonstrating turbulent reflux from the breach in the cortex (see accompanying online material). (**c**) PW measurement in the perforating vein. Only retrograde flow is visible, even during muscular systole Copyright: [Author]

down, the reflux flowed out of the bone into this perforating vein and then into the clinically visible varicose vein (presented at the Appenzell Conference 2007).

References

Cockett FB, Jones DE (1953) The ankle blow-out syndrome. Lancet 1:17

Delis KT, Husmann M, Kalodik E, Wolfe JH, Nicolafides AN (2001) In situ hemodynamics of perforating veins in chronic venous insufficiency. J Vasc Surg 33:773–782

Franceschi C (1993) Theory and Practice of the Conservative Haemodynamic Cure of Incompetent and Varicose Veins in Ambulatory Patients. Précy-sous-Thil (Armançon)

Franceschi C, Zamboni P (2009) Principles of venous hemodynamics. Nova Science Pub Inc., Hauppauge

Mendoza E (2013) Duplexsonographie der oberflächlichen Beinvenen. Springer, Berlin

Zamboni P, Gianesini S, Menegatti E, Tacconi G, Palazzo A, Liboni A (2010) Great saphenous varicose vein surgery without saphenofemoral junction disconnection. Br J Surg 97:820–825

Tributaries 10

Erika Mendoza and Christopher R. Lattimer

Chapter Summary
The scope of this chapter includes all the epifascial veins of the superficial venous system as well as the anterior and posterior accessory saphenous veins which run beneath the saphenous fascia in their proximal section. Varicose veins are tortuous and dilated veins. According to the UIP definition, these are defined as varicose if they exceed 3 mm in diameter. Spider or thread veins are flat, intradermal and impalpable and are different terms for the same condition. Reticular veins have a larger calibre and a profile with an intradermal component. Healthy veins are also included in this section.

10.1 Morphology

With few exceptions (Sect. 10.3.1), only those tributaries which are refluxive on duplex ultrasound have haemodynamic significance. Their morphology is very variable. They may be thin walled, have a large calibre, form tortuous networks or run a straight path over long stretches. When straight, they generally run parallel to the great saphenous vein. They may course through the leg uninterrupted from their origin to their drainage. Alternatively, they may be embedded in an extensively branched and refluxive venous network.

E. Mendoza, MD, PhD (✉)
Venenpraxis Wunstorf, Speckenstraße 10, Wunstorf 31515, Germany
e-mail: erika.mendoza@t-online.de

C.R. Lattimer, MD, PhD
Department of Vascular Surgery,
Josef Pflug Vascular Laboratory,
Ealing Hospital and Imperial College, London, UK

10.2 Examination Objectives

Answers should be sought to the following questions:

- Is the tributary refluxive?
- Where does it fill with reflux?
- Does the tributary have other inflow points like perforating veins, saphenous veins or tributaries?
- Does the tributary fill other tributaries refluxively?
- Does the tributary fill a saphenous vein refluxively?
- What are the drainage points: perforating veins, saphenous veins or tributaries?
- Is the tributary well or poorly drained (Sect. 3.2.3)?
- Is the tributary affected by superficial vein thrombosis (phlebitis)?
- Is it a secondary varicose vein which serves as a drainage point into the deep veins?

E. Mendoza et al. (eds.), *Duplex Ultrasound of Superficial Leg Veins*,
DOI 10.1007/978-3-642-40731-4_10, © Springer-Verlag Berlin Heidelberg 2014

10.3 Systematic Examination of Tributaries

The principal criterion for distinguishing between the saphenous trunks and a tributary is its relationship with the saphenous fascia (Fig. 10.1, see also Fig. 7.34 and Sects. 7.4.1 and 8.4.1). Tributaries do not run along this fascial compartment except for the last few millimetres where they cross beneath it to join the saphenous vein. As mentioned above, refluxive tributaries are the clinically visible, tortuous and dilated varicose veins which are the treatment focus for many patients.

10.3.1 Healthy Tributaries

The following tributaries should be examined routinely, even if they are healthy. These are the anterior and posterior accessory saphenous veins, which are automatically included in the examination of the junction and upper section of the great saphenous vein; the posterior arch vein, along which lie the perforating veins which are frequently pathologically dilated; and the upward extension of the small saphenous vein (vein of Giacomini or femoropopliteal vein). The latter, together with the posterior accessory saphenous vein, forms a connection between the great and small saphenous veins. The significance of this is shown in Sect. 10.5.

The above named tributaries can carry pathologically increased blood volumes to the saphenous veins, generally as exclusive reflux sources, but sometimes in addition to incompetent subterminal valves. If this is not diagnosed correctly and the saphenofemoral junction is simply ligated, then the patient will be incorrectly treated

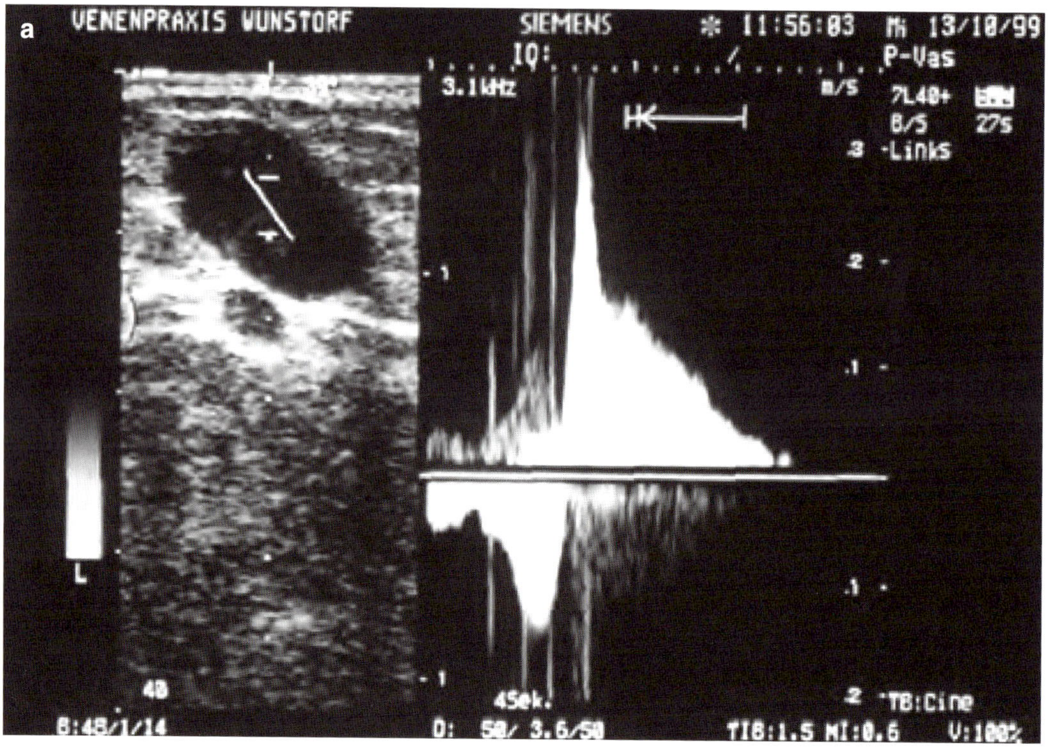

Fig. 10.1 (**a**) Transverse view through the inner thigh. A small-calibre competent great saphenous vein (*GSV*) is seen surrounded by its fascial compartment. There is a larger refluxive tributary running superficial to the great saphenous vein and its fascia. The PW curve of the tributary demonstrates relatively more reflux (*peak*) than antegrade flow (*trough*). (**b**) Longitudinal view of **a** distal to the point where the tributary branches off the great saphenous vein. A visible valve cusp is seen just below the branch point (*) before the great saphenous vein continues footwards. The great saphenous vein is thick walled and surrounded by fascia (**), whereas the tributary has no discernible wall Copyright: [Author]

Fig. 10.1 (continued)

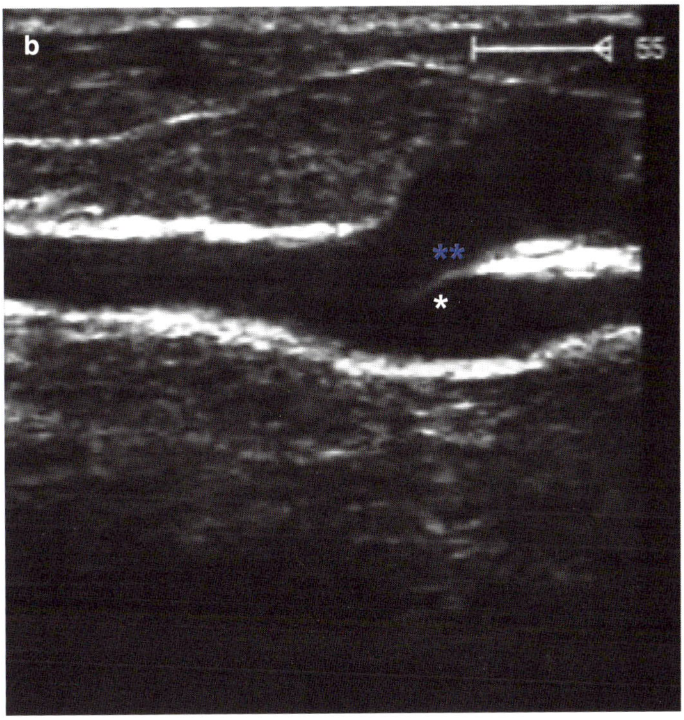

because the reflux source will remain. Early clinical **recurrence** is inevitable with **persistence** of the patient's symptoms.

10.3.2 Refluxive Tributaries

Refluxive varicose tributaries are the **cosmetic problem** for patients. An ultrasound examination of the saphenous veins will identify their refluxive tributaries (Sects. 7.4 and 8.4). The course of the saphenous trunks and all visibly refluxive tributaries are examined also for additional reflux sources.

Refluxive tributaries are sometimes not clearly visible in B scan, because they lie very close under the skin or form large convolutions where the flow on colour duplex is confusing (Fig. 10.2). It is not usually necessary to examine a varicosity down to its detail. However, it is important to establish where the refluxive blood comes from and where it drains by analysing the direction of flow and tracing this carefully with the probe. Identification of the reflux sources and drainage points is arguably the most common skill required in the ultrasound investigation of varicose veins.

The net flow direction in tributaries may reveal whether they are secondary varicose veins after deep venous occlusion. It may also determine the extent in which they contribute to the venous return (Chap. 15).

10.3.2.1 Important Drainage Points

The search for the inflow and drainage points of a varicose vein is difficult and tedious. The following technique can help by using either the CW probe or the duplex ultrasound probe in PW or colour mode. First, the probe is placed at the upper end of the vein to be examined. Next, the subject is told to raise and lower his toes (Wunstorf manoeuvre). In this way, reflux can be confirmed in this vein segment. Then the segment below the varicose vein is compressed with one finger and the subject is again asked to activate the muscle pump. If there is no drainage point between the probe and the point of digital compression, no reflux occurs in the first phase of muscular diastole. However, after the digital compression is released (top two curves, Fig. 10.3), reflux will resume. If a refluxive tributary branches off between the middle and lowest compression point Fig. 10.3, the waveform

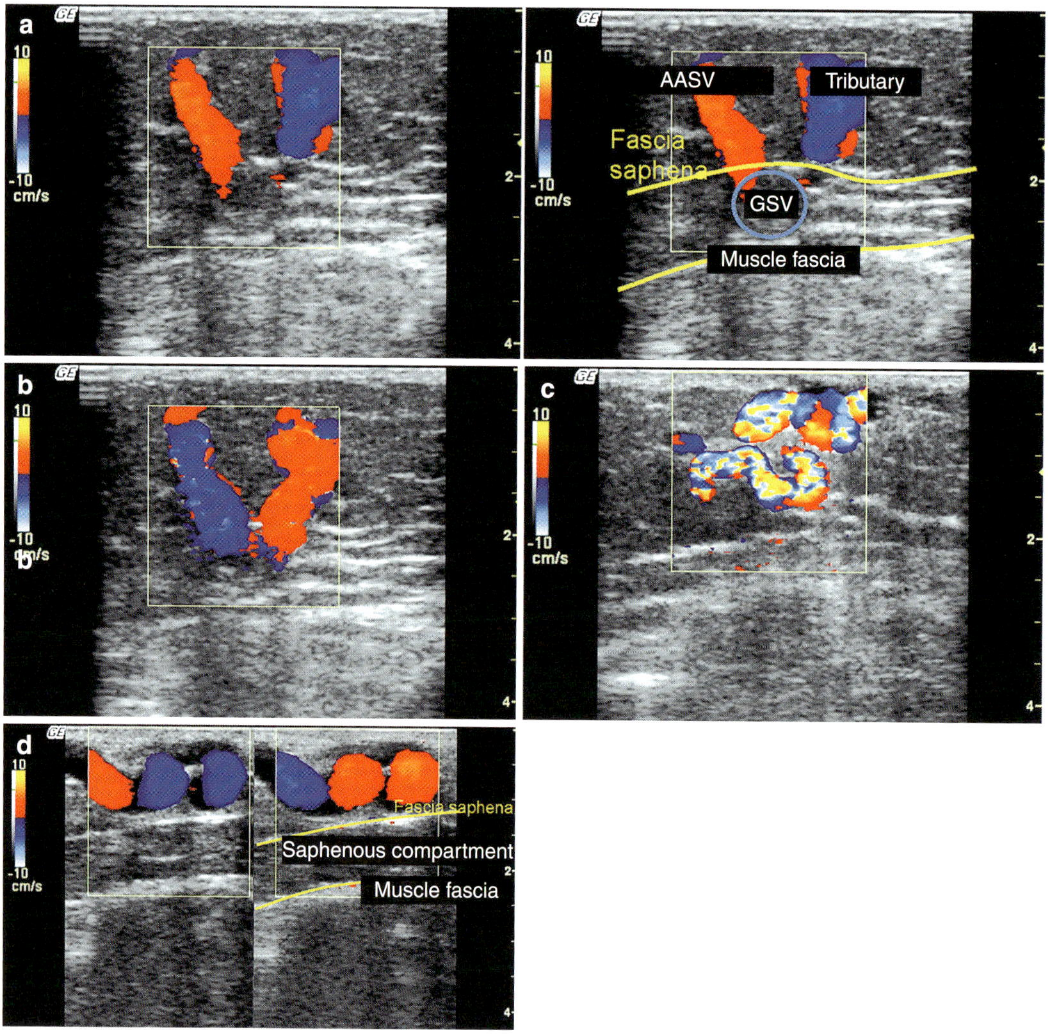

Fig. 10.2 Transverse view from the inner aspect of the right thigh demonstrating a refluxive anterior accessory saphenous vein (*AASV*) filling a great saphenous vein (*GSV*) from the lateral side, which is competent proximally and distally. Opposite, a medial tributary is seen refluxing out of the great saphenous vein. (**a**) Muscular systole; the blood flows upwards in the anterior accessory saphenous vein, towards the probe (*red*) and downwards from the medial tributary (*blue*). (**b**) Muscular diastole; the flow directions are reversed. The refluxive anterior accessory saphenous vein now fills the great saphenous vein which is inwards (*blue*), and the refluxive tributary carries the blood back to the surface (*red*) (see accompanying online material). (**c**) Refluxive tributary in the thigh. Turbulent flow is seen due to the multiple changes of direction in the vessel. The exact flow direction is difficult to determine. It is important to visualise whether there is a connection to the deep vein in this region like a high perforating vein of the adductor canal (formerly Dodd). (**d**) Longitudinal view of the inner thigh demonstrating a refluxive tributary in systole (*left*) and diastole (*right*). Confused colours are apparent due to the many changes in blood flow direction through the convolution Copyright: [Author]

changes. With digital compression at the lowest point, the reflux begins at the onset of muscular diastole which is independent of digital compression. This is because the refluxive volume is now drained by a tributary (bottom curve).

10.3.2.2 Important Reflux Source Points

Sometimes it is not obvious which vein is feeding a refluxive tributary. It is helpful in these cases to place the probe on the relevant segment, switch

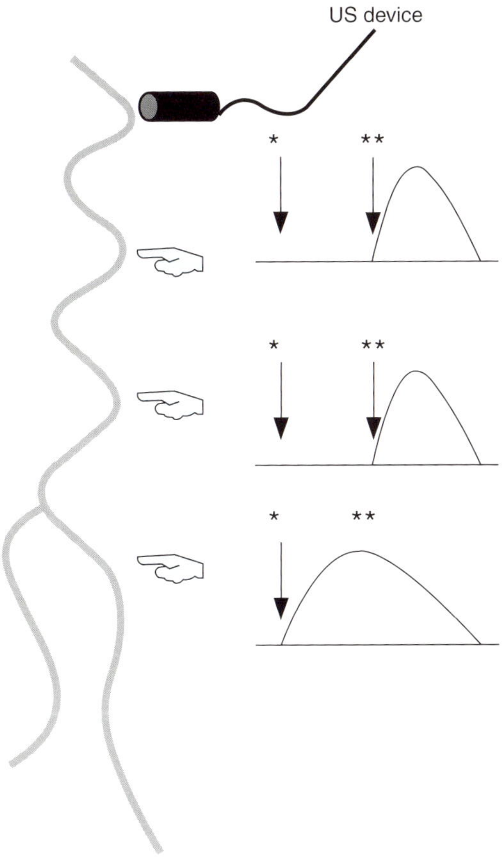

Fig. 10.3 Diagram of the examination technique used to determine the site of important drainage points. The probe is placed at the upper end and the hands indicate the points at which the vein is compressed with the finger. The curve on the right shows the velocity profile in each case after muscle contraction (raising the toes). * beginning of muscular diastole (lowering the toes), ** release of digital compression (see explanation in text) Copyright: [Author]

on colour duplex mode and tap the vein further up with one finger of the other hand or run it over the skin. If there is a **reflux source** further up, then a signal will be recorded in the vein.

10.4 Anterior Accessory Saphenous Vein

The anterior accessory saphenous vein joins the great saphenous vein in the region of the saphenofemoral junction. Rarely, it joins the common femoral vein directly (Fig. 10.4; see also Sect. 7.3.7). It courses downwards lateral to the great saphenous vein. Its first part is in the fascial compartment where it may lie in the same compartment as the great saphenous vein (Fig. 10.5a) or be separated from it by a layer of connective tissue (Fig. 10.5b).

After 15–20 cm of coursing interfascially, the anterior accessory saphenous vein usually surfaces from this compartment to follow the midline of the thigh. This configuration is relatively constant. A **communicating vein** often branches off the anterior accessory saphenous vein, connecting it to the great saphenous vein in this region.

If the anterior accessory saphenous vein is incompetent and filled refluxively from the common femoral vein through an incompetent terminal valve and competent preterminal valve, this communicating vein may carry the reflux further down the great saphenous vein causing it to become incompetent once more. This means that the great saphenous vein can have more than one incompetent segment separated by competent segments (Sect. 4.1.2.3).

On the other hand, only the lower part of the anterior accessory may be affected by reflux. This may occur in patients with reflux of the great saphenous vein to the thigh or an incompetent perforating vein of the adductor canal (formerly Dodd or Hunter). These provide reflux sources to the communicating vein which may fill the anterior accessory saphenous vein reflux ively further down the leg. For this reason, the anterior accessory saphenous vein, regardless of whether or not its origin is competent, should always be examined throughout its course.

The course of the anterior accessory saphenous vein between the groin and where it leaves the fascia is very constant. Its further course in the leg is only visible in very thin subjects or if it is incompetent. It forms part of a widely branched subcutaneous venous network travelling laterally. The course of a refluxive anterior accessory saphenous vein is very variable and tortuous. It frequently divides into several clinically visible refluxive tributaries. Possible courses are that it veers:

- Frequently laterally at knee height to fill veins on the lateral side of the calf. These

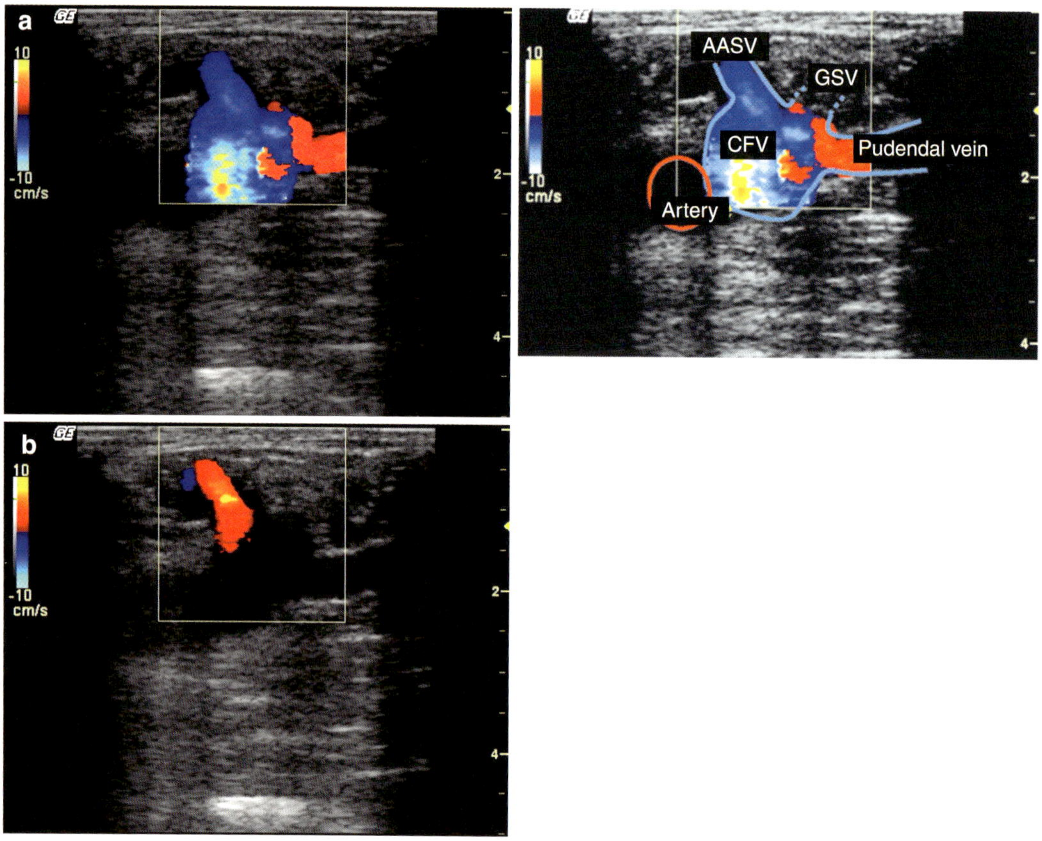

Fig. 10.4 (**a**) Transverse view through the right groin during muscular systole. Antegrade flow is seen in all the veins. The dilated pudendal vein carries blood towards the probe and therefore appears *red*. In this case, the junction between the pudendal vein and great saphenous vein is towards the probe, which is the reason it appears *red*. As the flow is only during systole and not diastole (see **b**), the pudendal vein is competent, even though it is dilated. The great saphenous vein joins around 2 mm further down. (**b**) Muscular diastole demonstrating reflux from the common femoral vein directly into the anterior accessory saphenous vein (see accompanying online material) Copyright: [Author]

may then remain lateral or veer posterior to the small saphenous vein or anterior to the tibial edge.

- Anterior with a refluxive tributary above the patella.
- Rarely medially with a refluxive tributary parallel to the great saphenous vein.

There is a series of **perforating veins** along the course of the anterior accessory saphenous vein which are invisible both clinically and on ultrasound. In its lateral course, a drainage point is common at the knee.

Identification of refluxive segments is predominantly clinical. Tortuous subcutaneous tributaries and areas of sudden increase in calibre usually indicate reflux. This can be confirmed using ultrasound. It is important to identify the reflux sources and drainage points prior to treatment in order to minimise recurrence.

10.4.1 Reflux Sources for the Anterior Accessory Saphenous Vein

With reflux arising from the deep system, varicose veins generally have a larger calibre, often as thick as a finger. Here, the reflux curve in PW duplex is short and fast. The further distal the drainage, the greater the possibility that this becomes damped and prolonged. With reflux not involving the deep veins, the reflux curve is slower with a gradual rise and a long-lasting flow. The branches are also smaller.

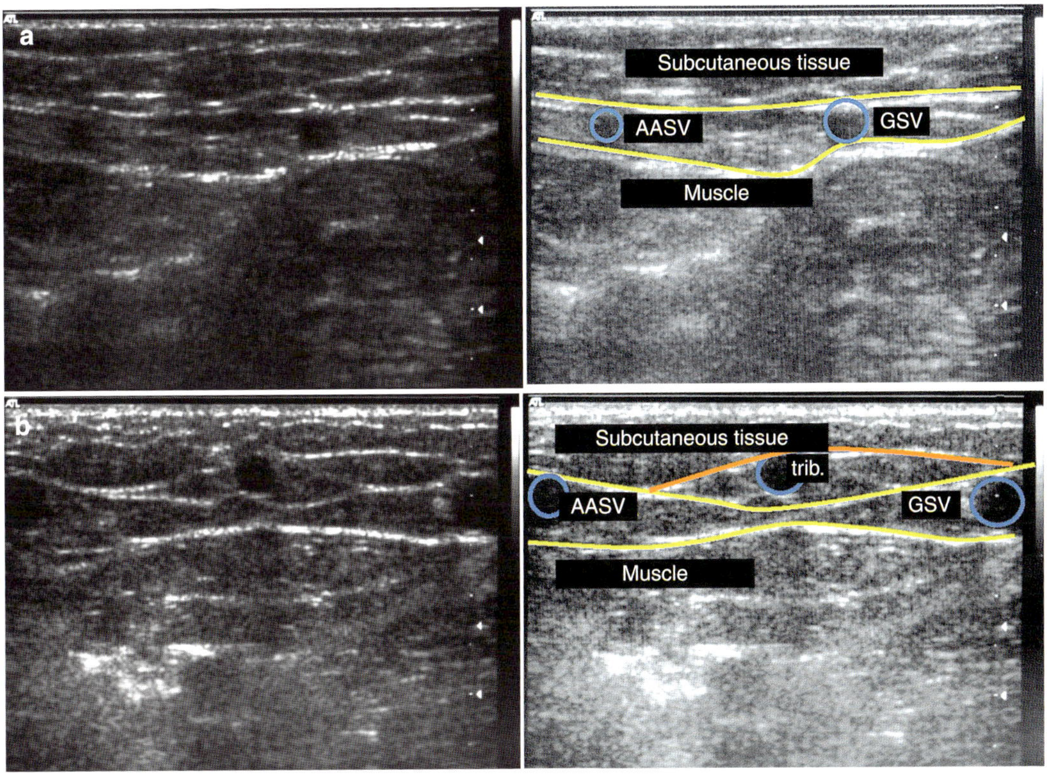

Fig. 10.5 Fascial compartment of the anterior accessory saphenous vein. (**a**) Transverse view through the right thigh 5 cm below the saphenofemoral junction. The great saphenous vein (*GSV*) and anterior accessory saphenous vein (*AASV*) are in the same fascial compartment (see accompanying online material). (**b**) Transverse view through the right thigh 10 cm below the saphenofemoral junction in a different leg. The great saphenous vein and anterior accessory saphenous vein have their own fascial compartments. In the middle of the image, there is a tributary which runs from the anterior accessory saphenous vein to the great saphenous vein where it has left the fascial compartment. However, it remains beneath a fascial remnant (*orange*) Copyright: [Author]

10.4.1.1 Reflux from Deep Veins

- **Incompetent saphenofemoral junction** (Fig. 10.6):
  - Incompetent terminal valve, competent preterminal valve and anterior accessory saphenous vein refluxive directly from the groin, the most common form in practice (Fig. 10.6a)
  - Incompetent terminal and preterminal valve, reflux only above the knee and anterior accessory saphenous vein filled refluxively through the communicating vein, common (Fig. 10.6b)
  - Incompetent terminal and preterminal valve, great saphenous vein refluxive above and below the knee and anterior accessory saphenous vein filled through the anterior arch vein in the calf region, less common (Fig. 10.6c)
- **Refluxive perforating vein of the adductor canal** (Fig. 10.7a) (formerly Dodd and Hunter):
  - The anterior accessory saphenous vein is filled through the communicating vein, rare.
- **Refluxive paratibial perforating vein** (Fig. 10.7b) (formerly Boyd):
  - The anterior accessory saphenous vein in the calf is filled through the anterior arch vein, rare.
- **Refluxive back thigh perforating vein** (Fig. 10.7c):
  - The anterior accessory saphenous vein is filled through tributaries in the back of the thigh which run laterally round the leg, rare.

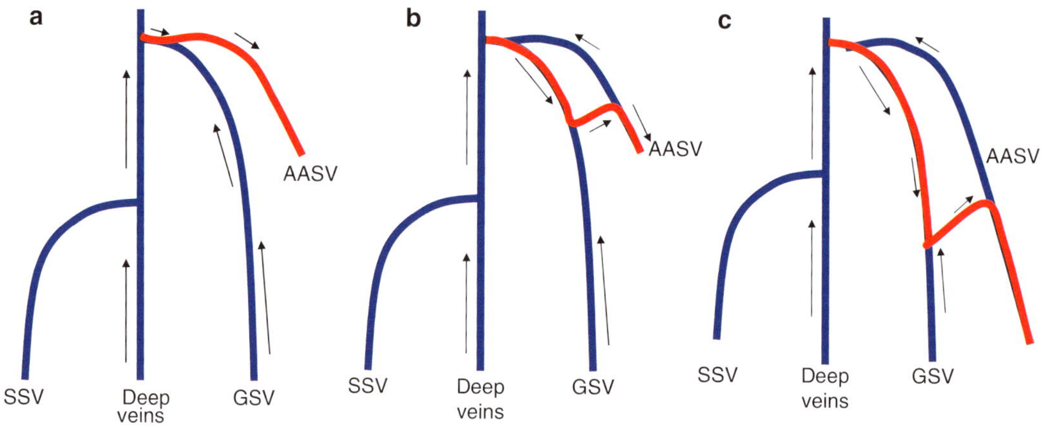

Fig. 10.6 Reflux in anterior accessory saphenous vein (*AASV*) with origin in the femoral vein and via the great saphenous vein (*GSV*). (**a**) Incompetent terminal valve, competent preterminal valve and reflux from great saphenous vein in anterior accessory saphenous vein at groin level (complete Hach I). (**b**) Incompetent terminal and preterminal valve, reflux in great saphenous vein above the knee (complete Hach II) and anterior accessory saphenous vein filled through communicating vein at thigh level. (**c**) Incompetent terminal and preterminal valve, reflux in great saphenous vein above and below the knee (complete Hach III) and anterior accessory saphenous vein filled at calf level

- **Refluxive unnamed perforating veins** in the course of the anterior accessory saphenous vein (Fig. 10.7d):
  – The anterior accessory saphenous vein is filled in its course from perforating veins, rare.
- **Refluxive small saphenous vein** (Fig. 10.8):
  – The anterior accessory saphenous vein in the calf is filled from refluxive tributaries of the small saphenous vein, relatively rare (Fig. 10.8a).
  – The anterior accessory saphenous vein is filled through the Giacomini anastomosis and great saphenous vein, very rare (Fig. 10.8b).
  – The anterior accessory saphenous vein is filled through refluxive tributaries of the Giacomini anastomosis through the outer side of the thigh, very rare (Fig. 10.8c).

10.4.1.2 Reflux Without Involvement of the Deep Veins

- **Refluxive network of superficial inguinal veins** (Fig. 10.9) with a competent saphenofemoral junction. The reflux originates in the organs of the pelvis and not from the deep veins:
  – The anterior accessory saphenous vein is filled directly in the groin from refluxive superficial inguinal tributaries, common (Figs. 10.9a and 10.11).
  – The anterior accessory saphenous vein is filled through the communicating vein from the great saphenous vein, which has a competent terminal valve and is filled through pelvic tributaries, less common (Fig. 10.9b).
  – The anterior accessory saphenous vein is filled in the calf through the posterior arch vein from a refluxive great saphenous vein. The great saphenous vein is filled from pelvic tributaries (competent terminal valve, incompetent preterminal valve) and is refluxive above and below the knee, less common (Fig. 10.9c).
- **Reflux through the epigastric vein** in the front of the thigh:
  – The anterior accessory saphenous vein fills through the subcutaneous vein network in the front of the thigh from the epigastric vein and anastomoses from the pelvis, common after crossectomy and stripping of the great saphenous vein (Fig. 10.9d).
- **Great saphenous vein with antegrade flow**, filling the anterior accessory saphenous vein refluxively:
  – The anterior accessory saphenous vein fills directly in the groin from the competent great saphenous vein, relatively common (Figs.10.10a and 10.11).

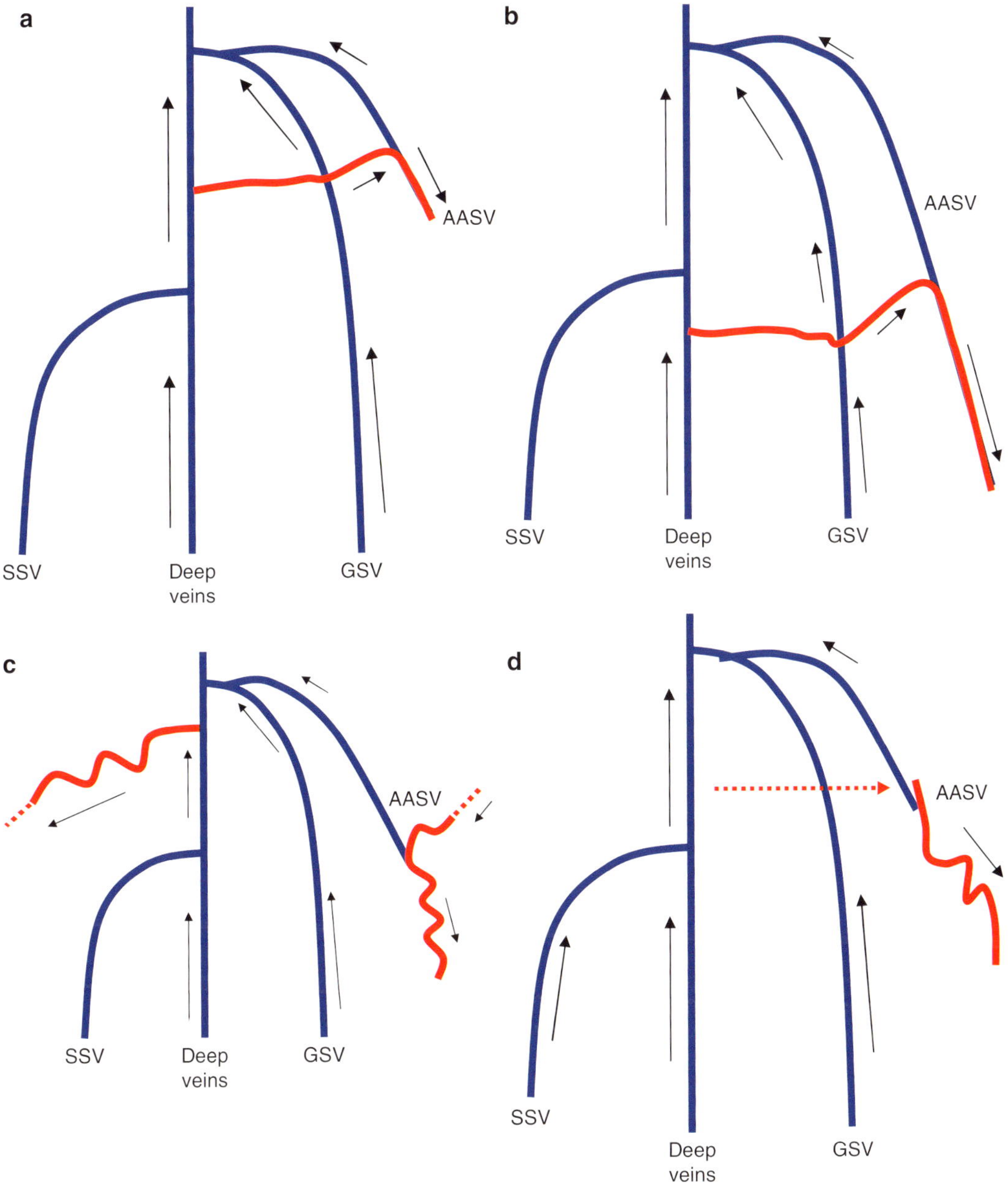

Fig. 10.7 Reflux in anterior accessory saphenous vein (*AASV*) originated in perforators. (**a**) Reflux from a perforator in the adductor channel into anterior accessory saphenous vein. (**b**) Reflux through a paratibial perforator and tributary in anterior accessory saphenous vein. (**c**) Reflux originating in perforator at back of high and filling the anterior accessory saphenous vein via the lateral plexus. (**d**) Reflux through no named perforator along the way of the anterior accessory saphenous vein

   – The anterior accessory saphenous vein fills through the communicating vein from the competent great saphenous vein, rare (Fig. 10.10b).

- **Reflux with no clear reflux source:** The anterior accessory saphenous vein fills from its many tributaries and its calibre increases continuously along its downward course (analogous to the situation described in Sect. 7.5.2 for the great saphenous vein). Since the anterior accessory saphenous vein has no valves, this situation often appears after crossectomy with or without stripping of the great saphenous vein. This occurs when there is

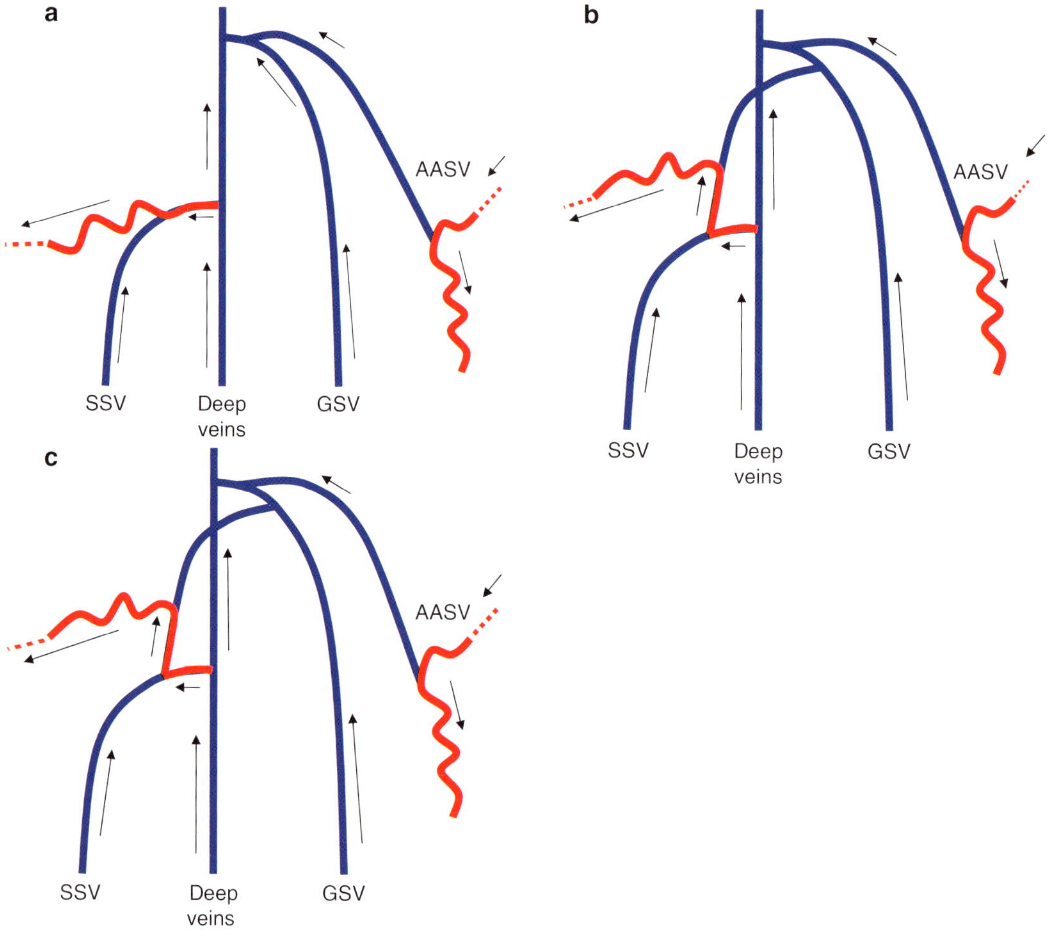

Fig. 10.8 Reflux in anterior accessory saphenous vein (*AASV*) originating in the deep venous system and taking the way through the small saphenous vein. (**a**) Reflux through saphenopopliteal junction and a tributary to the anterior accessory saphenous vein at the calf. (**b**) Reflux from the popliteal vein through small saphenous vein, Giacomini anastomosis and filling the great saphenous vein distal to the preterminal valve – then running through the communicans vein to the anterior accessory saphenous vein. (**c**) Reflux from the popliteal vein through small saphenous vein and Giacomini vein through a tributary to the anterior accessory saphenous vein

incompetence of the anterior accessory saphenous vein that was present preoperatively. In a standing subject, the blood in the tributaries will prefer the route of gravity through the dilated anterior accessory saphenous vein towards the foot, rather than through the network of smaller muscle perforating veins or the tiny veins along the route of the obliterated great saphenous vein (Fig. 10.10c).

10.4.2 Drainage Points of the Anterior Accessory Saphenous Vein

The anterior accessory saphenous vein forms part of the subcutaneous **venous network**, prominent in the thigh. Reflux from the anterior accessory saphenous vein often finds a communication into a healthy vein. These include the great saphenous vein or various small perforating veins in the

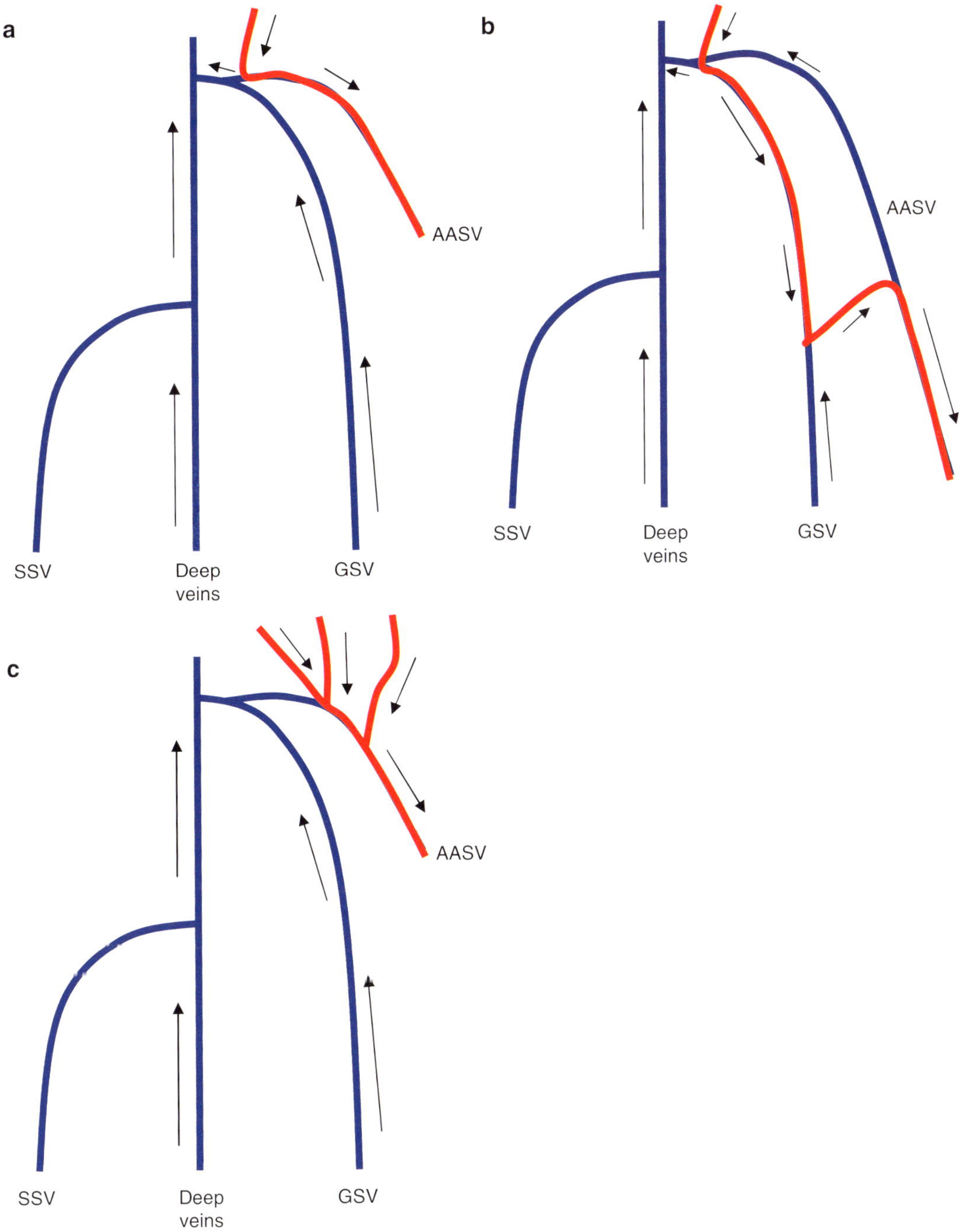

Fig. 10.9 Reflux in anterior accessory saphenous vein (*AASV*) with pelvic origin. (**a**) Reflux through a pelvic tributary filling the anterior accessory saphenous vein in the groin. (**b**) Reflux through a pelvic tributary filling great saphenous vein (*GSV*) (competent terminal valve, incompetent preterminal valve); the anterior accessory saphenous vein is filled through communicans at the thigh (incomplete Hach II). (**c**) Reflux of pelvic origin: competent terminal valve and incompetent preterminal valve in great saphenous vein; anterior accessory saphenous vein is filled at the calf (incomplete Hach III). (**d**) Reflux via subcutaneous tributaries originating in epigastric veins

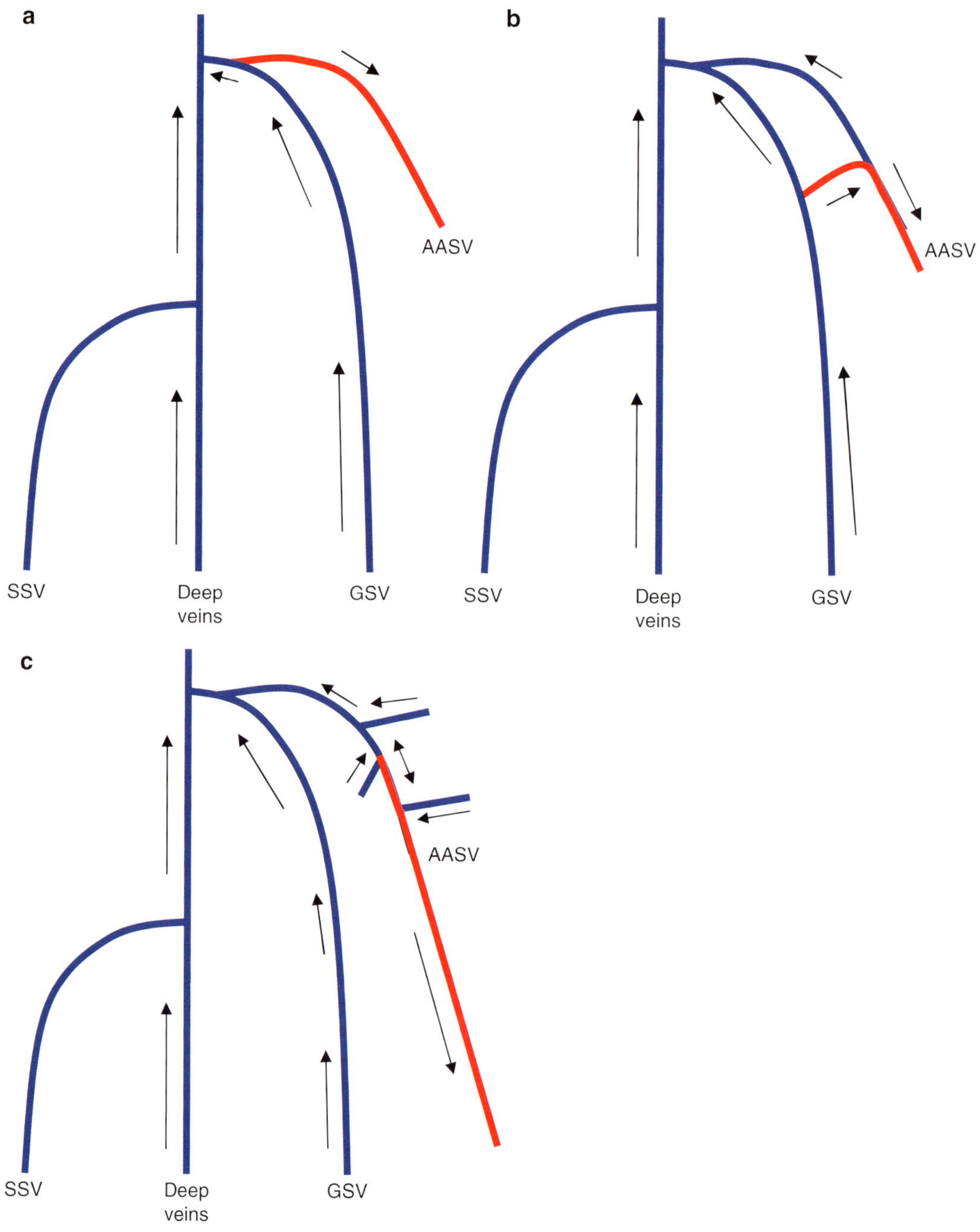

Fig. 10.10 Reflux in anterior accessory saphenous vein (*AASV*) with competent great saphenous vein (*GSV*) and small saphenous vein (*SSV*), as well as competent perforators. (**a**) Competent GSV fills the anterior accessory saphenous vein refluxively in the groin. (**b**) Anterior accessory saphenous vein filled through the communicating vein at the thigh. (**c**) Reflux without reflux source: anterior accessory saphenous vein filled through competent tributaries

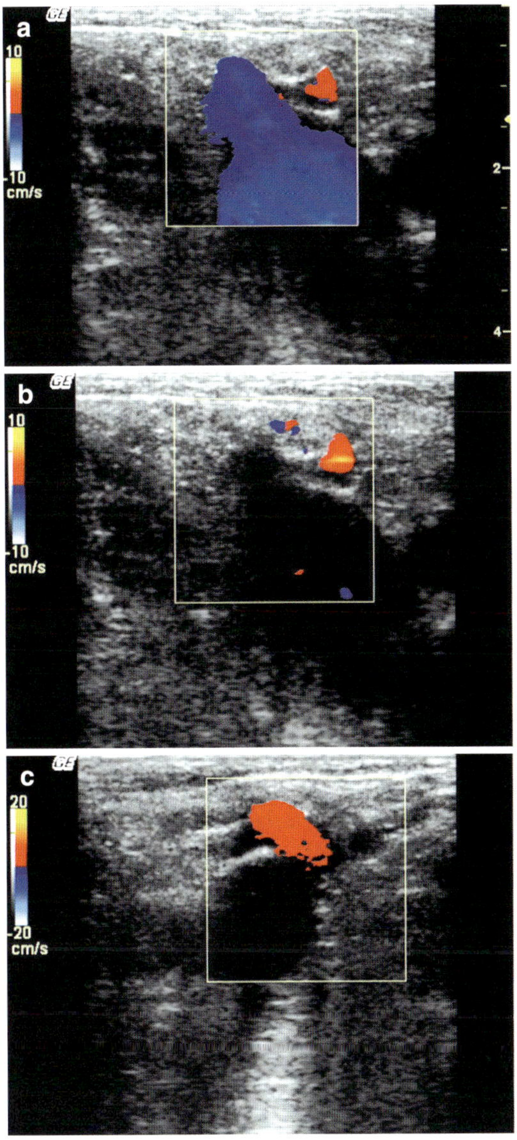

Fig. 10.11 Incompetence of the anterior accessory saphenous vein without reflux from the saphenofemoral junction. (**a**) Transverse view through the left groin. During muscular systole, there is antegrade flow up the great saphenous and common femoral veins (*blue*). The anterior accessory saphenous vein begins to fill refluxively during muscular systole (*red*). (**b**) During muscular diastole, there is reflux in the anterior accessory saphenous vein (*red*) without any reflux from the deep veins or the great saphenous vein. The reflux is slow and long-lasting (see accompanying online material). (**c**) Transverse view through the right groin of a different subject in muscular diastole. There is reflux from the great saphenous vein into the anterior accessory saphenous vein (*red*), but no involvement of the saphenofemoral junction Copyright: [Author]

musculature of the thigh. It is not always possible to identify individual drainage points on ultrasound. A dilated re-entry perforating vein is significant if the reflux curve is fast and short, but not if it is slow and long-lasting.

Examination of **re-entry points** is important for treatment. The techniques are described in Sect. 10.3.2. Possible re-entry points for reflux are (see accompanying online material):

- Communicating vein between the anterior accessory saphenous vein and the great saphenous vein. The reflux comes from the saphenofemoral junction down the anterior accessory saphenous vein to enter the great saphenous vein.
- Perforating vein lateral to the knee.
- Various perforating veins on the outside of the calf.
- Anterior accessory saphenous vein, which runs from lateral to posterior below the knee to drain into the small saphenous vein.
- Anterior accessory saphenous vein, which runs over the edge of the tibia below the knee to meet the great saphenous vein.
- In the course described above over the edge of the tibia, drainage of the reflux may also occur into the paratibial perforating veins.
- The reflux may also flow down the outside of the leg or the tibia edge to the ankle, where it flows into the veins on the back of the foot and thence into the deep vein system.

10.5 Posterior Accessory Saphenous Vein

The posterior accessory saphenous vein usually joins the great saphenous vein in the upper third of the thigh. Variations include a connection in the saphenofemoral junction or directly into the common femoral vein. It may also connect the great and small saphenous veins through the Giacomini anastomosis (Sect. 2.4.6 and Figs. 2.20, 2.21, and 2.22). The posterior accessory saphenous vein runs posterior to the great saphenous vein. The junction is always under the saphenous fascia (Fig. 10.12). A dilated posterior accessory saphenous vein or an increase in the calibre of the great saphenous vein in the

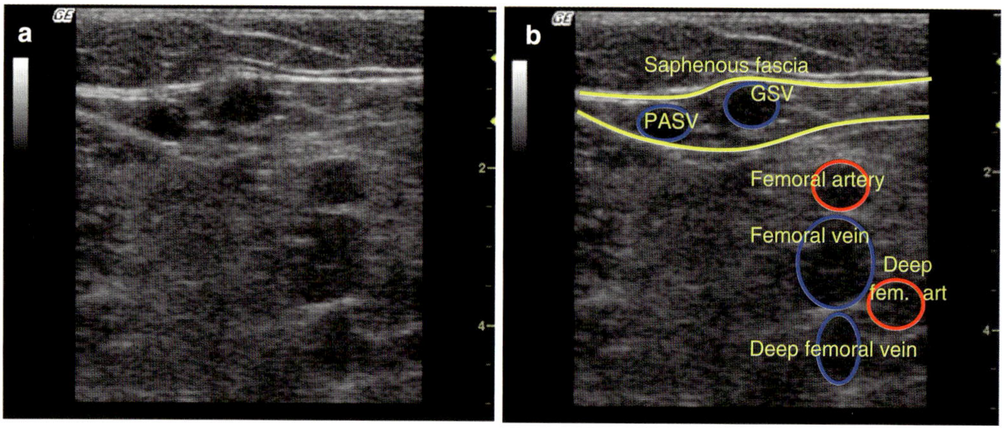

Fig. 10.12 Transverse view through the left thigh 10 cm below the groin demonstrating the posterior accessory saphenous vein. The great saphenous vein (*GSV*) increases in calibre above the communication with the posterior accessory saphenous vein (*PASV*) (see accompanying online material). The great saphenous vein is refluxive, while the posterior accessory saphenous vein is not. The femoral artery and vein and the deep femoral artery and vein can also be seen Copyright: [Author]

proximal thigh region indicates a pathological posterior accessory saphenous vein essential. A common cause for early recurrence after operations on the great saphenous vein is an overlooked reflux source from this vein.

The course of the posterior accessory saphenous vein from the great saphenous vein is around the inside of the thigh posterior and then to the popliteal region. Ultrasound is used to find the reflux sources for this vein. In B scan, tributaries can be seen coming from the pelvis which may fill the posterior accessory saphenous vein refluxively. Perforating veins can also fill this vein from the back of the thigh. Incompetence of the saphenopopliteal junction is frequently the cause of an incompetent posterior accessory saphenous vein, which then fills the great saphenous vein refluxively (Sect. 8.3.4 and Figs. 8.14a and 4.9a).

The flow direction in the Giacomini anastomoses connecting the great and small saphenous vein is **bidirectional**. Consequently, the **flow volume** in muscular diastole is used for assessing incompetence and not the direction of flow. Reflux from the small saphenous vein into its cranial extension and through the vein of Giacomini into the great saphenous vein is upwards. This pathological flow is apparent during calf muscle diastole. Its direction can confuse the beginner because reflux is normally associated with footward flow. Giacomini reflux is termed "antegrade" incompetence or ascending pathological reflux.

The following are sources for pathological filling of the posterior accessory saphenous vein:

- Great saphenous vein with reflux downwards towards the small saphenous vein.
- Small saphenous vein ("antegrade" incompetence) with reflux upwards towards the great saphenous vein.
- Reflux from a perforating vein on the back of the thigh. This may reflux downwards or upwards towards the great or small saphenous vein.
- Branches from the pelvis through the labia with reflux towards the great or small saphenous vein.

A pathologically filled posterior accessory saphenous vein may **drain** through the following veins:

- Epifascial tributaries in the thigh
- Posterior perforating vein
- Drainage through a competent saphenopopliteal junction via the small saphenous vein
- Drainage through the small saphenous vein filled refluxively
- Through the competent saphenofemoral junction via the great saphenous vein
- Refluxive filling of the great saphenous vein

10.6 Other Tributaries

10.6.1 Anterior Arch Vein

The tributaries which run anterolaterally to the great saphenous vein are known as the anterior arch veins. The main one is a tributary which joins the antegrade flow of the great saphenous vein below the knee. These veins are cosmetically unattractive because there is scarcely any subcutaneous tissue over the tibia.

The vein runs under the saphenous fascia, the first few centimetres below the connection with the great saphenous vein. It then emerges superficially medial to the tibia edge. Generally, the vein runs lateral to the tibia edge but may sometimes course over or run medially. The medial section may be filled by a refluxive paratibial **perforating vein**, or more rarely from a perforating vein more lateral. As a rule, perforating veins visible on ultrasound serve as drainage for arch veins.

10.6.2 Posterior Arch Vein

The posterior arch vein joins the great saphenous vein at the level of the paratibial perforating vein below the knee (formerly Boyd). Sometimes, it drains further up. Its usual course follows the **Linton Line** (Fig. 2.18). On ultrasound, it is generally only visible if it is part of a recirculation circuit.

With extensive varicose veins, it may be difficult to recognise the posterior arch vein as an independent vein in the varicose network. However, it is important to identify the perforating veins of the posterior tibial vein (formerly Cockett perforating veins) along its course and determine whether they are incompetent (Sect. 9.7 and Figs. 2.19 and 2.24).

10.6.3 Tributaries of the Small Saphenous Vein

The small saphenous vein may have several refluxive tributaries which can be identified using ultrasound. They are most commonly found in the middle third of the calf. However, tributaries may also be found in the popliteal and ankle regions.

10.6.4 Connections Between the Great and Small Saphenous Veins

The connection from the small saphenous vein to the great saphenous vein through the femoropopliteal vein has been described in Sect. 10.3. Another typical connection runs from the great saphenous vein at the knee medially to the small saphenous vein in the middle of the calf. If the small saphenous vein is examined above this tributary, a large volume of blood in antegrade flow makes it clear that the small saphenous vein is incompetent. As described in Sect. 3.4.3, this may be because the small saphenous vein is a drainage point for the great saphenous vein which becomes secondarily dilated. The valves then become incompetent and refluxive. Very often, the incompetence of the small saphenous vein in such patients recovers once the great saphenous vein has been treated.

In the calf, the blood flow in the connections between the great and small saphenous vein may be **bidirectional**. They must be examined thoroughly when either the great or small saphenous vein is incompetent. In either case, they may fill the other saphenous trunk refluxively. In the calf, this may result in below-knee incompetence of the great saphenous vein (Sect. 4.1.2.1) or incompetence in the small saphenous vein originating from the great saphenous vein (Sect. 4.1.3).

Superficial Vein Thrombosis 11

Erika Mendoza and Christopher R. Lattimer

Chapter Summary

Thrombus formation in the superficial venous system of the leg is usually referred to as phlebitis or inflammation of the veins. In ultrasound examination, a thrombus is invariably found in one or more superficial veins, very often with inflammatory changes of the surrounding tissue (periphlebitis). An up-to-date consensus statement on phlebitis by the international societies of angiology (UIA) and phlebology (UIP) exists (Kalodiki et al. 2012). It recommends the use of the term "superficial vein thrombosis (SVT)" instead of "phlebitis", to replace the suggestion of an infective aetiology with a thrombotic cause. Superficial vein thrombosis usually occurs in varicose veins; however, it can also develop in a healthy vein when there may be a more sinister aetiology.

Superficial vein thrombosis can also be indicative of thrombophilia or the hypercoagulable state of cancer.

The clinical importance of a diagnosis of superficial vein thrombosis must not be underestimated. Up to 25–33 % of patients with superficial vein thrombosis have an asymptomatic deep vein thrombosis (DVT), and up to 10 % have a pulmonary embolism (Decousus et al. 2010; Quéré et al. 2012). A history of confirmed superficial vein thrombosis is a risk factor for later thrombosis (increased risk 6.9 %) or pulmonary embolism (increased risk 3.9 %) (van Langevelde et al. 2011).

Classification of Superficial Vein Thrombosis

There are two ways of classifying superficial vein thrombosis (Kalodiki et al. 2012):

1. In the first, the aetiology is classified as primary (inflammation only in the vein and surrounding tissue) or secondary (inflammation resulting from inflammation elsewhere in the body, such as Buerger's disease, Behçet's disease, other vasculitides, chronic rheumatic syndrome of auto-immune origin or cancers).
2. In the second, the disease is classified by its location, aetiology and risk factors:
   - Superficial vein thrombosis of a varicose vein
     – Location: saphenous veins (great and small) and their varicose tributaries

E. Mendoza, MD, PhD (✉)
Venenpraxis Wunstorf, Speckenstraße 10, Wunstorf 31515, Germany
e-mail: erika.mendoza@t-online.de

C.R. Lattimer, MD, PhD
Department of Vascular Surgery, Josef Pflug Vascular Laboratory, Ealing Hospital and Imperial College, London, UK

E. Mendoza et al. (eds.), *Duplex Ultrasound of Superficial Leg Veins*, DOI 10.1007/978-3-642-40731-4_11, © Springer-Verlag Berlin Heidelberg 2014

    - Risk factors: alteration to the endothelium or haemodynamic impairment
    - Aetiology: trauma, iatrogenic (after endoluminal thermal vein ablation, CHIVA or foam sclerotherapy) or infection
- Superficial vein thrombosis of a non-varicose vein
    - Location: any superficial or saphenous vein
    - Risk factors/examples: thrombophilia in pregnancy, oral contraception, pre- or para-neoplastic conditions, alterations to the endothelium with vasculitis, Buerger's disease, Behçet's disease and Mondor's disease
- "Other" (in varicose or non-varicose veins)
    - Location: veins of the upper and lower extremities
    - Aetiology: posttraumatic, burns, iatrogenic (i.v. entry point, haemodialysis catheter) or sepsis

This classification is particularly important because it focuses on thrombosis in the absence of previously existing varices. This is more often found in conjunction with neoplasia or thrombophilia.

11.1 Acute Superficial Vein Thrombosis and Periphlebitis

Superficial vein thrombosis is associated with clot formation within the vein which may be accompanied by coexisting inflammation of the vein wall and surrounding tissue. These respective conditions may determine the presenting symptoms:

- **Localised hardness without pain**: Coagulum in the vein without associated periphlebitis usually presents with palpable hardness along the course of the vein. Occasionally the area has a brownish discolouration caused by the accumulation of haemosiderin in the skin with post-inflammatory hyperpigmentation. On ultrasound, echo-genic material is apparent partially or completely filling the vein. The vein is not compressible (Fig. 11.1).
- **Localised hardness with pain**: Characteristically there is a coagulum in the vein with inflammation of the vein wall. Clinically, the vein is indurated with a brownish discolouration and the course of the vein is painful when pressed. The brown areas may be accompanied by reddening confined to the course of the vein. The ultrasound image is similar to patients without pain (Fig. 11.1).
- **Superficial reddening with hardness and pain**: Coagulum in the vein with periphlebitis defines this condition. Severe pain occurs when the area is pressed. Examination is not easily tolerated and the skin appears red and inflamed. In the ultrasound image, the thrombosis is accompanied by loss of the typical structure of the subcutaneous fatty tissue which appears homogeneous (Fig. 11.2). Occasionally there is a surrounding inflammatory halo of oedema. Compression testing (Fig. 11.3) is very painful and should only be done to exclude thrombosis with extension into the deep veins (Fig. 11.4).

A characteristic of thrombus in the saphenous veins is that it can extend into the deep veins through several junctions. This condition is called **ascending superficial vein thrombosis**. The saphenous vein must be examined carefully up to its confluence with the deep vein. The end of the thrombus is best seen in longitudinal view (Fig. 11.4).

A superficial vein thrombosis may protrude into the deep veins where it becomes surrounded by flow without any attachment to the wall of the vein. This is called a **floating thrombus**. Until a few years ago, such a finding would have indicated immediate ligation of the saphenofemoral junction as an emergency. Today, more conservative measures are preferred which includes compression, therapeutic anticoagulation with low molecular weight heparin or oral anticoagulants (e.g. warfarin) and frequent check-ups as an

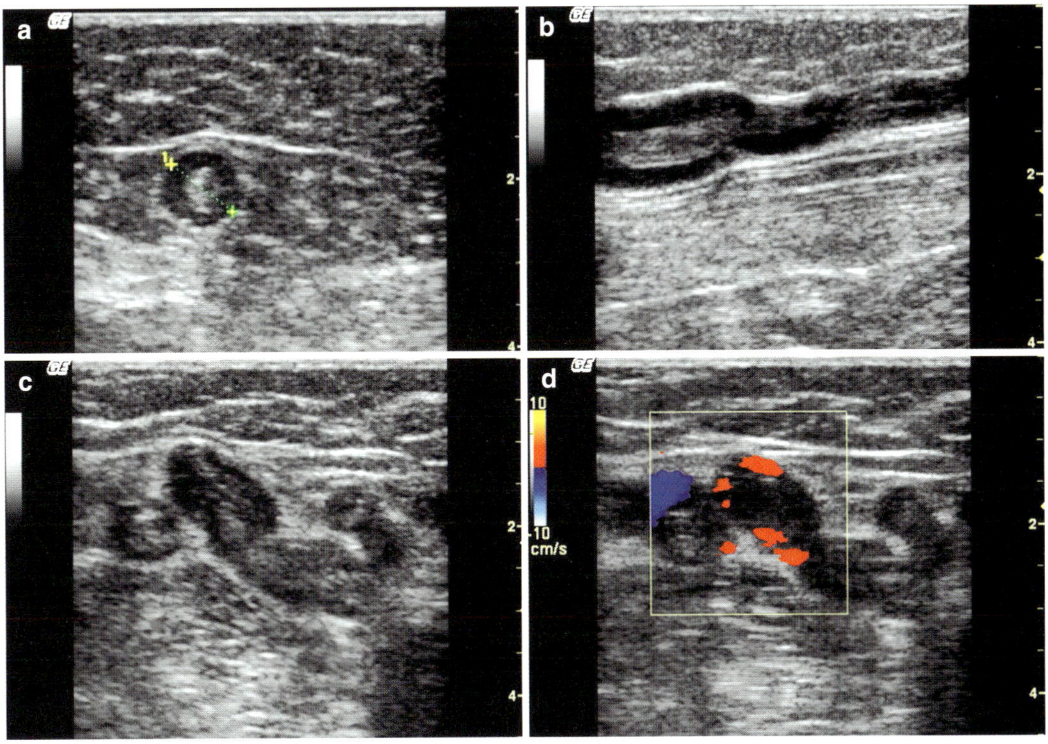

Fig. 11.1 (**a**) Thrombosis within the great saphenous vein in a transverse view through the thigh in a symptomless patient. There were no signs of periphlebitis. The fascial structures are recognisable as well as the connective tissue in the subcutaneous fat. (**b**) Thrombosis within the great saphenous vein in a longitudinal view in the same patient. (**c**) Transverse view through the thigh of the same patient further down the leg. Thrombus is seen in the great saphenous vein and a venous tributary which still lies deep to the fascia. It is important to determine if the superficial vein thrombosis within a perforating vein extends into the deep system. (**d**) Same position as (**c**) with colour duplex demonstrating partial flow around the thrombus Copyright: [Author]

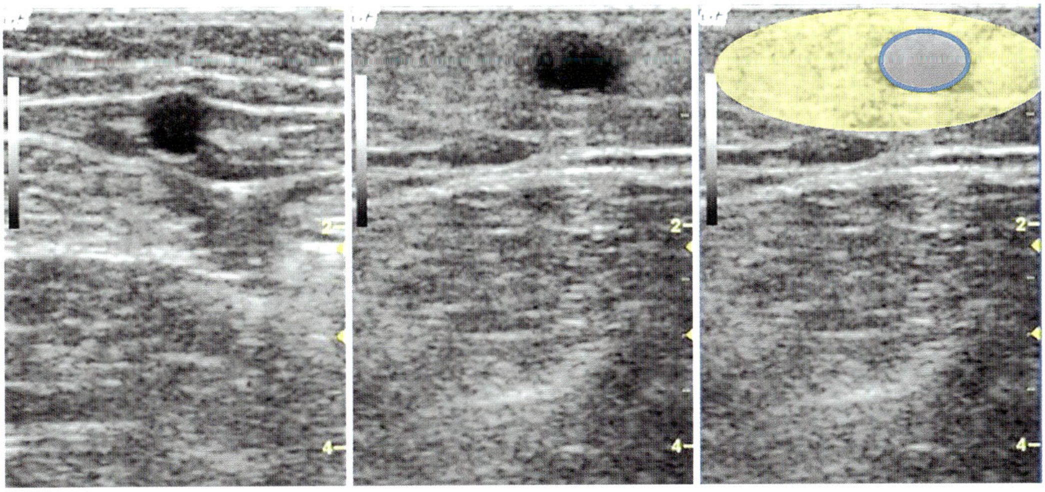

Fig. 11.2 Patient with pain and redness of the inner thigh. *Left*: transverse view of the mid-thigh above the painful area. The great saphenous vein is compressible and the fascial structures are preserved. *Middle*: transverse view further down and at the painful region. A thrombosed venous tributary is identified which is not compressible. The fascial structures in the subcutaneous tissue are no longer recognisable and the surrounding tissue appears grey and homogeneous. *Right yellow*: the subcutaneous fatty tissue has lost its architecture. *Blue*: thrombosed vein Copyright: [Author]

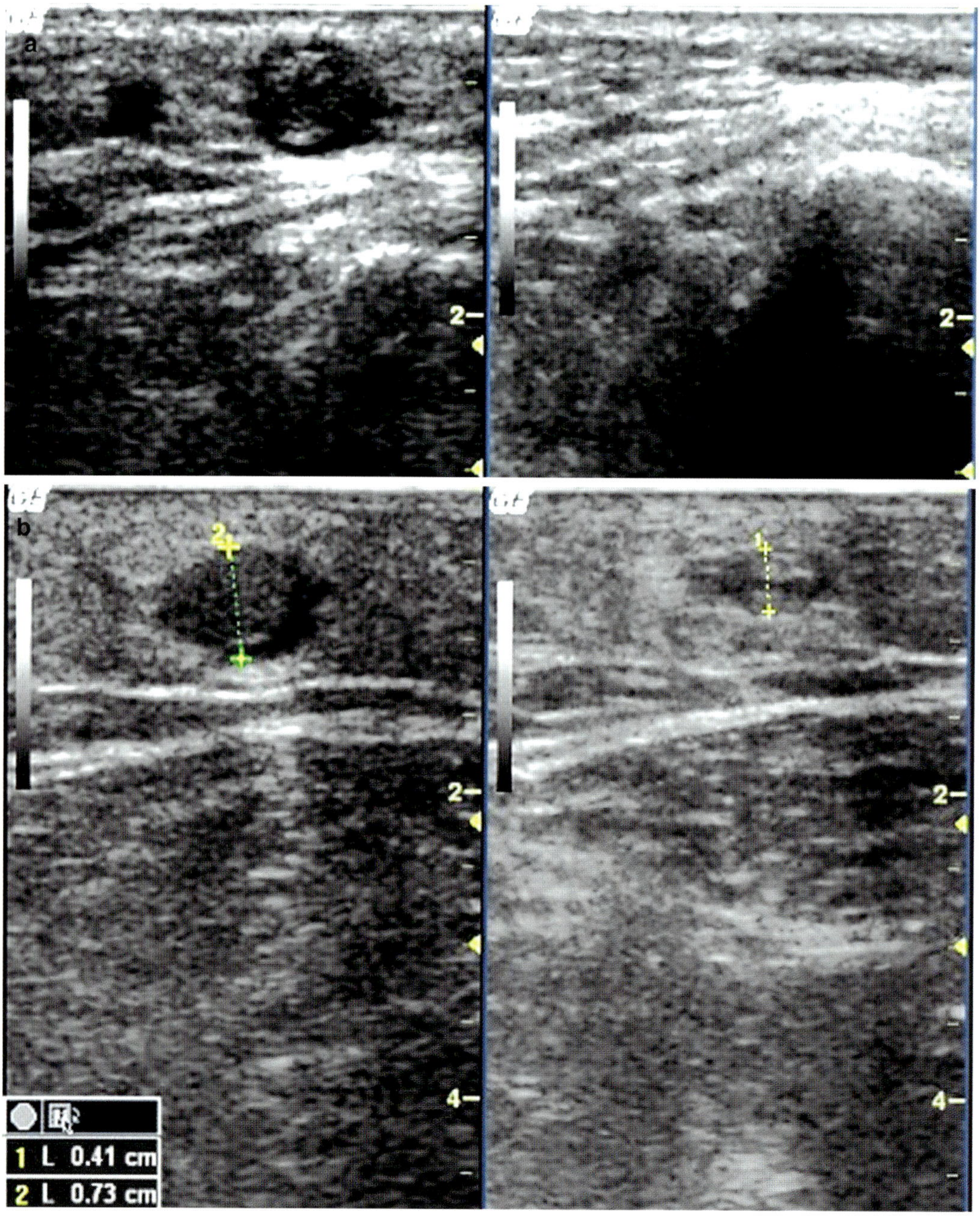

Fig. 11.3 Compression testing in superficial vein thrombosis. (**a**) Transverse view through the proximal section of the calf with an asymptomatic superficial vein thrombosis of the venous tributary, *left* without compression, *right* with compression: The great saphenous vein cannot be seen under compression. The venous tributary is smaller and only the echo-rich luminal material remains visible. There is preservation of the fascial architecture with no inflammation of the surrounding tissues (periphlebitis) (see accompanying online material). (**b**) Same patient as in Fig. 11.2 in transverse view through the thigh further down the leg. The coagulum appears more voluminous in the B-scan without compression than under compression. A periphlebitis is seen with loss of definition of the surrounding subcutaneous tissues. Compression is very painful (see accompanying online material) Copyright: [Author]

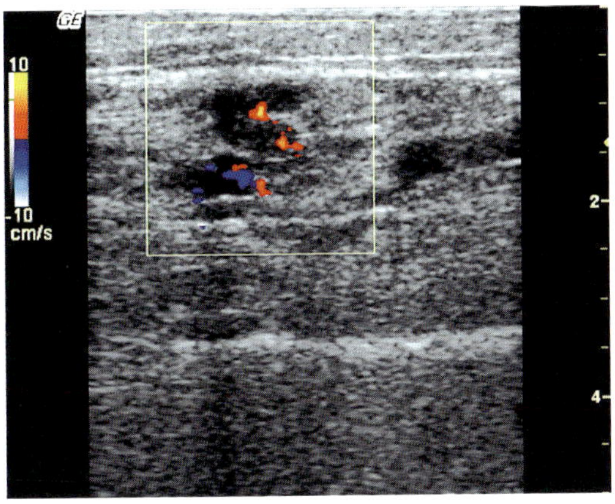

Fig. 11.4 Superficial vein thrombosis extending into a perforating vein. This occurred in a patient with pain in the inner calf after a football injury. Longitudinal view of the inner calf with a superficial vein thrombosis in a paratibial perforating vein demonstrating partial flow around the clot (see accompanying online material) Copyright: [Author]

outpatient. The patient must be told of the danger of a pulmonary embolism and is given the same information as outpatients who are treated for a deep vein thrombosis. Thrombus may also spread from the saphenous veins or, more frequently, from a venous tributary through perforating veins (Fig. 11.5e). Thrombotically altered veins must therefore be examined by ultrasound over their whole course and any perforation of the fascia should be tested with compression ultrasound for thrombotic material.

Clots in saphenous veins, especially in the thigh, are more frequently associated with deep vein thrombosis and pulmonary embolism than clots in venous tributaries. A further risk factor for deep vein thrombosis and pulmonary embolism is a superficial vein thrombosis in patients with no previous history of varicose veins (Kalodiki et al 2012).

Thrombophlebitis migrans or **saltans** is an exceptional situation. This is a recurrent superficial vein thrombosis which reappears repeatedly in different locations or is permanently present in a single region without any tendency to heal. It may be the expression of widely differing systemic diseases like polycythaemia, Buerger's disease, Behçet's disease and systemic lupus erythematosus. A mesothelioma can cause **Trousseau-Syndrome** which is recurrent superficial and deep vein thromboses with pulmonary embolism. Any patient with a non-resolving superficial vein thrombosis must therefore be investigated.

The following must be discriminated in saphenous superficial vein thrombosis:

- **Thrombosis without periphlebitis**: This is often a chance finding in an examination after CHIVA or incomplete stripping of the saphenous vein. The thrombosis is usually asymptomatic. The lumen of the great saphenous vein is partially or completely blocked by a thrombus (Fig. 11.1).
- **Thrombosis with periphlebitis**: Periphlebitis is characterised by the loss of connective tissue structures in the fascial compartment. It is sometimes impossible to distinguish muscle fascicles (Fig. 11.6). No external redness is seen and the pain reported by the patient is poorly localised. The pain tends to be muscular in nature because it is exacerbated during muscle activation. In the ultrasound image, a clot is seen in the saphenous vein (Fig. 11.1a) or sometimes simply a thickening of the vein wall, especially in the case of the small saphenous vein (Fig. 11.6). A hypoechoic inflammatory halo of oedema is occasionally seen around the vein.

In rare cases a thrombotically closed venous tributary may cause an incompetent saphenous vein to appear competent. This situation may occur if the venous tributary was responsible for draining the whole **reflux volume** from the saphenous vein. Consequently all reflux in the saphenous vein is abolished when this draining venous tributary is thrombosed (Fig. 11.7).

11.2 Natural History of Superficial Vein Thrombosis

A superficial vein thrombosis may resolve without any visible damage to the vein. However it is more common to find post-phlebitic changes:

- Small vessels may be completely **obliterated** by thrombosis. This usually corresponds to the "spontaneous healing" of a varicose tributary frequently reported by patients in the

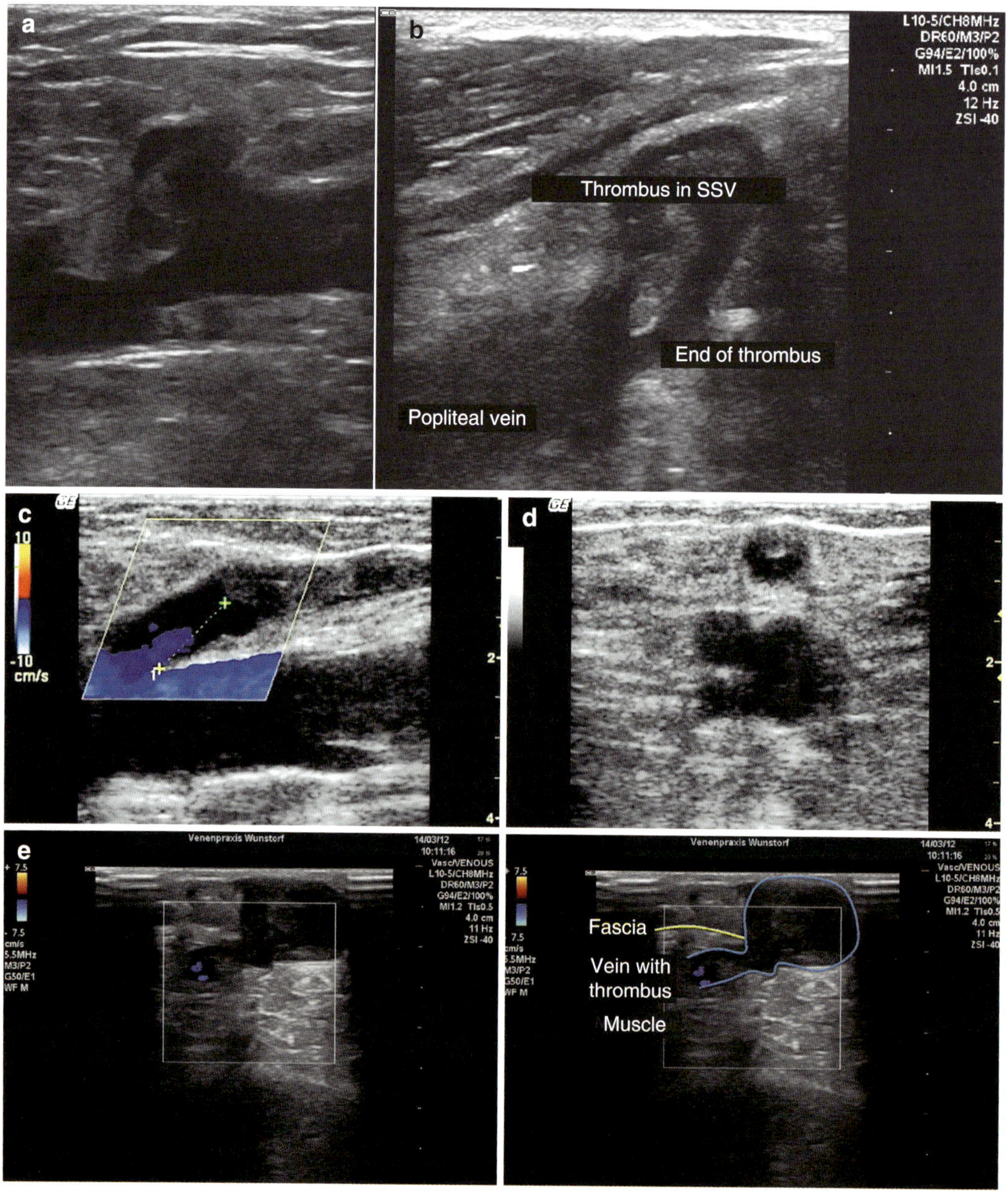

Fig. 11.5 Ascending superficial vein thrombosis. (**a**) Longitudinal view of the great saphenous vein through the left groin demonstrating thrombus protruding slightly into the common femoral vein. The thrombus appears interrupted because of flow draining the venous tributaries of the saphenofemoral junction. The image in the accompanying online material is further lateral showing the thrombus extending from the great saphenous vein into the deep vein. This is diagnosed as a partially occluding deep vein thrombosis. (**b**) Thrombus in the SPJ at 2 weeks. Longitudinal view through the popliteal region demonstrating thrombosis of the small saphenous vein. Flow is seen around the thrombus which is extending into the deep vein. The thin, longitudinal vein in the top part of the image beneath the fascia is the vein of Giacomini (see also Fig. 8.4 and accompanying online material). (**c**) Images of ascending superficial vein thrombosis of the anterior accessory saphenous vein (AASV) which almost reaches the saphenofemoral junction (SFJ). Longitudinal view of the saphenofemoral junction and anterior accessory saphenous vein. There is 11.9 mm between the termination of the thrombus and the saphenofemoral junction. Sequential compression images at the saphenofemoral junction and further down the leg with, including a longitudinal view, are shown on the accompanying online material. (**d**) Transverse view through the same groin demonstrating a visible thrombus in the anterior accessory saphenous vein. The great saphenous vein is not visible due to its small calibre. (**e**) A venous tributary superficial vein thrombosis is seen originating from a thrombosis of the small saphenous vein (**b**) with extension into the muscle veins through the fascia aperture via a perforating vein Copyright: [Author]

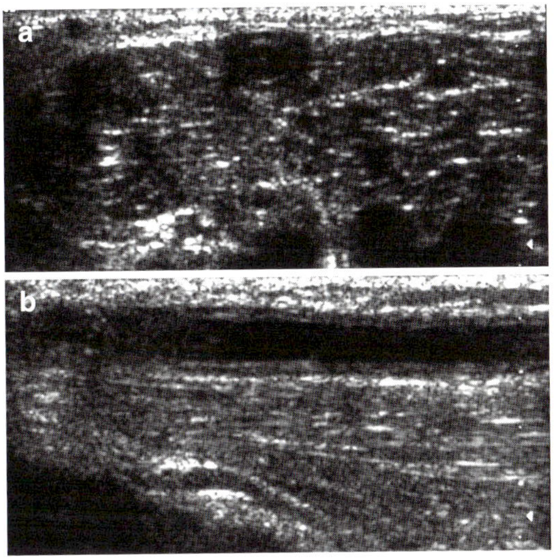

Fig. 11.6 Thrombosis of the small saphenous vein. (**a**) Transverse view through the calf in a patient with diffuse pain exacerbated by walking. The small saphenous vein is partially compressible and thickening of the wall can be seen with a double ring. The detail of the muscle fascicles beneath the vein is ambiguous. The image in the fascial compartment of the small saphenous vein is a homogeneous grey. Even in thin patients the tissue here is hard to assess. It is often easier to discriminate between normal and periphlebitic tissue clinically (see accompanying online material). (**b**) Longitudinal view through the same calf showing the thickening of the wall of the small saphenous vein Copyright: [Author]

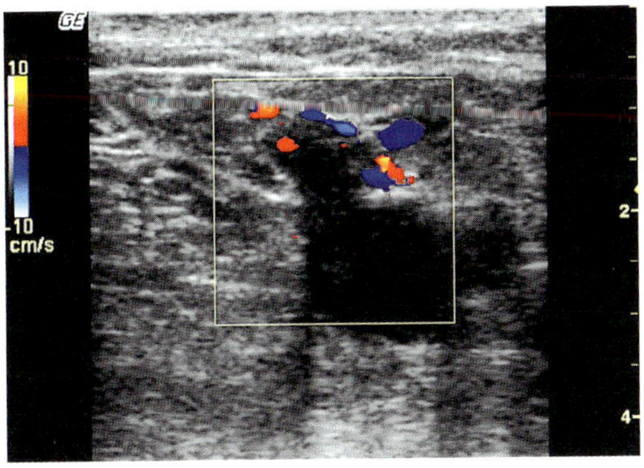

Fig. 11.7 Transverse view through the left groin in patient with known incompetence of the great saphenous vein which was refluxive down to the mid-thigh. Its drainage was through a lateral tributary. An acute superficial vein thrombosis of this venous tributary has occurred. Flow in the saphenous vein remains, but despite various manoeuvres, no reflux is seen in the proximal vein. It remains dilated and is therefore pathological (see accompanying online material) Copyright: [Author]

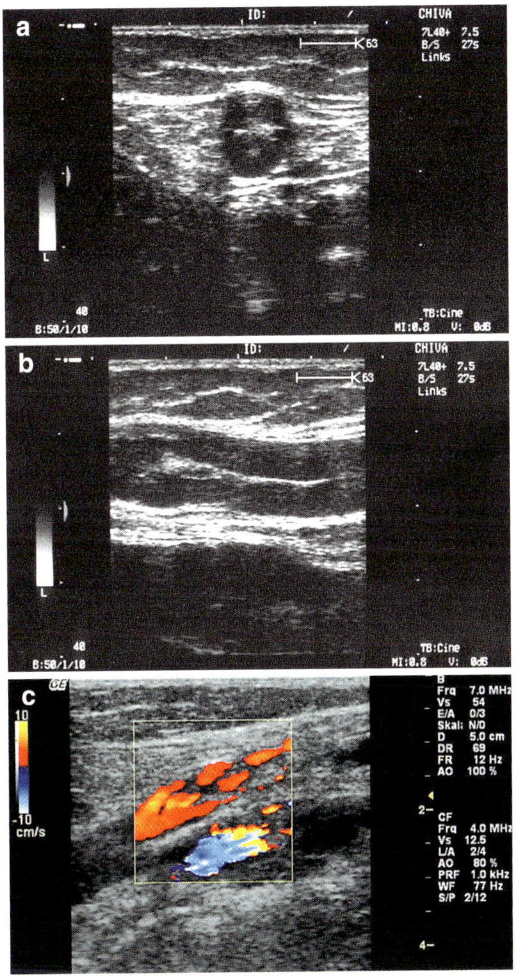

Fig. 11.8 (**a**) Transverse view through the thigh of a patient following a superficial vein thrombosis demonstrating changes within the great saphenous vein in its fascial compartment. The great saphenous vein diameter is over 1 cm in diameter with fibrotic tissue spanning across the lumen. (**b**) Longitudinal view through the thigh of the same patient demonstrating a septum. This extends for a considerable distance along the great saphenous vein and is reminiscent of the formation of "railway tracks" in the deep veins after thrombosis. (**c**) Post-thrombotic changes after a superficial vein thrombosis in the small saphenous vein demonstrating reflux as red in parts of the lumen during muscular diastole. It is partly recanalised and refluxive Copyright: [Author]

lateral calf region. Although, their lumen is no longer visible using ultrasound, their presence is indicated by a strong echo reflection.

- In similarity with deep veins, **septae** may develop across the lumen of the vein (Fig. 11.8).

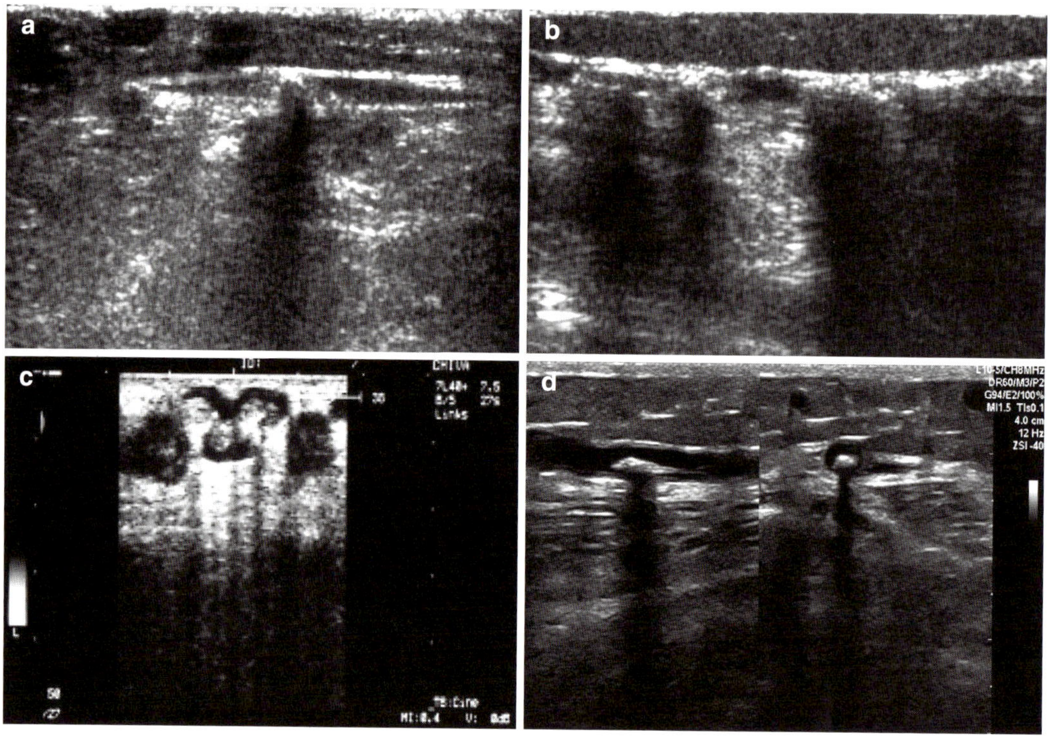

Fig. 11.9 Phleboliths. (**a**) Transverse view through the back of the calf of a patient who suffered recurrent attacks of superficial vein thrombosis years earlier. A strong echo-genic structure casting an acoustic shadow can be seen within the small saphenous vein compartment. (**b**) Longitudinal view of the same calf demonstrating a calcified small saphenous vein throughout its entire course. The characteristic acoustic shadow helps to differentiate between phleboliths and wall thickening caused by fibrosis (see accompanying online material). (**c**) Hardened structure in the inner thigh after a superficial vein thrombosis. The ultrasound image demonstrates echo-lucent areas with normal flow alternating with strong echo-genic areas representing calcification with prominent acoustic shadows. (**d**) Transverse and longitudinal views of the great saphenous vein in the calf after a superficial vein thrombosis with calcification and an acoustic shadow Copyright: [Author]

- Fibrosis of the vein wall following a thrombosis may become calcified giving rise to **phleboliths**. They return a strong echo in ultrasound and create a dense acoustic shadow (Fig. 11.9).
- The process of resolution may also cause destruction of previously competent valves, fibrotic strictures and areas of fresh echo-lucent thrombus, all visible on ultrasound.

Recommendations for Superficial Vein Thrombosis

The UIA and UIP consensus document mentioned above (Kalodiki et al. 2012) makes nine recommendations which are summarised below:

1. In every patient with superficial vein thrombosis in a non-varicose vein or with recurrent thromboses in varicose veins, the risk factors for superficial vein thrombosis should be extensively investigated. These include cancer and thrombophilia.
2. Clinical examination may underestimate the real extent of superficial vein thrombosis. Duplex ultrasound examination of the superficial and deep venous systems is therefore mandatory.
3. Duplex ultrasound should be performed on both the affected and the contralateral limb.

4. In patients with a saphenous vein thrombosis, the whole course of the vein must be examined together with the deep veins. This is especially true if the upper end of thrombus is less than 5 cm from the deep veins or if there is clinical worsening despite treatment.
5. All patients with superficial vein thrombosis should be treated with compression therapy.
6. Immediate mobilisation with elastic leg compression is mandatory. Patients should not be confined to bed.
7. If the superficial vein thrombosis is longer than 5 cm, the patient should take low molecular weight heparin in medium or therapeutic doses for 4 weeks. The dose and duration of the treatment will depend on risk factors and concomitant diseases.
8. Patients with superficial leg vein thrombi of more than 10 cm and additional risk factors for deep vein thrombosis and pulmonary embolism should take fondaparinux in prophylactic dose for 6 weeks.
9. Routine ligation of the saphenofemoral or saphenopopliteal junction to prevent extension into the deep leg veins is not indicated. However it is advisable to monitor the patient with elective treatment of their underlying varicose veins to avoid later complications.

References

Decousus H et al (2010) Superficial venous thrombosis and venous thromboembolism. Ann Intern Med 152: 218–224

Kalodiki E, Strvrtinova V, Allegra C, Andreozzi GM, Antignani PL, Avram R, Brkljacic B, Cadariou F, Dzsinich C, Fareed J, Gaspar L, Geroulakos G, Javien A, Kozak M, Lattimer CR, Minar E, Partsch H, Passariello F, Patel M, Pécsvárady Z, Poredos P, Rotocil K, Scuderi A, Sparovec M, Szostek M, Skorski M (2012) Superficial vein thrombosis: a consensus statement. Int Angiol 31:203–216

Quéré I, Leizorovicz A, Galanaud JP, Presles E, Barrellier MT, Becker F, Desprairies G, Guenneguez H, Mismetti P, Décousus H (2012) Prospective Observational Superficial Thrombophlebitis (POST) Study Investigators. J Vasc Surg 56(4):1032–8

van Langevelde K, Lijfering WM, Rosendaal FR, Cannegieter SC (2011) Increased risk of venous thrombosis in persons with clinically diagnosed superficial vein thrombosis: results from the MEGA study. Blood 118:4239–4241

Ultrasound in Varicose Vein Treatment

12

Erika Mendoza, Thomas M. Proebstle, Achim Mumme, Franz Xaver Breu, Nick Morrison, and Christopher R. Lattimer

Chapter Summary
Diagnosis is a prerequisite for all treatment strategies. Duplex ultrasound is the best diagnostic tool for varicose veins for all expressions of the disease (Nicolaides 2000). All types of intervention on varicose veins have their own special demands on ultrasound. Ultrasound-guided vein mapping on the skin is very helpful prior to saphenous stripping (See Sect. 12.1), and it is absolutely indispensible for CHIVA (See Sect. 12.2). In endovascular thermal therapies (See Sect. 12.3) or foam sclerotherapy of trunk veins (See Sect. 12.4), ultrasound is an essential part of the treatment process. The actual procedures will only be explained here in relation to ultrasound.

E. Mendoza, MD, PhD (✉)
Venenpraxis Wunstorf,
Speckenstraße 10, 31515 Wunstorf, Germany
e-mail: erika.mendoza@t-online.de

T.M. Proebstle, MD, PhD
Hautklinik und Poliklinik, Universitätsmedizin der Johannes Gutenberg-Universität Mainz,
Langenbeckstraße 1, 5131 Mainz, Germany
e-mail: thomas.proebstle@web.de

A. Mumme, MD, PhD
Klinik für Gefäßchirurgie,
St. Josef-Hospital, Universitätsklinikum,
Gudrunstraße 56, 44791 Bochum, Germany
e-mail: achim.mumme@ruhr-uni-bochum.de

F.X. Breu, MD
Praxis für Gefäßmedizin am Tegernsee,
Tegernseer Straße 101, 83700 Rottach-Egern, Germany
e-mail: f.x.breu@t-online.de

N. Morrison, MD
Morrison Vein Institute,
Suite 223, 8575 E. Princess Dr., Scottsdale, AZ, USA

C.R. Lattimer, MD, PhD
Department of Vascular Surgery,
Josef Pflug Vascular Laboratory,
Ealing Hospital and Imperial College, London, UK

12.1 Ultrasound in Varicose Vein Removal

For 90 years, trunk veins were removed without utilising ultrasound. However, the treatment benefits are significant if the surgeon has access to detailed information obtained by preoperative duplex ultrasound (Nicolaides 2000; Coleridge-Smith et al. 2006).

In the event of complete insufficiency of the great saphenous vein, the saphenofemoral junction is always treated concurrently. It is helpful for the surgeon to know the anatomy of the region in advance (Sect. 7.3):

1. Is the saphenofemoral junction located in the groin or, as is very often the case, higher up?
2. What is the course of the great saphenous vein in relation to the other two long veins: the anterior accessory saphenous vein and the posterior accessory saphenous vein?

E. Mendoza et al. (eds.), *Duplex Ultrasound of Superficial Leg Veins*,
DOI 10.1007/978-3-642-40731-4_12, © Springer-Verlag Berlin Heidelberg 2014

3. Is the anterior accessory saphenous vein also dilated or refluxive, a frequent cause of early recurrence after crossectomy?
4. Does the patient have a venous aneurysm?
5. Does the patient have any anatomical particularity, for example, a great saphenous vein or anterior accessory saphenous vein termination between the femoral and deep femoral arteries?

More important is the preoperative duplex mapping of the termination of the small saphenous vein, usually followed by marking the configuration on the skin. This is often located above the joint space (Sect. 8.3) in which case it lies very close to the peroneal nerve (Sect. 17.6) which might be damaged during the operation. The following information is also helpful to the surgeon:

1. Relative position of the knee joint space, also best marked on the skin
2. Relative position of the peroneal nerve
3. Depth of the confluence of the small saphenous vein and the popliteal vein, in centimetres
4. Relative position of the musculature of the thigh (is the confluence covered by muscle?)
5. Presence of a vein of Giacomini or thigh extension, its morphology and hemodynamics (refluxive or not)
6. Presence of one or more muscle veins in the region of the confluence

Stripping of the saphenous vein assumes that the distal end of reflux is known, termed the distal insufficiency point, according to Hach (Sect. 4.1.3). If applicable, this should be marked on the skin. It is likewise helpful to identify hypoplastic segments of the great saphenous vein. In this situation the stripping probe must not be forced into the anatomical continuation within the fascial compartment, but carefully directed into the side branch. If the hypoplastic section is marked on the skin, the probe can usually be manipulated into the epifascial side branch by external compression.

Enlarged perforating veins are often interrupted during varicose vein avulsions, regardless of whether or not they are refluxive. Preoperative marking of these on the skin makes them easier to find and allows a smaller incision to be made.

Phlebectomies do not require duplex ultrasound for marking because these veins can be felt and marked directly on the standing patient.

12.2 Ultrasound with the CHIVA Method

Before the CHIVA method is selected as the surgical strategy, recirculation must be analysed exactly and the type of shunt established (Sect. 4.2). The difference between shunt types I and III or IV and V is especially important, since these represent the commonest forms of recirculation. They are treated completely differently (Sect. 4.2.9). The CHIVA technique involves surgically interrupting haemodynamically critical vein connections whilst leaving other connections that may be beneficial (Franceschi 1988 in Appendix 2; Mendoza 2002 in Appendix 2).

Apart from operations on the saphenofemoral junction in the groin, where marking is not necessary, the ligation and transection points are marked on the skin with an indelible ink marker. This simplifies the operation, which is usually carried out under local anaesthetic. It also minimises the pain which the patient may suffer if the operator has to dissect to search for the veins.

When treating the saphenofemoral junction, it must be established whether the saphenofemoral junction is refluxive or the saphenofemoral junction tributaries are refluxive or whether both are responsible for the reflux. The operator will decide on his own judgement whether to carry out a classic crossectomy at the saphenofemoral junction, ligation of the great saphenous vein only at the level of femoral vein (crossotomy) or a short ablation using endoluminal devices distal to the terminal valve.

1. In the case of reflux from the deep veins through an incompetent terminal valve, ligation of the saphenofemoral junction may be carried out exclusively (crossotomy).
2. In the case of additional reflux through pudendal, epigastric or circumflex veins (Fig. 12.1a, b), reflux will persist after ligation of the saphenofemoral junction at the terminal valve (Fig. 12.1c). For this reason these incompetent tributaries must also be interrupted.
3. In the case of a competent terminal valve and incompetent preterminal valve, interruption of

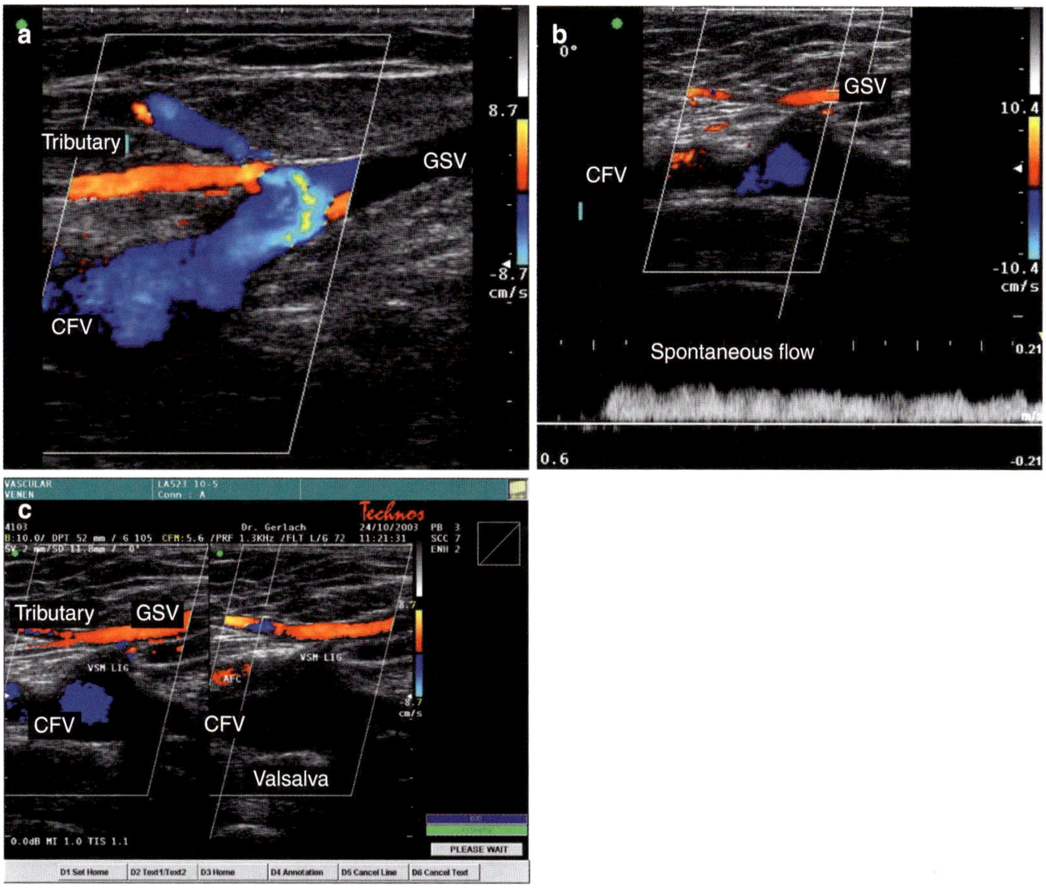

Fig. 12.1 Refluxive saphenofemoral junction tributaries. (**a**) Antegrade flow (*blue*) across the saphenofemoral junction during muscular systole. The epigastric vein (EV) is shown in red demonstrating blood which is refluxing into the saphenofemoral junction tributaries (see online material). (**b**) Spontaneous flow in the great saphenous vein (great saphenous vein) in the same patient standing. The slow, drawn-out, long-lasting reflux is typical of reflux originating in refluxive saphenofemoral junction tributaries. (**c**) Flow in the great saphenous vein after ligation of the saphenofemoral junction without ligation of the refluxive saphenofemoral junction tributaries. The reflux in the great saphenous vein persists unchanged (CFV – common femoral vein, VSM lig = ligated GSV) (Dr. Horst Gerlach, Mannheim; by kind permission) Copyright: Dr. Horst Gerlach, Mannheim

the saphenofemoral junction leaving the tributaries untouched does not have a significant effect on saphenous reflux. In this case the classic crossectomy (interruption of saphenofemoral junction and all tributaries) or the ablation with endoluminal devices distal to the confluence of the refluxive side branches is proposed.

In the presence of a shunt type III, the doctor must decide according to the ultrasound findings whether or not a CHIVA 2 strategy can be used. CHIVA 2 is ligation and transection of the tributaries of a saphenous trunk, with preservation of the saphenofemoral junction. With this strategy the refluxive great saphenous vein remains in continuity with the common femoral vein. Here there is a risk that a post-operative saphenous thrombosis might extend into the deep veins. The following preoperative duplex ultrasound criteria may help in the decision whether to use CHIVA 2 in order to lessen the chance of this complication.:

1. Diameter of the great saphenous vein 15 cm from the groin greater than 10 mm: do not use CHIVA 2 strategy but operate directly on the saphenofemoral junction.
2. Aneurysmal enlargement of the great saphenous vein in the region of the saphenofemoral junction: do not use CHIVA 2 strategy but operate directly on the saphenofemoral junction.

3. Diameter of the great saphenous vein between 6 and 10 mm: administer low molecular weight heparin in prophylactic dose for 10 days with CHIVA 2 strategy.
4. Diameter of great saphenous vein less than 6 mm: CHIVA 2 strategy may be followed without administration of low molecular weight heparin.

Perforating veins are only treated when they constitute the point of insufficiency. They are examined following the criteria mentioned in Chap. 9. A perforating vein should only be interrupted if it is found to be refluxive during calf diastole. This is very seldom the case in the first intervention.

12.3 Ultrasound in Endovenous Treatment of Varicose Veins with Thermal Procedures

Endovenous obliteration for the treatment of varicose veins has gained a firm place in varicose trunk vein therapy in the last 10 years. In particular, thermal procedures have reached clinical maturity in recent years. Their ablative effects are controllable in comparison to foam sclerotherapy which has also become widely practised. The two competing thermal procedures are endovenous radiofrequency ablation (Proebstle et al. 2011) and endovenous laser ablation (Schwarz et al. 2010; Prince et al. 2011). In both procedures the treatment can be controlled using ultrasound. The same is true for the newer procedures of mechanochemical ablation (Elias and Raines 2012) and endovenous cyanoacrylate glue embolization (Almeida et al. 2013).

The principal technical steps for all endoluminal procedures are:

1. Setting up access to the vein
2. Introduction of a catheter or laser fibre
3. Peri-venous injection of a tumescent or local anaesthetic solution
4. Release of the thermal energy during withdrawal of the fibre

All these steps are usually performed under continuous ultrasound control.

12.3.1 Prerequisites

An ultrasound machine which can be part of the standard operating room equipment is a prerequisite for continuous preoperative monitoring. Portable, space-saving, laptop-size machines are particularly suitable. The machine must have a data storage facility and documentation function. It should also be fitted with a linear probe which should ideally be able to work at frequencies between 8 and 15 MHz. The system should include functions which allow a duplex ultrasound image to be recalled as needed at any time during the operation. The first priority is an excellent quality B-scan, in which the anatomical structures and the catheters and fibres in use can be clearly recognised in all phases of the operation.

The operating doctor can ensure complete ultrasound sterility throughout the operation by using the following:

1. Sterile latex or plastic cover for the transducer
2. Sterile ultrasound gel
3. Sterile plastic keyboard cover

12.3.2 Interventions for Trunk Vein Insufficiency

12.3.2.1 Choice of the Most Suitable Entry Point into the Vein

The first step to the endoluminal treatment is the introduction of the needle into the vein. With duplex the optimal point is to be found. One possibility is to use the most distal point of reflux as the point of entry into the vein to be treated. In the case of the great saphenous vein, this is usually found in the proximal lower leg or the distal thigh. In general, all the entry locations can be chosen on the inner side of the leg, so long as this is consistent with the pathological findings. In very obese patients, where the vein lies too deep, an alternative is to choose an entry point via a more superficial venous tributary provided it is below the distal end point of reflux. Alternatively, if the vein calibre permits, this can be accessed further distally. There are very few entry problems with

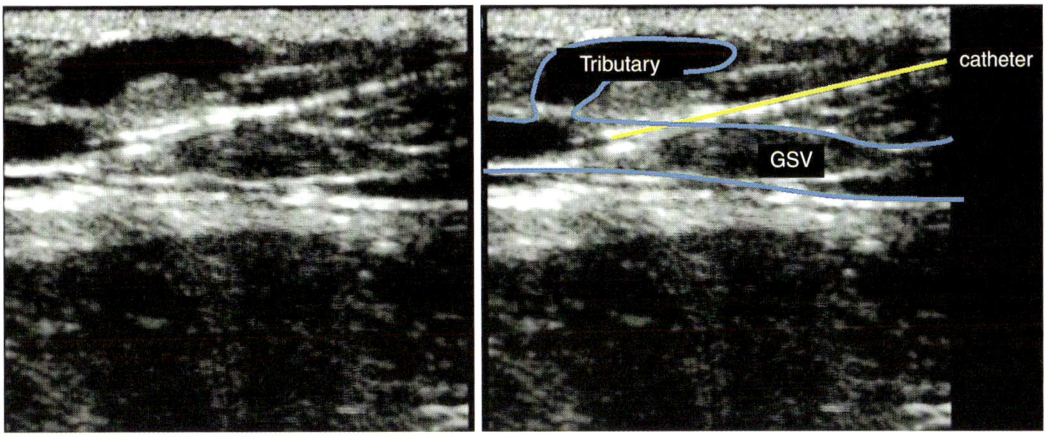

Fig. 12.2 Axial representation of the great saphenous vein (great saphenous vein) in the proximal lower leg region during introduction of an 18G, 40 mm long, peripheral venous catheter Copyright: [Author]

the small saphenous vein on account of its relatively superficial position. Puncture of the vein at the ankle may be hampered by bony prominences like the lateral malleolus.

12.3.2.2 Venous Access in Practice

Endovenous obliteration procedures are usually performed via a percutaneous puncture. Entry into the vein through a cutdown or using a phlebectomy hook is a possibility; however, it detracts from the minimally invasive nature of the operation and experience with the procedure will generally render these techniques obsolete. Insertion of a peripheral venous catheter or needle followed by a guidewire is performed under ultrasound control. During puncture, the transducer head can be oriented transversally or longitudinally to the axis of the vein, according to the operating doctor's personal preference (Fig. 12.2).

The following measures facilitate ultrasound-guided percutaneous venous access:

1. Achieving a vein diameter as large as possible at the puncture site by:
   1. Placing the patient in the reverse Trendelenburg position, with the legs angled downwards approximately 15°–30°
   2. Maintaining a warm operating room temperature to avoid cold-induced venospasm
   3. Occasionally by inflating a tourniquet proximal to the puncture point
2. Technical tips on achieving successful cannulation:
   1. Stretching the skin at the intended puncture site. In patients with slack skin or obesity, manual stretching is recommended, if necessary with the help of an operating room assistant. This stabilises the vein and prevents it from yielding during attempted puncture.
   2. In patients with thick skin, an initial puncture with a pointed blade helps to maintain a sharp needle. It also reduces any friction between the skin and needle which helps to prevent cutaneous recoil and subsequent needle displacement out of the vein.
   3. Cannulation with the bevel of the needle downwards is preferred into small superficial veins when a shallow approach is used. With deeper punctures and a steeper angle of entry, an upward-directing bevel is more likely to lie across the lumen.

12.3.2.3 Introduction of the Laser Fibre or Radiofrequency Catheter

Whether the treatment method is radiofrequency, endoluminal laser ablation or one of the newer procedures, a suitable diameter tube or angiography catheter is then slid over the introduced guidewire. Once the guidewire is removed, this will allow the introduction of the laser fibre, radiofrequency catheter or other endovenous

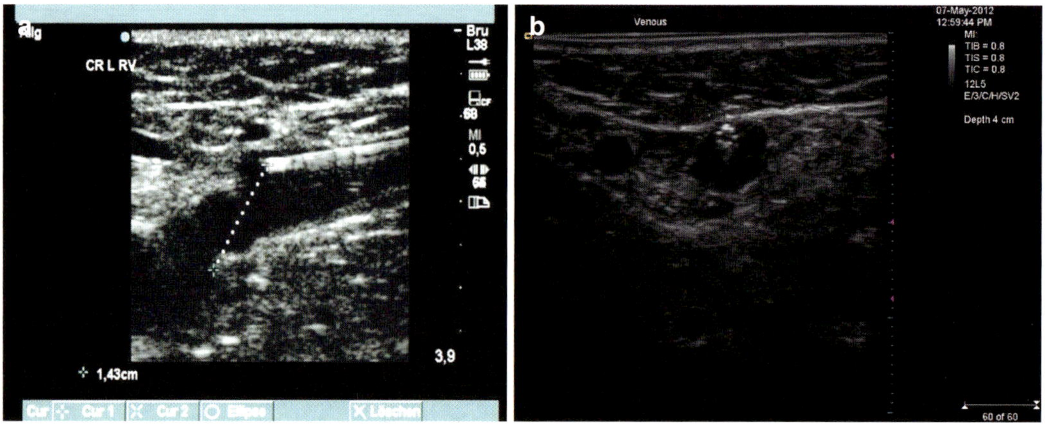

Fig. 12.3 (**a**) Longitudinal view through the groin demonstrating the termination a laser fibre before the saphenofemoral junction. (**b**) Transverse view of the patented 4 F Teflon catheter from the acrylic cement system. The eight microscopic air channels in the catheter wall at its termination make it very easy to identify on ultrasound Copyright: [Author]

ablative device. With bare laser fibres, the use of a sheath of the same length as the vein to be treated is recommended. This reduces the risk of perforation since an unprotected bare laser fibre, when advanced, can lodge into the vein wall. The process of introducing the tube or catheter need not necessarily be controlled by ultrasound, so long as the wire and catheter advance easily and without resistance.

However, the final resting positioning of the end point of the endoluminal ablation device close to the deep vein system requires precise ultrasound control. This location must be documented in relation to the distance from the saphenofemoral or saphenopopliteal junction; knee flexion must be avoided as this can cause a change in the final position. If the tip of the endovenous ablation device is positioned too close to the deep vein system, this can lead to thrombus extension into deep veins. This is true for all endovenous procedures. For this reason the point of the catheter or laser fibre must not be positioned less than 1–2 cm from the saphenofemoral junction (Fig. 12.3a). If a cyanoacrylate glue deployment catheter is used, this distance should be 5 cm in order to avoid unintentional introduction of the cement applicator into the deep vein system (Fig. 12.3b). In treatment of the small saphenous vein, the catheter or fibre should be positioned up to the point where the vein lies directly under the crural fascia which is just as it turns down towards the popliteal vein.

However, the use of ultrasound support may be advisable, and in some cases indispensible, during positioning of the guidewire, particularly if the wire cannot be advanced without resistance. Possible reasons for this might be a previously undiscovered segment of hypoplasia which can occur in up to 25 % of patients; Sect. 2.4.4). Other impediments include marked tortuosity which occurs in 1–2 % of patients or calibre variations in around 7 % of patients (Ricci and Caggiati 1999). With complete vein occlusion, a second puncture proximal to the occlusion is required in order to ablate the remaining segment. With very tortuous veins, some passages may be impossible to navigate. When it proves difficult to push the wire forward, the course of the vein is first analysed in three dimensions using ultrasound. The passage where the hindrance occurs is very often S-shaped. In such cases, it is sometimes possible to advance the wire by stretching the course of the vein using digital pressure on the skin at the affected region (Fig. 12.4) or by simply straightening the leg.

12.3.2.4 Application of Local Anaesthetic (Tumescence)

The principal advantage of carrying out the operation under tumescent anaesthesia, as compared to general or regional anaesthesia, is that peri-venous structures can be protected from the effects of the heat generated by radiofrequency or laser. In particular, with tumescent anaesthe-

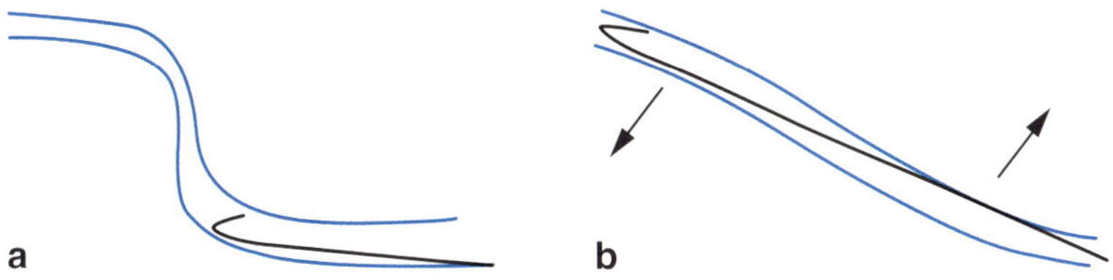

Fig. 12.4 Diagram of how to advance through a tortuous vein by manipulating the course of the vein. (**a**) Original course. (**b**) The vein is straightened using manual traction of the skin and subcutaneous tissue Copyright: [Author]

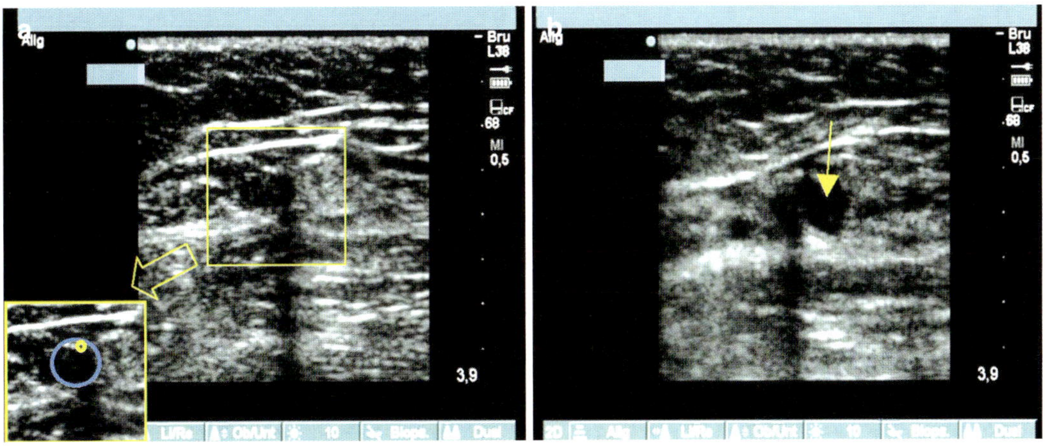

Fig. 12.5 (**a**) Transverse view of a great saphenous vein in the thigh with the laser fibre in the vein demonstrating an acoustic shadow caused by the laser fibre (see detail). (**b**) Immediate peri-venous injection of the tumescent solution (echo-poor, *arrowed*), which only partially compresses the great saphenous vein. The laser fibre can be visualised to the side with its characteristic acoustic shadow Copyright: [Author]

sia, the patient can inform the operating doctor if there is any heat damage to the principal nerves. For example, if radiating pain occurs in the heel area due to irritation of the sural nerve, the energy source can quickly be turned off and the catheter repositioned a few millimetres along. Tumescent anaesthesia seems not to be required in mechano-chemical ablation or acrylic cement deployment.

Tumescent anaesthetic is injected into the peri-venous space, preferably in a slight Trendelenburg position (Fig. 12.5). In this way the analgesic effect is obtained immediately, and the operation can be started directly after the injection. The use of an automated roller pump is easier than using direct injections by hand. Both injection of the tumescent solution and the Trendelenburg position lead to a significant reduction of the vein diameter. This means that a smaller volume of blood is present in the vein around the catheter. In endovenous laser ablation, a small amount of remaining blood results in better energy transfer to the vein wall because it facilitates the formation of steam bubbles and convection currents. This is in contrast to radiofrequency closure where the operator applies additional manual pressure over the catheter point to try to expel the remaining blood from the vein lumen. This is because radiofrequency works by conductive heat transfer making the presence of blood unnecessary or counterproductive. In contrast to peri-venous injection fluid constrained within the saphenous compartment, tumescent solution around a superficial vein disperses more easily. Therefore, care must be taken to ensure an adequate volume of tumescence remains between the skin and vein. This will avoid thermal damage to the dermis and consequent hyperpigmentation.

12.3.2.5 Energy Transfer During Treatment

During radiofrequency ablation, ultrasound monitoring is superfluous, since the principal

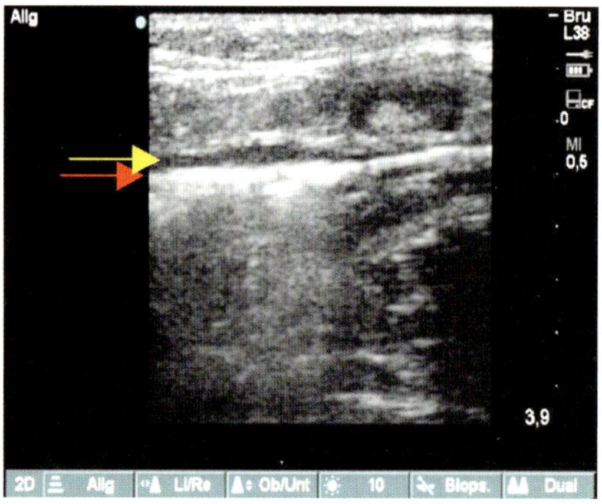

Fig. 12.6 Longitudinal view of the proximal great saphenous vein. Release of laser energy from a 600 μm diameter fibre (30 W, 940 nm) demonstrating steam bubbles. The strong echo reflection in the vein (*red arrow*) stands out from the surrounding echo-poor tumescent anaesthetic (*yellow arrow*) Copyright: [Author]

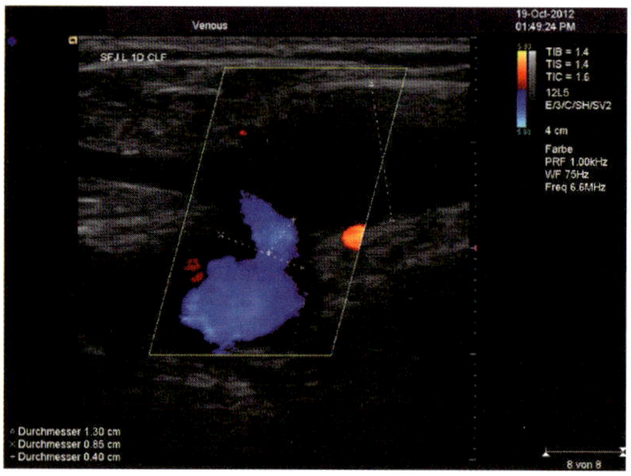

Fig. 12.7 Typical ultrasound findings one day after ClosureFast® treatment. The superficial inferior epigastric vein is patent with preservation of drainage into the saphenofemoral junction. The distance between the confluence and the closure of the great saphenous vein is 8 mm Copyright: [Author]

focus of the operator is on maintaining the target temperature at the catheter point. This temperature is easier to maintain if the operator applies pressure over the catheter point. This is considerably easier using manual compression applied directly with the hand than with the ultrasound probe.

In contrast to radiofrequency ablation, manual pressure over the laser fiber tip should be avoided. This is especially true when a bare fibre is used, because this action may facilitate vein wall perforation. Furthermore, residual blood is needed to obtain a better, more regular transfer of laser energy to the vein wall. This takes place through convection currents or, more accurately, via a turbulent flow of steam bubbles and blood (Fig. 12.6). Continuous ultrasound monitoring of the endovenous laser process in case of bare fibres allows the formation and spreading of steam bubbles to be observed and in particular allows significant perforations of the vein wall to be recognised in time. This is identified when steam and gas bubbles spread into the surrounding tissues during an extraluminal release of laser energy. In this event lasering is stopped and the fibre is withdrawn a few millimetres, after which normal endovenous ablation can be resumed.

12.3.2.6 Ultrasound Surveillance

Duplex ultrasound examination of the ablated vein should be performed within one week after the operation. In ideal circumstances, a duplex assessment should take place on the first postoperative day. This is mainly to confirm closure of the vein throughout the whole treated section. In all cases the following are documented: the new anatomical and haemodynamic configuration at the junction with the deep vein system, the proximal end of the treated vein, the maximum diameter of the obliterated vein and the distance of any thrombus from the deep veins (Fig. 12.7).

The event of an extension of thrombus into the deep veins is termed an endovenous heat-induced thrombosis (EHIT). Treatment involves anticoagulation with low molecular weight heparin with frequent duplex assessments until resolution. Although strictly speaking this is a deep vein thrombosis, this phenomenon usually follows a benign clinical course until the thrombus resolves by breaking off or retracting.

If there is severe pain along the treated vein in the post-operative interval of around 1–3 weeks, the ultrasound examination often demonstrates a characteristic halo of peri-phlebitic oedema. Nonsteroidal anti-inflammatory drugs are the preferred treatment. Ultrasound monitoring is rarely required.

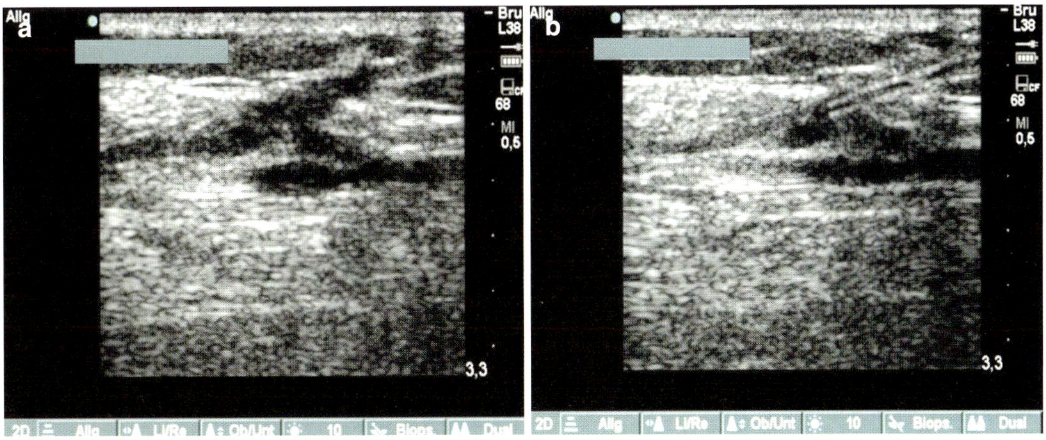

Fig. 12.8 Laser obliteration of a posterior tibial perforating vein (formerly Cockett). (**a**) Longitudinal view through the calf showing the posterior tibial perforating vein. (**b**) An 18G peripheral venous catheter introduced just below the fascia Copyright: [Author]

12.3.3 Treatment of Incompetent Perforating Veins

Thermal closure of incompetent perforating veins by radiofrequency or laser has now been accepted as a standard technique for endovenous therapy. It is rarely used for treating early venous disease but more common for CEAP $C_{4\text{-}6}$ clinical states. Percutaneous ablation of perforating veins (PAPS) is significantly less discussed in the literature than saphenous vein ablation. The procedures are similar to those used in trunk vein treatment in that they involve continuous ultrasound monitoring. However, greater practical dexterity is required by the operator. The following practicalities must be considered in the treatment of incompetent perforating veins:

1. When puncturing the perforating vein, a 16G or 18G peripheral venous catheter (PVC) must first be positioned so that when the laser fibre or RF catheter is introduced into the PVC, it is in the correct place for energy release (Fig. 12.8). The preferred location is within the perforating vein just below the point where it penetrates the fascia.
2. Puncturing requires a particularly precise technique because of the restricted space available for manoeuvring. Careless technique results in bruising around the perforating vein which is associated with failure of thermoablation.
3. Injection of local anaesthetic and release of thermal energy are both monitored using ultrasound. This must be carried out with great care due to the proximity of deep veins, particularly at the distal medial lower leg.

12.4 Duplex Ultrasound in Extraluminal Valvuloplasty

Incompetence of the great saphenous vein at the saphenofemoral junction is associated with dilatation of the vessel wall. If the vein diameter measured 1 cm distal from the saphenofemoral junction is greater than 7 mm, then valve incompetence is nearly always present. If the diameter is less than 6 mm, however, pathological reflux is rare. This observation is the principle behind venous valve reconstruction using extraluminal valvuloplasty. The dilated vein is reduced to a physiological diameter of less than 6 mm by the use of an external sheath or plication. The valve leaflets, which had become separated, regain contact and are thus able to carry out their closure function (Fig. 12.9).

Degenerative changes in venous valves always accompany the development of trunk vein insufficiency. As the disease develops, the valve leaflets become fibrotic and immobile and are eventually resorbed. Gross vein degeneration

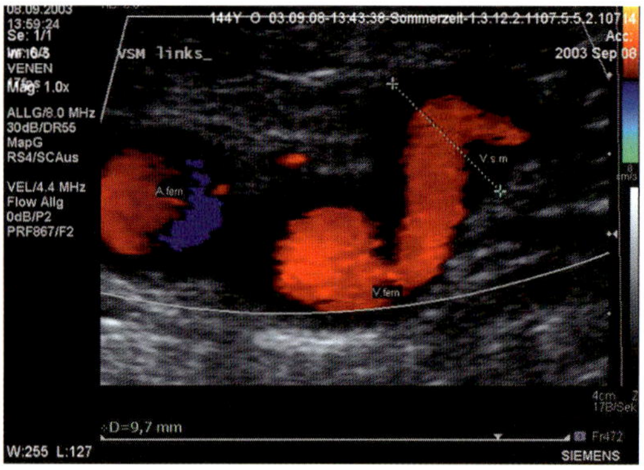

Fig. 12.9 Saphenous dilatation at 10 mm at the terminal valve. The separated valve leaflets can be seen with intervening reflux provoked using a Valsalva manoeuvre Copyright: [Author]

seldom occurs with vein diameters of less than 10 mm (Yamaki et al. 2002). Severe damage to venous valves is predominantly observed with greater vein diameters.

To determine the suitability of venous valve reconstruction, duplex ultrasound examination of the standing patient is obligatory. This must include routine imaging of the whole course of the great saphenous vein together with a Brightness Flow Mode image of the saphenofemoral junction. This examination is preferred to an image in colour mode because it provides greater detail of the valve leaflets when observed during a Valsalva manoeuvre. However, in machines without B-Flow Mode, B-scan can be used after prolonged standing. Here it is possible to see the flow of erythrocytes through the valve opening streaming in the centre of the vein. Here the pressurised jet stream of reflux through the separated valve leaflets can be seen more clearly than in colour mode because colour overlaps are avoided (see also Fig. 7.6).

12.4.1 Preoperative Duplex Ultrasound

The main questions necessary to assess treatment suitability are as follows:

1. Are the leaflets of the terminal valve and the first subterminal valve visible and mobile?
2. Is the maximum diameter of the saphenofemoral junction less than 10 mm in women or 12 mm in men?
3. Can degenerative changes in the trunk section of the vein be excluded, for example, post-thrombotic changes, marked tortuosity or aneurysmal dilatation?

If the answers to all three questions are positive, then the patient is suitable for an extraluminal valvuloplasty from an ultrasound perspective.

12.4.2 Intra-operative Checking of Venous Valve Functioning

Venous valve function is normally checked intra-operatively by testing whether a collapsed great saphenous vein demonstrates retrograde filling during a Valsalva manoeuvre. This check can also be carried out using a 5–10 MHz transducer covered with ultrasound gel and placed in a sterile plastic cover. The probe is placed against the inner side of the thigh, and the flow in the great saphenous vein is measured during the Valsalva manoeuvre. If the patient is under a general anaesthetic, pressure over the abdomen or hyper-insufflation of the lungs by the anaesthetist can substitute as a Valsalva manoeuvre.

If the valvuloplasty is correctly performed, there should be no reflux.

12.5 Ultrasound-Guided Foam Sclerotherapy

According to the recommendations of the 1st and 2nd European Consensus Meeting on Foam Sclerotherapy at Tegernsee, the use of duplex ultrasound is expressly recommended during puncture and foam injection in the sclerotherapy of saphenous veins, perforating veins and veins in or close to the groin or the popliteal region, as well as in recurrent varices (Breu et al. 2008). Apart from the ultrasound-guided sclerotherapy procedure itself, duplex ultrasound has a firmly established role in pre-sclerotherapy diagnosis, monitoring therapy and in follow-up. It can be used for:

1. Locating invisible incompetent veins, such as the great saphenous vein in the thigh
2. Determining the best puncture point

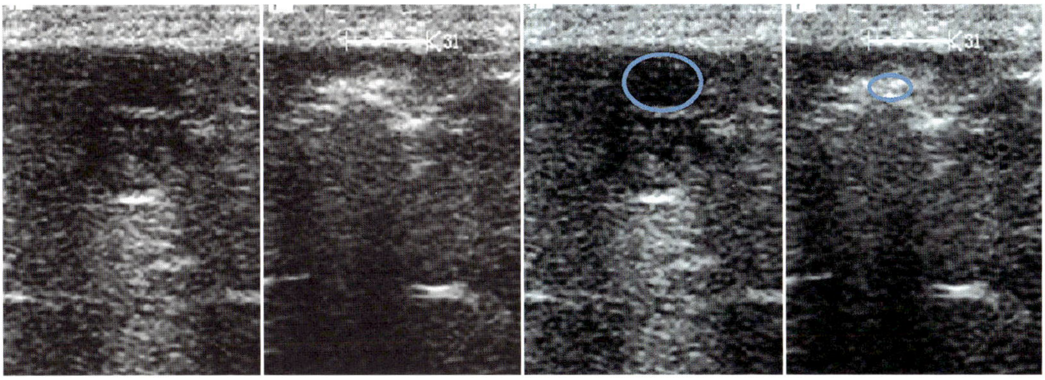

Fig. 12.10 Transverse view through the front of the thigh demonstrating the anterior accessory saphenous vein (*blue ring*): left with no foam and a poor acoustic shadow and right with echo-rich foam and a strong acoustic shadow. Sclerosing foam is seen spreading along a vein (see accompanying online material) Copyright: [Author]

3. Distinguishing veins from neighbouring arteries
4. Determining the depth of the vein in order to select the right length cannula or Braun catheter
5. Procedural visualisation of the point of the cannula or catheter
6. Procedural visualisation of the luminal spread of migrating foam
7. Advancing the foam cannula into the area to be treated
8. Recognising vasospasm
9. Documentation of the details of the sclerotherapy procedure

12.5.1 Ultrasound Imaging of Foam in Veins

The strong echogenesis provoked by gas in human tissue leads to an echo-rich delineation of foam from adjacent structures. Foam strongly reflects ultrasound waves and produces a characteristic acoustic shadow. A B-scan of a vein demonstrates poor or non-existent echoes from the intraluminal structures and a poor acoustic shadow. In contrast, foam is echo-rich, with a prominent acoustic shadow (Fig. 12.10).

It should be noted that the layer of foam bubbles closest to the probe, which rise to the surface in a horizontal vein, will also cause echogenic effects, even if the vein is not completely filled with foam. If the layer of floating foam on the surface is only thin or discontinuous, or the foam is mixed with the blood in the form of individual bubbles, the echo-richness of the foam is diminished resulting in a weakening of the acoustic shadow. This is because there is a reduced reflection off the gas (Fig. 12.11). In this case, the foam appears as a heterogeneous echo-generating structural mass, with only a few, scattered, ultrasound shadows. Even days or weeks after treatment, occasional enclaves of gas are found in the newly formed sclerothrombus, visualised as echo-rich structures.

The strong ultrasound reflection off the gas boundary surfaces means that colour-coded imaging of blood flow is no longer possible. On the other hand, because sclerosing foam is also a contrast medium, it can be used to mark the course of the vessels. This is useful because the site of action and the extent of spread of foam can both be visualised making foam travel more or less controllable by the operator.

Foam echogenicity is dependent on its structure (Foam property; Fig. 12.10). Foam consisting of large bubbles is "thinner" and produces fewer echoes than firmer foam with smaller bubbles which is more compact and stiffer. Foam produced according to the Montreux method generates large bubbles in contrast to microfoam with smaller bubbles. Small-bubbled foam is also known as "dry" foam and can be produced according to Tessari's method or modified from Wollmann's produced foam (Breu et al. 2008; Wollmann 2002 in Appendix 2).

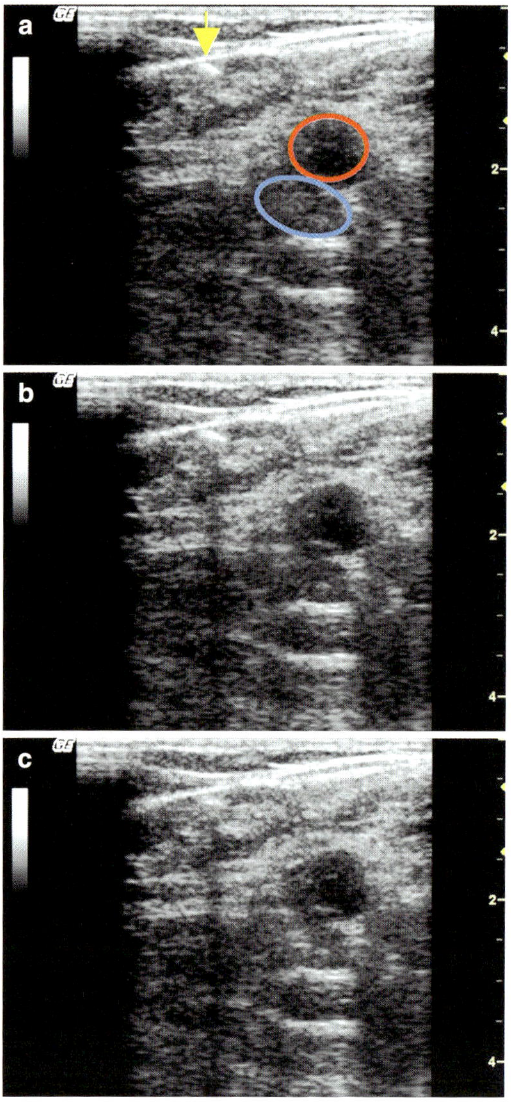

Fig. 12.11 Transverse view through the groin. Sclerosant foam is seen mixed with blood in the common femoral vein 10 (**a**), 20 (**b**) and 30 s (**c**) after injection into the anterior accessory saphenous vein (*arrow*) Common femoral vein: *blue circle*, common femoral artery: *red circle*. (see online material) Copyright: [Author]

12.5.2 Ultrasound Puncture Control in Sclerotherapy

With deep-lying epifascial and transfascial veins, selecting the best puncture point is only possible using ultrasound. The first objective of sclerotherapy in most cases is to "seal" the proximal insufficiency point, which is identified during

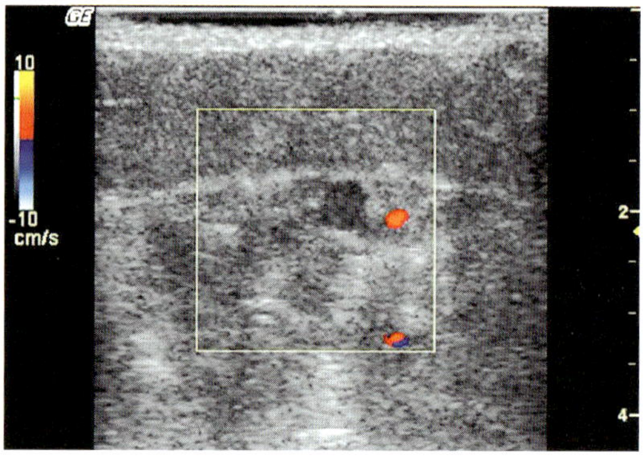

Fig. 12.12 Transverse view through the back of the calf below the popliteal region. An artery is seen immediately adjacent to the small saphenous vein (see accompanying online material) Copyright: [Author]

pretreatment mapping and confirmed immediately before the first injection.

The special value of duplex ultrasound is its ability to distinguish adjacent arterial vessels which must not be inadvertently punctured. The course of the small saphenous vein, in particular, is intimately related to accompanying arteries (Fig. 12.12).

The length of the introducer needle is selected according to the travel distance. This is the measured distance to the deepest part of the vein, i.e. the vein wall furthest from the probe to the skin surface. Using the needle technique, it has been found that the needle length selected should be only 5 mm longer than the travel distance. This procedure prevents the risk of overshoot by crossing the walls of the vein with the needle (Partsch 2004 in Appendix 2) (Fig. 12.13).

The technique of vein puncture with a needle and cannula is best seen using B-scan ultrasound. This is ideal for varices and refluxing veins which are not visible to the naked eye and can be felt only with difficulty or not at all. This is normally the case with an incompetent great saphenous vein or small saphenous vein. The metal of the introducer needle and the plastic cannula both produce strong echoes comparable to bone. When the vein of a lying patient is cannulated, the probe is placed on the skin lengthwise or at right angles to the course of the vein, with the lumen of the vein positioned exactly in the middle of the ultrasound field. The cannula or Braun catheter is inserted at an angle of between 45°

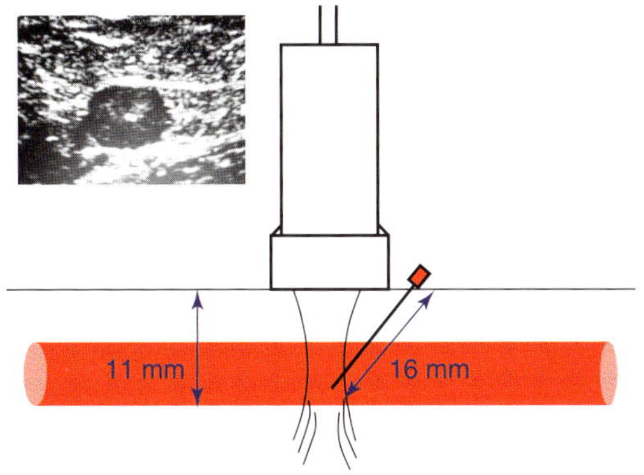

Fig. 12.13 Principle of ultrasound-guided vein puncture. The ultrasound image shows a transverse view of the great saphenous vein with a needle correctly positioned within the vein lumen (Bernhard Partsch, Vienna; by kind permission) Copyright: Bernhard Partsch, Vienna

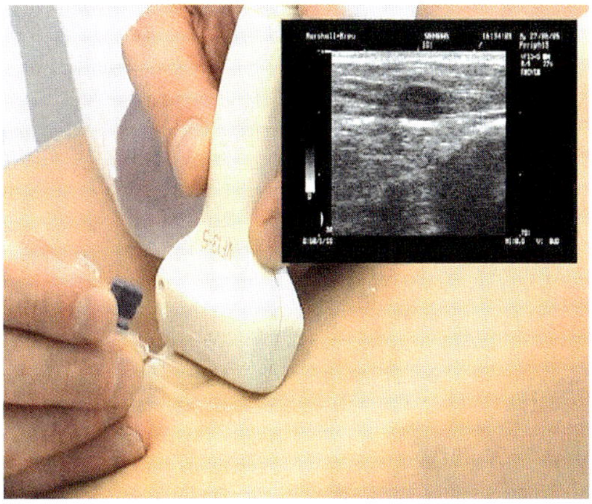

Fig. 12.14 Transducer position during great saphenous vein puncture with a Braun catheter. The needle has been partially withdrawn and is not seen in the image Copyright: [Author]

and 60° to the skin surface, exactly next to the centre of the transducer (Fig. 12.14).

The author prefers to have the vein shown in transverse view because of the advantages this offers in guiding and correcting the line of insertion if the vessel yields slightly. The direction of insertion, proximal or distal, and the insertion point, proximal or distal from the probe, are optional. A left-handed operator will probably prefer to hold the probe in the right hand and the cannula in the left.

The actual puncture should be done slowly, so as to monitor the advance of the point of the cannula through the tissue, since it produces a strong echo. Depending on the quality and calibration of the equipment, thinner needles are more difficult or sometimes impossible to see in B-scan. Therefore "thicker" needles or Braun catheters are preferred for ultrasound-guided punctures (e.g. 21G needles) (Partsch 2004 in Appendix 2). As the point of the needle reaches the vein, a dent can be seen on the vein wall closest to the probe. The dent should be symmetrical and should exactly overlie the vessel axis. If the dent is eccentric, either lateral or medial, it is necessary to withdraw the cannula slightly and correct the line of insertion. If the line of insertion hits the vein axis exactly the vessel wall nearest to the probe reassumes its normal position once the point of the cannula has penetrated the lumen (Fig. 12.13). With the open needle technique, blood appears in the cannula base. With the closed needle technique, blood can be aspirated to confirm successful access. In the author's experience, short catheters (Braun catheters) sit more firmly in the vein than cannulas which can be easily dislodged by slight movements of the leg or subsequent injections. Learning ultrasound-guided vein puncturing on a dummy, as we practise in our sclerotherapy seminars, has proved successful.

A high-definition probe should be used to control the puncturing process, although a 7.5–13 MHz transducer is ideal, monitoring can also be done with a 5 MHz probe. A tilt bed having the patient lying at a slight angle during puncture results in better venous filling. The veins are clearly seen in the image and easier to puncture.

In techniques using long-line catheters, as carried out by some work groups, the point of the catheter can also be clearly seen in the ultrasound image, allowing it to be positioned in the proximal great saphenous vein or small saphenous vein.

12.5.3 Ultrasound Monitoring of Foam Travel and Spread

The ultrasound image allows the operator to observe and control the spread of the sclerosing foam in the vein segment to be treated (Fig. 12.15, see also Fig. 12.11). It is of primary significance to note which part of the vessel contains the

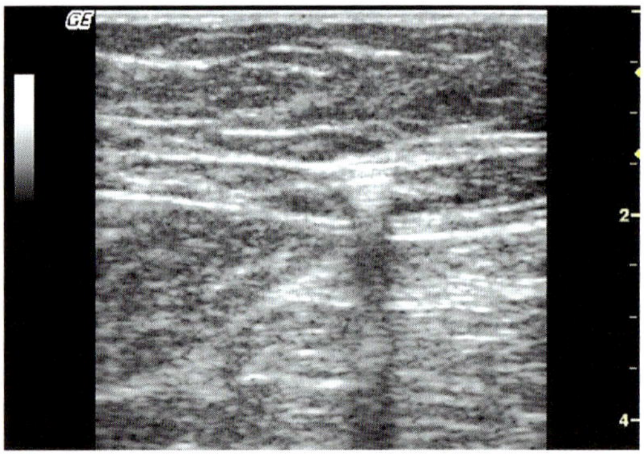

Fig. 12.15 Transverse view through the inner thigh showing the initial spreading of foam within the great saphenous vein (see accompanying online material) Copyright: [Author]

greatest concentration of foam and into which regions the foam spreads spontaneously. The foam column can be steered into neighbouring regions by skin manipulation or by altering the patient's position because foam floats in blood and tends to travel against gravity. In the same way it could be shown that foam travels with blood and is found in the right atrium seconds after injection in the leg. As sclerosing agents are inactivated seconds after getting in contact with blood collateral damage is prevented.

The injection of a small quantity of foam immediately after the vein is punctured is a wise first move because it allows the correct position of the cannula to be confirmed by ultrasound before the therapeutic foam is injected. It may also be checked with saline or aspiration prior to foam application if there remains a doubt. If the cannula is outside the vein, this is identified immediately because intraluminal spreading does not occur (Fig. 12.15).

The total volume of foam can also be administered in sequential doses with continuous or repeated ultrasound monitoring. The appropriate volume of foam can be determined by ultrasound observation of the early reaction of the vessel (Sect. 12.5.4). Some work groups use ultrasound monitoring of the spreading of the foam to determine the moment for compression of transfascial connections and especially the confluence of the great saphenous vein. Compression with the probe or by hand should prevent the foam from spreading into the deep vein system too early or in excessive volume (Wildenhues 2005 in Appendix 2). If a long catheter is used, the great saphenous vein confluence can be blocked with a balloon and this can also be controlled by ultrasound. In the light of recent research, blocking of the great saphenous vein confluence is no longer recommended, since when the block is removed, the sudden release of too large a bolus of foam into the pelvic vein may produce side effects, which should be avoided. The recommended practice today is to obtain a slow, continuous flow of foam rather than to precipitate any bolus displacements into deep veins which may occur after release of any compression or occlusion techniques (Hill 2008). Aspiration of the foam through the catheter can also be monitored by ultrasound.

12.5.4 Ultrasound Evaluation of the Sclerosant Reaction

The first sclerosant reaction which can be seen in the ultrasound image is venospasm. This normally occurs within 10–30 s after foam injection, although in some cases it is only seen after several minutes (Fig. 12.16). There is no consensus as to whether the magnitude of the venospasm correlates with the quality of the sclerosing foam (Hamel-Desnos 2003). Usually, the venospasm is so intense that it compresses the foam column causing an even spread along the incompetent vein segment.

One day later, a poor to moderate echo-generating sclerothrombus can usually be seen which may still contain echo-rich gas bubbles. The vein wall becomes oedematous, typical of fresh thrombus, with fluid separation of the wall structures (Fig. 12.17). At this stage the vessel

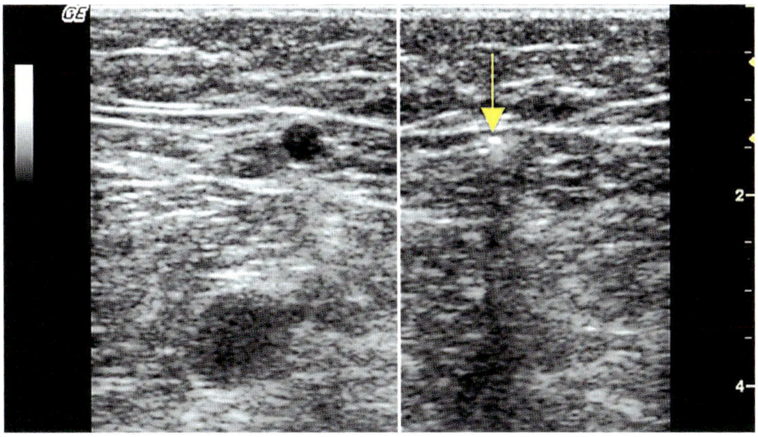

Fig. 12.16 Vasospasm in a great saphenous vein: left before injection of the sclerosing foam and right one minute afterwards (*arrow*). The ultrasound shadow is caused by the sclerosing foam Copyright: [Author]

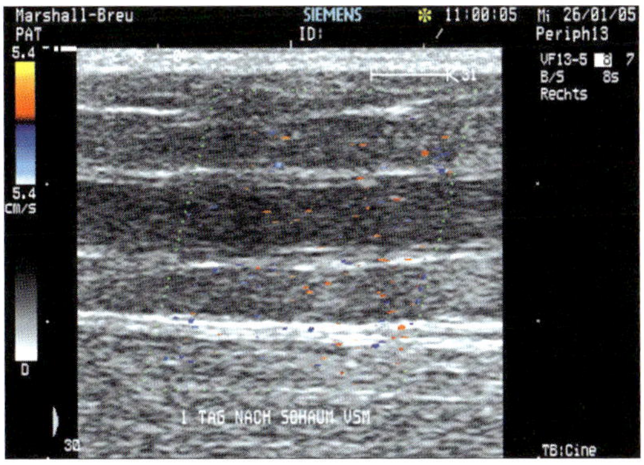

Fig. 12.17 Longitudinal view of the inner thigh showing the great saphenous vein 1 day after sclerotherapy. The vein wall appears oedematous demonstrating a double echo-generating outline. There is no flow in the lumen Copyright: [Author]

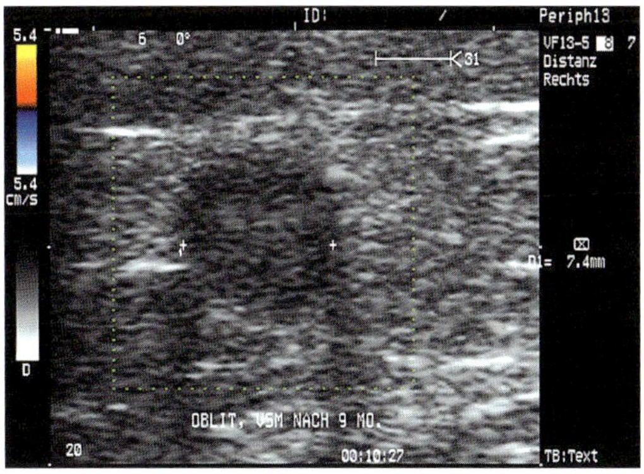

Fig. 12.18 Transverse view through the inner thigh showing the great saphenous vein 9 months after sclerotherapy. There is no blood flow in the great saphenous vein, the vein is no longer compressible and the vein wall cannot be seen. This vein has been successfully ablated Copyright: [Author]

still has a residual degree of compressibility. It can be compressed with the probe by about 30 %. After 4–6 weeks the proximal end of the sclerothrombus can be evaluated and documented. This is important for long-term prognosis and in indicating whether further treatments are necessary (Figs. 12.18 and 12.19).

Efficiency criteria

Reflux phenomena in patent tributaries no longer appear as varices after sclerotherapy of the trunk veins and can only be detected using ultrasound. These should be imaged and evaluated as they are important for planning further treatment. Incomplete sclerosis with partial vein closure, either lengthwise or transversely, or rapid recanalisation can be detected early with ultrasound (Fig. 12.20). Other ultrasound criteria for treatment efficiency after obliteration include calibre reduction of the target vein, absent reflux and possibly antegrade flow (Breu et al. 2008; Lattimer et al 2012). Ideally, a fibrous, heavily echogenic segment should be found as a later reaction after 1 year, which is difficult to distinguish from surrounding structures (Fig. 12.18).

12.5.5 Ultrasound Diagnosis of Complications in Sclerotherapy

The most important question which can be answered by ultrasound in the context of sclerotherapy is the diagnosis of thrombosis, which

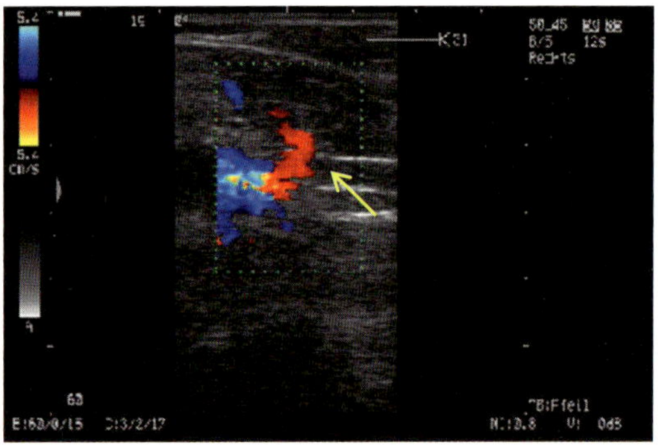

Fig. 12.19 Longitudinal view through the great saphenous vein confluence one day after sclerotherapy. This demonstrates ideal treatment with the proximal end of the sclerothrombus distal to the confluence of the superficial epigastric vein. The great saphenous vein (*arrow*) is closed and the fascia demonstrates a strong echo reflection (for a case of thrombus extending into the deep leg vein, see accompanying online material) Copyright: [Author]

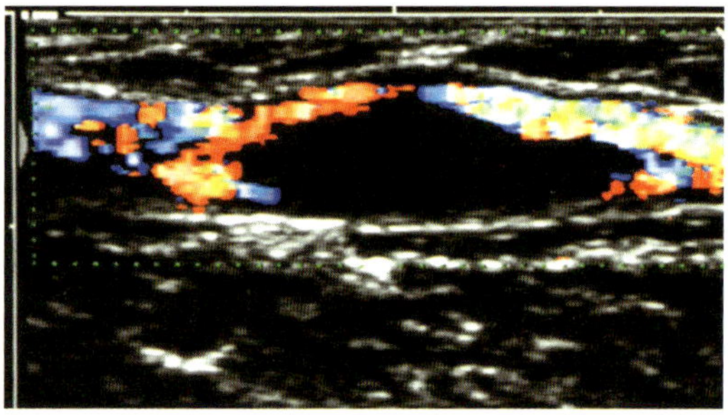

Fig. 12.20 Longitudinal view of the back of the calf. The small saphenous vein has recanalised and with only partial sclerosis Copyright: [Author]

occurs very occasionally in the deep and muscle veins. After the application of sclerosing foam, we have occasionally seen thrombosis of the calf muscle veins and very occasionally thrombosis of the deep veins (Fig. 14.12, online material). All the same ultrasound criteria applicable to fresh vein thrombosis must be observed in such cases (Chap. 14).

Possible thrombus extension into the deep veins must be detected early by frequent monitoring. The same ultrasound criteria are applicable in the case of thromboses which develop independently of the sclerosis reaction and may present a threat of propagation or ascension. In case of sclerotherapy of the great saphenous vein, a sclerothrombus up to the saphenofemoral junction is desired and progression into deep veins should be excluded by ultrasound or treated with immediate anticoagulation. In case of sclerotherapy of tributaries, an ascending thrombosis in great saphenous vein may occur. This should be diagnosed and treated as described in Chap. 11 (Fig. 11.5). Foam extravasation appears as an irregular-shaped, echo-rich structure with a broad acoustic shadow outside the vein. Haematomas look like sharp or ill-defined regions of an echo-poor mass in the subcutaneous tissues (Fig. 17.13a). Posttreatment lymphoedema is a secondary lymphoedema which can be recognised by a thickening of the subcutaneous region with typical echo-free gaps that cannot be compressed with the probe (Chap. 16).

12.5.6 Foam Sclerotherapy with Tumescence

This is a technique designed to improve the efficacy of foam sclerotherapy by surrounding the saphenous trunk with fluid. This tumescence is performed in exactly the same way as for endovenous laser ablation or radiofrequency ablation, but local anaesthesia is not required. The objective is to compress the saphenous vein internally (peri-venous) so that its calibre is reduced and less blood remains in the lumen. Long-line catheters are used to ensure foam delivery at the intended site of action. They also discourage flow and promote venospasm further reducing the required foam volume. Once an initial bolus is received into the upper part of the great saphenous vein, the remaining foam is deployed along the length of the catheter as it is withdrawn (Thibault 2005) (Fig. 12.21a, b).

12.6 Ultrasound of Veins in the Assessment of a Bypass Conduit

Veins are frequently used as a bypass material in patients with coronary heart disease or arterial occlusive disease. Since the introduction

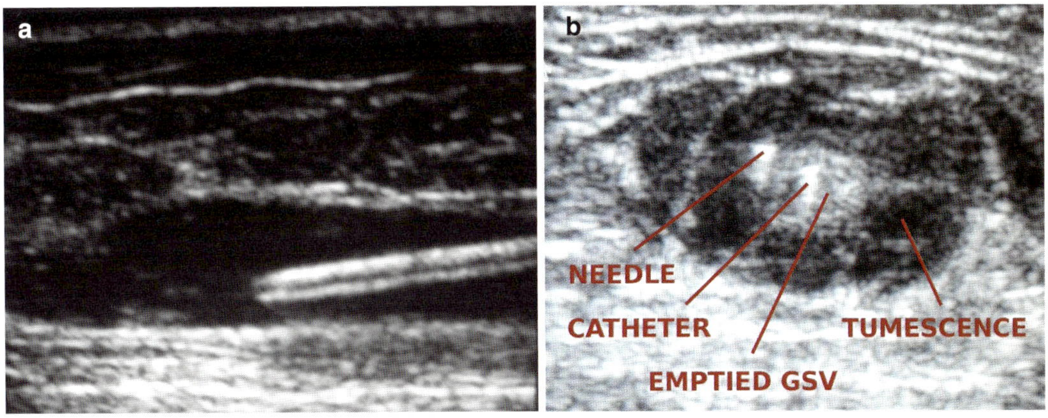

Fig 12.21 (**a**) Longitudinal view of the upper thigh. A long-line catheter is seen within the great saphenous vein, before tumescence the foam is injected. (**b**) Transverse view of the mid-thigh. The tumescence needle, intravenous catheter and peri-venous fluid are seen causing internal peri-venous compression of the great saphenous vein prior to foam injection

of ultrasound, it has been possible to check the quality of a vein conduit by ultrasound prior to harvest.

Their special morphology, with a strong muscular sheath, makes trunk veins particularly suitable for use as a bypass material. They have to be identified by ultrasound throughout their course in the saphenous compartment (Sects. 2.4.2 and 7.4.1). The great saphenous vein is the only leg vein to present an increasing accumulation of muscle cells in the media of the wall from the foot to the groin. The vein in the calf is therefore ideal for artery replacement.

Veins planned for use as bypass material should not demonstrate any calcification or postphlebitic alterations in their wall (Chap. 11), nor should they be fibrotic which may occur after trauma or an operation (Sect. 13.4.4). If the great saphenous vein is hypoplastic in its part, the epifascial accessory branch may be used, but it is a second choice because the wall does not have as many muscle cells in the media. Saphenous, basilic or cephalic veins less than 3 mm in diameter in the standing patient are not ideal as an arterial bypass conduit.

The small saphenous vein can also be used as a bypass material. However, for technical reasons, simultaneous excision during cardiac or arterial dissection is often very cumbersome and therefore rarely performed.

However, despite the above, veins which have previously been refluxive and now have a reduced calibre as the result of previous surgery have all been used successfully as a bypass material in coronary and peripheral arterial surgery (J. Juan, Barcelona, verbal communication 2009).

12.7 Ultrasound Monitoring of Compression Therapy

Ultrasound can also be used to examine veins through a compression stocking and even demonstrate flow signals. The stocking must first be thoroughly saturated with ultrasound gel to prevent the presence of air bubbles impeding the propagation of sound. Although the image appears to be seen through a grey veil, most structures can still be recognised (Fig. 12.22). Indications for ultrasound in these conditions usually relate to studies on the use of compression. Occasionally, ultrasound can be used in this way to convince patients of the effectiveness of their stocking.

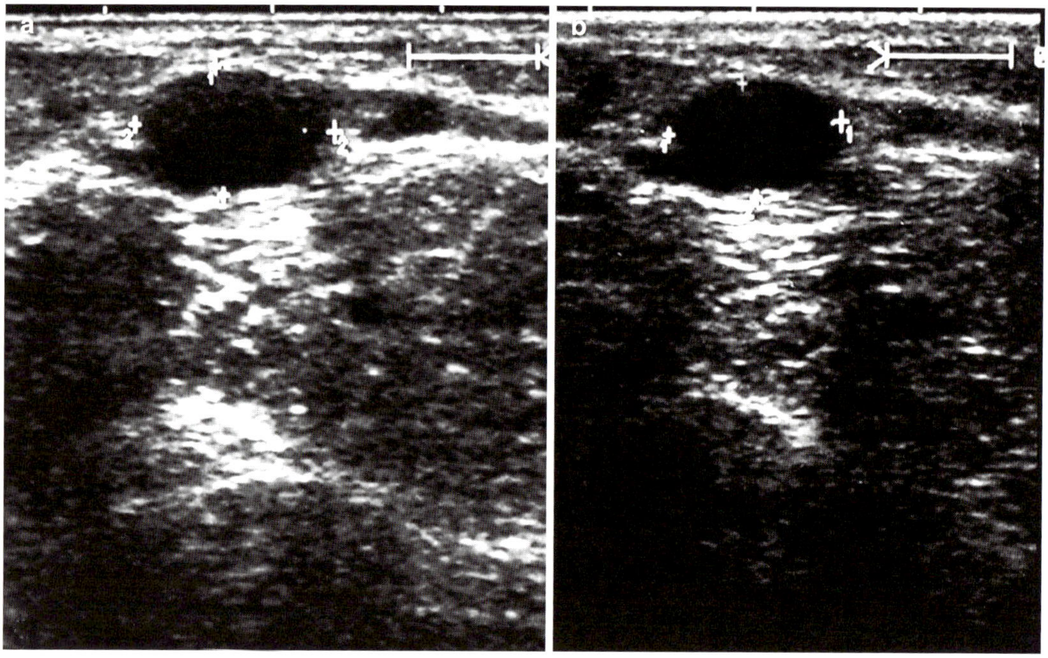

Fig. 12.22 Transverse view through the back of the calf in a standing patient with incompetence of the small saphenous vein: (**a**) without a compression stocking, (**b**) wearing a compression stocking. The diameter measurements without compression are 11.8 mm horizontal (*2*) and 7.4 mm vertical (*1*). Wearing compression they are 9.6 mm horizontal (*1*) and 5.8 mm vertical (*2*) Copyright: [Author]

References

Almeida JI, Min RJ, Raabe R, McLean DJ, Madsen M (2011) Cyanoacrylate adhesive for the closure of truncal veins: 60-day swine model results. Vasc Endovascular Surg 45:631–635

Breu FX, Guggenbichler S, Wollmann JC (2008) 2nd European Consensus Meeting on foam sclerotherapy 2006, Tegernsee, Germany. Vasa 37(Suppl 71):1–29

Coleridge-Smith P, Labropoulos N, Partsch H, Myers K, Nicolaides A, Cavezzi A (2006) Duplex ultrasound investigation of the veins in chronic venous disease of the lower limbs-UIP consensus document, Part I. Basic Principles. Eur J Vasc Endovasc Surg 31:1–10

Elias S, Raines JK (2012) Mechanochemical tumescentless endovenous ablation: final results of the initial clinical trial. Phlebology 27:67–72

Hamel-Desnos C (2003) Evaluation of the efficacy of polidocanol in the form of foam compared with liquid form in sclerotherapy of the greater saphenous vein. Dermatol Surg 29:1170

Hill D, Hamilton R, Fung T (2008) Assessment of techniques to reduce sclerosant foam migration during ultrasound-guided sclerotherapy of the great saphenous vein. Journal of Vascular Surgery 48(4): 934–939

Lattimer CR, Azzam M, Kalodiki E, Shawish E, Trueman P, Geroulakos G (2012) Cost and effectiveness of laser with phlebectomies compared with foam sclerotherapy in superficial venous insufficiency. Early results of a randomised controlled trial. Eur J Vasc Endovasc Surg 43:594–600

Nicolaides AN (2000) Investigation of chronic venous insufficiency – a consensus statement. Circulation 102:126–163

Prince EA, Soares GM, Silva M, Taner A, Ahn S, Dubel GJ, Jay BS (2011) Impact of laser fiber design on outcome of endovenous ablation of lower-extremity varicose veins: results from a single practice. Cardiovasc Intervent Radiol 34:536–541

Proebstle TM, Alm J, Göckeritz O, Wenzel C, Noppeney T, Lebard C, Pichot O, Sessa C, Creton D, European Closure Fast Clinical Study Group (2011) Three-year European follow-up of endovenous radiofrequency-powered segmental thermal ablation of the great saphenous vein with or without treatment of calf varicosities. J Vasc Surg 54:146–152

Ricci S, Caggiati A (1999) Echoanatomical patterns of the long saphenous vein in patients with primary varices and in healthy subjects. Phlebology 14:54–58

Schwarz T, von Hodenberg E, Furtwängler C, Rastan A, Zeller T, Neumann FJ (2010) Endovenous laser ablation of varicose veins with the 1470-nm diode laser. J Vasc Surg 51:1474–1478

Thibault P (2005) Internal compression (peri-venous) following ultrasound guided sclerotherapy to the great and small saphenous veins. Aust NZ J Phlebol 9:29–32

Yamaki T, Nozaki M, Sasaki K (2002) Alternative greater saphenous vein-sparing surgery: valvuloplasty combined with axial transposition of a competent tributary vein for the treatment of primary valvular incompetence – 18-month follow-up. Dermatol Surg 28:162–167

Ultrasound After Venous Intervention

13

Erika Mendoza, Achim Mumme,
Andreas Hildebrandt, Nick Morrison,
and Christopher R. Lattimer

Chapter Summary
Ultrasound is indispensible for checking success and detecting complications during and immediately after intervention. These changes after endoluminal procedures, foam sclerotherapy and stripping have already been described in Sects. 12.3 and 12.4. This chapter discusses complications, follow-up and nature of recurrences using duplex ultrasound with pertinent points on documentation.

E. Mendoza, MD, PhD (✉)
Venenpraxis Wunstorf, Speckenstraße 10,
31515 Wunstorf, Germany
e-mail: erika.mendoza@t-online.de

A. Mumme, MD, PhD
Klinik für Gefäßchirurgie, St. Josef-Hospital,
Universitätsklinikum, Gudrunstraße 56,
44791 Bochum, Germany
e-mail: Achim.Mumme@ruhr-uni-bochum.de

A. Hildebrandt, MD
Ullsteinhausklinik GmbH,
Mariendorfer Damm 3, 12099 Berlin, Germany
e-mail: ahildebrandt1@me.com

N. Morrison, MD
Morrison Vein Institute,
Suite 223, 8575 E. Princess Dr., Scottsdale, AZ, USA

C.R. Lattimer, MD, PhD
Department of Vascular Surgery,
Josef Pflug Vascular Laboratory,
Ealing Hospital and Imperial College, London, UK

13.1 Ultrasound of Complications

Early post-operative complications can be identified by ultrasound if the clinical picture suggests their presence. Swelling under the skin may be caused by **bruising** (violet-blue skin colour), a lymphatic fistula (clear discharge from the wound) or an **abscess** (inflammation, reddening). Ultrasound is useful for assessing the extent and size of a collection over time. If there is bruising ultrasound can differentiate between diffuse bruising and the presence of a collection, (Fig. 17.13a), circumscribed accumulations of blood of different echogenicity (Fig. 17.13b) and lymphatic collections and fistulae (Fig. 17.13c).

Injuries to the peroneal nerve in the popliteal region are difficult to see in cicatrised tissue (Sect. 17.6); however, an experienced user can detect them (Kaps et al. 2004).

Ultrasound of superficial vein thrombosis (phlebitis) is described in Chaps. 11 and 14.

13.2 Post-operative Scar Tissue

Fresh scar tissue appears as a homogeneous area with a relatively strong echo. The very echo-rich connective tissue septa can no longer be distinguished from the echo-poor fatty tissue. If a fascia is opened, it becomes less echogenic until it is replaced by homogeneous scar tissue (Fig. 13.1).

Recurrences can be detected early in scar tissue (de Maeseneer et al. 2005). It is therefore important to examine this tissue using colour duplex ultrasound (Fig. 13.2).

E. Mendoza et al. (eds.), *Duplex Ultrasound of Superficial Leg Veins*,
DOI 10.1007/978-3-642-40731-4_13, © Springer-Verlag Berlin Heidelberg 2014

After a time, which may vary between 2 and 6 months in different patients, the original configuration of connective tissue is re-established. In this case this can only be recognised at the site of an operation if non-resorbable sutures or clips were used (Fig. 13.3a). Either an acoustic shadow is identified or the suture material is recognised directly as an echo-generating structure (Figs. 13.3b, d).

Documentation of the scar at early follow-up serves as proof that the target structure has been treated. This is relevant for CHIVA since with saphenous conservation treatments in the event of recurrence, the suspicion might arise that the vein was never touched (see below).

13.3 Post-intervention Follow-Up

13.3.1 Ultrasound After Stripping

In check-up examinations weeks to months after saphenous stripping, the following should be assessed and documented:

- Operation at the junctions:
  - Is there a stump of great saphenous vein after an incomplete flush ligation (Figs. 13.4 and 13.8d)?
- Is there neovascularisation with reflux from deep veins (Fig. 13.2)?
  - Are there refluxive sapheno-femoral venous tributaries which form a tangle in the groin without necessarily bringing reflux from the deep leg veins? Later, these might reconnect and come into contact with refluxive epifascial veins.
  - Has the fascia in the popliteal fossa been closed?
- Removal of the vein along its course:
  - Has the saphenous vein been removed between the intervening scars?
  - Is there a remaining vein within the fascial compartment or is the fascial eye empty (Fig. 13.1c)?
- Interruption of perforating veins:
  - Are the formerly incompetent perforating veins still visible in the image?
  - Has any flow within these areas been documented using colour duplex?
- Venous tributaries (treated or not):
  - Are areas of thrombosis found in the remaining venous tributaries (Chap. 11)?
  - Has any flow at the avulsion sites been documented using colour duplex?

13.3.2 Ultrasound After CHIVA

An ultrasound check-up examination is indispensable 6–12 weeks after CHIVA treatment since up to 20 % of patients require a supplementary operation before the treatment can be considered closed. This decision is based on clinical and ultrasound evidence.

Saphenous vein **flow and diameter** are documented and compared to their pre-operative findings. After ligation of the sapheno-femoral junction, there is a short-term retrograde flow during calf diastole (Fig. 13.5a). This is caused by drainage of the venous tributaries via the saphenous trunk and then into the deep veins

Fig. 13.1 Scar tissue. (**a**) Transverse view through the calf 6 weeks after interruption of a venous tributary of the small saphenous vein (CHIVA 2). *Left*, proximal to the scar; *right*, at the level of the scar. It is obvious that the fascia has been opened and the saphenous fascia is not visible. The "scar cloud" (*arrow*) reaches the small saphenous vein where the muscle fascia was not opened. (**b**) Transverse view through the inner thigh 8 weeks after ligation of a venous tributary of the great saphenous vein. *Left* above, *right* at the level of the scar where the saphenous fascia is interrupted, but the muscle fascia remains intact. (**c**) Transverse view through the calf 2 months after stripping of the small saphenous vein up to the interrupted soleus perforating vein (formerly May). *Left*, empty fascial eye above the scar; *centre*, scar tissue where both fascias were opened; *right*, small saphenous vein in the fascial compartment distal from the scar. (**d**) Four months after stripping of the great saphenous vein. Transverse view through the inner thigh at a skin scar. *Left* slightly above; *middle* slightly below; *right* at the scar. *Left*, an echo-generating region with a weakened acoustic shadow visible in the intact fascial compartment which may correspond to a suture; *middle*, distal to the scar the remaining small saphenous vein can be seen in its compartment; *right*, shows how the scar tissue slowly degenerates and no longer generates as strong an echo as in (**a–c**) and the recovering connective tissue septa within the region of the scar (*MV*, muscle vein) Copyright: [Author]

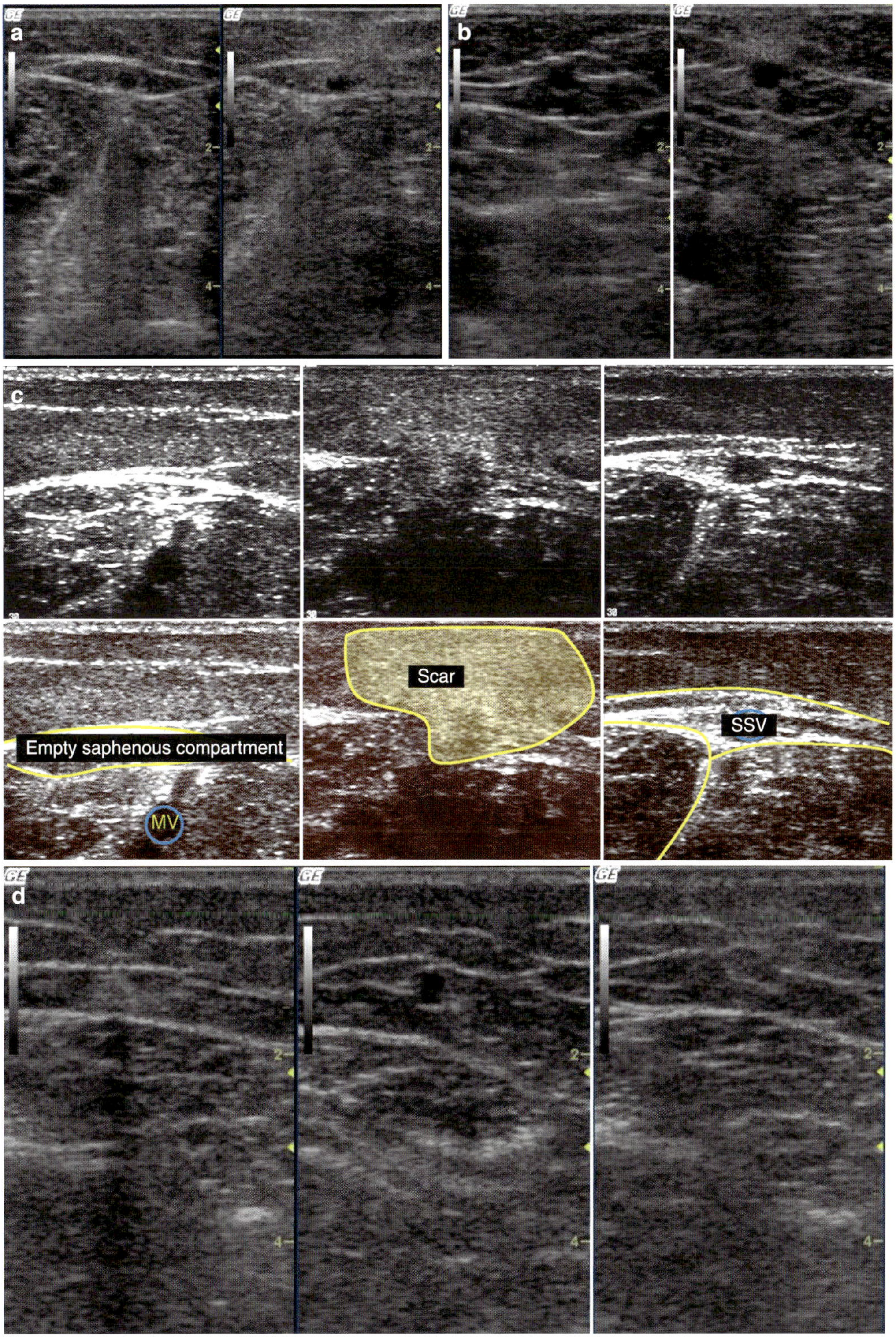
a
b
c
Empty saphenous compartment
MV
Scar
SSV
d

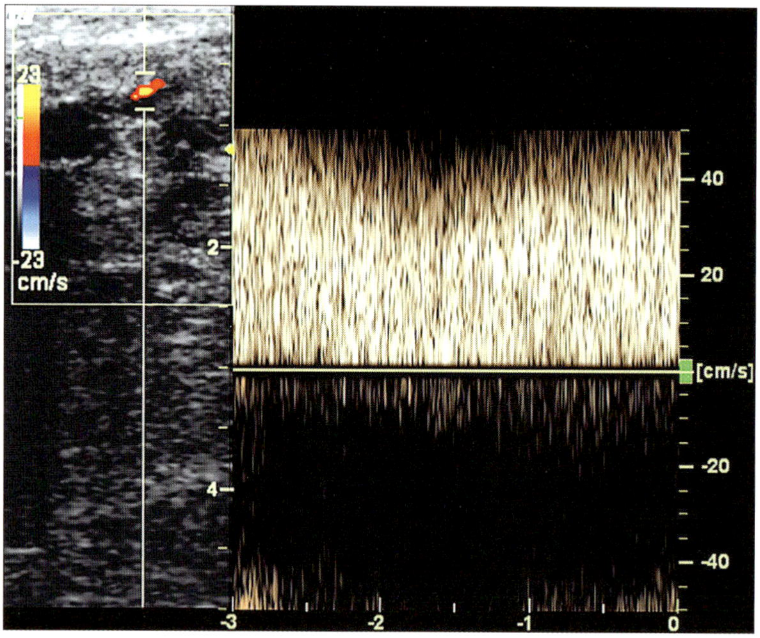

Fig. 13.2 Reflux from a sapheno-femoral junction venous tributary 2 months after crossectomy and stripping of the great saphenous vein in a 45-year-old man. He suffered with pains in the groin region with the appearance of new reticular varices in the outer thigh. A very small sapheno-femoral junction venous tributary is seen with high-velocity reflux in the region of the scar. This fills the anterior accessory saphenous vein which is dilated with very slow flow (see accompanying online material) Copyright: [Author]

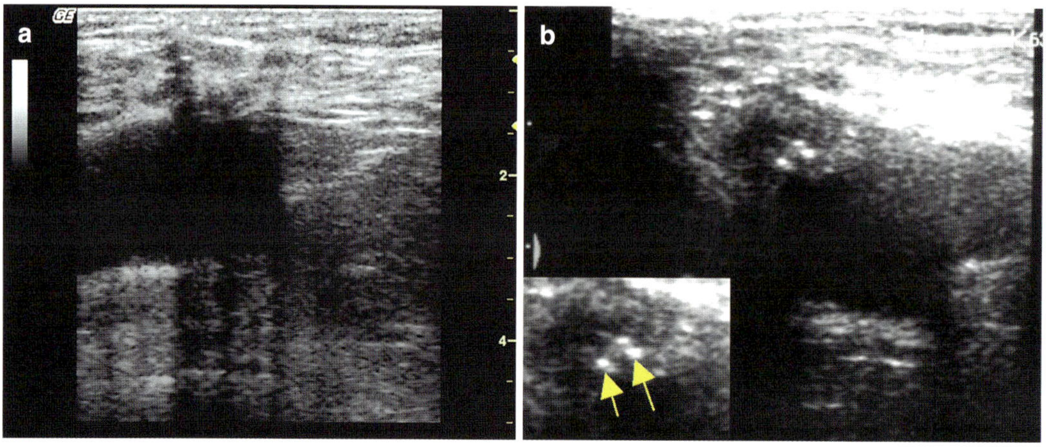

Fig. 13.3 (**a**) Longitudinal view through the groin 3 years after crossectomy showing the femoral vein and the completely re-established subcutaneous connecting tissue structures. Suture material can be identified indirectly by the resulting acoustic shadow. (**b**) Transverse view through the left groin 2 years after ligation of the sapheno-femoral junction which is magnified in the lower image. The non-resorbable suture can be recognised as two white points indicated by *arrows*. Suture material can obscure the colour signal with their sound shadow (see accompanying online material) Copyright: [Author]

through a distal perforating vein. After CHIVA 2 antegrade flow can be measured during calf systole (Fig. 13.5b). In cases of persisting great saphenous vein reflux, retrograde flow may be similar to or less than that documented prior to the operation. In this case a new perforating vein

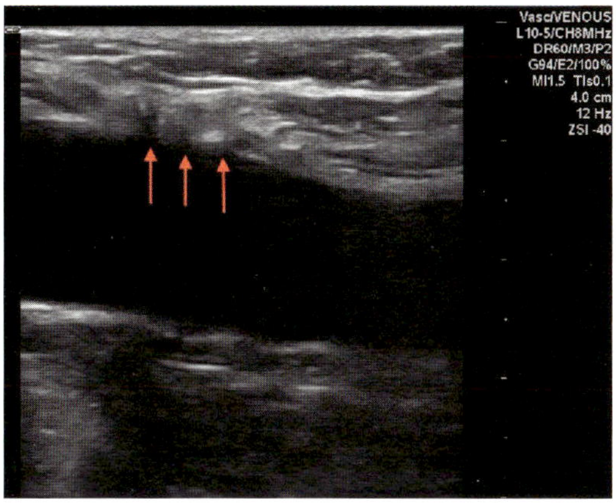

Fig. 13.4 Ultrasound of the sapheno-femoral junction after stripping. Longitudinal view through the groin showing the common femoral vein with the interruption point (*arrowed*) in the front wall. The front wall of the vein is smooth indicating a flush ligation (online material: image with flow) Copyright: [Author]

or venous tributary re-entry point must be found, and treatment of the sapheno-femoral junction may be indicated.

In general, venous tributaries and saphenous veins must be examined for superficial thrombosis. Although this is usually asymptomatic after CHIVA, it delays the volume reduction in the tributaries. That means possible discomfort and a longer time until the final cosmetic result is achieved.

After ligation or crossectomy of the sapheno-femoral junction, post-operative flow in the groin must be monitored with special care and the absence or presence of a stump must be clarified (Fig. 13.6). The problem of a refluxing venous tributary at the sapheno-femoral junction which was not identified pre-operatively has already been discussed in Sect. 12.2 (Fig. 13.6b).

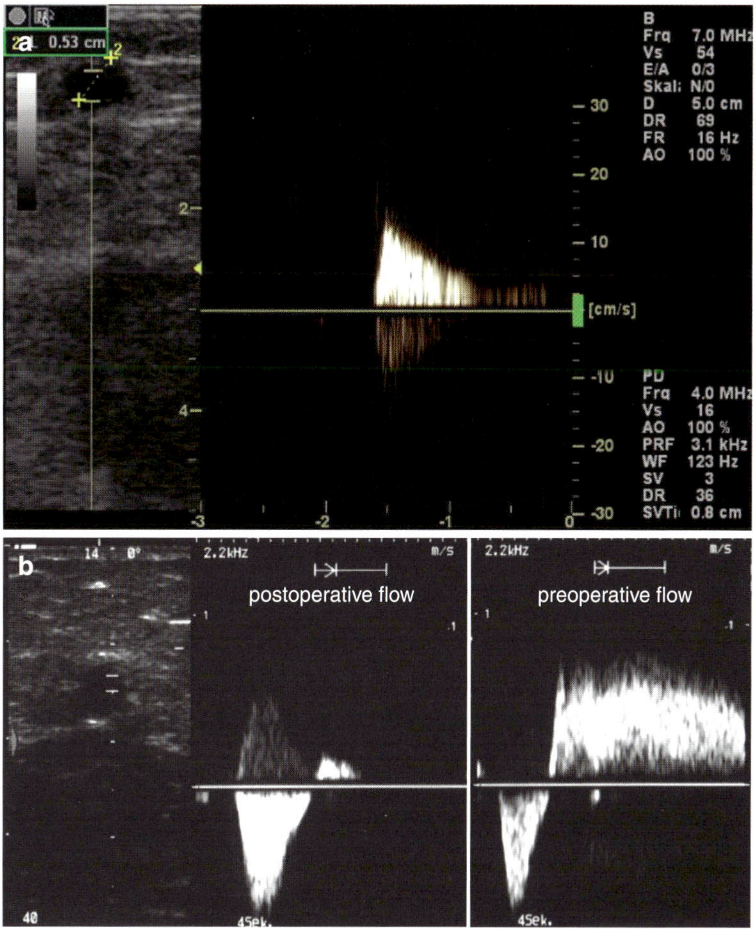

Fig. 13.5 Venous flow after CHIVA. (**a**) Flow during calf diastole in the great saphenous vein after ligation of the sapheno-femoral junction. The great saphenous vein diameter has reduced from 8.8 mm prior to the operation to 5.3 mm. (**b**) After CHIVA 2: *left velocity profile* at a subsequent examination demonstrating antegrade flow during calf systole and a limited short return flow until valve closure lasting approximately 300 ms and *right velocity* profile demonstrating a pre-operative comparison with antegrade flow during calf systole followed by reflux Copyright: [Author]

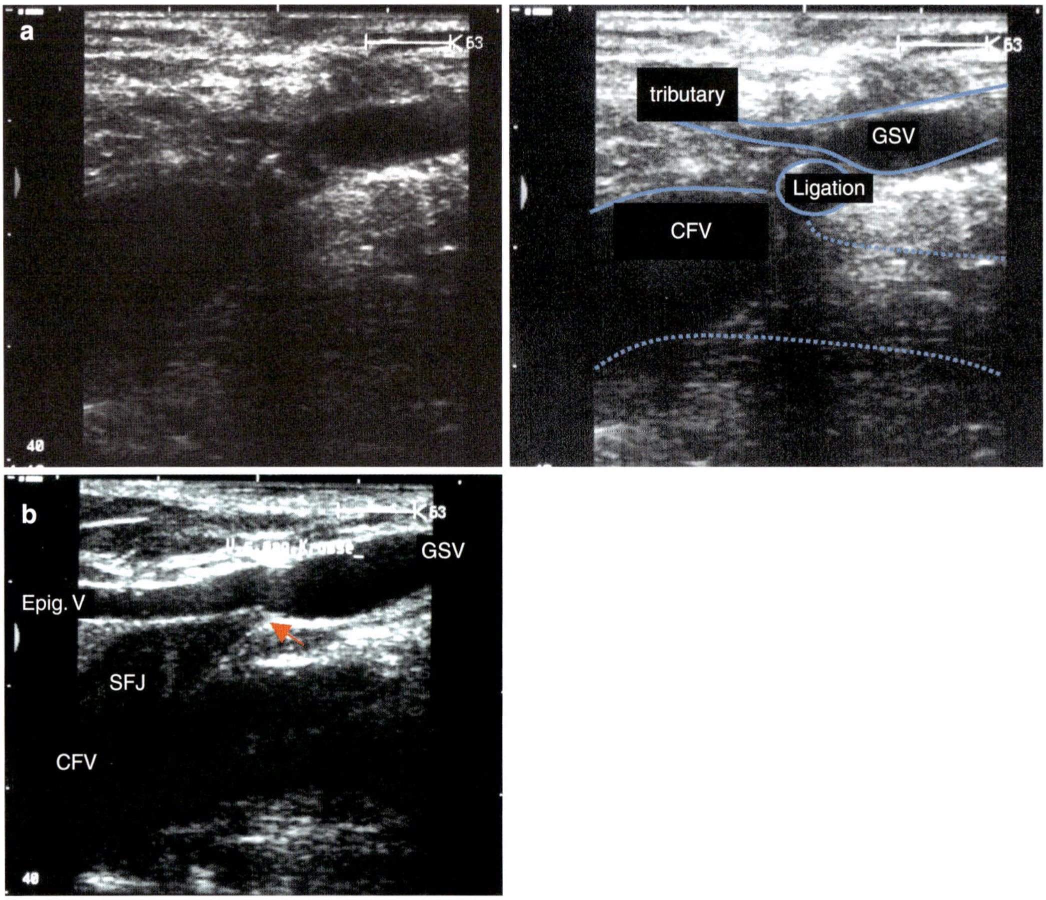

Fig. 13.6 Longitudinal view through the groin after ligation of the sapheno-femoral junction. (**a**) Correctly carried out double ligation appears as an oval, echo-poor element lying between the common femoral and great saphenous veins. The great saphenous vein receives a minimal antegrade flow from a competent venous tributary of the sapheno-femoral junction (Fig. 13.5a and c.f. Fig. 12.1). (**b**) Incorrect interruption of the sapheno-femoral junction. A single ligation has been performed directly below the junction of the superficial epigastric vein with the great saphenous vein at a distance of approx. 1 cm from the femoral vein (*arrowed*). The epigastric vein is pathological with continuous drainage into the great saphenous vein (see online material and c.f. Fig. 12.1) Copyright: [Author]

A closed sapheno-femoral junction should be documented (Fig. 13.6a). A minimal drainage of the venous tributaries of the sapheno-femoral junction into the great saphenous vein is desirable as it prevents thrombus forming in the saphenous vein. If pre-operative reflux exists in the venous tributaries of the sapheno-femoral junction, this paves the way for a groin recurrence. This occurs through newly formed anastomoses 8 weeks after operation with the development of a long-term pathological reflux from the sapheno-femoral junction venous tributaries into the distal great saphenous vein.

After CHIVA 2 with ligation of a venous tributary for flow reversal in the saphenous vein, the operator must decide during post-operative examination whether the treatment has been completed (Sect. 12.2). If reflux persists, the stump must be reexplored. As in conventional sapheno-femoral junction ligation operations, a stump or a venous tributary can lead to recurrence (Fig. 13.7).

In post-operative duplex ultrasound evaluations, the venous flow of remaining venous tributaries must be examined. If they present a high-volume, long-lasting reflux, an incompetence

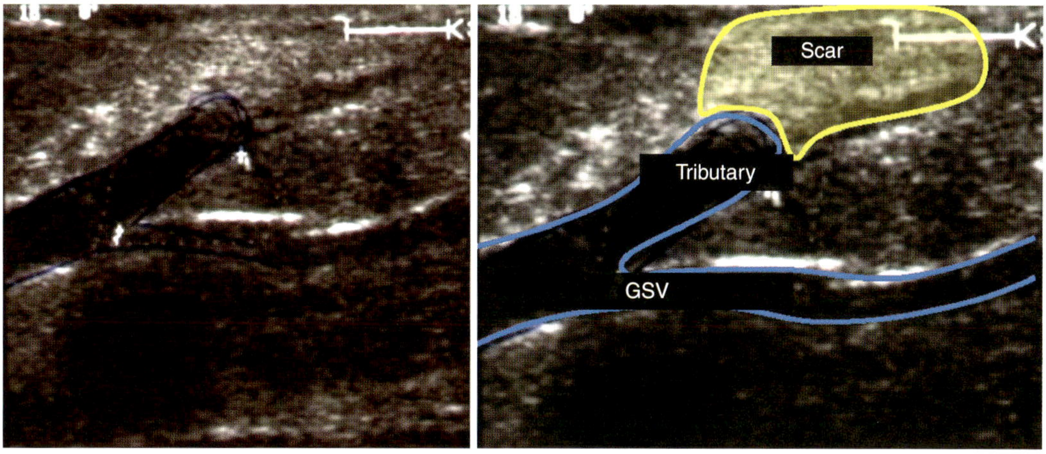

Fig. 13.7 Unsuccessful CHIVA 2 treatment with a great saphenous vein stump 1 cm long. Recanalisation and recurrent reflux are seen at this point (see accompanying online material) Copyright: [Author]

point must be sought. If the venous tributaries are only dilated but not refluxive, it may be concluded that the walls lack tone. They can be removed or treated by sclerotherapy.

13.3.3 Ultrasound After Extraluminal Valvuloplasty

Post-operative check-ups serve to ensure that the venous valve in the groin is functional. The check-up should be done between 2 and 4 weeks after surgery. Older valvuloplasty implants returned a strong echo making it impossible to take direct measurements in the confluence area. The image was completely obscured by acoustic shadowing. The new implants, available since 2007, are almost ultrasound neutral and allow haemodynamic measurements to be taken.

As with the old implants, the competence of the new venous valve in or below the groin must be tested using a Valsalva manoeuvre. The diameter of the great saphenous vein is determined at predefined points usually 5 cm below from the junction and 5 cm above the knee joint space. These measurement points were used for follow-up. In most cases the vein regained its competence with a reduction in diameter. In approximately 40 % of valvuloplasties, oscillating flow, backwards and forwards, is observed in the saphenous vein section after calf compression and release. This finding only defines true failure when, in addition, a positive reflux is found at the sapheno-femoral junction during a Valsalva manoeuvre.

13.4 Recurrence After Surgery on Varicose Veins

Recurrence of visible varicose veins after treatment is classically designated as recurrence. The REVAS classification was developed to describe this recurrence (Perrin et al. 2000). The cause of recurrence can be distinguished from the site of recurrence as listed below.

- The cause of recurrence may be influenced by:
  1. Technical error
  2. Tactical error
  3. Neovascularisation
  4. Progression of the disease
  5. A combination of two or more of the above
  6. Unclear
- The site of recurrence may be:
  1. Remaining stump of the great or small saphenous vein
  2. Pathological perforating veins (regardless of whether these were present previously or were treated)
  3. Remaining incompetent saphenous veins
  4. Development of incompetence in remaining veins which previously were competent

If visible varicose tributaries reoccur in a patient after a varicose vein operation, the diagnosing doctor must find the sources of reflux and treat them if appropriate. Duplex ultrasound is agreed in the international consensus document to be the best method (Nicolaides 2000). The clinically visible vessels must be examined by ultrasound to find the sources of reflux. The hidden course of the veins at the point of visible recurrence should be evaluated, especially in the region of surgical scars.

The work of Carandina et al. 2008 compared 54 legs in which the great saphenous vein was treated by stripping to 70 legs treated with CHIVA. The reflux visible on ultrasound was reported at 10 years and subsequently classified in Table 13.1.

13.4.1 Recurrence After Sapheno-femoral Junction Surgery

Recurrence at the sapheno-femoral junction can be divided into two groups:

1. Reflux from deep veins
2. Reflux from the sapheno-femoral junction venous tributaries without deep vein connections

13.4.1.1 Reflux from Deep Veins

During calf diastole or a Valsalva manoeuvre, reflux is seen originating from the deep vein (Fig. 4.2). The deep vein displays red colour or retrograde flow. There are three possibilities:

- **Reflux through a remaining stump:** The junction of the great saphenous vein is clearly visible and occasionally the first subterminal valve (Fig. 13.8). It is called the "stump" because of the remaining piece of great saphenous vein which ends close to the common femoral vein. Connections from this sometimes develop to a venous tributary, often the anterior accessory saphenous vein, which convolutes in part of the course of the removed great saphenous vein and subcutaneous tissue. Alternatively, connections may develop directly into the great saphenous vein if this has not been removed. In the 1960s–1980s, the great saphenous vein was often interrupted in the proximal thigh resulting in recanalisation which is a common cause of recurrence (Fig. 13.9). In these patients the length of the stump together with the flow velocity should be documented because this may influence the selection of treatment. With slow flow sclerotherapy can be used, while fast flows may be treated better with repeat crossectomy or an endoluminal procedure. However, this is controversial with some practitioners treating all recurrences with foam sclerotherapy. A remaining stump which presents no reflux is not a cause of recurrence.

Table 13.1 Analysis of recurrence after stripping and CHIVA according to Carandina et al. (2008)

Sources of reflux	Frequency after stripping (%)	Frequency after CHIVA (%)
Reflux through the sapheno-femoral junction or sapheno-popliteal junction after interruption, with or without removal of the saphenous vein either via the remnant stump or by neovascularisation (Sects. 13.4.1 and 13.4.2)	5.5	2.9
Reflux from pelvic veins not connected to the common femoral vein	3.7	1.4
Reflux from a perforating vein which was not noticeably refluxive before the treatment	7.4	0
Reflux into a venous tributary from the great saphenous vein via the sapheno-femoral junction, a pelvic vein or healthy proximal venous tributaries	0	18.5
Reflux into venous tributaries of diameter greater than 5 mm with no connection to a visible source of reflux	22	0
Total	*35*	*18.5*

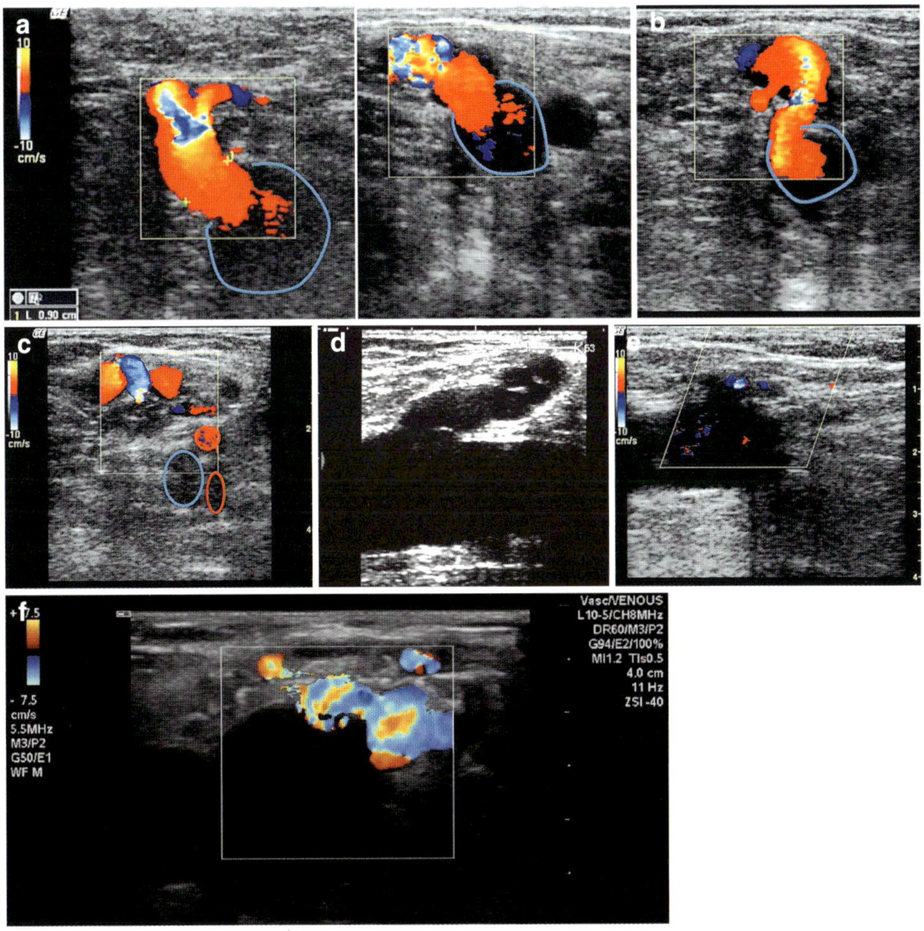

Fig. 13.8 Typical findings in recurrence. (**a**) *Left,* after a redo crossectomy in the groin, a gaping, refluxive junction of the great saphenous vein is seen of 9.0 mm in diameter; *right*, recurrence through a great saphenous vein stump from which a bundle of small vessels are seen filled in multiple colours (*blue*, *yellow* and *red*). The common femoral vein is outlined in blue (see accompanying online material). (**b**) Recurrence through the stump which fills the newly developed anterior accessory saphenous vein which enters the fascial compartment (see **c** and accompanying online material). As in (**a**) the reflux arises from the common femoral vein (*outlined in blue*). (**c**) The same patient as in (**b**), 3 cm further down demonstrating reflux into this newly developed vein which has formed in the compartment of the great and anterior accessory saphenous veins. (**d**) After ligation of the great saphenous vein approximately 2 cm distal to the sapheno-femoral junction with stripping. The valve can be seen at the sapheno-femoral junction with the formation of convoluted venous tributaries arising from the distal end of the stump. (**c**) Longitudinal view through the groin after a successful crossectomy and stripping of the great saphenous vein. A stump is visible demonstrating antegrade flow during calf diastole from the remaining sapheno-femoral junction tributaries via the stump and into the common femoral vein. No reflux is observed (see accompanying online material). (**f**) Recurrence with bunches of small veins. There is no stump and no reflux or flow from the deep leg veins during calf diastole. Instead, flow in the bunch originates from the sapheno-femoral junction venous tributaries and not from the deep veins. This is shown in the accompanying online material that after crossectomy there is no stump and no neovascularisation Copyright: [Author]

- **Neovascularisation** is the new formation of a tangle of very small vessels which fill from deep veins through one or more connections (Fig. 13.10). It has been demonstrated that some patients have a propensity to develop neovascularisation where new veins may be seen in the region of the sapheno-femoral junction as early as 6 months (de Maeseneer et al. 2005).

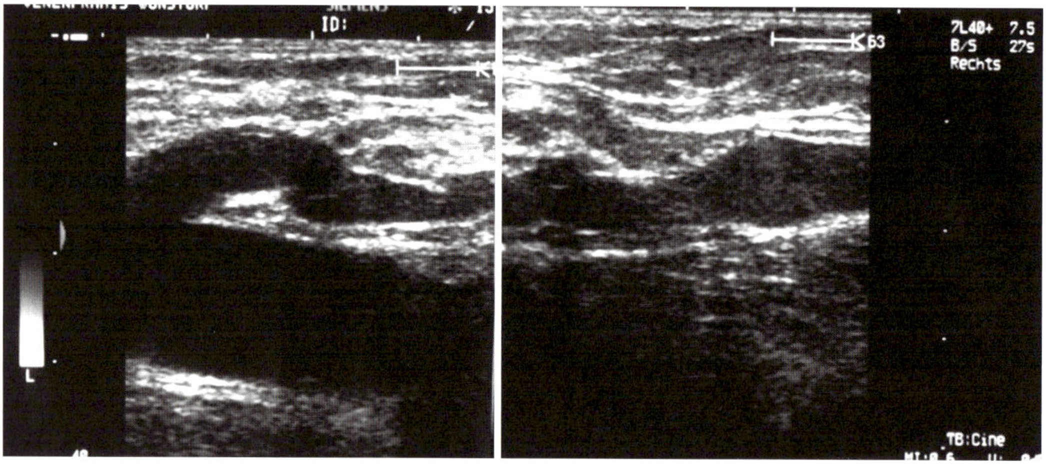

Fig. 13.9 After ligation and interruption of the great saphenous vein approximately 12 cm below the groin in the mid-1980s. Recanalisation and renewed reflux is seen in the distal great saphenous vein (see accompanying online material) Copyright: [Author]

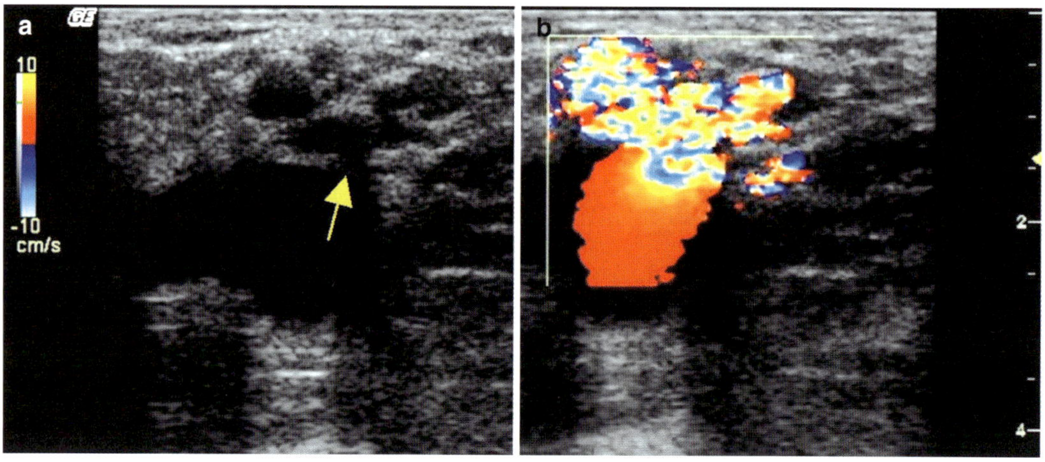

Fig. 13.10 Neovascularisation with no stump. (**a**) Even without colour it can be seen that there is flow from the deep vein through a tiny connecting vein (*arrow*). (**b**) The flow in the small veins is turbulent and very fast (see accompanying online material) Copyright: [Author]

- **Recurrence through atypical connections** to the deep system can occur especially between the femoral and deep femoral arteries (Fig. 13.11).

13.4.1.2 Reflux from the Sapheno-femoral Junction Tributaries Without Deep Vein Connections

Reflux arising from the pelvic vein occurs in 11 % of patients with incompetent saphenous veins (Mendoza 2002 in Appendix 2). Some of these patients have additional reflux from the femoral vein through the sapheno-femoral junction. After a classic crossectomy with interruption of the sapheno-femoral junction, venous tributaries recurrence may still occur through tiny vessels in the region of the groin scar which continue to be fed from refluxive pelvic veins. In this situation there is no connection with the deep veins with the absence of retrograde flow through the common femoral vein into the superficial veins during a Valsalva or calf muscle provocation manoeuvre (Fig. 13.12) (Carrandina et al. 2008).

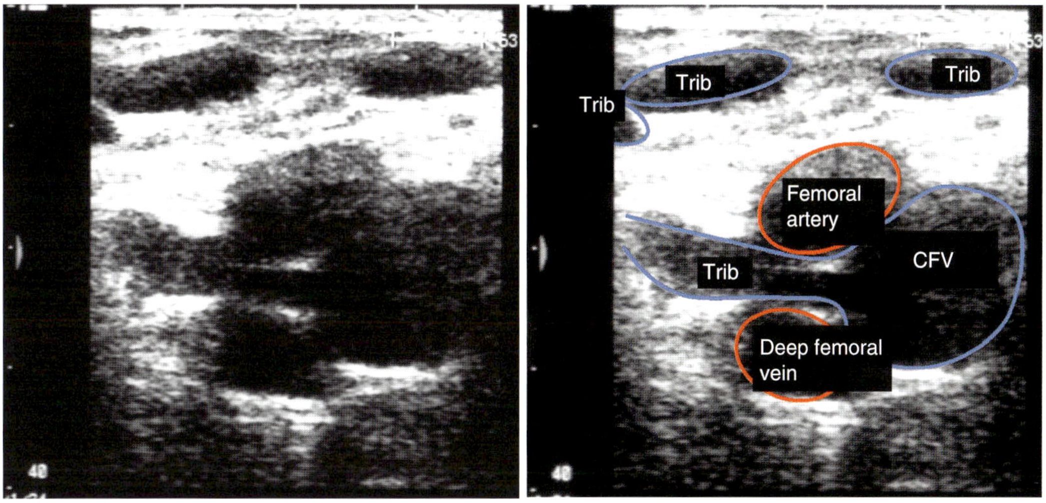

Fig. 13.11 After crossectomy and stripping of the great saphenous vein in the right leg, recurrence has occurred through an atypical connecting vessel. Reflux is seen arising directly from the common femoral and into the lateral accessory saphenous vein between the femoral artery (formerly superficial) and the deep femoral artery (see accompanying online material) Copyright: [Author]

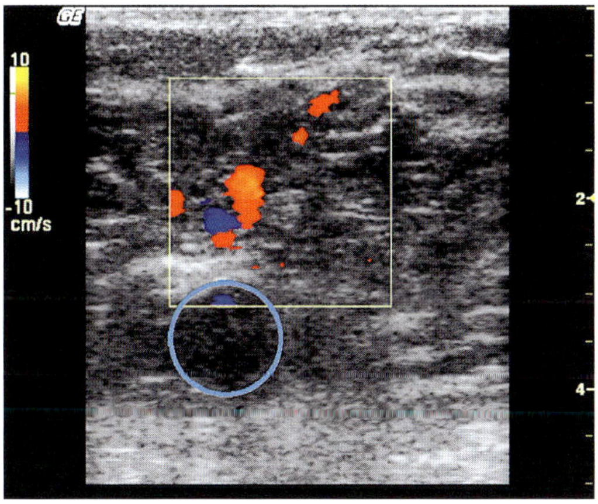

Fig. 13.12 Recurrence with visible venous tributaries in the left thigh after crossectomy and stripping of the great saphenous vein 5 years previously. Reflux arises from the sapheno-femoral junction venous tributaries without reflux from the common femoral vein (*blue ring*) (see accompanying online material) Copyright: [Author]

The different patterns of recurrence are very valuable for planning further treatment. The first group can be treated relatively easily, but it is still useful for the surgeon to know whether he will find a sapheno-femoral junction stump or a neovascularisation and reexploration should be required. When reflux arises from the pelvic veins, it is futile to perform a groin exploration because the reflux source is much higher.

After a correctly executed crossectomy with no recurrence, the anterior vein wall of the common femoral vein is smooth (Fig. 13.4 and Film 13.8 online material).

13.4.2 Recurrence After Sapheno-popliteal Junction Surgery

The termination of the small saphenous vein with the deep vein is quite variable (Sects. 2.5.1 and 8.3). Operating on the sapheno-popliteal junction is not as standardised as operating on the sapheno-femoral junction. Dissection down to the termination into the deep vein with a flush ligation always used to be required; however, if the confluence was above the popliteal region, the preferred option was interruption of the small saphenous vein at knee level with distal stripping which is technically easier. Today, ultrasound

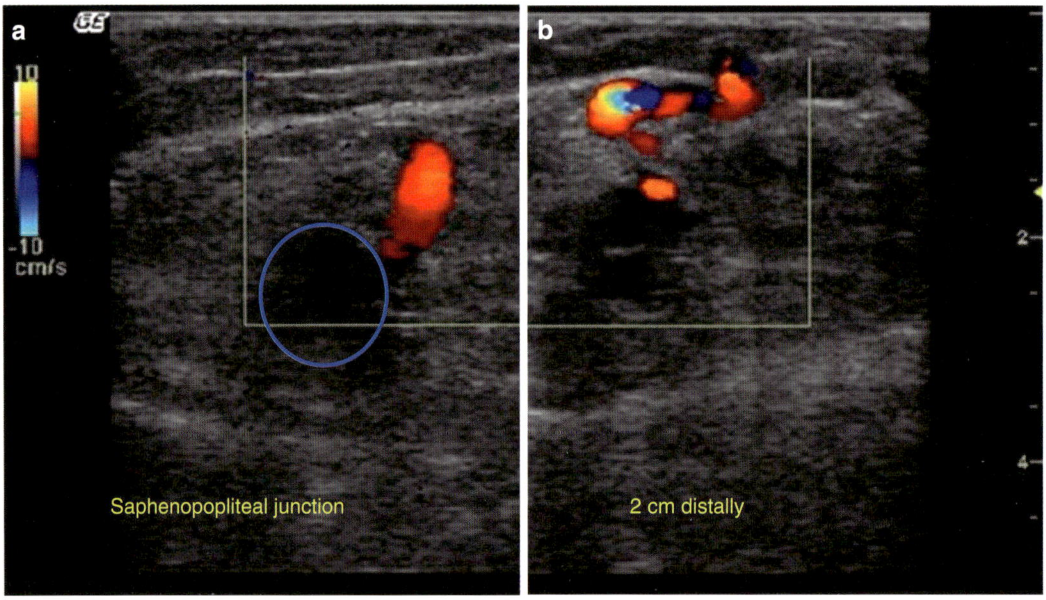

Fig. 13.13 Recurrence at the sapheno-popliteal junction. (**a**) Stump of the small saphenous vein and popliteal vein (*circled in blue*). (**b**) Reflux is seen arising from the stump into epifascial venous tributaries in the popliteal region (see accompanying online material) Copyright: [Author]

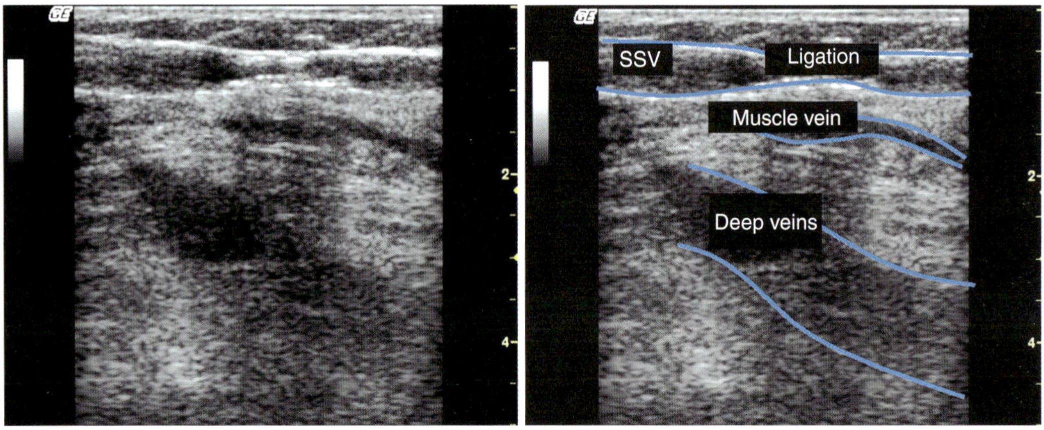

Fig. 13.14 Recurrence after ligation and interruption of the small saphenous vein. According to the operation report, a crossectomy was performed. Longitudinal view through the knee and upper part of the calf. The calibre is reduced at the ligation point, but blood can still pass. The small saphenous vein remains refluxive (see accompanying online material) Copyright: [Author]

diagnosis makes it possible to decide on the exact level of interruption of the small saphenous vein which is usually below its termination and also below a competent muscle vein.

In recurrences arising from a remaining small saphenous vein stump, this can be demonstrated on ultrasound as an abrupt termination in the popliteal fossa with sprouting convoluted venous tributaries (Fig. 13.13). These cross the fascia of the popliteal fascia and continue as visible epifascial tributaries. A subfascial location of these convoluted veins can occasionally be seen in the image. Remaining stumps without reflux are not a cause of recurrence.

After ligation of the small saphenous vein without removal, it is very common to find incompetence in at least one segment of the remaining vein (Fig. 13.14).

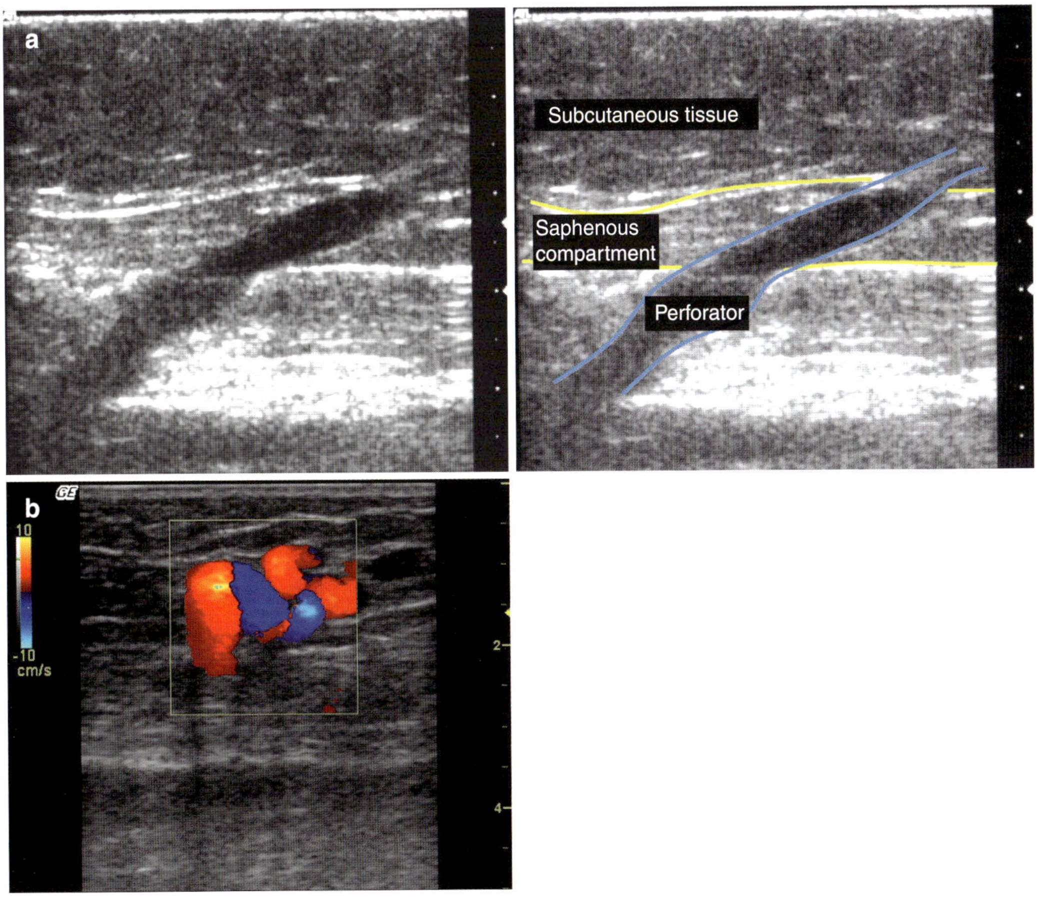

Fig. 13.15 Recurrence in the perforating veins. (**a**) Longitudinal view of recurrence in the inner thigh after stripping of the great saphenous vein. A perforating vein seen in the adductor canal penetrating the empty fascial compartment and filling a venous tributary. (**b**) Longitudinal view of the inner thigh after stripping of the great saphenous vein. The perforating vein in the adductor canal fills a convolution of small veins in the fascial compartment, from which it soon exits (see accompanying online material). (**c**) Blowout of a paratibial perforating vein after stripping. When the patient is standing still, there is little flow; however, strong oscillating flow back and forth is observed using provocation manoeuvres Copyright: [Author]

Other variants of new refluxes in the popliteal fossa are also possible such as the formation of a popliteal neovascularisation where it is often difficult to define a feeding point. Recurrent reflux can also arise directly from a perforating vein into a convoluted venous tributary.

13.4.3 Recurrence from a Perforating Vein

Perforating veins are very often sources of recurrence after the removal of saphenous veins. These include the perforating vein in the adductor canal (formerly Dodd) in thigh recurrences and the group consisting of the posterior tibial (formerly Cockett) and paratibial perforating veins in calf recurrences (Fig. 13.15). These may fill remaining segments of the great saphenous vein or result in a tangle of veins in the fascial or more often in the epifascial compartment.

The post-operative evaluation must include an assessment at the typical perforating vein locations before pathological feeding points can be excluded. Ideally, an accurate pre-operative documentation of the state of these perforating veins should be carried out. This will help assess their residual or recurrent contribution as a cause of recurrence at a later date.

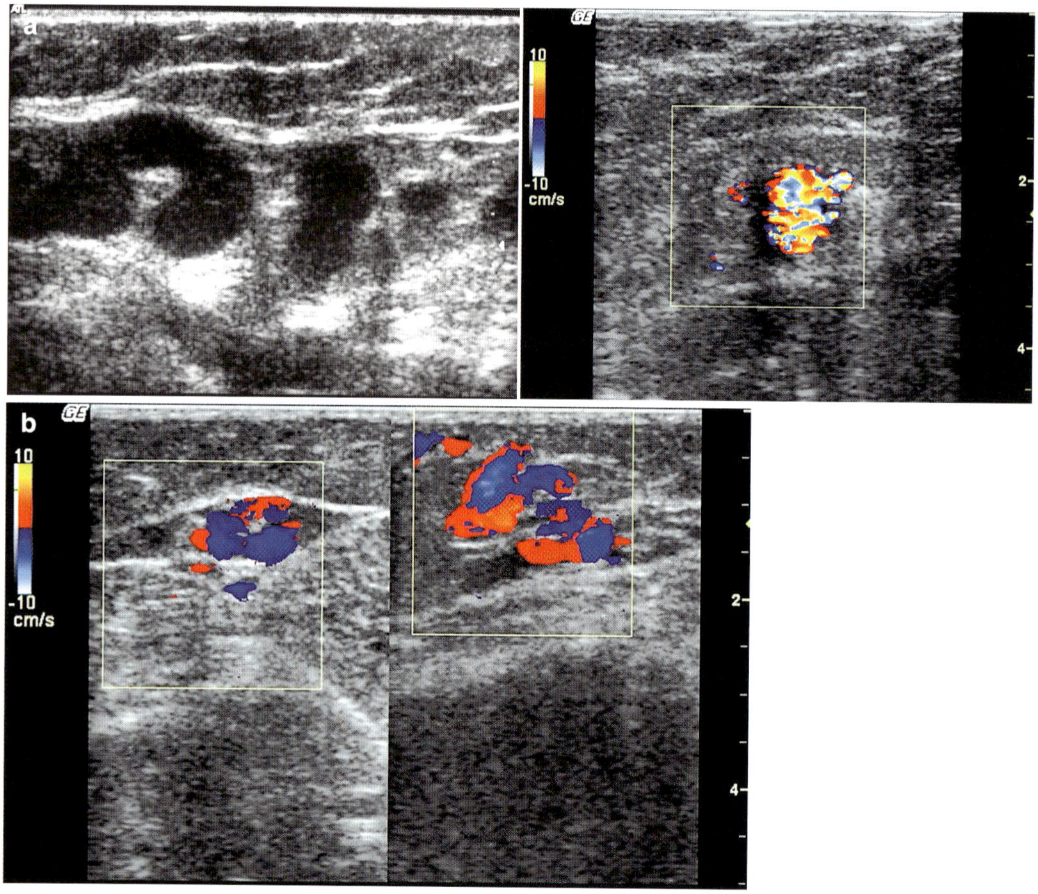

Fig. 13.16 Recurrence in the saphenous fascial compartment. (**a**) Longitudinal view of the inner thigh after stripping of the great saphenous vein with clinical recurrence in the inner calf. A convoluted vein has formed in the saphenous compartment which probably arose from the original *vasa vasorum* of the great saphenous vein (transverse view see accompanying online material). (**b**) Transverse view through the inner thigh demonstrating recurrence after stripping of the great saphenous vein in B-scan. A vein is shown in the compartment. In colour flow this can be seen to consist of several small lumina with turbulent reflux (see accompanying online material). (**c**) Recurrence after stripping of the small saphenous vein in transverse view through the back of the calf. *Left*, upper third demonstrating a convoluted vein in the saphenous compartment; *right*, middle third demonstrating reflux in venous tributaries in the subcutaneous tissue arising from this convolution (see accompanying online material). (**d**) The saphenous compartment after "complete" stripping. The ultrasound is aligned from proximal to distal. The great saphenous vein suddenly appears as if it had not been removed. It is not refluxive, and after a few centimetres, it joins a minimally refluxive venous tributary which drains blood out of the vein. Below this point the saphenous compartment is empty once more Copyright: [Author]

13.4.4 Recurrence in the Tract of a Stripped Saphenous Vein

A recurrent or remaining vein may be found in the saphenous compartment after stripping. These can be distinguished easily by their morphology.

Recurrent Vein

These rarely occur after stripping of the saphenous vein. However, they sometimes form bizarre convolutions within the saphenous compartment (Fig. 13.16a, c), and occasionally bundles of tiny veins which at first glance look like normal veins. However, when assessed using colour duplex, it can be seen that there is turbulent flow in a number of small lumina (Fig. 13.16b).

Saphenous Veins Remaining After Operation

These segments look like untreated veins and must be examined by ultrasound to see whether or not they are refluxive. Prior to the operation there was probably reflux in various accessory veins which were cannulated during stripping. Consequently, these refluxive extrafascial veins were then stripped leaving a normal competent great saphenous vein in situ. Juan established that these segments are not involved in the development of recurrence (Juan et al. 2002 in Appendix 2).

13.4.5 Recurrence Without Connections to the Deep Veins

Juan et al. (2002 in Appendix 2) showed retrospectively that in 12 % of clinical recurrences after stripping, the newly formed visible veins presented no connection to the deep veins. They postulated that as these new veins are located in the subcutaneous tissues, they lost their drainage due to stripping. Therefore, blood within them drains in a retrograde fashion.

Carandina et al. (2008) showed prospectively that in 22 % of cases of recurrence after stripping, there is the presence of venous tributaries without a source of reflux from the deep veins. Reticular veins are usually involved which drain into large or small diameter veins that are visible and clinically distressing. If ultrasound is used to look for the source of the reflux, it will not be found. Typically, these veins become increasingly thin and branched and finally no longer visible if the source of the reflux is looked after. The velocity profile in PW-mode is slow and long lasting. These authors also postulate that retrograde flow from the subcutaneous veins within the fatty tissue is involved which can no longer be drained through the saphenous vein.

13.5 Recurrence After Sclerotherapy

Ultrasound examination after sclerotherapy can be onerous. This is particularly true when the great saphenous vein has been treated with hypertonic saline, which was a method popular in Germany in 1980–2000. During examination of the course of these veins, they may suddenly disappear without a draining visible venous tributary, only to reappear further down. It is almost impossible to look for sources of reflux in a venous tributary, as described in Sect. 10.3. When recanalisation occurs after sclerotherapy of saphenous veins, irregularities may appear similar to those found after superficial vein thrombosis (Chap. 11, Sect. 12.4). This results in heterogeneous image patterns which are often difficult to interpret (Fig. 13.17). Flow may be so slow, so that power duplex is necessary to visualise it. Occasionally adjuvant foam can also be used as feedback because it is also a contrast medium which can be used to determine retrospectively whether recanalisation had taken place or whether a particular vein was patent.

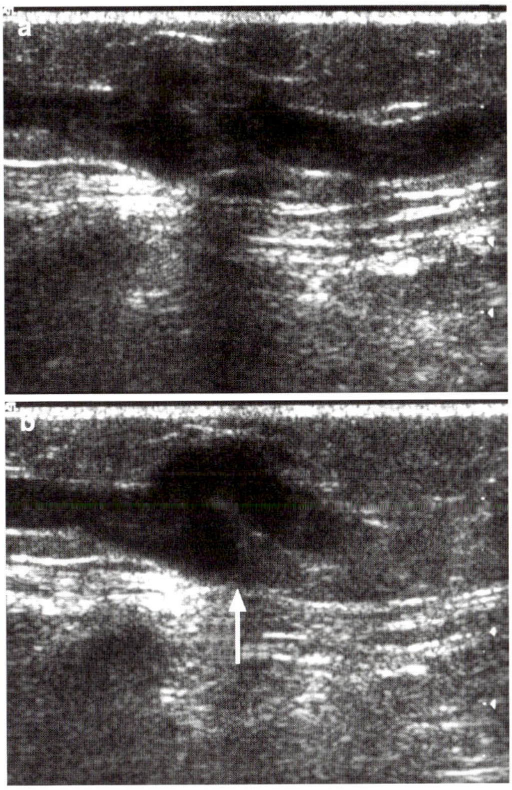

Fig. 13.17 (**a**) Longitudinal view through the inner thigh after sclerotherapy of venous tributaries of the great saphenous vein in the calf. The great saphenous vein has an irregularity in its normally smooth course and it is totally refluxive. (**b**) The same finding as in **a**, with the transducer held at an angle. At one point the course of the great saphenous vein is completely interrupted (*arrow*) with a distended venous tributary bridging the area of occlusion Copyright: [Author]

13.6 Recurrence After Endoluminal Procedures

After a successful endoluminal procedure, regular ultrasound monitoring is required. The following intervals are recommended:

- **1st check-up:** 24–72 h after surgery. In this early check-up it is especially important to recognise signs of unsuccessful therapy and to exclude deep venous thrombosis. No conclusion can be reached at this stage on a closure operation at the sapheno-femoral junction because swelling and thrombosis from endothermal injury may cause the region to appear to be closed. Therefore, the treated saphenous vein may be erroneously interpreted as closed. Failure with patency and reflux is much easier to recognise.
- **2nd check-up:** 3–4 months after intervention. The post-operative changes will have disappeared allowing a confident assessment of closure on the length of the treated vein.
- **3rd check-up:** over 1 year. If a relatively long refluxive sapheno-femoral junction stump (>0.5–1 cm) is found, the patient should be examined annually by ultrasound in order to identify any clinically relevant early recurrence.

Nomenclature and Classification

By definition a recurrence at the sapheno-femoral junction occurs if there has been a previous operation or intervention in the region. This should be mentioned particularly in the context of thermal ablation procedures since it was common practice to leave a stump as a matter of course. The "rule" was that thermal ablation should take place no closer than 1–2 cm from the sapheno-femoral junction or treatment should begin below the confluence of the superficial epigastric vein. More recently with the introduction of radial laser fibres, there has been a change in the method. Now some operators are trying more and more to close the region of the sapheno-femoral junction as close as possible to the femoral vein. In this way relevant venous tributaries in the region will also be treated and in particular the anterior accessory saphenous vein (Fig. 13.18).

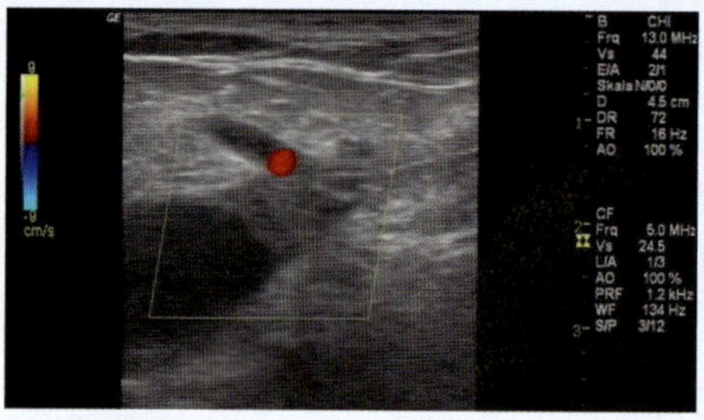

Fig. 13.18 Examination of the sapheno-femoral junction on the first day after endoluminal surgery with abolition of flow down to the deep vein. This treatment is analogous to a surgical crossectomy. **Oblique** view through the right groin with the great saphenous vein closed up to the drainage of the tributaries (see online material). The upper part is open and perfused (*red* in colour duplex) Copyright: [Author]

When discussing recurrence after treatment of an incompetent saphenous vein, it is important to differentiate between an ultrasound finding, like the sapheno-femoral junction stump with or without reflux, and the occurrence of new and clinically relevant varicose veins with reflux arising from the previously treated region. There is a consensus document known as the REVAS document (Perrin et al. 2000), which classifies and evaluates recurrent varicose veins after surgery. This is now undergoing revision to encompass endovenous treatments.

Over 60 % of recurrence after stripping of the great saphenous vein is caused by a long sapheno-femoral junction stump remaining after treatment (Geier et al. 2008). The REVAS group classified these recurrences as technical errors (Perrin et al. 2000). For this reason an exact description of the sapheno-femoral junction stump is required, if present. This is an important indication for colour-coded duplex ultrasound.

The REVAS document (Perrin et al. 2000) distinguishes the following causes of recurrence:

- Technical or tactical error usually from a long remaining sapheno-femoral junction stump
- Neovascularisation
- Both of the above

The length of the sapheno-femoral junction stump may be assumed to be significant for prognosis because of the likelihood of recurrence arising from venous tributaries which join the great saphenous vein in this region. For this reason a detailed preoperative evaluation is particularly important in minimising the risk of recurrence after endoluminal treatment.

It has been shown (Mühlberger et al. 2007) that there is a consistent relationship in the distance between the drainage of the venous tributaries and the level of the terminal valve of the common femoral vein. In our duplex ultrasound examinations of 126 control subjects with healthy veins, it was found that in almost 50 % of the sapheno-femoral junctions examined, the anterior accessory saphenous vein was the highest venous tributary, with no further tributary between anterior accessory saphenous vein and deep vein joining the great saphenous vein. It was lateral in location and joined the great saphenous vein between 0–7 mm below the terminal valve. In almost 70 % of cases, the course of the anterior accessory saphenous vein was interfascial. This highest lateral venous tributary was very frequently erroneously described as the superficial epigastric vein. The termination of the superficial epigastric vein into the great saphenous vein at the level of this venous tributary was shown in only 27 % of legs, whilst the rest drained further away of the sapheno-femoral junction as compared to the first tributary (Sect. 7.3.9). As in Mühlenberger's anatomical study in over 70 % of legs, the distance from the drainage of the venous tributaries to the sapheno-femoral junction was between 10 and 15 mm. If left untreated this confluence might affect the result of an endoluminal procedure.

After endoluminal thermal ablation, recurrence may occur from two principal sources:

1. Recurrence in the treated section of saphenous vein
2. Recurrence arising from the sapheno-femoral region

13.6.1 Recurrence in the Treated Section of Saphenous Vein

At follow-up the treated vein segment may appear as follows:

- Initially not closed or partially closed when it is filled with fibrinothrombotic material around which there is continuous flow confirming unsuccessful treatment
- Initially completely closed but later presenting as recanalisation
- Invisible to ultrasound in the long term
- Fibrosis within the former saphenous compartment

Initially Not Closed or Partially Closed

Depending on how the vein has responded to treatment, the ultrasound image may demonstrate a varying range of appearances. A completely untreated vein wall may be observed. Occasionally, irregularities of the wall are seen similar to the aftermath of a phlebitis. The vein may also be coated with highly echogenic material. In colour duplex ultrasound the image shows flow in one or more segments with widely varying vein diameters. Sometimes only a residual lumen of 1–2 mm is identifiable in which flow can only be detected in power duplex mode. This outcome can easily be corrected with foam sclerotherapy (Fig. 13.19).

Recanalisation

This is frequently observed on ultrasound after using bare laser fibres with short wavelength

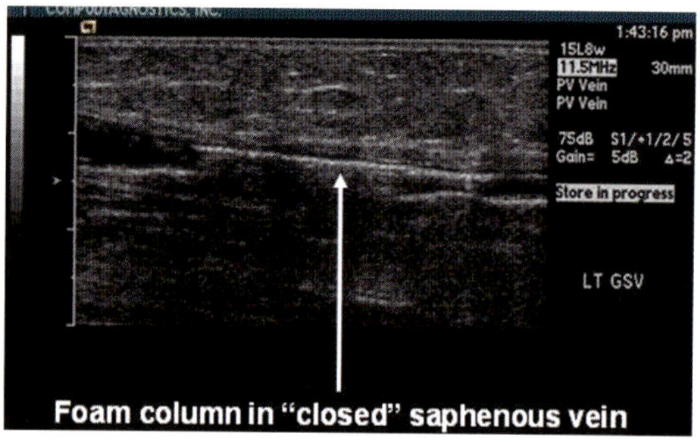

Fig. 13.19 Longitudinal image of the great saphenous vein closed at the inner thigh by endoluminal treatment. No flow or reflux is visible in colour-coded duplex ultrasound (not shown). Note that a large quantity of foam entered this "closed" great saphenous vein during foam sclerotherapy of a venous tributary. This is direct evidence that a lumen persisted in the vein. Retrospectively, power duplex might have shown the flow and thus could have explained the apparently inexplicable recurrence after vein "closure" (Nick Morrison, USA, by kind permission) Copyright: [Author]

lasers. With this technique the heated blood in the vein leads indirectly to the thermal effect on the vein wall. The denatured blood usually occludes the vein. If insufficient energy is applied, only a modest degree of contraction and shrinkage is observed on ultrasound. If a radial laser fibre with a longer wavelength is used, over twice the shrinkage of the saphenous vein is found and no significant lumen remains. This of course assumes that a sufficient energy dose per cm was applied to the treated vein.

The optimum energy dose per cm of treated saphenous vein has been established for laser and radio frequency treatment. With laser it should be between 70 and 90 J per cm in lower wavelength lasers, while in higher wavelength lasers, the requirement is 40–60 J per cm. Adhering to this dosage complete thermal eradication of the treated vein should be achieved in almost 100 % of cases today. In Germany, most short wavelength bare laser fibres have been replaced with radial lasers with longer wavelengths. Cases of unsuccessful ablation with the same anatomical and pathological findings before and after treatment are uncommon. If they occur it is usually attributable to user error or equipment failure.

13.6.2 Recurrence Arising from the Sapheno-femoral Region

This can occur irrespective of whether the sapheno-femoral junction was directly treated endothermally or left alone. After conservative thermal ablation of the great saphenous vein with a remaining stump or a complete endoluminal ablation up to the sapheno-femoral junction, recurrence may occur directly from the sapheno-femoral region. The following ultrasound findings have been recorded most frequently in our patients:

1. A sapheno-femoral stump 1.5–2 cm long with no reflux.
2. Reflux in the sapheno-femoral stump from the common femoral vein or an inguinal venous tributary with formation of new venous tributaries from the lateral side which existed prior to the first intervention (see Fig. 7.13) (Fig. 13.20).
3. A remaining lateral and sometimes medial segment including the upper two venous tributary terminations with no reflux.
4. Reflux drainage from above into the lateral segment to below with continuation into the anterior accessory saphenous vein. This occurs when the course of the vein is interfascial.

In many cases a short segment of refluxive great saphenous vein may be found above the termination of the lateral segment. This segment has a narrow, thread-like lumen which is either completely closed or cannot be seen in the ultrasound

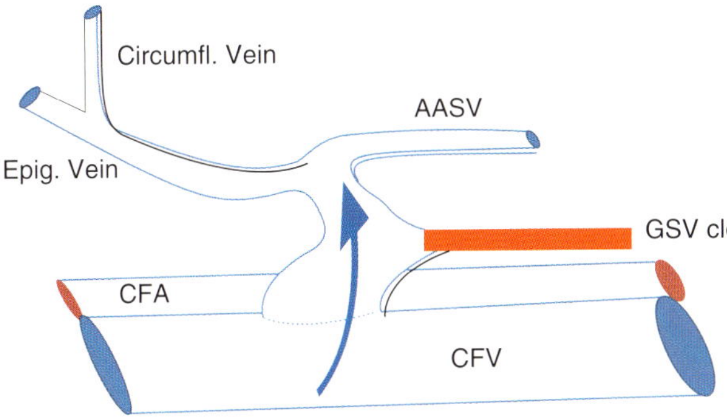

Fig. 13.20 Diagram showing reflux from the common femoral vein through the remaining lateral segment into the anterior accessory saphenous vein (see also Fig. 7.13). A closed great saphenous vein seen in orange (*CFV*, common femoral vein; *SCIV*, superficial circumflex iliac vein; *SEV*, superficial epigastric vein; *GSV*, great saphenous vein; *AASV*, anterior accessory saphenous vein Copyright: [Author]

Table 13.2 Main morphological and haemodynamic duplex ultrasound findings after endovenous ablation of a saphenous trunk

Morphology

(a) Obliteration of the vein: total incompressibility and absence of colour flow; the vein can be classified as visible or nonvisible

(b) Partial patency of the vein: partial compressibility and presence of colour flow in a part of the lumen

(c) Total patency of the vein: complete compressibility and presence of colour flow in the totality of the lumen

(d) Outer diameter of the residual vein

(e) Inner diameter of the residual lumen in case of partial or total patency

(f) Segmental obliteration/patency: length of the obliterated, partially or completely patent segment(s)

Haemodynamics

(a) Absence of flow with both principal manoeuvres (Valsalva, compression/release)

(b) Antegrade flow during compression manoeuvre

(c) Retrograde flow >0.5 s during one or both manoeuvres

From de Maeseneer et al. (2011)

Table 13.3 Proposed classification of duplex findings at the junction (J) and at the treated trunk (T) after endovenous ablation

J for SFJ or SPJ:

- J0: no patent stump
- J1, J2, J3, J4, etc.: junction with patent stump of 1, 2, 3, 4 cm, etc.

R+, reflux; R−, no reflux

T for GSV/AASV/SSV trunk:

- Ti: invisible trunk
- To: obliterated trunk (diameter, mm)
- Tp: completely or partially patent trunk (diameter, mm)
- To/Tp or Tp/To: segmental obliteration/patency or patency/obliteration (length of patent segment, cm; diameter of residual lumen, mm)

R+, reflux; R−, no reflux

From de Maeseneer et al. (2011)

image. De Maeseneer (de Maeseneer et al. 2011) stratified the recurrences after physical or chemical endoluminal treatments as shown in Tables 13.2 and 13.3.

Recurrence After Endoluminal Treatment

Short-term results exist following treatment with the radial laser fibre. In the comparative study between crossectomy and stripping of the great saphenous vein versus radial laser (Rasmussen et al. 2011), it was shown that significantly more sapheno-femoral stumps, both with and without reflux, were found after endovenous laser ablation. The natural history of these sapheno-femoral stumps will presumably only be seen in the next 4–6 years.

An increasing number of case descriptions are being published of clinically relevant recurrences at the sapheno-femoral junction after thermal ablation of the great saphenous vein. An increase has also been experienced in our practices. The tendency among many users of thermal procedures is to position the fibre ever closer to the sapheno-femoral junction to avoid possible later recurrences at the sapheno-femoral junction bearing in mind that this may increase the risk of endoluminal heat-induced thrombosis (EHIT) complications. However, an evidence-based recommendation cannot be made until after the completion of an appropriate comparative study.

References

Carandina S, Mari C, De Palma M, Marcellino MG, Cisno C, Legnaro A, Liboni A, Zamboni P (2008) Varicose vein stripping vs haemodynamic correction (CHIVA): a long term randomised trial. Eur J Vasc Endovasc Surg 35:230–237

De Maeseneer MG, Vandenbroeck CP, Hendriks JM, Lauwers PR, van Schil PE (2005) Accuracy of duplex evaluation one year after varicose vein surgery to predict recurrence at the sapheno-femoral junction after five years. Eur J Vasc Endovasc Surg 29:308–331

De Maeseneer M, Pichot O, Cavezzi A, Earnshaw J, van Rij A, Lurie F, Smith PC (2011) Duplex ultrasound investigation of the veins of the lower limbs after treatment for varicose veins e UIP consensus document. Eur J Vasc Endovasc Surg 42(1):89–102

Geier B, Stücker M, Hummel T, Burger P, Frings N, Hartmann M, Stenger D, Schwahn-Schreiber C, Schonath M, Mumme A (2008a) Residual stumps associated with inguinal varicose vein recurrences: a multicenter study. Eur J Vasc Endovasc Surg 36: 207–210

Juan J, Escribano JM, Maeso J (2002) Hämodynamik des Varizenrezidivs nach Strippingoperationen. Abstractband Jahreskongress 2002 der DGG: 35 (nachzulesen unter www.chiva.info)

Kaps M, von Reutern GM, Stolz E, von Büdingen HJ (2004) Ultraschall in der Neurologie. Thieme, Stuttgart/New York

Mühlberger D, Morandini L, Brenner E (2007) Frequency and exact position of valves in the saphenofemoral junction. Phlebologie 36:3–7

Nicolaides AN (2000) Investigation of chronic venous insufficiency – a consensus statement. Circulation 102:126–163

Perrin MR, Guex JJ, Ruckley CV, dePalma RG, Royle JP, Eklof B, Nicolini P, Janet G and the REVAS group (2000) Recurrent varices after surgery (REVAS), a consensus document. Cardiovasc Surg 8:233–245

Rasmussen LH, Lawaetz M, Bjoern L, Vennits B, Blemings A, Eklof B (2011) Randomized clinical trial comparing endovenous laser ablation, radiofrequency ablation, foam sclerotherapy and surgical stripping for great saphenous varicose veins. Br J Surg 98:1079–1087

14 Deep Leg Veins

Hans-Joachim Kruse, Erika Mendoza, Nick Morrison, and Christopher R. Lattimer

Chapter Summary

Treatment of the superficial leg veins invariably requires examination of the deep leg veins. This is because any pathology identified in the deep veins may influence the treatment strategy. Since this book focuses on superficial veins, only an elementary description of the subject is presented. This includes the basics in the diagnosis of thrombosis and the ultrasound appearances observed in patients with the post-thrombotic syndrome.

H.-J. Kruse, MD, PhD (✉)
Praxis für Gefäßmedizin, Gabelsbergerstraße 3, 09405 Zschopau, Germany
e-mail: hjkruse@gmx.de

E. Mendoza, MD, PhD
Venenpraxis Wunstorf, Speckenstraße 10, 31515 Wunstorf, Germany
e-mail: erika.mendoza@t-online.de

N. Morrison, MD
Morrison Vein Institute, Suite 223, 8575 E. Princess Dr., Scottsdale, AZ, USA

C.R. Lattimer, MD, PhD
Department of Vascular Surgery, Josef Pflug Vascular Laboratory, Ealing Hospital and Imperial College, London, UK

14.1 Anatomy

Leg veins can be divided into three systems and two compartments. The systems are the (1) superficial veins, (2) deep veins and (3) perforating veins which connect them. The compartments are (1) superficial and (2) deep. These are separated by the muscle fascia (Caggiati et al. 2002). The deep system consists of veins which run **inside the muscle fascia**. These are the following:

- Muscle veins
- Three calf veins, namely, the anterior and posterior tibial veins and peroneal veins
- Popliteal vein
- Femoral vein
- Common femoral vein
- Deep femoral vein
- Deep parts of the numerous perforating veins (Figs. 14.1, 2.25, 2.26, 2.27, 2.28, and 2.29)

It must be emphasised that the term "superficial femoral vein" has been replaced by "femoral vein" (Caggiati et al. 2002). The term "communicating veins" is reserved for linking veins within the same system.

The deep veins of the leg accompany the arteries of the same name and are generally paired in the calf. However, their junctions are not paired and their locations are variable. In the context of diagnosing a deep vein thrombosis, the posterior tibial and peroneal veins are the most frequently affected.

The posterior tibial veins arise in the deep calf compartment and join the peroneal veins. They are joined also by perforating veins from the posterior arch veins and the great saphenous vein (Chaps. 2

E. Mendoza et al. (eds.), *Duplex Ultrasound of Superficial Leg Veins*,
DOI 10.1007/978-3-642-40731-4_14, © Springer-Verlag Berlin Heidelberg 2014

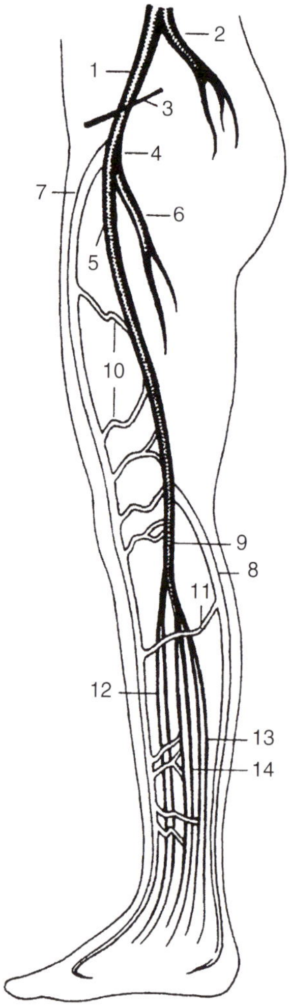

Fig. 14.1 Anatomy of the deep and superficial vein systems of the leg: *1* external iliac vein, *2* internal iliac vein, *3* inguinal ligament, *4* common femoral vein, *5* femoral vein (formerly superficial), *6* deep femoral vein, *7* great saphenous vein, *8* small saphenous vein, *9* popliteal vein, *10* perforating veins, *11* superficial communicating vein, *12* anterior tibial vein, *13* posterior tibial vein, *14* peroneal vein (From Strauss (1995)) Copyright: Springer

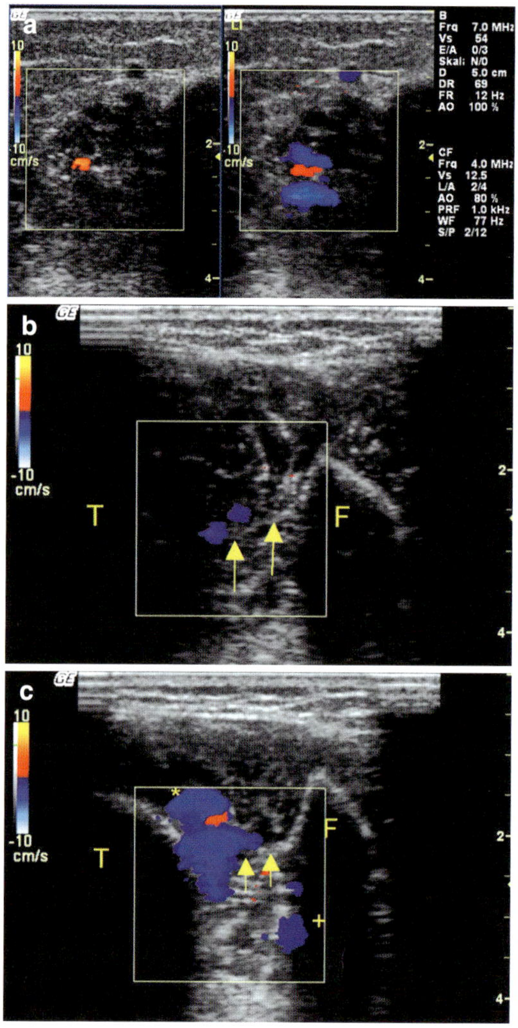

Fig. 14.2 (**a**) Transverse view through the distal and middle thirds of the calf in a standing patient. The posterior tibial artery is shown with its accompanying veins. *Left*, at rest. The tibial artery (*red*) is seen between two veins (*black*). The great saphenous vein is seen at the top of the colour duplex window. *Right*, during muscular systole. The posterior tibial veins demonstrate antegrade flow (*blue*). (**b**) Transverse view through the front of the calf in a standing patient. The probe has been placed lateral to the edge of the tibia. The paired anterior tibial veins are shown during muscular systole (*blue*) between the tibia (*T*) and fibula (*F*) but anterior to the interosseous membrane (*yellow arrows*). (**c**) Transverse view lateral to the edge of the tibia during muscular systole. The anterior tibial veins are shown with the anterior tibial artery in the centre (*). In addition, the peroneal veins (+) can be seen on the posterior side of the interosseous membrane (*yellow arrows*) Copyright: [Author]

and 9). Using ultrasound they are best visualised from the medial side. In the lower third of the calf, their course is relatively superficial where they are easily noticeable. This is apparent especially in the standing patient because of their paired position in relation to a central artery (Fig. 14.2a).

The anterior tibial veins are usually small so they cannot be always identified with certainty. They run anterior to the interosseous membrane and are best shown by positioning the probe transversely and

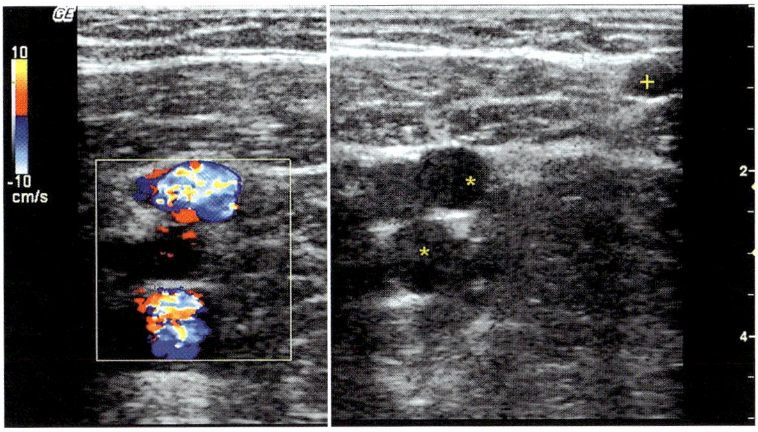

Fig. 14.3 Transverse view through the thigh demonstrating duplication of the common femoral vein (*) during muscular systole (*left*) and in B scan (*right*). Approximately 5 cm further down the great saphenous vein (+) is also visible in the image (on the online material there are further examples of duplicate femoral and popliteal veins with thrombi in one of the two lumens) Copyright: [Author]

lateral to the edge of the tibia (Fig. 14.2b, c). In the upper third of the calf, they pierce the interosseous membrane and run posterior where they join the posterior tibial and peroneal veins at a variable level to form the popliteal vein.

The *peroneal veins* run upwards on the anterior side of the interosseous membrane just medial to the fibula. In their course in the upper part of the calf, they receive blood from the muscle veins. They are best identified higher up in the calf where they form large calibre calf veins. On ultrasound they are best seen from a posterior viewpoint.

The gastrocnemius and soleus veins are the most clinically significant muscle veins in the calf. They have a large lumen in the standing patient, and they are often the point of origin of a deep vein thrombosis. The gastrocnemius veins join the popliteal vein either in isolation or together with the small saphenous vein at an acute angle (Sect. 2.5 and Figs. 8.14, 8.15, 8.16, and 8.17).

Knowledge of the variations in this region is important for diagnosing thrombosis. In one study (Kubik 1985 in Appendix 2), a single popliteal trunk vein was found in the popliteal fossa in only 55 % of legs. In 40 % there were two trunk veins which joined the femoral vein, generally together to form a single femoral vein. However, in around 2 % of cases, duplicate trunk veins join duplicate femoral veins. In 5 %, three or more trunk veins are present in the popliteal fossa. In addition, the small saphenous vein and its cranial extension (vein of Giacomini) may run through the popliteal fossa (Chap. 8).

In the **thigh**, the upward extension of the popliteal vein from the adductor hiatus to its junction with the deep femoral vein is known as the femoral vein (Caggiati et al. 2002). The term superficial femoral vein should no longer be used in order to avoid potentially dangerous confusion with superficial veins in clinical treatment decisions. For example, superficial vein thrombosis (phlebitis) may be a thrombosis of the great saphenous vein, but it usually does not involve the "superficial" femoral vein, or a diagnosis of superficial femoral vein thrombosis may indicate to some less experienced practitioners a thrombus in a superficial vein rather than the very significant deep venous thrombosis that actually is present. The femoral vein courses upwards, winding medially around the femur to reach an anterior position in the groin. Around 2–7 cm below the skin crease of the groin, it is joined by the deep femoral vein. At this point it becomes the common femoral vein (Fig. 7.20). A deep vein thrombosis can be missed easily if only one of the limbs of a duplicate femoral vein is involved (Fig. 14.3).

The *deep femoral vein* can generally only be seen on ultrasound near its junction with the femoral vein from the posterolateral aspect (Fig. 7.20).

The *common femoral vein* is only a few centimetres long. It is joined by the great saphenous vein and some other tributaries which enter it directly in the region of the saphenofemoral junction. The term saphenofemoral junction is preferred to synonyms like "crosse" or "confluence of superficial inguinal veins". The common femoral vein then runs cranially under the inguinal ligament where it becomes the external iliac vein.

Table 14.1 Stages of deep vein thrombosis

Description	Location	Proximal limit
One level	Limited to the calf veins	Below the popliteal vein
Two levels	Calf and popliteal veins	Popliteal vein
Three levels	Calf, popliteal and thigh veins	Femoral vein or common femoral vein
Four levels	Calf, popliteal, thigh and pelvic veins	Iliac vein

14.2 Deep Leg Vein and Muscle Vein Thrombosis

14.2.1 Definition of Deep Vein Thrombosis

In clinical practice deep vein thrombosis is a thrombus formation in the deep veins of the leg.

In most cases the **proximal extent** of a thrombosis is easily visualised and well delimited. Thus, a calf vein thrombosis is termed when the proximal end of the thrombus is below the popliteal vein. In calf and popliteal vein thrombosis, the proximal end of the thrombus ends in the popliteal vein. If the femoral vein is thrombosed up to the inguinal ligament, this is described as a calf, popliteal and femoral vein thrombosis. A further stage may involve a thrombosis of the iliac vein. Here the proximal end of the thrombus remains in the iliac vein, below the junction with the inferior vena cava (Table 14.1).

Deep vein thrombosis may **ascend** in an ordered fashion from the calf upwards involving the upper segments in sequence. Less frequently they may develop in a localised segment within the thigh, and rarely, they may descend from the iliac vein (Sect. 14.2.4). Thrombosis is a dynamic process with concurrent propagation, detachment, resolution and recanalisation occurring in varying degrees.

14.2.2 Diagnostic Techniques

The historical technique for diagnosing a deep vein thrombosis used to be with **CW Doppler** ultrasound. Its diagnostic value is limited because of incomplete imaging and a diagnosis based on exclusion. For example, if there is duplication a wrong diagnosis may result. Thrombosis of one limb may not be recognised because of incomplete imaging, and the patent remaining limb may give the false reassurance of a negative diagnosis. Furthermore, the diagnostic criteria using CW Doppler ultrasound are very dependent on the experience and technique of the examiner. This leads to a high risk of misinterpretation. Whilst the safety of a diagnosis in the proximal veins is quite good, with a maximum sensitivity of 80–85 % and a specificity of 85 %, the sensitivity and specificity in the calf are unacceptably low.

Now that **B scan** and **duplex ultrasound** are generally available, these techniques should be used exclusively for diagnosing thrombosis. They have greater diagnostic precision. For decades ascending phlebography was the gold standard test in the diagnosis of a deep vein thrombosis. However, venous compression ultrasound, and its systematic use in the technique of complete compression ultrasound (CCUS), has now pushed phlebography into the background (Schellong et al. 2009). Other points in favour of compression ultrasound are its non-invasive nature and the practical advantage of a rapid on-the-spot diagnosis. This is because of the portability of the ultrasound machine in everyday clinical use. Furthermore, the simultaneous use of B scan ultrasound may help in the differential diagnosis. These include recognition of a ruptured Baker's cyst, torn or bruised muscle fibres, an aneurysm, compartment syndrome or a tumour. Tissue ultrasound also makes it possible to determine the location and extent of oedema. The above factors have led to a considerable increase in examination frequency as compared to phlebography. High-quality compression ultrasound is now readily available in most hospitals.

The few remaining indications for conventional **phlebography** are when the ultrasound findings do not yield a clear diagnosis or for monitoring and research purposes. Descending phlebography is helpful in assessing the level and

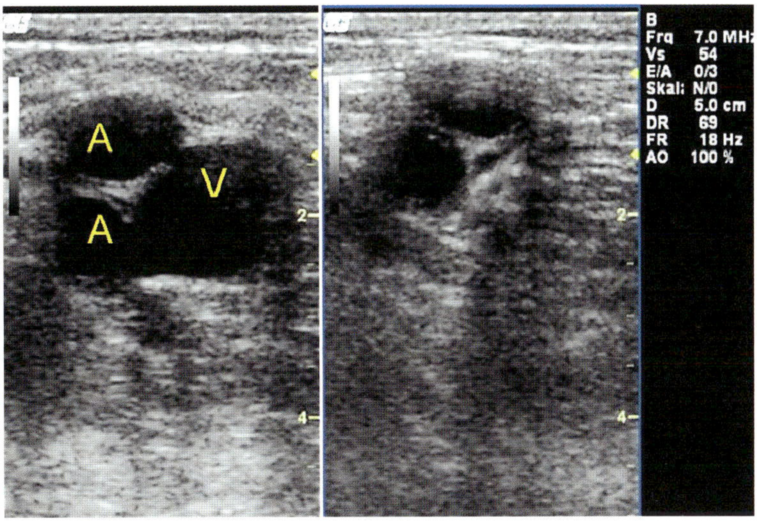

Fig. 14.4 Transverse view through the right groin demonstrating a normal femoral vein (*V*) in the supine patient without (*left*) and with compression (*right*). Artery (*A*). In the supine patient the vein can be compressed easily, and the lumen of the arteries is unaffected by the pressure. In the standing patient (not shown), the vein is fuller and greater pressure is required for vein compression. Occasionally, the arteries may narrow or even close under this pressure (see online material) Copyright: [Author]

grade of deep venous reflux as a pre-operative assessment for deep venous valve repair. Computerised tomographic venography (CTV) with direct contrast injection into the femoral vein and intravenous ultrasound (IVUS) may both assist in the evaluation of post-thrombotic obstruction of the external and common iliac veins and vena cava.

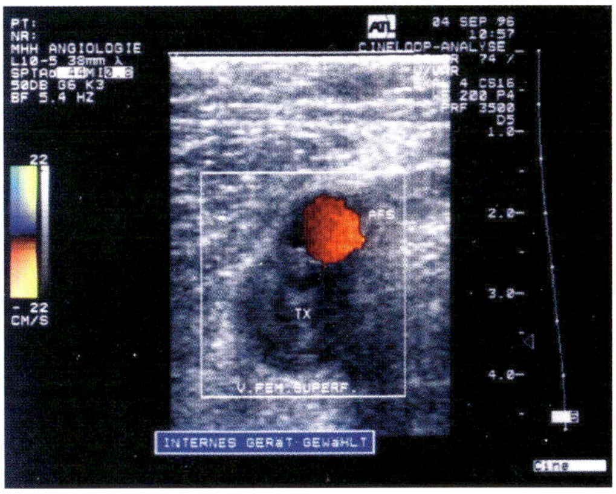

Fig. 14.5 Transverse view through the left groin demonstrating a fresh thrombus of the femoral vein. The vein diameter is much larger than that of the accompanying artery (*red*). In a supine patient the femoral vein is normally smaller (Fig. 5.3a, b) Copyright: [Author]

14.2.3 Ultrasound Criteria for Thrombosis

The essential, scientifically proven, **exclusion criterion** for thrombosis is complete compressibility of the vein when the probe is placed across the course of the vein in B scan (Figs. 14.4 and 5.10). The disappearance of the colour signal under pressure is not a strict requirement for exclusion. Any hindrance to complete compressibility of a vein segment caused by an intraluminal defect must be reproducible. This can be achieved by varying the position of the probe or the direction of compression.

If the visibility in B scan is not optimal, the addition of **colour coding**, in combination with manual compression below the probe, can improve the diagnostic yield by accelerating the flow. The junctions of the great and small saphenous vein with the deep veins should be examined also in longitudinal section. This is because ascending thrombus arising from the saphenous veins and emerging into the deep veins can be seen with greater clarity, despite apparent compressibility of the deep vein (Chap. 11). The echogenicity of a thrombus is not a reliable indication as to its maturity.

It is prudent to use additional **ultrasound criteria** to support the diagnosis even if they are not sufficiently validated. These include:

- The vessel diameter in acute thrombosis, which should be measured and compared with the adjacent artery in the supine patient (Fig. 14.5).

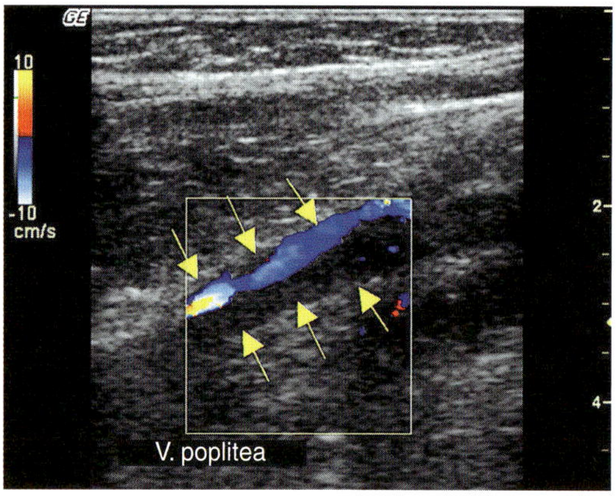

Fig. 14.6 Longitudinal view through the popliteal fossa during muscular systole demonstrating a thrombosis of the popliteal vein (*arrowed*). This has existed for 6 weeks. The popliteal vein has partly recanalised Copyright: [Author]

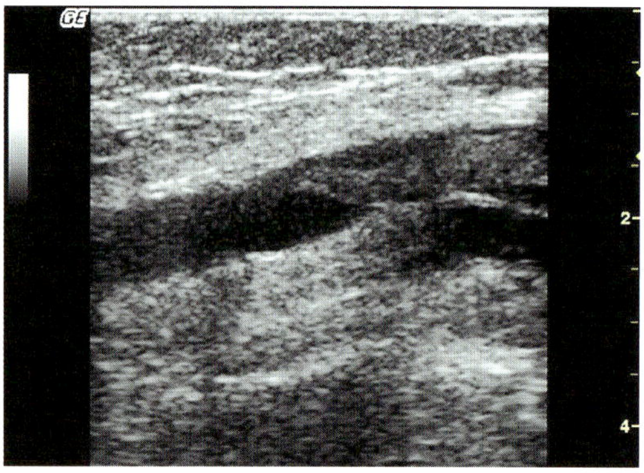

Fig. 14.7 Longitudinal view through the back of the distal thigh showing the proximal extent of a thrombus within the popliteal vein (*right*), just prior to where it becomes the femoral vein Copyright: [Author]

- The echo-rich patterns within an old thrombus in the vein lumen (Fig. 14.6) with changes in the flow direction in collateral vessels.
- The proximal extent of an acute thrombus in longitudinal view (Fig. 14.7). Although the end of the thrombus is free floating, this has no proven value in influencing the likelihood of a detachment and subsequent pulmonary embolism (Aschwanden et al. 2001).
- Loss of the normal respiratory modulation of flow with partial or complete obstruction in a proximal vein. In deep veins further distal, there may be an antegrade continuous linear flow unaffected by stimulation manoeuvres (Figs. 14.8 and 6.7).

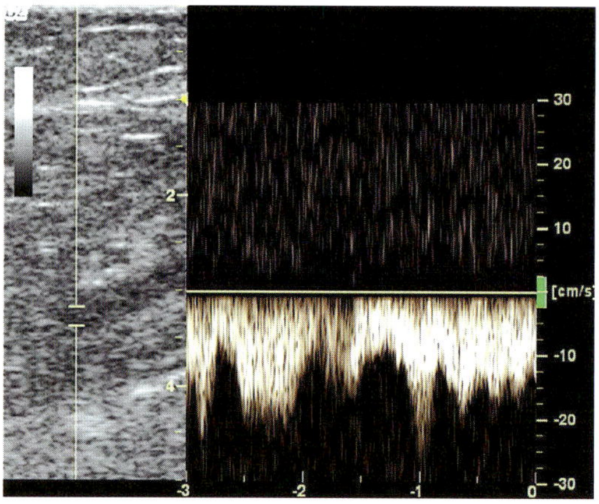

Fig. 14.8 A constant antegrade flow pattern in the popliteal vein when the femoral vein is obstructed (on online material, flow in the healthy leg is shown for comparison). This flow is not modulated by respiration nor is it accelerated by stimulation manoeuvres Copyright: [Author]

14.2.4 Standard Examination, Choice of Probe and Patient's Position

National and international guidelines offer standardised algorithms for the ultrasound examination in patients with a suspected diagnosis of a deep vein thrombosis. The examination must include the common femoral, femoral and popliteal veins as well as the saphenofemoral and saphenopopliteal junctions, as well as the iliac, deep femoral and calf veins. The examination should proceed from proximal to distal. We have to differentiate between patients that developed their thrombosis after surgery who remain in bed and those with an ambulatory-acquired thrombosis. The former should be kept lying during the examination because of a theoretical (unproven) risk that mobilisation may precipitate a pulmonary embolism. The latter may be investigated lying, sitting or standing.

The deep veins in the **thigh** are examined with the patient lying down, the trunk raised and the leg turned slightly outwards using a 4–7 MHz ultrasound probe. Starting at the groin, the vein segments to be examined are mapped with a continuous transverse image whilst compressing the vein periodically against the femur. The femoral

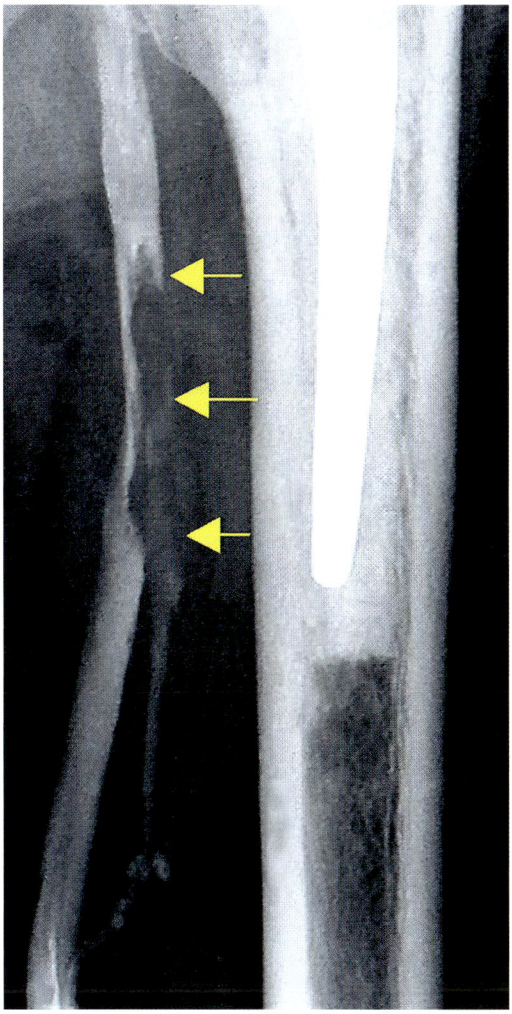

Fig. 14.9 Phlebographic image of a segmental thrombosis of the femoral vein after a hip operation Copyright: [Author]

vein can be examined more easily in the region of the adductor canal if the examiner compresses it with his free hand from the posterior side, against the probe, rather than directly with the probe. The *deep femoral vein* should also be examined at its junction with the femoral vein in transverse and longitudinal views. This is because a thrombosis can originate at this level, especially after hip operations (Fig. 14.9).

The best position for examining the *popliteal vein* is with the patient lying prone and, if necessary, with a support under the feet, or from the side. If the patient is immobile, then the examination can take place supine with the knees bent. The probe is positioned in the popliteal region and moved up and down. The aim is to achieve sufficient overlap with the distal femoral vein. This is difficult with the patient sitting.

The preferred position for examination of the **calf veins** is with the patient sitting and the legs hanging dependently. Thromboses in the calf are most often found in the peroneal and posterior tibial veins. Isolated thromboses in the anterior tibial veins are rare. With more localised pain or pain under pressure, thrombosis of a perforating vein or a muscle vein should be suspected (Sect. 14.2.6 and Chap. 9).

If thrombosis is suspected in an ambulatory patient, strict rest is contraindicated. The patient should be examined standing and sitting. Thrombosis-free veins distend whilst standing and are easier to find, especially in the calf. The disadvantage of standing is that the muscle tension may hamper the compression ultrasound test. A combination of sitting and standing is therefore recommended.

The contralateral leg should also be examined. It has been shown that the **contralateral leg** of a proven thrombosis has a coexisting thrombosis in up to 20 % of patients. Some recommendations are to compress the common femoral vein and the popliteal vein at only two points during the examination with the aim of shortening the examination time. However, this strategy is at the cost of a high risk of overlooking segmental thromboses (Fig. 14.10) or thrombi extending out of the perforating veins into the deep system. A limited examination strategy is not advised (Badgett et al. 2000).

A high specificity of >90 % can be achieved in the diagnosis of calf vein thrombosis using compression ultrasound. A thorough examination of the lower leg to exclude thrombosis should be included in all patients with medical conditions where a deep vein thrombosis is suspected (Lindhoff-Last 2011).

After a thorough compression ultrasound investigation, a 3-month incidence of deep vein thrombosis after initial negative investigation

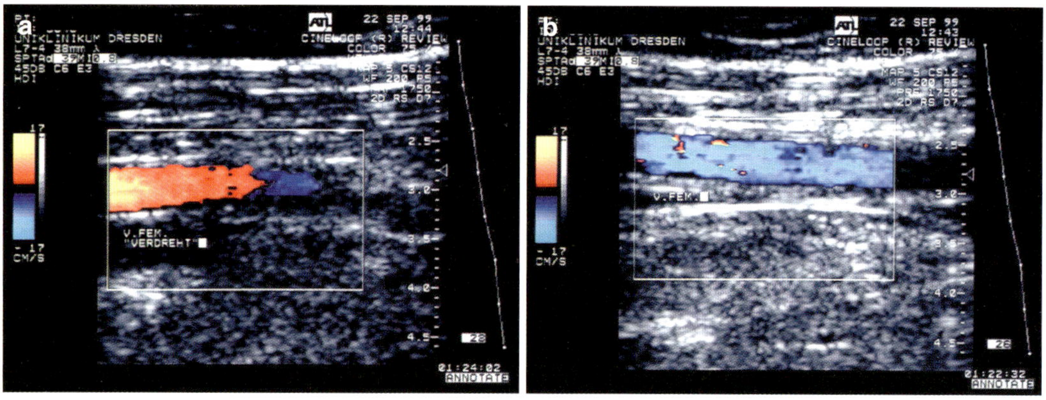

Fig. 14.10 A common pitfall may occur when examining the femoral vein in longitudinal view. Thrombotic closure is suggested because the course of the vein is not straight (**a**). A uniform uninterrupted sound signal can only be seen when the position of the probe is corrected (**b**) Copyright: [Author]

was 0–0.8 % (95 % CI 0.1–1.6) (Schellong et al. 2009; Elias et al 2003; Gottlieb et al 2003).

14.2.5 Possible Errors

With a **very fresh thrombosis,** the vein may still be compressible by strong pressure from the probe. The soft thrombotic material is unable to resist the deformation forces produced by the probe. Furthermore, **non-thrombosed vein segments** in strong muscles with unfavourable angles of compression may appear uncompressible. The femoral vein at the adductor canal or the peroneal group of veins are often hard to compress.

If the probe is positioned **longitudinally** when examining the femoral vein and it is moved off the vessel's axis because the vessel does not run straight, thrombotic closure may be suggested. This error can be avoided by placing the probe in a transverse position (Fig. 14.10).

Venous valves may be confused with intraluminal threads of thrombus. This can be clarified by changing the angle of insonation and the imaging axis (Fig. 14.11a) and also by adding colour (Fig. 14.11b) and by using compression.

Small thromboses in the calf veins can easily be overlooked, especially if they are only present in one segment, for example, in only one of the posterior tibial veins (Fig. 14.12).

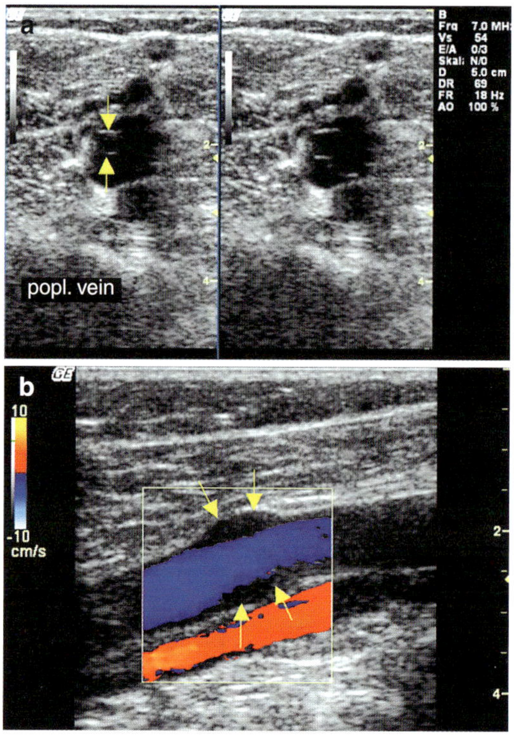

Fig. 14.11 (**a**) Transverse view through the popliteal fossa showing the popliteal vein with echo-producing structures in the lumen (*arrowed*) (longitudinal view and film sequence on online material). (**b**) Longitudinal view of the popliteal fossa during muscular systole. The blood flow shown in blue is not occupying the full diameter of the popliteal vein (*arrowed*). In B scan it was shown that this flow pattern was caused by valve cusps (online material) Copyright: [Author]

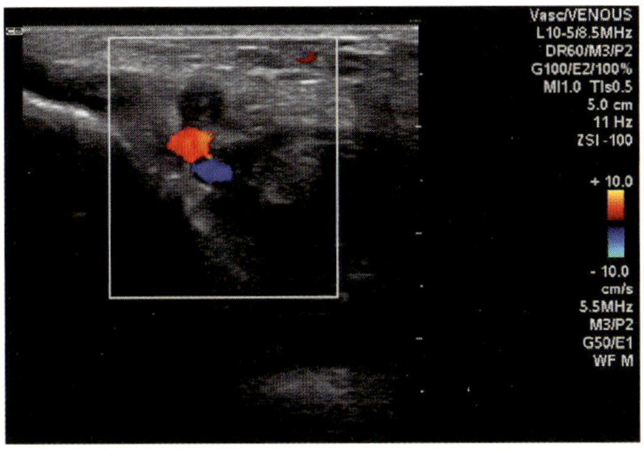

Fig. 14.12 Thrombosis in one of the distal posterior tibial veins at the ankle. Compression ultrasound on online material Copyright: [Author]

14.2.6 Muscle Vein Thrombosis

Thromboses frequently occur in the muscle veins of the calf. Therefore, they should always be included in the routine examination protocol. Muscle veins should be regarded as a distinct venous group because of their special haemodynamic situation as the outflow of the calf muscle pump. They differ from other veins because of the presence of numerous valves and the rapid dilatation of the trunk vessel from the convergence of numerous inflow veins.

Muscle vein thromboses in the lower leg refer principally to thromboses of the **soleus** and **gastrocnemius vein systems**. As with deep vein thrombosis, muscle vein thrombosis is excluded using compression ultrasound (Fig. 14.13). Their examination does not differ from the ultrasound process used for deep veins. Muscle vein thrombosis can be diagnosed also using tissue harmonic imaging (THI) or an ultrasound CT technique (cross beam) as well as with pure B scan. Any clear advantages using these techniques have yet to be evaluated in practice (Sect. 1.3).

14.3 Ultrasound Changes After a Deep Vein Thrombosis

After a deep vein thrombosis, the affected vein segment may present **post-thrombotic changes**. These include permanent closure, partial recanalisation with residual thrombus on the walls, or simply wall irregularities. Alternatively, there may be no identifiable changes to suggest a previous deep vein thrombosis. The presence of thrombotic residua is associated with an increased risk of recurrence. The remaining thrombotic mass can be documented in percent of obstructed versus recanalised vein in transverse view or in millimetres of uncompressible lumen. These changes as well as the site of an occlusion or obstruction may influence the duration of anticoagulation treatment for secondary prevention (Lindhoff-Last 2011).

Permanent post-thrombotic valve incompetence may develop after a deep vein thrombosis. This is seen as a pathologically retrograde refluxive flow occurring spontaneously or under stimulation. This can be evaluated qualitatively and quantitatively by colour duplex ultrasound. In a standing patient, the blood in any vein should flow out of the leg. The concept of **chronic venous insufficiency** indicates any degree of diminution of the venous return to the heart ranging between outflow obstruction and deep venous reflux. Reflux in a vein segment generally leads to venous hypertension in the region of venous drainage. The clinical symptoms are caused by the local manifestations of venous hypertension. In pathophysiological terms, three separate groups of causes of chronic venous insufficiency can be defined:

1. Obstruction of the venous flow by thrombotic occlusion or compression of proximal vein segments.
2. Reflux in the deep veins after a recanalised deep vein thrombosis. This is caused by direct valve destruction or by the long-term effects of volume overloading from recirculation.
3. Hindrance of the calf-muscle pump with restricted dorsal extension and/or flexion of the foot.

The presence of reflux and obstruction results in chronic venous hypertension which forms part of the duplex manifestations of the **post-thrombotic syndrome**.

Duplex ultrasound is useful for showing **old thrombotic changes** after a deep vein thrombosis which helps to differentiate the post-thrombotic syndrome from primary varicose

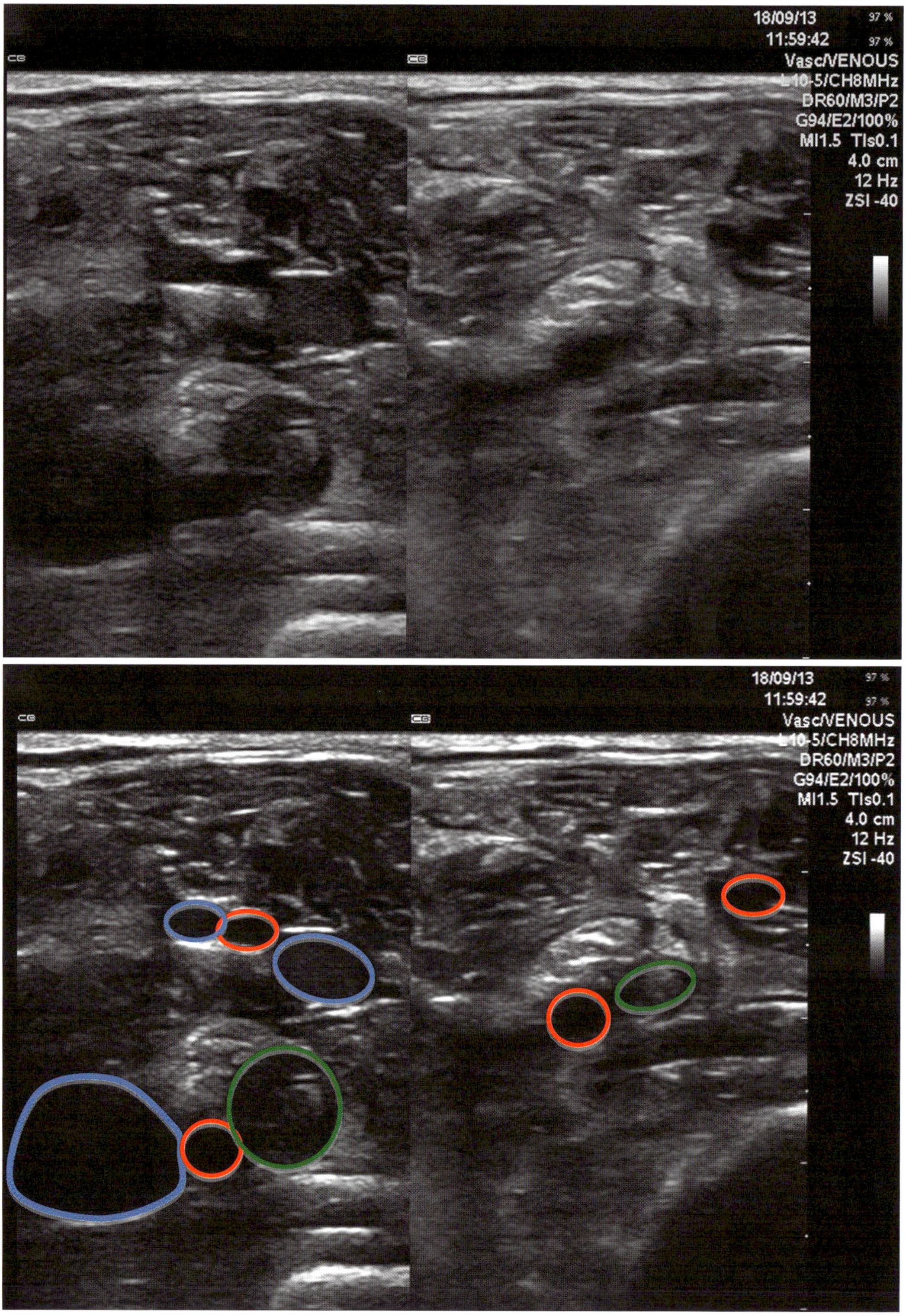

Fig. 14.13 Compression ultrasound image of a venous thrombosis in the gastrocnemius muscle without (*top*) and with (*bottom*) compression (see online material). In *blue* are muscle veins, in *green* is the one with a thrombus and in *red* are arteries. The thrombus in one muscle vein (*green*) and the arteries are seen in the *right image* under compression Copyright: Erika Mendoza

veins. In practice, reflux is assessed by examining the most accessible segments and those which can be imaged most reliably. These are the femoral, popliteal, peroneal and posterior tibial veins. However, a deep vein thrombosis can be missed if the entire system is not thoroughly examined.

The Valsalva manoeuvre is useful only for checking the closure capacity of venous valves in the groin. It is harder to evaluate venous valves in more peripheral vein segments when stimulation manoeuvres are required. This can be achieved manually by calf compression or by using pneumatic cuffs. However, muscle activation by the patient is a more physiological stimulation manoeuvre (Chap. 6).

The presence of pathological venous **reflux** is defined as reflux lasting more than 0.5 s in superficial veins and >1 s in deep veins. In the popliteal vein, the maximum speed of reflux in post-thrombotic syndrome correlates with the clinical picture with a specificity of 95 % and a sensitivity of 92 %. With the standardisation of compression and relaxation manoeuvres, it is possible to use reflux speed as a quantitative measurement (Wuppermann 2002 in Appendix 2). However, in practice the assessment of reflux is limited to its description.

Duplex ultrasound images seldom show dilated collateral vessels (Fig. 14.14). If there are no thrombotic remains or echogenic wall irregularities present in a person without a primary varicose vein condition, then these collateral veins may be a sign of the post-thrombotic syndrome. This can be evaluated if necessary using phlebography since this may reveal recanalised deep veins which were unremarkable on duplex ultrasound.

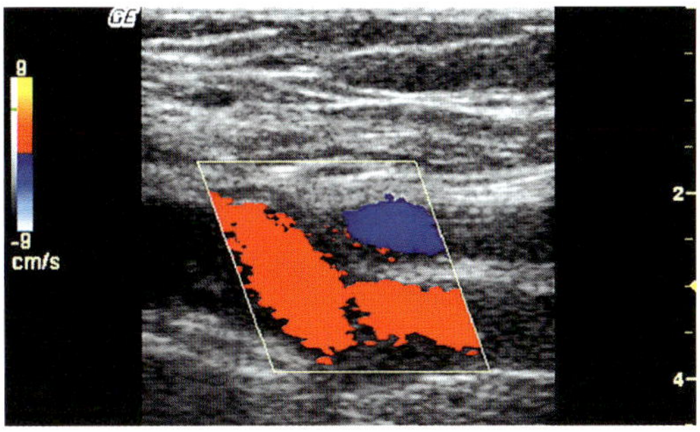

Fig. 14.14 Longitudinal section through the groin showing a dilated deep femoral vein (*red*) after thrombosis of the femoral vein which has now recanalised (*blue*). This is because the deep femoral vein (profunda femoral vein) has become the main drainage vein of the leg (axialisation). In both veins the flow is now antegrade (online material) Copyright: [Author]

14.4 Secondary Deep Vein Insufficiency

This term was coined by Hach for dilated deep leg veins in patients with **primary varicose veins** (Hach in Appendix 2); (see also Sect. 4.1.1). At first the deep leg veins are dilated by the recirculation volume. As the volume increases, the vein starts to dilate even further becoming tortuous until the valve becomes incompetent. This was originally demonstrated as a phlebographic finding, but this can now be shown by ultrasound particularly well in the region of the popliteal vein.

It is important to distinguish the post-thrombotic syndrome from secondary deep vein insufficiency. Elongation and increasing tortuosity of the popliteal vein usually indicates secondary deep vein insufficiency, as do trunk and tributary varices with large recirculation volumes. Secondary deep vein insufficiency, especially in the early phase of a failing valve, is generally reversible after treatment of the varicose veins.

14.5 Documentation and Description of Findings

The following procedure should be followed for documenting examination findings:

- In the **proximal leg veins** (common femoral vein and femoral vein, plus the popliteal vein if applicable), the transverse view of the thrombotic segment should be documented individually, both in the normal state and under compression with the probe.

- In the **lower leg veins**, the transverse view of the corresponding veins at the maximum point of thrombosis should likewise be documented individually, both in the normal state and under compression with the probe.
- To **describe the findings**, a textual description or a diagram of the vessel is required to show the extent and mobility of the thrombus, as well as recording the degree of pain caused by pressure.
- Individual documentation of the thigh and leg veins examined in diagnosing thrombosis (including by exclusion) should show the transverse view in the normal state and under compression with the probe (longitudinal view of iliac vein). It is advisable to show the two images side by side.

In **post-thrombotic syndrome** individual documentation of the longitudinal view through the femoral vein in the middle of the thigh is recommended, as well as the popliteal vein. The velocity profile under spontaneous flow conditions and under compression/decompression manoeuvres and/or the Valsalva manoeuvre should be provided.

References

Aschwanden M, Labs KH, Engel H (2001) Acute deep vein thrombosis: early mobilization does not increase the frequency of pulmonary embolism. Thromb Haemost 85:42–46

Badgett DK, Comerota MC, Khan MN, Eid IG, Kerr RP, Comerota AJ (2000) Duplex venous imaging: role for a comprehensive lower extremity examination. Ann Vasc Surg 14:73–76

Caggiati A, Bergan JJ, Gloviczki P, Jantet G, Wendell-Smith CP, Partsch H (2002) Nomenclature of the veins of the lower limbs: an international interdisciplinary consensus statement. J Vasc Surg 36:416–422

Elias A, Mallard L, Elias M et al (2003) A single complete ultrasound investigation of the venous network for the diagnostic management of patient with a clinically suspected first episode of deep venous thrombosis of the lower limbs. Thromb Haemost 89:221–227

Gottlieb RH, Voci SL, Syed L et al (2003) Randomized prospective study compaing routine versus selective use of sonography of the complete calf in patients with suspected deep venous thrombosis. Am J Roentgenol 180:241–245

Lindhoff-Last E (2011) Risk assessment of recurrence of venous thromboembolism. Hamostaseologie 31:7–12

Schellong S, Gerlach H, Hach-Wunderle V et al (2009) Diagnosis of deep vein thrombosis: adherence to guidelines and outcomes in real-world health care. Thromb Haemost 102:1234–1240

15 Examination of Superficial Veins in the Presence of Deep Venous Disease

Erika Mendoza and Christopher R. Lattimer

Chapter Summary

Deep venous disease may lead to secondary pathologies in the superficial veins and vice versa. A patient with existing incompetence in a superficial vein may also develop deep vein thrombosis and deep venous reflux. In this case two pathologies can occur in the same leg, namely, the aftermath of a deep vein thrombosis plus pre-existing disease in the superficial system. Regardless of the chronological order of disease and the mechanisms giving rise to them, special care must be taken when examining the superficial vein system in the presence of deep venous pathology. This is of particular importance when choosing the appropriate surgical treatment.

In functional terms, there are two possible ways in which the deep venous pathology may cause abnormalities in the superficial system:

1. The deep veins are no longer able to drain the leg in the presence of obstruction.
2. The deep veins are refluxive with retrograde flow in addition to antegrade flow.

E. Mendoza, MD, PhD (✉)
Venenpraxis Wunstorf,
Speckenstraße 10, 31515 Wunstorf, Germany
e-mail: erika.mendoza@t-online.de

C.R. Lattimer, MD, PhD
Department of Vascular Surgery,
Josef Pflug Vascular Laboratory,
Ealing Hospital and Imperial College, London, UK

15.1 Superficial Veins with Deep Venous Obstruction

The deep vein system may be occluded by thrombosis without recanalisation. Other causes include injuries to the deep veins, for example:

- Direct puncture of the leg veins in non-sterile conditions for intravenous drug consumption resulting in sepsis and abscess formation
- Injury to the vessels in neonates due to repetitive cannulation of the common femoral vein
- Injuries to the deep leg veins in major trauma

Complete obstruction (occlusion) of a deep vein due to tumour infiltration (e.g. sarcoma) occurs but is rare in everyday practice. Congenital atresia of the vena cava hampers the venous drainage of the legs with the development of huge collateral veins.

In a standing patient, **complete valve incompetence** of the deep leg veins may produce a condition similar to occlusion with failure of the venous return.

During examination of the superficial veins, large diameter saphenous trunks will be noticed. The flow in these veins is antegrade in the early stages of the disease (Fig. 15.1a, b). It is remarkable that a very large blood volume flow is observed during calf-muscle systole. During diastole the flow is also antegrade and generally constant and slow. Over the course of time, the excessive volume load will cause failure of valve closure in the superficial veins. This will lead to diastolic reflux and the formation of refluxive venous tributaries (Fig. 15.1c, d).

E. Mendoza et al. (eds.), *Duplex Ultrasound of Superficial Leg Veins*,
DOI 10.1007/978-3-642-40731-4_15, © Springer-Verlag Berlin Heidelberg 2014

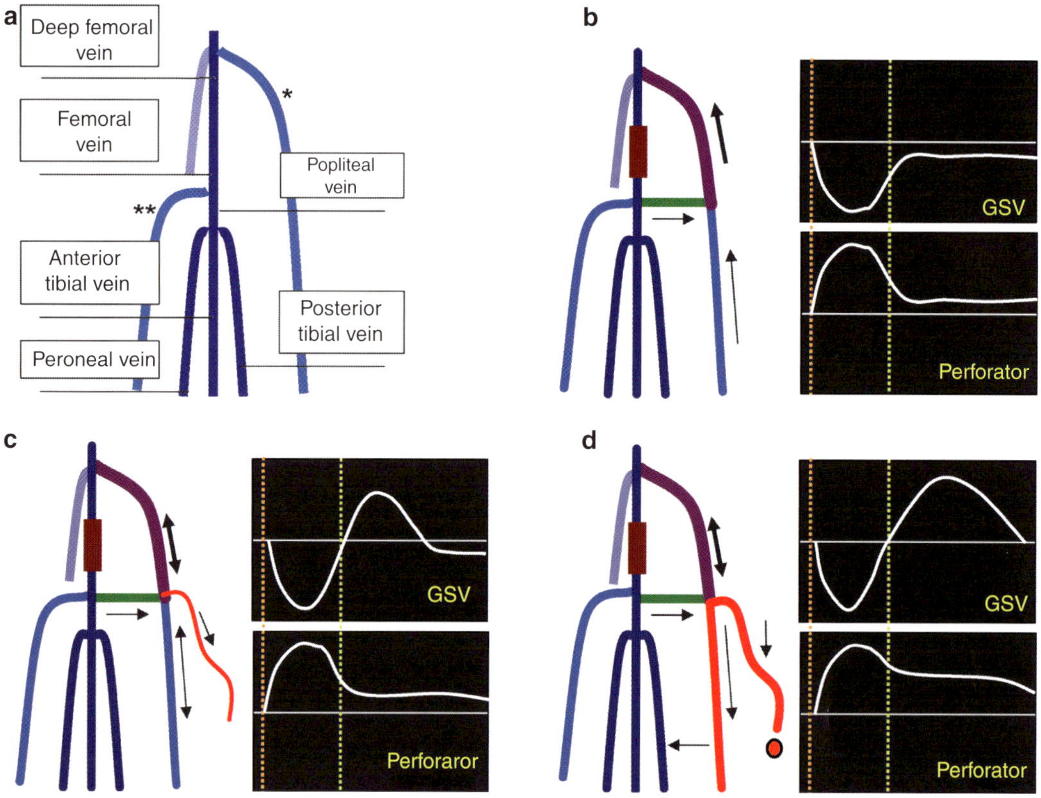

Fig. 15.1 (**a**) Diagram of the deep veins in the previously used scheme of the superficial leg veins with great saphenous vein (*) and small saphenous vein (**). (**b**) Development over time of flow in the great saphenous vein (*VSM*) with an occluded femoral vein (formerly superficial). *Dark red*, vertical obstruction; *orange dotted line*, beginning of muscular systole (toes raised); *yellow dotted line*, beginning of muscular diastole (toes lowered). The blood flows from the distal calf through a paratibial perforating vein (formerly Boyd; *green*). The flow is antegrade at first into the great saphenous vein causing its dilatation (*violet*). (**c**) Commencement of oscillating volume flow as valve closure starts to fail in the over-dilated great saphenous vein. Furthermore, a deep to superficial drainage flow develops within this segment of refluxive great saphenous vein. This drainage during calf systole can occur either via an incompetent great saphenous vein or an incompetent venous tributary. (**d**) Refluxive venous tributaries are seen receiving flow volumes from the great saphenous vein. Although the vein is technically refluxive, the considerably large volume of blood with antegrade flow is remarkable. Meanwhile, several refluxive venous tributaries have formed, and the lower part of the great saphenous vein has yielded and become refluxive. This reflux volume fills the deep system at the ankle during muscular diastole. As a result of this increased flow and pressure, the perforating vein dilates and an outward flow may also be recorded in the perforating vein during calf systole Copyright: [Author]

The flow of blood leaves the deep vein system through a perforating vein. The blood flow in this vein is retrograde, refluxive and outwards. It brings blood from deep to superficial veins (Fig. 15.2) and serves to drain the lower segments of the deep veins because they no longer have a drainage route due to higher obstruction.

Blood will flow upwards in the superficial veins and then re-enter the deep veins above the point of closure. This occurs usually after femoral vein (formerly superficial) occlusion through the saphenofemoral junction. This pathway is called an open compensatory (vicarious) shunt (Franceschi and Zamboni 2010).

When the common femoral vein or the iliac vein is blocked, the blood finds a way to the contralateral pelvic veins through an anastomosis via the saphenofemoral junction. Large calibre veins can be seen above the pubic bone which drain into the saphenofemoral junction of the contralateral leg. Drainage of the diseased leg takes place through the contralateral saphenofemoral

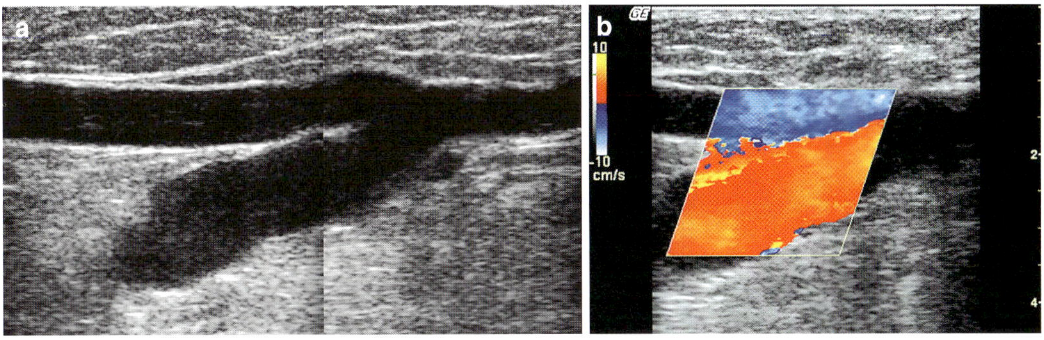

Fig. 15.2 The aftermath of occlusion of the common femoral vein in the right leg due to an abscess in an iv heroin abuser. Dilated perforating veins are seen in the adductor canal (formerly Dodd). These carry blood outwards into the great saphenous vein. This increase in flow causes saphenous dilatation in an attempt to bypass the femoral occlusion. Although most of the blood in the upper part flows antegrade, the lower segment also becomes refluxive which can give rise to several refluxive venous tributaries. (**a**) Longitudinal view of the inner thigh. Dilated perforating vein in the adductor canal (formerly Dodd) which drains into the great saphenous vein. *Right*, in the picture, refluxive lower segment of great saphenous vein; *left*, dilated great saphenous vein with antegrade flow. (**b**) The same leg in colour duplex during calf-muscle systole. Outward flow is seen in the perforating vein with antegrade flow up to the great saphenous vein. See accompanying online material Copyright: [Author]

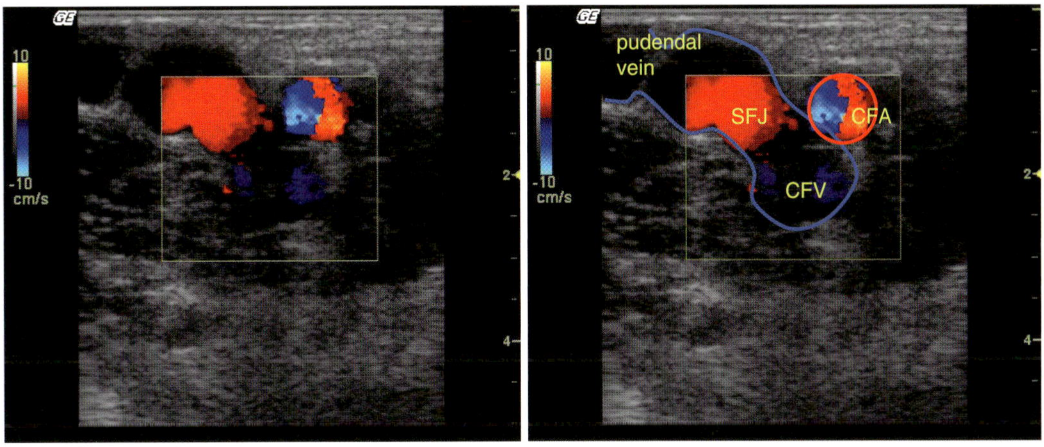

Fig. 15.3 Flow in the saphenofemoral junction with a spontaneous Palma shunt. This occurs several days after a thrombosis with occlusion of the left iliac vein and common femoral vein. The femoral vein (formerly superficial) is partly recanalised. Drainage of the diseased left leg occurs through the right side. Blood is bypassed to the right side via the ipsilateral pudendal vein. Here it reaches the contralateral pelvic veins through the confluence of the great saphenous vein (*GSV*). See accompanying online material Copyright: [Author]

junction into the contralateral common femoral vein. These cross-pelvic collaterals are often called as **spontaneous Palma shunt** (Fig. 15.3).

15.2 Superficial Veins with Deep Venous Reflux

A refluxive deep system after the destruction of valves by thrombosis is more common than a permanent occlusion. When blood is pumped upwards during calf-muscle systole, a part will leave the leg while a part will reflux back into the deep vein system. This results in oscillating flow patterns back and forth in the deep veins like a see-saw.

This increases the pressure during muscular diastole which impedes the superficial to deep drainage pathway (Sect. 3.1.2). The result is a permanent dilatation of the perforating and superficial veins whose valve leaflets no longer meet. The ensuing reflux is termed **secondary** incompetence (Fig. 15.4a).

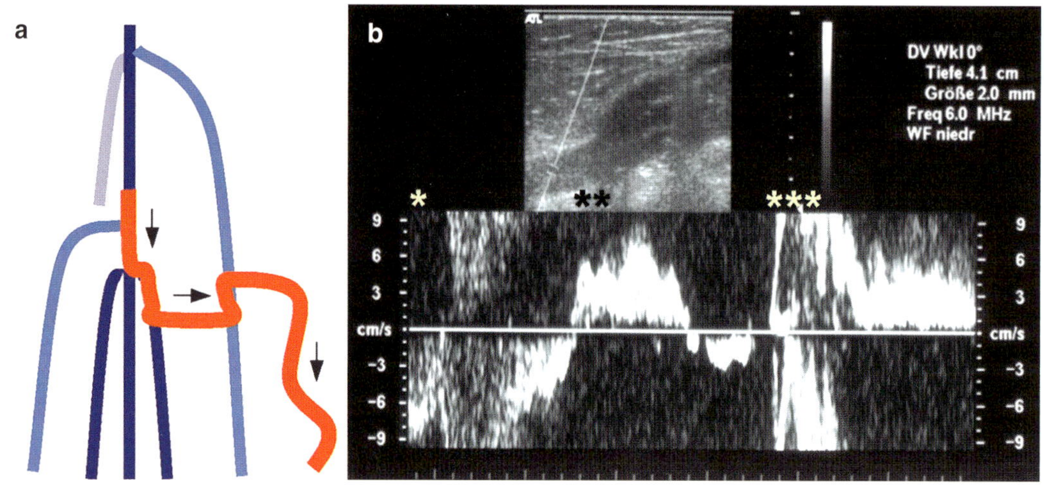

Fig. 15.4 (**a**) The aftermath of a thrombosis of the posterior tibial vein. Reflux is seen descending from the popliteal vein down to the posterior tibial and the paratibial perforating veins (formerly Boyd) and then into the great saphenous vein. Blood then refluxes from the great saphenous vein into varicose tributaries. (**b**) Longitudinal view through the popliteal vein using PW duplex with digital occlusion of the refluxive perforating vein. The reflux pathway is temporarily abolished (* toes raised, ** toes lowered, *** pressure on perforating vein released). See accompanying online material Copyright: [Author]

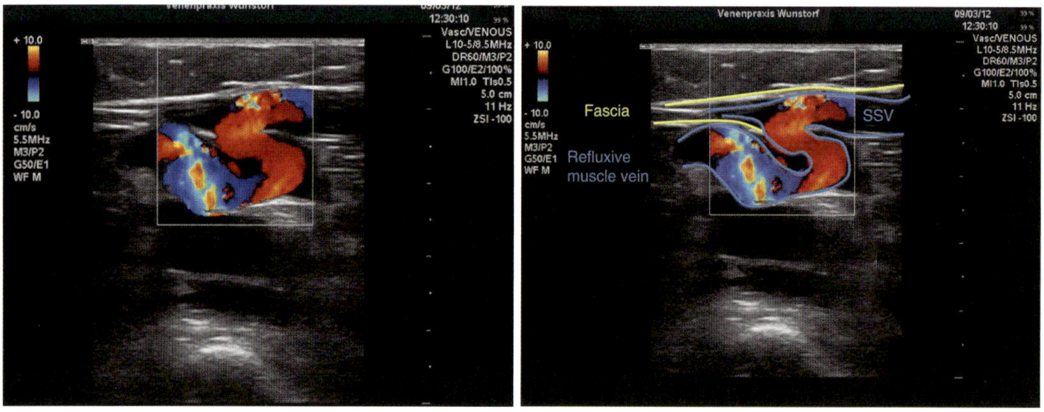

Fig. 15.5 Reflux is seen arising from a post-thrombotic muscle vein and into the small saphenous vein. This remains competent at its upper end but becomes refluxive at the point of entry of the perforating vein Copyright: [Author]

As the number of secondary varicosities increases, this has the effect of increasing the venous volume and varicose reservoir. The resulting pressure in the deep and superficial veins can no longer be eased by the calf-muscle pump. This leads to the post-thrombotic syndrome and **chronic venous insufficiency** (see also Sect. 14.4). The influence of the individual perforating veins on the volumes of reflux in the deep vein system (and thus also the prospects for clinical success in interrupting the perforating veins) can be established semi-quantitatively by digital compression of the perforating veins during examination in PW mode (Fig. 15.4b).

A common **special form** of secondary varicose veins is found in post-thrombotic valve destruction of a muscular vein. This results in retrograde flow with reflux outwards via a perforating vein and then into the small saphenous vein (Fig. 15.5, see also Figs. 8.15 and 8.17). The small saphenous vein becomes secondarily refluxive.

15.3 Duplex Ultrasound as a Tool to Direct Treatment

In the presence of an existing pathology of the deep veins, the diagnosing doctor must decide whether treatment of the superficial veins will improve the haemodynamic condition of the leg. In such a situation, ultrasound is preferable to phlebography (Nicolaides 2000). One axiomatic rule must be followed.

If a superficial vein serves to drain the deep system, it must never be interrupted or removed.

The following **ultrasound criteria** will help to determine whether a superficial vein serves to drain the deep system:

- Dilated superficial vein with large antegrade systolic blood volumes irrespective of the presence of reflux
- Distally located perforating vein which fills the superficial vein from the deep vein system, in other words antegrade superficial flow via an outward perforating vein during calf systole (Fig. 15.2b)

Additional Criteria

- Worsening of findings in volume measurement methods like air plethysmography. If the calf-muscle pump ejection fraction and the outflow fraction reduce on digital occlusion of targeted veins, they should not be removed.
- A blue-red discolouration of the leg with pain of the vein on digital compression in the standing patient.

On the other hand, refluxing superficial veins which also fill the leg in a retrograde flow will act to increase the calf-diastolic pressure in the ankle region (Sect. 15.2). These veins should be treated only if their contribution to symptoms from reflux is much greater than their potential role as a deep drainage pathway. This evaluation requires much skill and experience. The venous filling index of air plethysmography is a useful test which may help because it can quantify the degree of reflux (Lattimer et al. 2012). Perforating veins should be interrupted if they do not contribute to drainage and are shown to increase the volume of reflux in the deep veins (Fig. 15.4b).

If the volume of reflux in the deep vein system is diminished in pulsed-wave mode (PW mode) under compression of the perforating vein, interruption should be considered (Fig. 15.4).

Exclusively refluxive tributaries must always be treated to reduce the venous reservoir as should refluxing saphenous veins which do not have a drainage function.

References

Franceschi C, Zamboni P (2010) Principles of venous haemodynamics. Novapublishers, New York

Lattimer CR, Azzam M, Kalodiki E, Geroulakos G (2012) Venous filling time using air-plethysmography correlates highly with great saphenous vein reflux time using duplex. Phlebology. PMID: 230350010. [in print]

Nicolaides AN (2000) Investigation of chronic venous insufficiency – a consensus statement. Circulation 102:126–163

16 Differential Diagnosis of Leg Oedemas of Venous and Lymphatic Origin

Erika Mendoza and Christopher R. Lattimer

Chapter Summary
Patients are often referred to the phlebologist or vascular surgeon suffering with leg swelling of uncertain origin. This is usually accompanied by a request to confirm or exclude venous insufficiency. Standard duplex ultrasound is useful for a primary haemodynamic evaluation. However, high-resolution ultrasound may distinguish between different types of oedema.

16.1 Definitions

Lymph is the tissue fluid which bathes cells. It has a filtration system that is so fine that it is not visible to the naked eye or ultrasound. Lymph flows in the pre-lymphatic canals, passing from the lymph capillaries and pre-collectors, which have a diameter of approximately 0.1 mm. Next, it flows into lymph collectors with diameters of 0.5 mm and then into the lymphatic channels of 2 mm diameter. The thoracic duct and the right lymphatic duct take the lymph from these channels where it drains into the venous system via the brachiocephalic veins. Only the lymphatic channels are visible on ultrasound. If they become obstructed, the lymph collector may dilate, in which case it also becomes visible (see below).

The classic **lymphatic oedema** or **lymphoedema** is caused by a disturbance of lymphatic drainage. This may be primary with no identifiable cause or due to congenital dysplasia or hypoplasia of the lymphatic channels. Secondary lymphoedema is usually caused by compression of the lymphatic channels from a tumour or destruction after an infection, operation or radiotherapy. Cellulitis and erysipelas are common features of clinical infection. The location and nature of the impediment to drainage is usually evaluated clinically. Further information and diagnostic thresholds can be established by lymphoscintigraphy. The clinical sign is swelling of the leg down to the foot. The oedema is pitting at first which becomes firm and very hard later. A positive *Stemmer sign* confirms lymphoedema when the skin on the dorsal surface of the toes cannot be lifted up into a fold. A hump on the dorsal surface of the foot with transverse skin creases at the bases of the toes with squaring of the toes themselves is also characteristic (Fig. 16.1). The skin colour is pale at first but becomes browny with advancing disease when the condition is termed dermatoliposclerosis. The appearance of hyperkeratosis, hyperpigmentation, verrucae, papillomas and fungal infections are also characteristic skin changes of advanced disease.

E. Mendoza, MD, PhD (✉)
Venenpraxis Wunstorf,
Speckenstraße 10, Wunstorf 31515, Germany
e-mail: erika.mendoza@t-online.de

C.R. Lattimer, MD, PhD
Department of Vascular Surgery,
Josef Pflug Vascular Laboratory,
Ealing Hospital and Imperial College, London, UK

E. Mendoza et al. (eds.), *Duplex Ultrasound of Superficial Leg Veins*,
DOI 10.1007/978-3-642-40731-4_16, © Springer-Verlag Berlin Heidelberg 2014

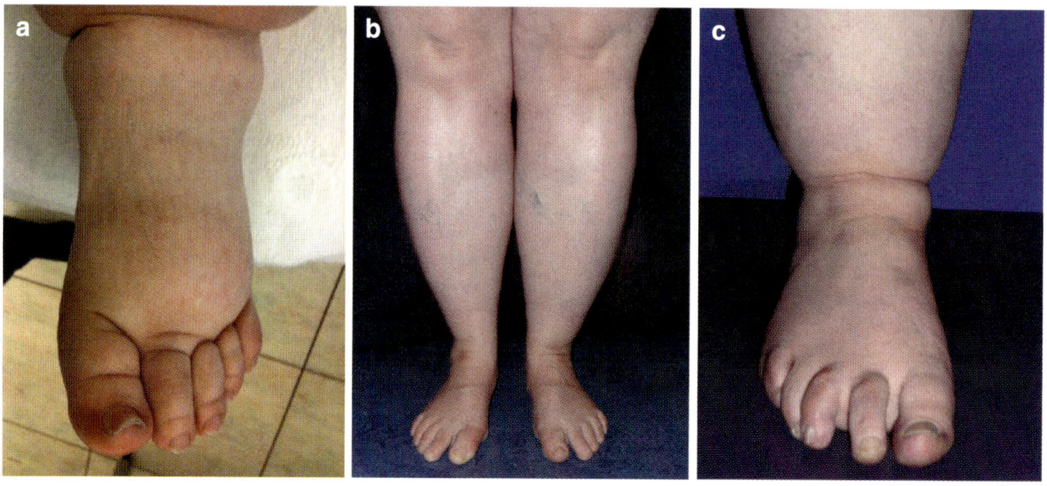

Fig. 16.1 Clinical features of oedema: (**a**) lymphoedema of the foot with swollen toes and transverse creases on the distal part of the dorsal surface of the foot. (**b**) Lipoedema with a slender foot and ankle. The oedema is symmetrical and starts above the gaiter area which gives the appearance of a constriction. (**c**) Lipolymphoedema with classic broadening of the calf and slender ankle as with lipoedema. Note the secondary lymphatic oedema on the dorsal surface of the foot Copyright: [Author]

Phleboedema is part of chronic venous insufficiency. With this condition the venous capillaries distend from the raised ambulatory venous pressure. This itself is caused by a reduced venous filling time and raised venous filling index (Lattimer et al. 2013). The increased intravascular pressure leads to extravasation of fluid by the Starling mechanism. The extravasation of blood components like haemosiderin stimulates melanin release, and the whole process causes hyperpigmentation, induration and fibrosis of the gaiter area. This typical brown skin discolouration is termed dermatoliposclerosis. Circumferential venous ulcers can result in a secondary lymphoedema of the foot.

Lipohyperplasia and **lipoedema** may occur independently of lymphoedema or phleboedema and is sometimes familial. In these conditions there is a symmetrical thickening of the subcutaneous fatty tissue, starting in the supramalleolar region (gaiter area) and extending to the thigh. Lipohyperplasia is the first phase of the disease and is painless. Later, pain sets in as the pressure increases. It is a *fat distribution dysfunction* or lipodystrophy. It is not a form of obesity because the cell count in the subcutaneous fatty tissue is abnormally high. This is in contrast to adiposis which is the accumulation of fat into a constant number of cells. The clinical picture is limited

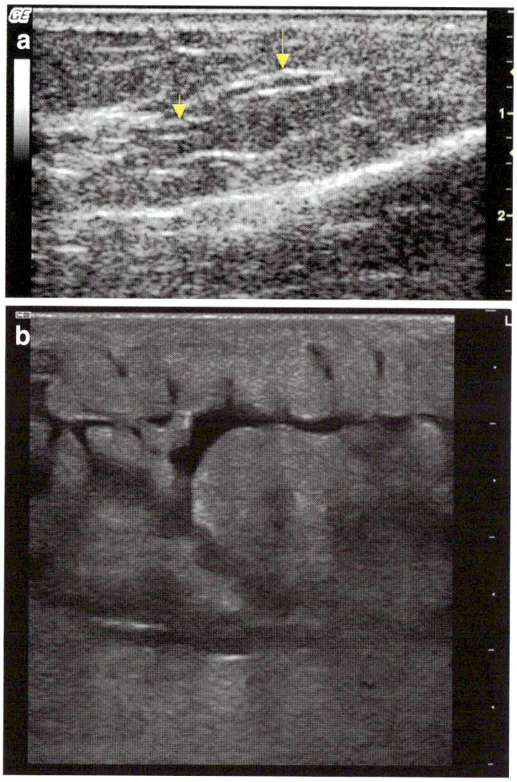

Fig. 16.2 (**a**) Longitudinal view through the inner calf in lymphatic oedema demonstrating sclerosed collectors with thickened walls (*arrowed*). (**b**) Acute lymphatic oedema with free fluid between islands of fatty tissue and stretched collecting ducts Copyright: [Author]

Table 16.1 Systemic causes for oedemas in the extremities

Cause	Clinical picture
Renal	Glomerulonephritis, nephrotic syndrome
Cardiac	Right ventricular failure
Hepatic	Cirrhosis of the liver
Vascular	Acute tissue ischaemia, oedema after revascularisation
Intestinal	Ulcerative colitis, enteropathy, malabsorption
Thyroid disease	Hyper- or hypothyroidism
Iatrogenic	Medications including antihypertensives, nonsteroidal anti-inflammatory drugs, steroids, proton-pump inhibitors, hormones, ciclosporin, immunosuppressive agents
Nutritional	Protein deficiency, malnutrition
Infectious	Cellulitis, borreliosis, filariasis
Pregnancy and hormones	Cyclical oedema, eclampsia and pre-eclampsia

initially to calf, thigh and pelvic oedema, but the foot remains unaffected (Fig. 16.2) (Cornely 2011 in Appendix 2). In its further course, lipoedema may obstruct the lymphatic drainage due to increased pressure in the tissue giving rise to mixed forms of lipolymphoedema with pain and involvement of the foot and toes.

Many systemic diseases may cause secondary **oedemas in the extremities** (Table 16.1).

Sonoelastography can measure the compressibility of the subcutaneous fatty tissue by applying pressure with the ultrasound probe. The distance between the skin surface and the muscle fascia is measured with and without compression. In healthy persons, the subcutaneous fatty tissue can be compressed by approximately 40 % (Marshall and Breu 2005 in Appendix 2).

16.2 Ultrasound Appearances of Lymphoedema

Under ultrasound, oedema is characterised by an unordered, three-dimensional, linked **build-up of fluid** in the subcutaneous fatty tissue throughout the affected region (Figs. 16.2a, b and 1.16). These are not specific for lymphoedema but oedema in general.

Clinical examination provides complementary information for diagnostic assistance. The clinical findings of importance for a diagnosis of lymphoedema include a hump on the dorsal part of the foot, Stemmer sign or a distally distributed oedema in an extremity. If the ultrasound appearances described above are present on one side only, then this is characteristic of a lymphatic oedema (Table 16.2).

Atypical lesions or signs of discrete skin constriction will suggest lymphatic oedema due to self-harm (*Secretan's syndrome*). Extensive homogeneous areas of oedema are visualised on ultrasound. Dermal thickening, typical of lymphoedema, is absent in the early stages.

In the acute situation of new lymphatic oedema or deterioration of pre-existing oedema, large collections of lymph are often visualised between islands of fatty tissue (Fig. 16.2b). With chronic oedema, echo-free longitudinal "canals" appear in the subcutaneous tissues. These are lined with a characteristic echo-rich wall indicative of sclerosis (*lymphangiosclerosis*). These "canals" are likely to represent stretched lymphatic collectors. The skin and subcutaneous tissues are usually equally echogenic with a strong echo pattern (Fig. 16.3). Their thickness reflects the clinical picture. In advanced lymphatic oedemas, there is reduced compressibility which can be demonstrated by sonoelastography.

16.3 Lipohyperplasia and Lipoedema

Pure lipohyperplasia and pure lipoedema demonstrate characteristic morphological findings on ultrasound. This is important for differential diagnosis and to differentiate this condition from lymphatic oedema. In lymphoedema or lymphatic oedema, there is the presence of a thickened dermis in keeping with the clinical appearance. An increased homogeneous echo pattern called a "snowstorm" is typical. There are prominent subcutaneous septae with a total lack of echo-free gaps. This finding is especially specific in the medial ankle region, since here the subcutaneous tissues are usually no more than

Table 16.2 Differential diagnosis of three different types of oedema

Symptoms	Lymphoedema	Lipoedema	Phleboedema
Manifestation	Primarily in one leg with differences between the sides	Primarily symmetrical and almost exclusively in women	Oedema concurrent with evidence of venous disease
Location		Lower leg, thigh, hips (foot typically not affected)	Predominantly at the ankle and dependent in nature
Swelling	Hump on dorsal surface of foot. Loss of the leg contours	Collar-like, supramalleolar fat accumulation	Initially retromalleolar, then ascending. Foot rarely affected
Colour	Body colour but may darken with chronicity	Body colour	Brownish discolouration from haemosiderin and melanin
Induration	Pitting in the early stages but non-pitting later. Stemmer sign positive	Firm but Stemmer sign negative	Hard but the pitting nature persists. Eventually becomes woody
Temperature	Cool	Normal to cool	Warm
Sensation	Painless	Painful under pressure in later stages	Painful, itching and throbbing
Heaviness	Evening time	Evening time	Evening time
Complications	Erysipelas, cellulitis, athletes foot, exudation of lymph	Intertrigo, cellulitis, athletes foot	Venous ulcer, superficial vein thrombosis, haemorrhage
High-resolution ultrasound	Subcutaneous tissues in the region of the oedema are thicker and more echogenic. Characteristic echo-free gaps and canals	Supramalleolar subcutaneous tissues are thicker and very echogenic. Prominent echogenic septae	Non-specific oedema. Venous disease findings of reflux, thrombosis, obstruction and occlusion within veins

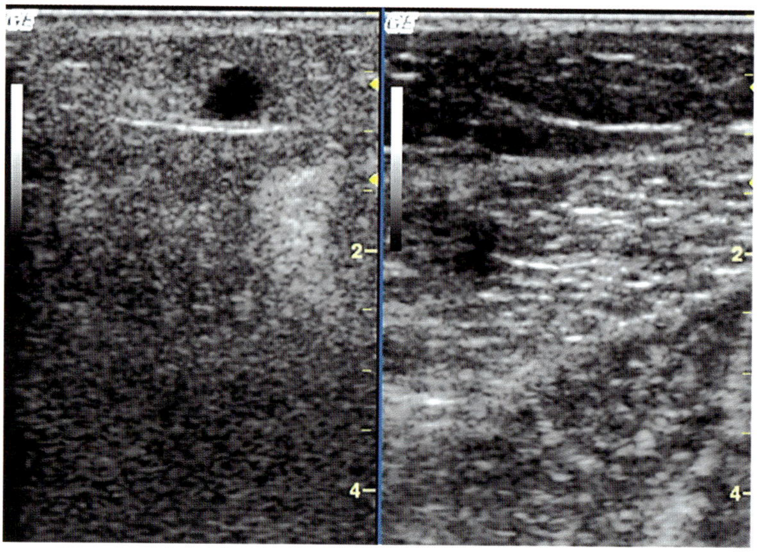

Fig. 16.3 Phleboedema. *Left*, transverse view through the medial right lower leg of a patient with chronic venous insufficiency. The subcutaneous tissue and muscles are structurally altered appearing as a homogeneous shade of grey with white spots. An ectatic venous tributary is visible. *Right*, transverse view of a healthy left leg. Note the clear differentiation of the fascia in the subcutaneous fatty tissue and the well-defined muscle structure Copyright: [Author]

Table 16.3 Correlation between the thickness of the subcutaneous tissues and the clinical diagnosis of lipoedema

Subcutaneous thickness measured approximately a hand's breadth above the medial malleolus in cm	Confidence of diagnosing lipoedema
1.2–1.5	Slight
1.5–2.0	Moderate
>2.0	Certain
>3.0	Clinically obvious

10–12 mm thick, even in obesity (Table 16.3). With lipoedema there is an absence of dermal thickening which looks normal on ultrasound. When the typical clinical features are taken into consideration (Fig. 16.1b), ultrasound provides a confident diagnosis.

In lipohyperplasia, which is an early form of the disease, an additional finding may consist of

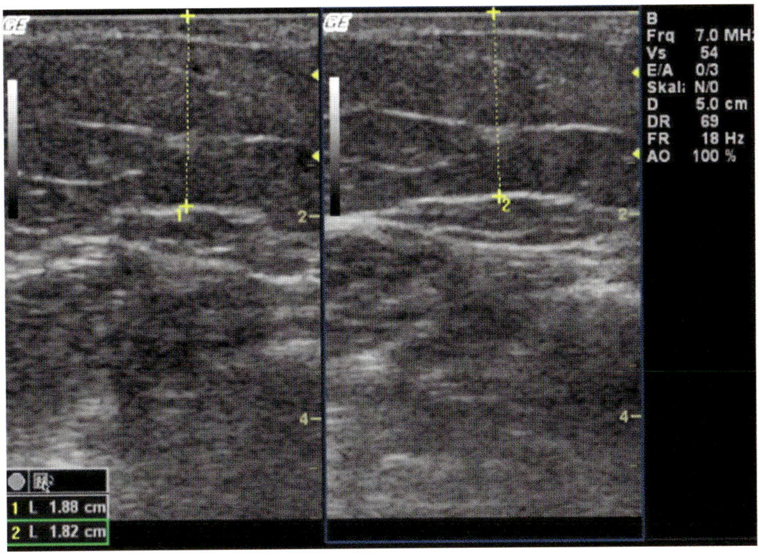

Fig. 16.4 Sonoelastography in advanced lipoedema which is usually painful. The tissue is homogeneous with a "snowstorm" appearance. The septae appear echo-rich and the subcutis is barely compressible. *Left,* without compression at 18.8 mm; *right,* with compression at 18.2 mm (3 % compressibility) Copyright: [Author]

good compressibility of the subcutis using sonoelastography at approximately 40 %. With a painful lipoedema, the compressibility is much less at approximately 10 % (Fig. 16.4).

If the two diseases described above coincide, the condition is called lipolymphoedema or lympholipoedema. Characteristic mixed images occur among the findings described above.

Reference

Lattimer CR, Kalodiki E, Azzam M, Geroulakos G (2013) Reflux time estimation on air-plethysmography may stratify patients with early superficial venous insufficiency. Phlebology 28:101–108

Incidental Findings During a Venous Examination of the Leg

17

Erika Mendoza, Hans-Peter Weskott, Helmut Kopf, and Christopher R. Lattimer

Chapter Summary

One of the advantages of ultrasound over phlebography is that the surrounding tissues can be evaluated during the examination. These are comprised of the subcutaneous tissue, fascia, muscles, arteries, nerves, lymph nodes and bone contours. This chapter describes the features and pathology of these which may be noticed during a venous examination. The examiner should be alerted to incidental findings in order to carry out further investigations, if appropriate. This may also help in the differential diagnosis of the painful leg.

Arterial pathologies are not covered in detail other than a few characteristic duplex appearances and urgent findings requiring further evaluation.

Examination of the nerves of the leg is addressed separately (Sect. 17.6).

E. Mendoza, MD, PhD (✉)
Venenpraxis Wunstorf,
Speckenstraße 10, 31515 Wunstorf, Germany
e-mail: erika.mendoza@t-online.de

H.-P. Weskott, MD
Klinikum Siloah – Zentrale Sonographie,
Roesebeckstr. 15, 30449 Hannover, Germany
e-mail: hans-peter.weskott@krh.eu

H. Kopf, MSc
Institut für diagnostische und interventionelle
Radiologie Wilhelminenspital Wien,
16, Montleartstrasse 37, 1171 Wien, Austria
e-mail: helmut.kopf@wienkav.at

C.R. Lattimer, MD, PhD
Department of Vascular Surgery,
Josef Pflug Vascular Laboratory,
Ealing Hospital and Imperial College, London, UK

17.1 Findings in the Groin and Thigh

Lymph nodes are frequently found around the saphenofemoral junction. Normal lymph nodes are up to 0.5 cm in size and have an oval or slightly triangular shape with a smooth perimeter. Their **echo characteristics** are an important criterion for differential diagnosis:

- Normal: strong echo generation with a thin, echo-lucent edge
- Chronic inflammation: homogeneous, strong echo generation (Fig. 17.1a, b)
- Acute inflammation: large, homogeneously echo lucent (Fig. 17.1c, d)
- Malignant: large, heterogeneous, echo-lucent areas with absence of an internal structure (Fig. 17.1e)

After groin surgery **a lymphatic collection** may develop. Occasionally this erupts as a cutaneous lymph fistula. On B-scan this appears as an echo-lucent structure separating the other tissues or forming a smooth-edged lymphatic cyst. On colour duplex there is no flow (Fig. 17.2a).

Lymphatic cysts are round, smooth-edged structures with a strong acoustic shadow. They

E. Mendoza et al. (eds.), *Duplex Ultrasound of Superficial Leg Veins*,
DOI 10.1007/978-3-642-40731-4_17, © Springer-Verlag Berlin Heidelberg 2014

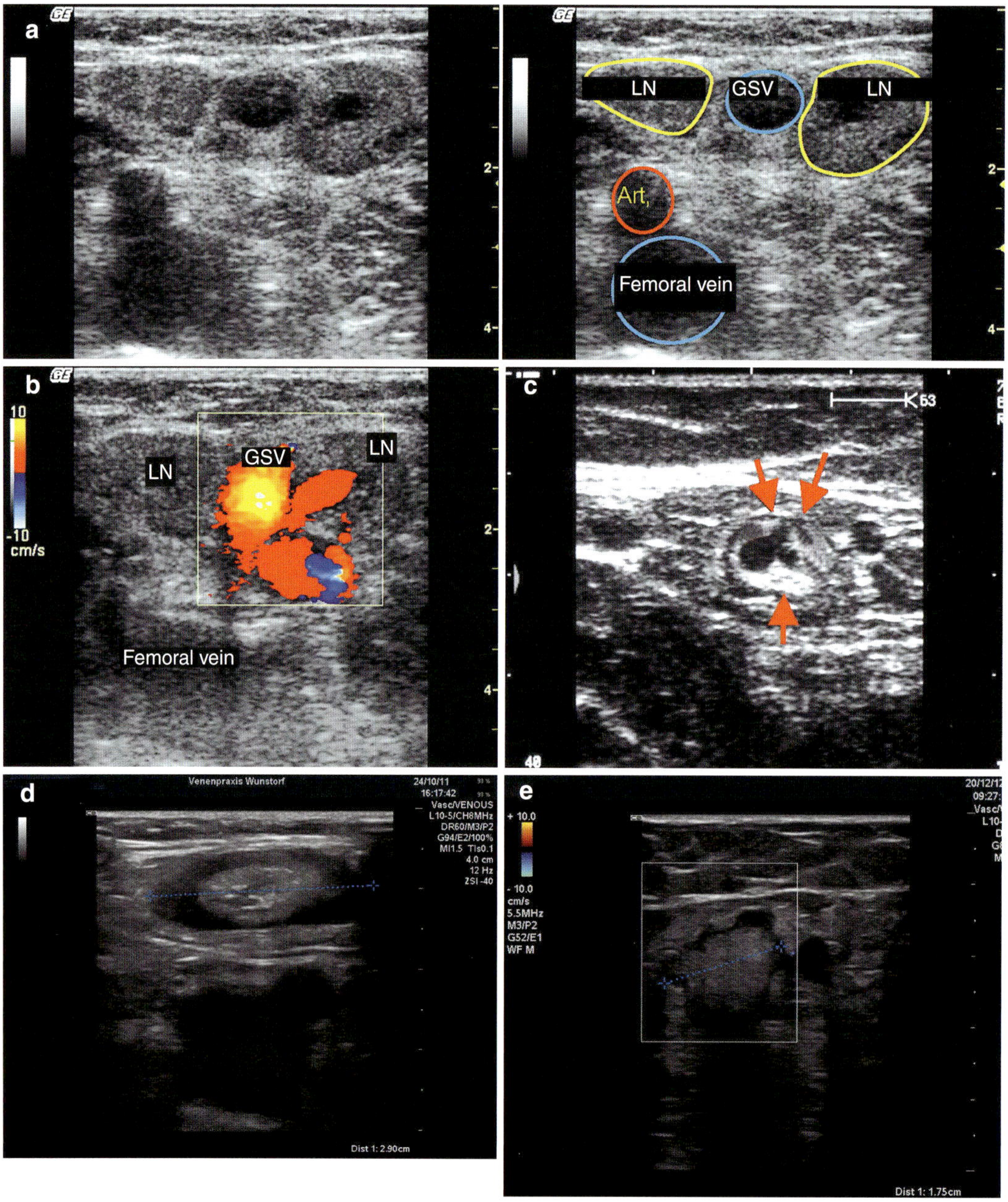

Fig. 17.1 Lymph nodes. (**a**) Transverse view through the right groin demonstrating enlarged lymph nodes (*LN*). (**b**) Transverse view 0.5 cm further distal during muscular diastole in colour duplex. The lymph node is in contact with the refluxive vein which may even flow through the node (see accompanying online material). (**c**) Transverse view through the right groin in a patient with a venous ulcer: the lymph node (*red arrows*) lies between the great saphenous vein and the anterior accessory saphenous vein (unlabelled). Both veins are refluxive on colour duplex. The contours of the lymph node are smooth which lessens their chance of being malignant. The node demonstrated has mixed areas of chronic and acute inflammation. (**d**) Transverse view of a large, acutely inflamed lymph node in the left groin due to erysipelas. Note the wide echolucent (*black*) border. (**e**) Longitudinal view of a malignant lymph node in the left groin. This patient presented with increasing swelling of the left leg for 4 weeks. Multiple lymph nodes are demonstrated with irregular borders that are partially inseparable from the surroundings Copyright: [Author]

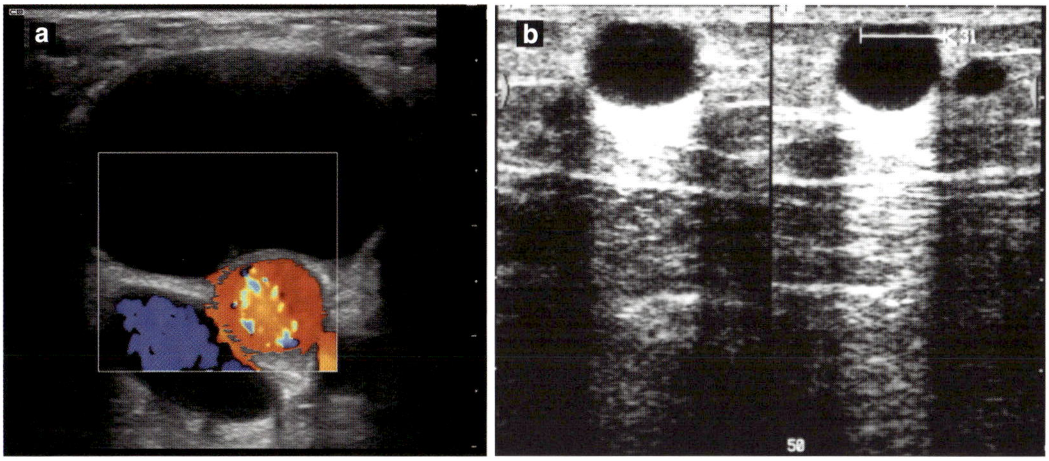

Fig. 17.2 (**a**) Lymphatic cyst in the left groin 3 months after cannulation of the femoral artery for cardiopulmonary bypass. Lymphatic cysts with arteries and/or veins flowing through them have a smooth border. Those without have an echo reinforcement (see accompanying online material). (**b**) B-scan of the thigh at the level of the adductor canal (*left*, longitudinal; *right*, transverse). A great saphenous vein tributary was ligated 8 weeks previously. The patient had a painful, tender, indurated area in the region of the scar. A lymphatic cyst appears as an echolucent expansion with a strong acoustic shadow, 11 × 13 × 10 mm in size. In transverse view the great saphenous vein tributary is visible Copyright: [Author]

may develop after trauma or from iatrogenic causes like previous surgery (Fig. 17.2b).

Occasionally a Valsalva manoeuvre may interfere with the ultrasound view of the saphenofemoral junction because of the descent of an **inguinal hernia**. Reducible hernias can be controlled with groin pressure by the patient in order to facilitate the examination.

Calcifications of the arterial wall appear as white, usually irregular alterations to the wall with a prominent acoustic shadow. They represent dystrophic calcification in a degenerative arterial wall which indicates **arterial disease** (Fig. 17.3a).

The diameter of arteries enlarges with age. An excessive generalised dilatation is termed arteriomegaly. Saccular or fusiform dilatation is called an **aneurysm**. Their walls are often calcified with turbulent flow (Fig. 17.3b) and laminated thrombus (Fig. 17.5) in the lumen.

After interventions requiring femoral artery cannulation, an expansible, pulsatile swelling may develop. It gradually increases in size causing discolouration of the overlying skin with eventual rupture. It is caused by blood leaking from the puncture site and is termed a **false aneurysm**. Rupture into an adjacent vein results in an **arteriovenous fistula**, which is common in IV drug abuse (see Fig. 6.2). These expansible lesions differ from lymphatic cysts because they demonstrate flow in the region of the echo-lucent space. Furthermore, an extensive visible subcutaneous haematoma is usually present. They can be sealed by direct compression (30 min to hours) with the ultrasound probe, surgical repair or by a percutaneous injection of thrombin under ultrasound guidance.

Occluded arteries are visible as an echo-poor structure without flow on colour duplex. After an arterial **bypass**, the blood flow can be seen in the bypass graft just as easily as in the native vessel. If the volume flow diminishes, then the patient is advised to seek urgent advice from a vascular surgeon. Areas of increased velocity are usually indicative of a stenosis.

The ultrasound appearances of **thromboangiitis obliterans** (von Winiwarter-Buerger's disease) consist of arterial as well as venous wall changes typically in men <40 years. Atherosclerosis is identified in the arteries with characteristic corkscrew-like collateral vessels attempting to bypass arterial occlusions.

17.2 Findings in the Popliteal Fossa

A **Baker's cyst** is an echo-lucent fluid collection which accumulates behind the knee. It is an expansion filled with synovial fluid. It typically occurs

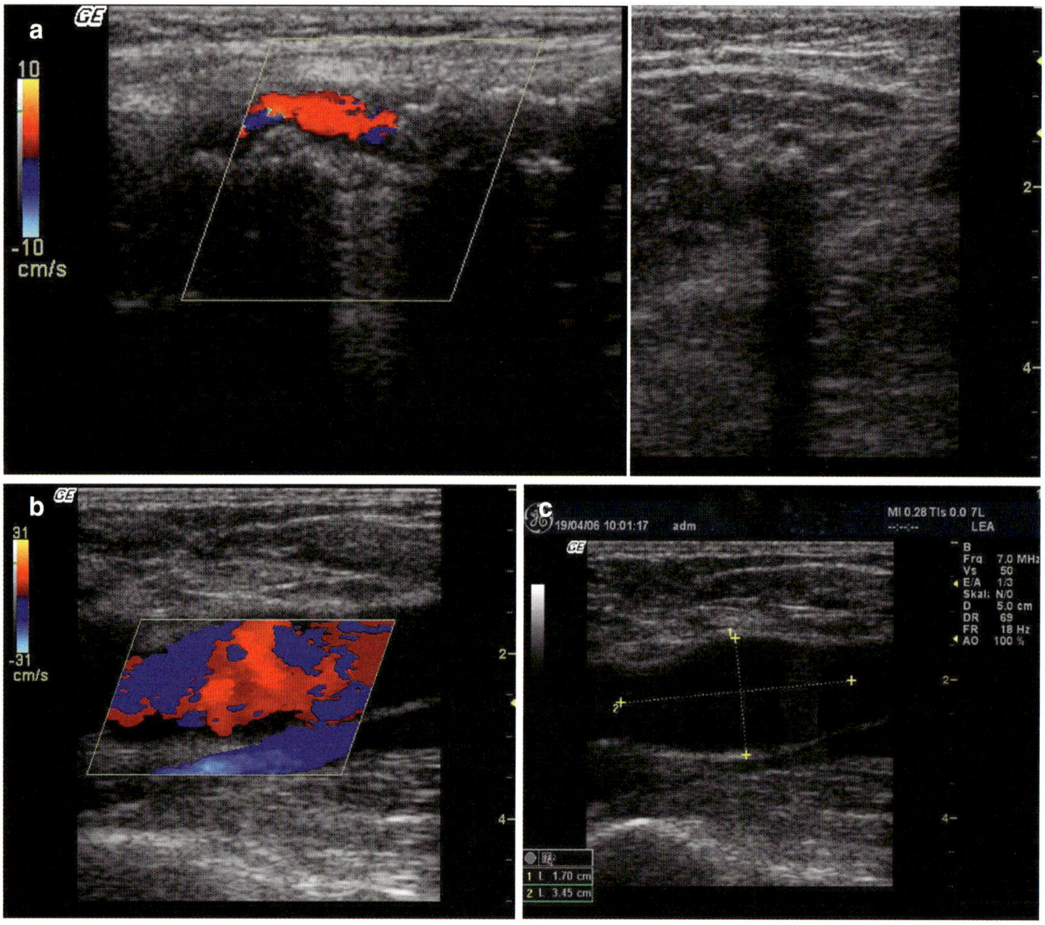

Fig. 17.3 (**a**) Calcification of the femoral artery. *Left*, longitudinal view through the groin showing a completely calcified common femoral artery with a prominent acoustic shadow. Blood flow is visible within a narrowed lumen. *Right*, transverse view through the inner thigh demonstrating a calcified femoral artery casting an acoustic shadow. (**b**) Longitudinal view of a common femoral artery aneurysm with turbulent flow (see accompanying online material). (**c**) The diameter of this aneurysm is 17 mm Copyright: [Author]

in the popliteal fossa but can also appear laterally or medially. A communication with the knee joint is suspected because the cyst runs towards it in a wedge shape (Fig. 17.4a, b). However, a Baker's cyst can also be completely round (Fig. 14.6c), haemorrhagic or divided into chambers. In the two latter cases, the internal echo is not homogeneous (Fig. 17.4c, d). A Baker's cyst may be asymptomatic or it may compress surrounding structures, especially veins and nerves, and sometimes cause pain due to pressure (Fig. 17.4e). Rupture causes severe acute pain with swelling in the calf and reddening of the skin.

Patients with an acute rupture of a Baker's cyst are often referred with a suspected deep vein thrombosis because the clinical appearance of the leg is similar. A ruptured cyst can be monitored in B-scan. Black, echo-lucent bands of fluid can be seen separating the layers of tissue. The tissues become oedematous with similar appearances as the surrounding oedema characteristic of the inflammation of a periphlebitis (Figs. 17.4d and 11.2). A ruptured Baker's cyst is a common finding in the event of an acute pain in the knee or calf. The more serious condition of a deep vein thrombosis should always be excluded.

Baker's cysts are usually part of an arthritic process which may undergo repeated rupture and haemorrhage as well as inflammation and scar formation. Over time, this results in a hard

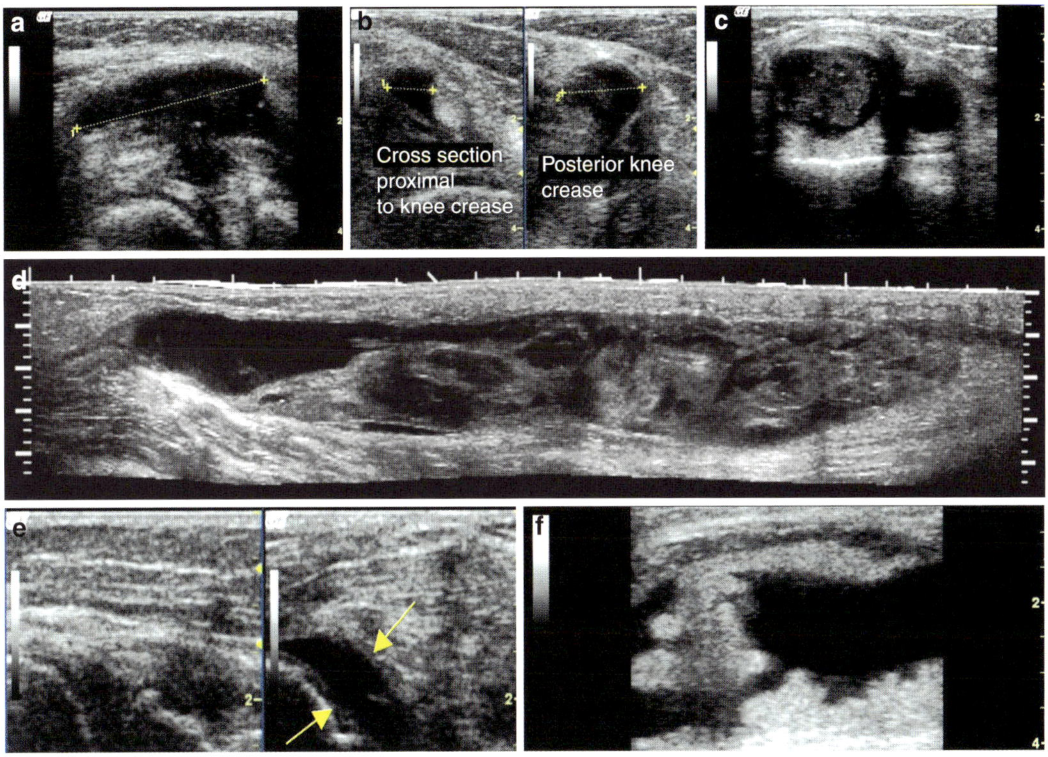

Fig. 17.4 Baker's cyst. (**a**) Longitudinal view through the right popliteal region. Baker's cyst measured at a length of 3.6 cm. The cyst points towards the knee joint (see accompanying online material). (**b**) Transverse view of the same knee. The left half of the image shows the proximal, rather narrower section of the cyst which corresponds to the left half of the previous image. The right half of the image shows the transverse view through the joint with the communication as mentioned above (see accompanying online material). (**c**) Longitudinal view through the medial popliteal region of the right leg of a patient with a painful, expanding tumour that has been increasing throughout the last 6 months. A partially solid, partially liquid-filled neoformation can be seen. It is not compressible and has no flow on colour duplex. The tumour seems to be adjacent to the bone, and the first idea was a malignant neoformation. Further examination using high-resolution ultrasound (in a clinic) resulted in a mistaken diagnosis of malignancy. The clinical history of intermittent expansion and partial resolution over 4 years confirmed the correct diagnosis of a Baker's cyst with old haemorrhagic complications that organise and solidify over time (see accompanying online material). (**d**) Ruptured Baker's cyst. Although the clinical diagnosis can be difficult, the ultrasound appearances are usually able to make the diagnosis. Using panoramic ultrasound a fluid-filled sinus is seen in the calf extending over 23 cm, 3 days after the clinical event. (**e**) Knee joint effusion after fall demonstrating free fluid separating the sides of the joint (*arrowed*). (**f**) Longitudinal view of the thigh just above the patella demonstrating chronic retropatellar bursitis. There is fluid extension into the thigh (*right side*) with internal echoes representing joint debris (see accompanying online material) Copyright: Fig. d: Dr. Weskott

expanding lesion with heterogeneous internal echoes and irregular margins. This can be differentiated from a malignant tumour by the presence or absence of flow on colour duplex. A tumour has a pathological circulation, whilst a mature Baker's cyst consists of scarring and old haematoma (Fig. 17.4c). Synovial fluid accumulation may occur also at the head of the fibula or subcutaneously which may be seen to communicate with the joint.

Popliteal artery aneurysms are visualised easily using ultrasound (Fig. 17.5). Colour duplex confirms they have not thrombosed since thrombosis may be a cause of acute limb ischaemia. They occur frequently on both sides. A maximum wall to wall diameter of 2.5 cm indicates the need for surgical repair. Popliteal artery aneurysms may progressively occlude the calf arteries or embolise into the calf and foot. Rupture is rare.

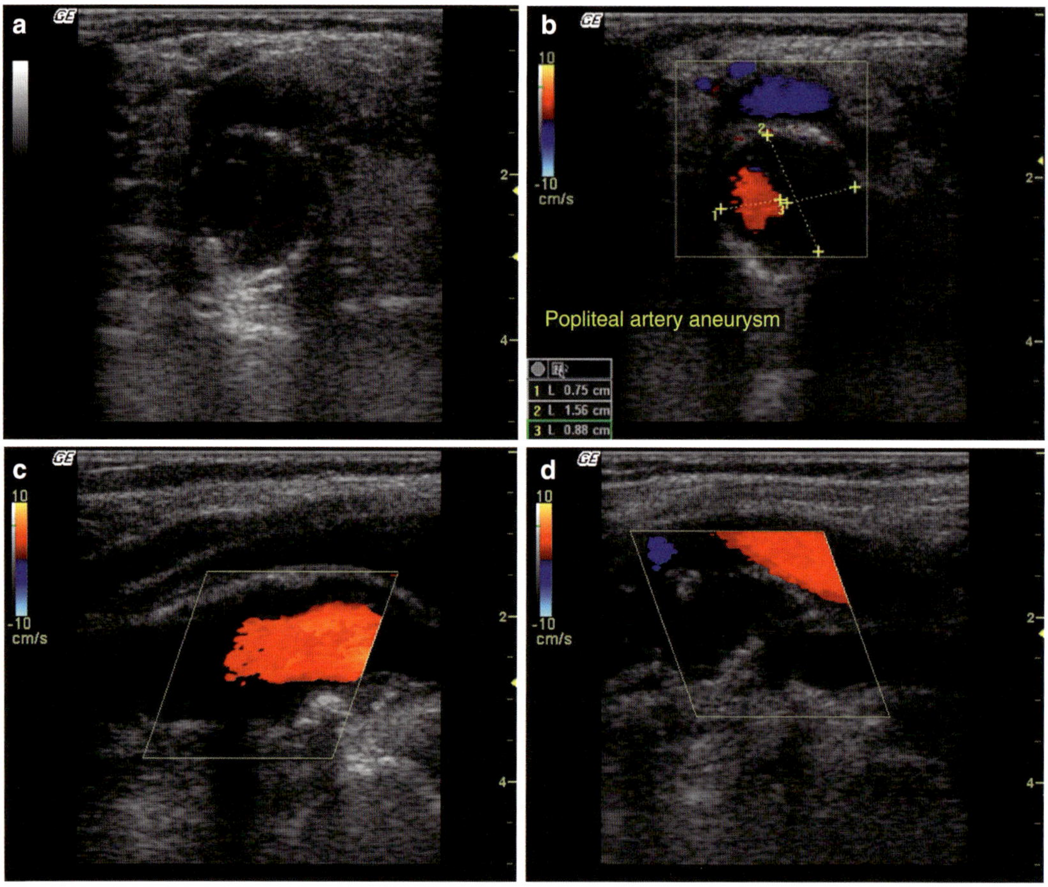

Fig. 17.5 Popliteal artery aneurysm. (**a**) Transverse B-scan through the popliteal aneurysm of the right leg containing a mural thrombus. The popliteal vein is compressed by the aneurysm (see accompanying online material). (**b**) Colour duplex demonstrates the remaining luminal area. (**c**) Longitudinal section through the same aneurysm (see accompanying online material). (**d**) Longitudinal view through the aneurysm demonstrating a tortuous lumen with irregular contours (see accompanying online material) Copyright: [Author]

Cystic adventitial disease of the popliteal artery is rare, occurring in young men and presenting with intermittent claudication. The wall of the popliteal artery appears irregular in places with adjacent cystic areas compressing the lumen.

17.3 Findings in the Calf and Foot

Muscle hernias present as discrete superficial bulges which develop along the lateral part of the leg muscles when standing. They look like venous blow outs and can be confused with a varicose vein. These muscular hernias are usually easily differentiated clinically from a varicosity by having the patient stand with his weight on the ipsilateral leg, then with the weight off that leg, which should then make the bulge disappear. If there is still doubt, this can be resolved by duplex ultrasound. On ultrasound an interruption of the muscle fascia is seen with protruding muscle tissue. They can be caused by an overzealous phlebectomy, but they do not require treatment (Fig. 17.6).

With an under- or overactive thyroid gland (**hypo- or hyperthyroidism**), calf oedema may occur (Chap. 16). It presents between the muscles and is deep to the muscular fascia (Fig. 17.7).

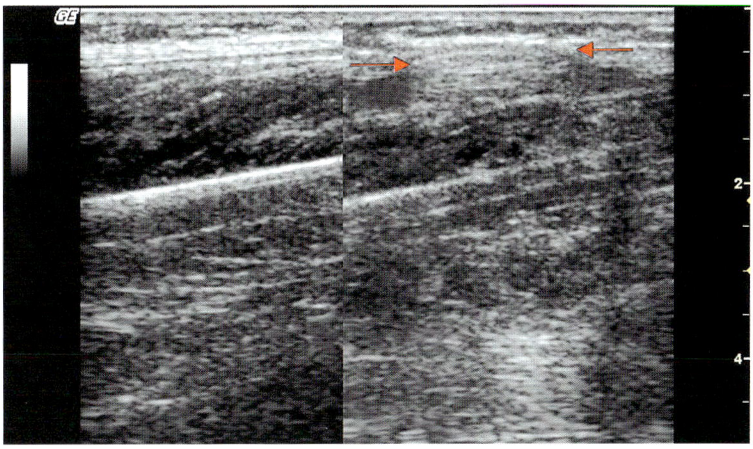

Fig. 17.6 Muscle hernia. Longitudinal view at the middle third of the calf in a standing patient just lateral to the tibia. *Left*, fascia and muscle are clearly delineated; *right*, a little further lateral the fascia is interrupted, and the muscle hernia appears as a spindle-shaped protrusion (*arrows*) Copyright: [Author] see online material

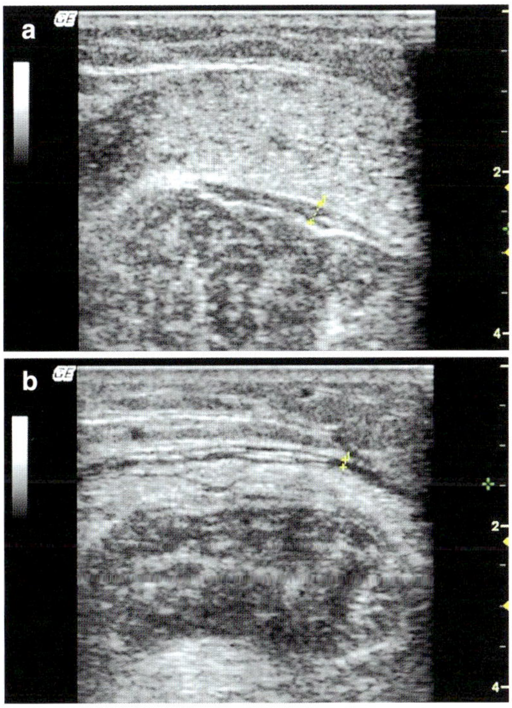

Fig. 17.7 Intermuscular oedema in a patient with thyrotoxicosis. (**a**) Transverse view through the calf with an echo-poor layer of oedema between the soleus and gastrocnemius muscles. This may also occur in hypothyroidism. (**b**) Transverse view through the same calf further up demonstrating another echo-poor layer of oedema between the muscle fascia and the gastrocnemius muscles (see online material) Copyright: [Author]

Muscle veins including the **soleal sinusoids** may distend with thick "erythrocyte sludge" which gives the appearances of discrete lesions within the calf muscle. Compression or contraction of the calf should flush the veins and clarify the diagnosis (Fig. 17.8).

Inflammation of a tendon sheath in the foot or ankle is part of the differential diagnosis of painful oedema. A normal tendon appears as a strong echogenic structure without an echo-free halo. When inflammation occurs there is an echo-free build-up of oedema in the tendon sheath surrounding the echogenic tendon. The only echo-free structures that are normally seen at this location are the posterior tibial artery and accompanying veins (Fig. 17.9). Part of the differential diagnosis is a thrombus in the lumen of the posterior tibial vein. Unlike a patent vein it is incompressible without flow on colour duplex. Furthermore, the posterior tibial artery and vein are located antero-medially in relation to the Achilles tendon (see accompanying online material). Inflammation of the Achilles tendon results in a thicker tendon when compared to the contralateral side (Fig. 17.10).

A **bone lesion** may be found incidentally during the examination. The bone edge normally produces a strong echo which is completely extinguished deeper and beyond. It can be followed along the whole length of the bone as an unbroken line. If there is a lesion, this line appears interrupted. Patients can present with a painful calf or an oedema of uncertain origin. A bone lesion is part of the differential diagnosis (Fig. 17.11).

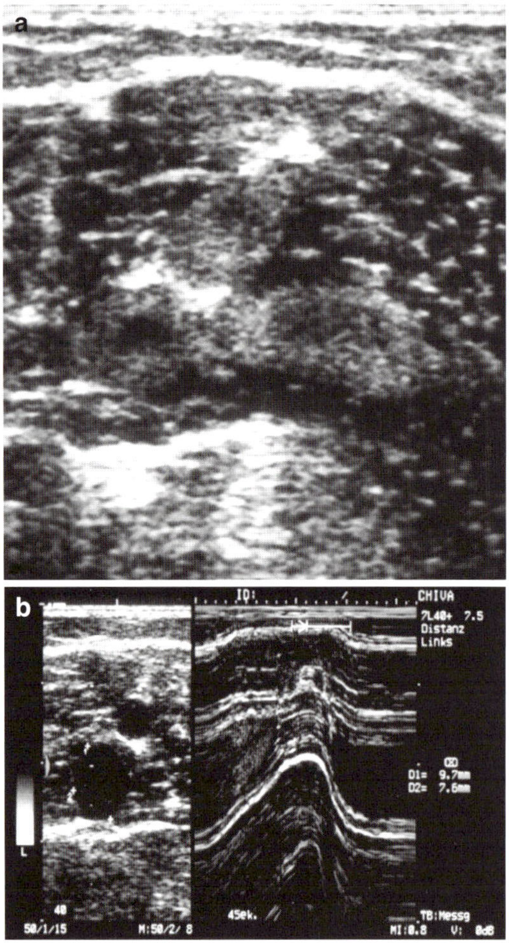

Fig. 17.8 Soleal sinusoids distended with "erythrocyte sludge". (**a**) Transverse view through the calf with homogeneous areas in the muscle suggestive of a fatty or fibrous tumour. (**b**) Compression of the calf flushes the muscle veins from "erythrocyte sludge" which becomes echo lucent after compression. In M mode (*right*) the veins are filled with echogenic material beforehand which clears after compression Copyright: [Author]

17.4 Generalised Findings

Muscle normally has an echo-poor internal structure with regular stripes in longitudinal view. With neurological and myogenic disease, **muscular atrophy** is a frequent finding. Muscle fibres are replaced by fat and connective tissue. On ultrasound, a nonhomogeneous structure with a stronger echo can be observed especially if a bilateral comparison is possible

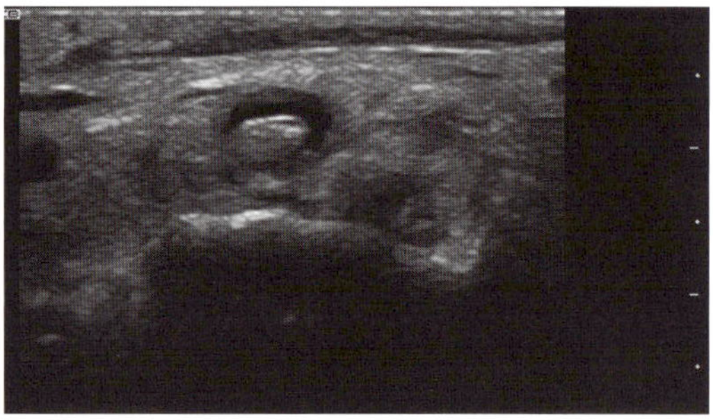

Fig. 17.9 Inflammation of the synovial sheath of a tendon on the medial side of the tibia at the ankle. An echo-free halo of fluid is seen around the otherwise strongly echogenic tendon (see accompanying online material) Copyright: [Author]

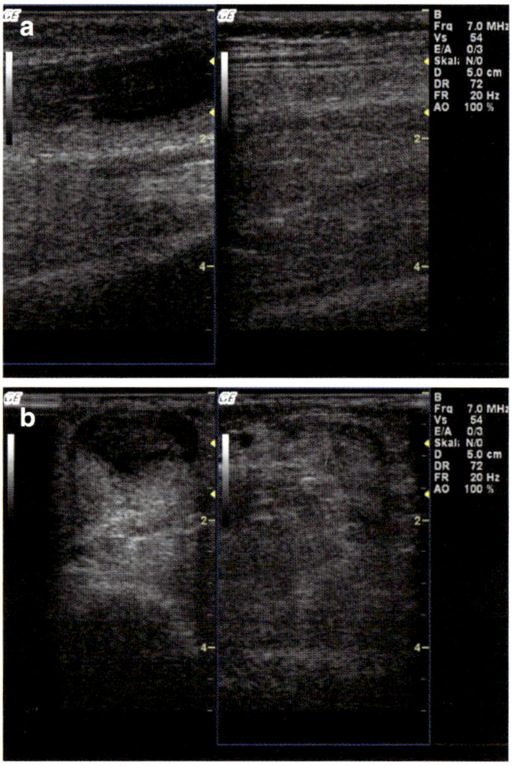

Fig. 17.10 Inflammation of the Achilles tendon in patient with renal failure compared to the normal contralateral side. (**a**) Longitudinal view, (*left*) echo poor, thickened Achilles tendon, (*right*) normal demonstrating a thin Achilles tendon with a strong echo. (**b**) Transverse view, (*left*) thickened, echo-poor profile of the Achilles tendon, (*right*) normal Copyright: [Author]

(Fig. 17.12a, b). When both calves demonstrate atrophy, the musculature should be compared with the thigh.

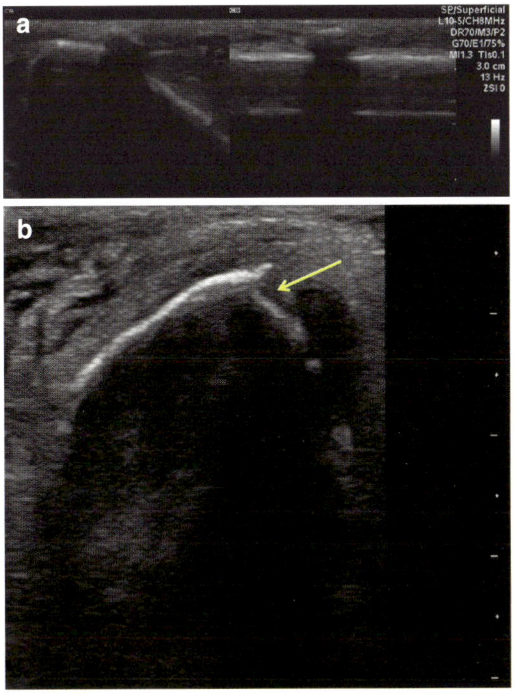

Fig. 17.11 Bone injury. (**a**) Bone splinter on the edge of the tibia: *left*, transverse view; *right*, longitudinal view. (**b**) Fracture on the inner part of the distal end of the fibula (*arrowed*). Both patients presented with a painful oedema of unknown origin Copyright: [Author]

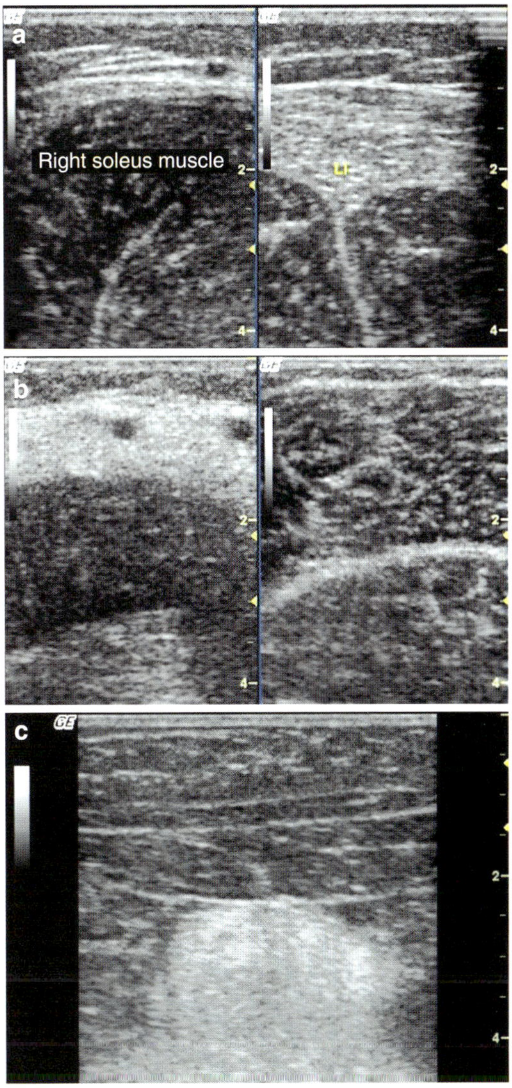

Fig. 17.12 (**a**) Transverse view of normal right (*left*) and left (*right*) calves in B-scan. Clear echo images of the soleus muscles are seen. *LI* stands for left. (**b**) Muscular atrophy of the right leg (*left*) in a patient with poliomyelitis depicting a soleus muscle completely replaced by connective tissue. The left side (*right*) is normal. (**c**) Transverse view through inner thigh in a patient with congenital myopathy depicting an accentuated, echo-rich muscle (see accompanying online material) Copyright: [Author]

Subcutaneous/epifascial **haematomas** are generally visible externally. When they diffuse into the tissues, these bruises give an appearance similar to phlebitis, namely, a homogeneous, echo-rich layer (Fig. 17.13a). In haematomas with fluid segments, the homogeneous grey region is interspersed with echo-poor layers or areas. A fluid haematoma or subcutaneous build-up of blood appears echo-free in the centre with occasional echo enhancement around the margins (Fig. 17.13b).

Penetrating post-traumatic injury can result in a communication between an artery and vein. This is known as an arteriovenous fistula (**AV fistula**). The vein becomes distended with pulsatile flow (Fig. 6.3). In early stages or with a minor fistula, this discreet pulsatile flow can easily be overlooked.

Benign or malignant tumours of various origins can be found in the subcutaneous tissue or vessels. Ultrasound serves as a guide, but the final diagnosis is usually reached by histology (Fig. 17.14).

The appearance of scar tissue on ultrasound is described in Chap. 13.

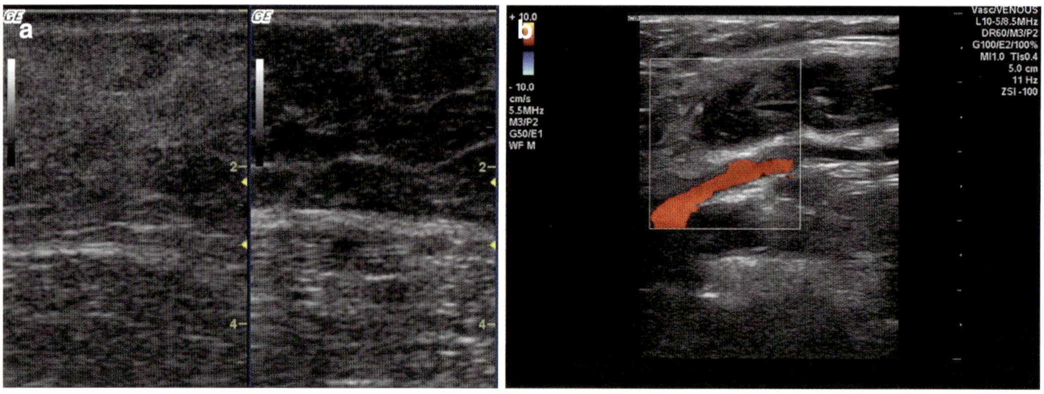

Fig. 17.13 (**a**) Subcutaneous infiltrating haematoma after a fall on the right thigh. *Left*, transverse view with a haematoma seen as a *grey*, homogeneous area; *right*, transverse view through the unaffected left thigh at the same height (see accompanying online material). (**b**) Longitudinal view of a haematoma of the gastrocnemius muscle. Flow is seen only within an underlying artery. Compression ultrasound is helpful in distinguishing this from a fresh deep vein thrombosis (see accompanying online material) Copyright: [Author]

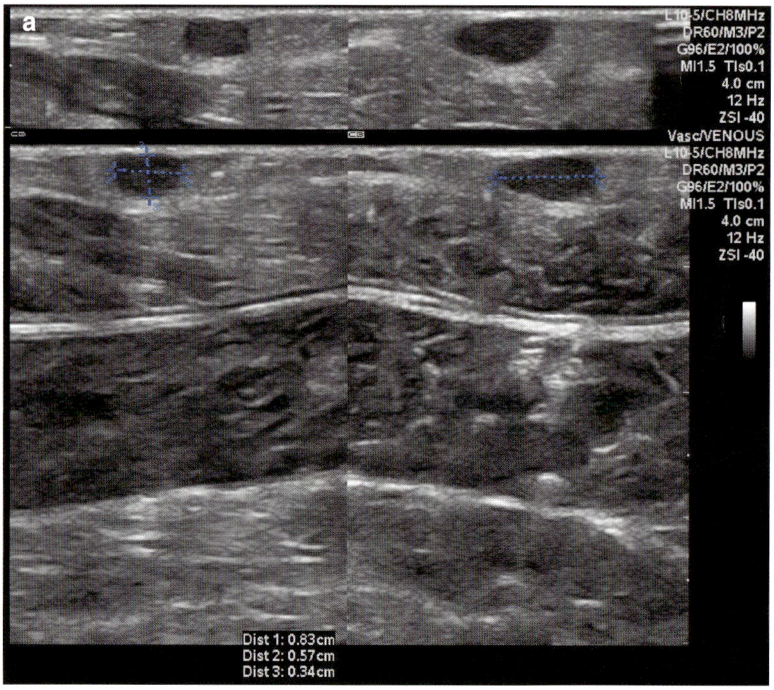

Fig. 17.14 Tumours. (**a**) Transverse and longitudinal views of fibromata in the subcutaneous tissue of the calf (see accompanying online material). (**b**) Pilomatrixoma in the subcutaneous fat of the calf with slightly irregular edges and a tendency to calcify. (**c**) Transverse and longitudinal views of a lipoma in the thigh in a patient with multiple lipomata (see accompanying online material). (**d**) Longitudinal view above the popliteal region demonstrating a polycystic tumour of unknown origin penetrating the thigh muscles. This was confirmed as a neurofibroma on histology (see accompanying online material). (**e**) Longitudinal view demonstrating that these neurofibromas are in close contact with the popliteal vein which is compressed further up (see accompanying online material). (**f**) A fluid-filled swelling on the inner calf which turned out to be an abscess after its surgical removal. The net-like intraluminal filling defect on the left side of the image represents debris Copyright: [Author]

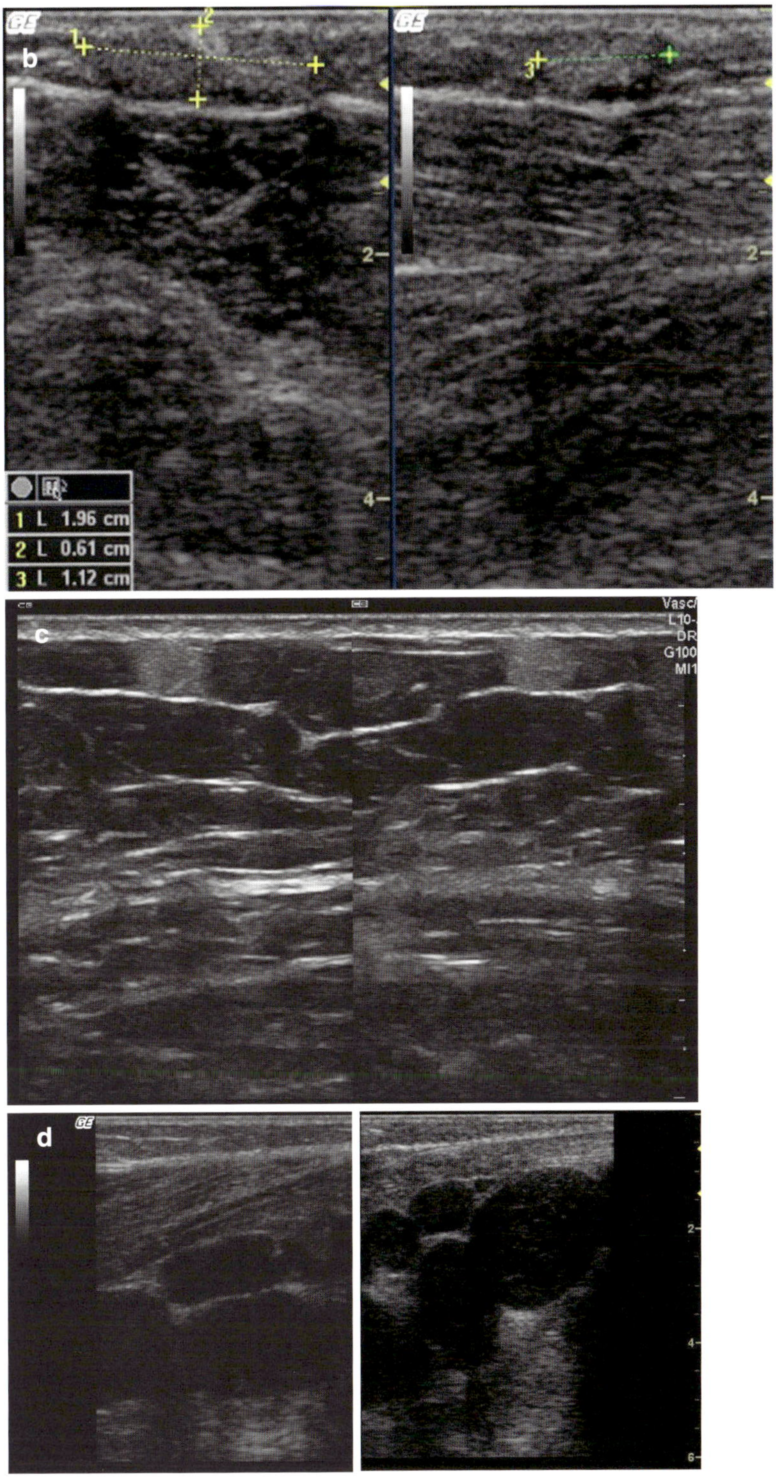

Fig. 17.14 (continued)

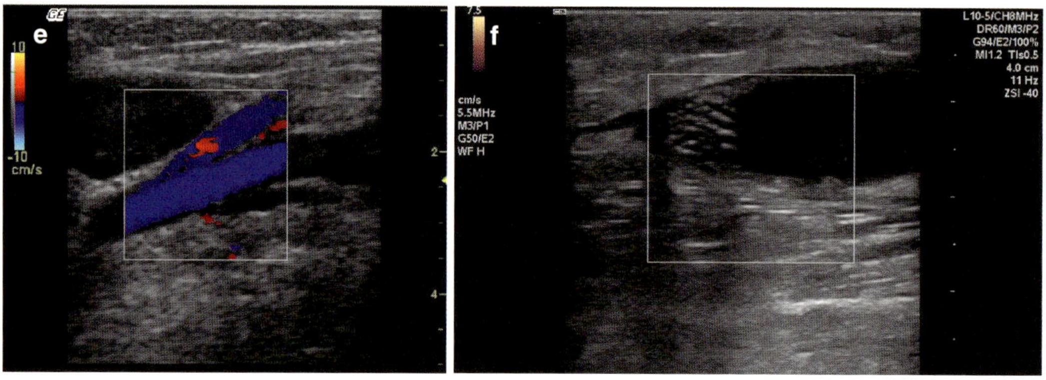

Fig. 17.14 (continued)

17.5 Findings with Right Heart Failure

Venous flow character is modulated by the change of the atrial and intrathoracic pressure. Doppler ultrasound spectral curves even reflects little pressure changes as during respiration or patient's posture. With deep inspiration the intra-abdominal pressure increases, thus causing a reduction in venous return flow to the heart. An increase of intra-abdominal pressure like in the presence of ascites might change the flow character in the veins of the lower limb as well.

When assessing the venous condition of a lying patient, the variations in flow velocity caused specifically by respiration can easily be recognised. On inhalation the velocity reduces; on exhalation it increases. Respiration-dependent variations in flow and velocity can also be used to assess valve function (Sect. 6.3).

Physiological blood flow in the **large veins close to the heart** has a three-phase, W or M-shaped flow pattern in Doppler ultrasound. It reflects variations in venous pressure during atrial and ventricular systole and diastole. During atrial systole a short venous reflux into the vena cava can be registered after the p-wave of the ECG. This is called the a-wave which is also seen as a pressure peak during right heart catheterisation. Ventricular systole and diastole cause the x- and y-waves. The inflection point between the x- and y-wave is the v-wave (Fig. 17.15).

In the deep veins of the leg the variations in cardiac pressure are usually not recognizable in colour or pulse wave Doppler ultrasound. This is due to damping and the low pressure gradients of the right heart. In contrast, in veins closer to the heart, like in the subclavian vein, a cardiac modulated pulsatile flow pattern is a normal finding. If this pulsatile flow is absent it may be an indirect sign of a central venous obstruction, especially when compared to the normal waveform of the other side. In pulmonary hypertension or right heart stress from tricuspid valve incompetence, high retrograde flow occurs which is recognisable as an unusually high a-wave. Pronounced cardiac modulation of venous flow indicates an underlying cardiac and/or pulmonary disease (Fig. 17.16). The pulsatility of the flow diminishes as the vein calibre diminishes towards the periphery.

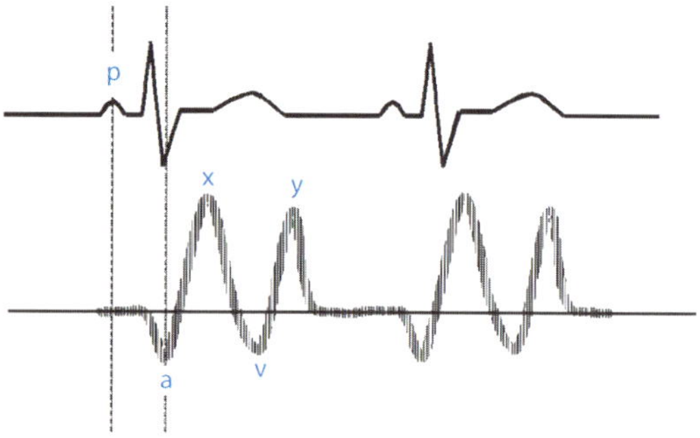

Fig. 17.15 Relationship between electrocardiogram (*above*) and spectral Doppler curve (*below*) with right heart stress. The distance between the vertical cursor lines marks the time lapse between the *p*-wave in the electrocardiogram and the a-wave in the Doppler curve Copyright: [Author]

Heaviness of the legs or oedema may occur bilaterally or unilaterally, in varying degrees of

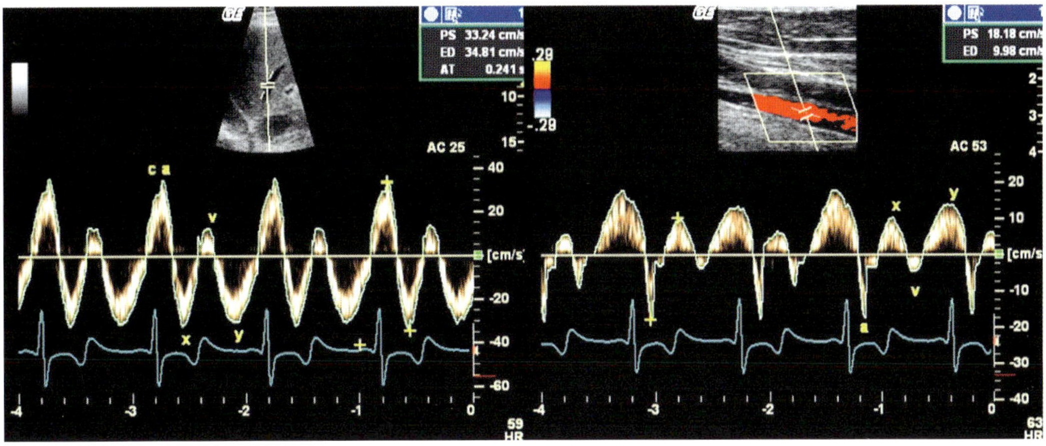

Fig. 17.16 Spectral curves from the right liver vein (*left*, 3.5 MHz curved array ultrasound probe) and the superficial femoral vein (*right*, 10 MHz linear ultrasound probe) in a patient with leg oedemas from a dilated cardiomyopathy. Note the pronounced cardiac modulation of the venous velocity profile. The concurrent electrocardiogram makes ordering the velocity peaks easier Copyright: [Author]

severity. If there is unilateral leg swelling a DVT should be excluded using ultrasound. Since venous, cardiac and pulmonary diseases frequently coexist, especially in elderly patients, their haemodynamic effects may cause oedema. Venous valve insufficiency will augment oedema in the extremities. Colour Doppler, and especially PW Doppler, in peripheral veins will show an increased pulsatility with high a-wave and x-wave, thus mirroring the pressure changes of the right heart.

Doppler ultrasound is of great value in the diagnosis of a unilateral or bilateral leg swelling. A pronounced oedema in one leg may be due to a greater degree of valve incompetence. Using colour Doppler a switch in colour between red and blue corresponding with the cardiac cycle, suggests cardiac disease This high pulsatile flow pattern may protect the veins from stasis and a resulting deep vein thrombosis. Figure 17.17 shows examples of cardiac modulation of the flow in the deep leg veins.

Note of the Editors: The high pulsatile flow pattern may correspond to arterial drive through from microcirculatory failure (see Sect. 7.5.3) (Lattimer et al. 2012).

Using high-frequency probes subcutaneous soft tissue oedema can easily be seen especially towards the feet (Chap. 16 and Figs. 1.16 and 1.17). Important differential diagnoses are inflammatory oedema like erysipelas or phebitis. Both these conditions are usually accompanied by inflamed and swollen, local or regional lymph nodes.

17.6 Peripheral Nerves in Relation to Leg Veins

Inadvertent damage to peripheral nerves during venous interventions may lead to paresis, dysaesthesia or chronic pain. This can be lessened by a detailed pre-operative ultrasound examination and a careful operation or intervention with a full understanding of the ultrasound anatomy and pathology of the peripheral nerves (Kopf et al. 2011). Unusual features of the nerves may be noted during the venous examination which can lead to an alternative diagnosis of leg discomfort.

17.6.1 The Healthy Peripheral Nerve

The healthy peripheral nerve consists of several parallel fascicles of differing thicknesses. Each fascicle is formed from several nerve fibres, which in turn is composed of numerous axons with myelin sheaths and Schwann cells. The individual nerve fibres are enclosed in an endoneurium, and

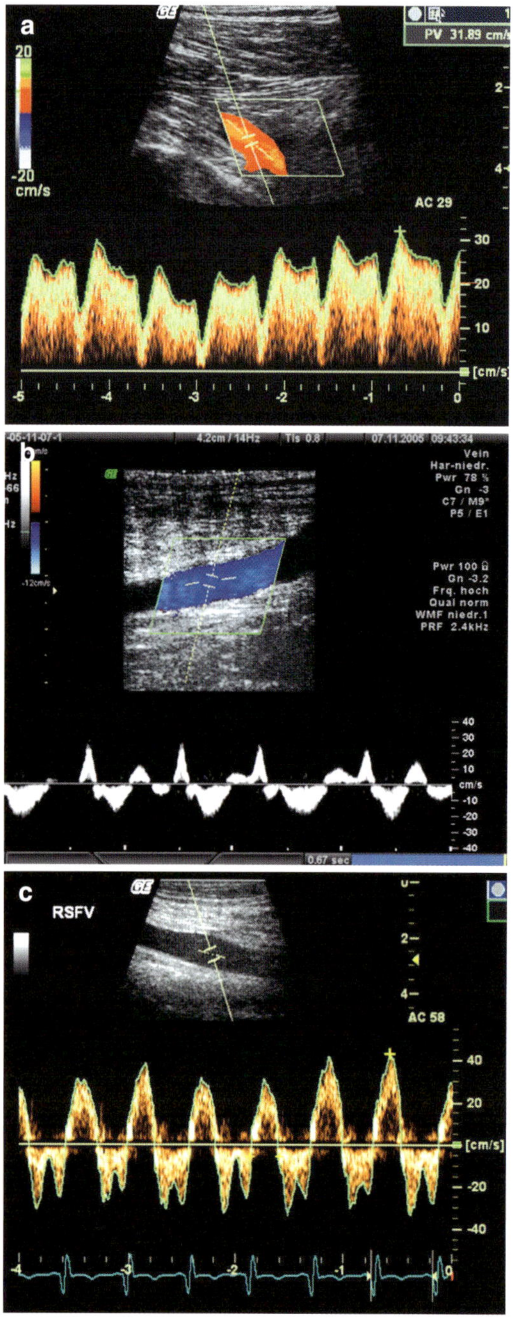

Fig. 17.17 Pathological flow profiles with right heart stress in failure patients with a unilateral discrepancy in their clinical expression of oedema. (**a**) M-shaped flow profile with no atrial return flow. (**b**) Pronounced cardiac modulation of flow in the popliteal vein with a short atrial return flow. Inverting the spectrum makes a comparison to the waveform of the hepatic veins easier. (**c**) When the Doppler spectrum is inverted, there is a marked W-shaped flow spectrum with high atrial return flow Copyright: [Author]

the fascicles are enveloped in epineurium which is a sheath of connective tissue rich in fat and collagen. The epineurium enclosing the individual fascicles is called the interfascicular epineurium, and the epineurium enclosing all the fascicles thus ensheathing the nerve is called the outer or epifascicular epineurium. The epineurium also contains the vasa nervorum (Fig. 17.18a, b).

This fascicular architecture of the peripheral nerves can be clearly recognised using a linear broadband ultrasound probe >12 MHz with soft tissue contrast-enhancing software. Care must be taken to ensure that the equipment is set to obtain the maximum soft tissue contrast. The settings for a venous examination are generally not suitable for showing nerves.

In transverse view the nerve has an oval to round shape with an echo-rich outline corresponding to the epineurium. The echo texture has a typical honeycomb pattern in which the echo-poor "cells" are the individual fascicles and the echo-rich "cell walls" are the interfascicular epineurium (Silvestri et al. 1995) (Fig. 17.19a and accompanying online material).

In longitudinal view the peripheral nerve appears as an echo-lucent, cable-like strand contrasting with the surrounding soft tissue, which has a slightly stronger echo. Within it are wavy, echo-rich strands, corresponding to the interfascicular epineurium (Fig. 17.19b).

In contrast to nerves, **tendons** have a fine, fibrillar texture, with a strictly parallel arrangement. Multidirectional ultrasound can be used for differentiating tendons from nerves. **Anisotropy** means that the tissue under examination has directionally dependent properties. If ultrasound is applied to parallel boundary surfaces which are offset from a true right angle, then the law of reflection (angle of incidence = angle of reflection) dictates that a large proportion of the reflected sound waves escape the examination field and therefore are not detected by the probe. Sections of tendon or nerve which do not run at right angles to the probe will return a weaker echo. As tendons contain many more parallel boundary surfaces than nerves, anisotropy is greater in tendons (Fig. 17.20).

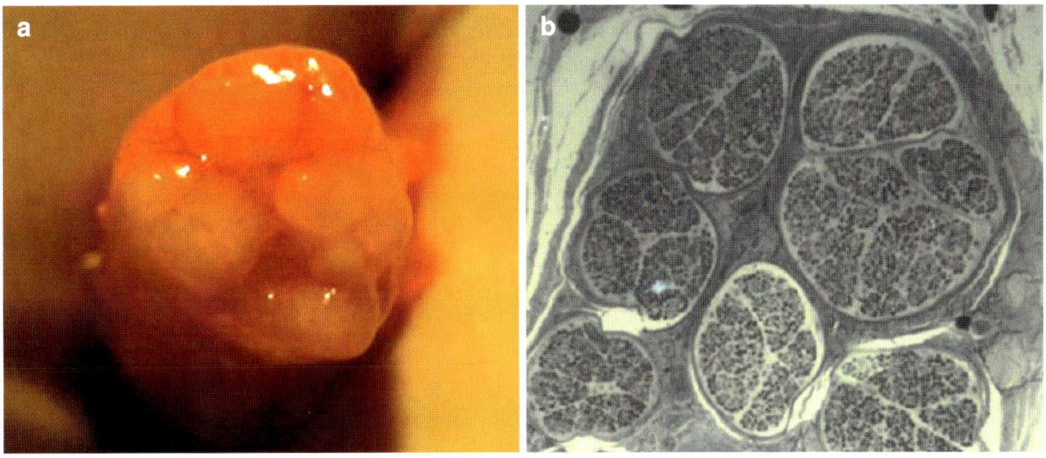

Fig. 17.18 Macroscopic (**a**) and microscopic (**b**) transverse views through a peripheral nerve. With the naked eye the individual fascicles can be recognised easily with their sheath, the interfascicular epineurium. On microscopy the fascicles are seen consisting of several nerve fibres which are formed of numerous axons, surrounded by the endoneurium Copyright: [Author]

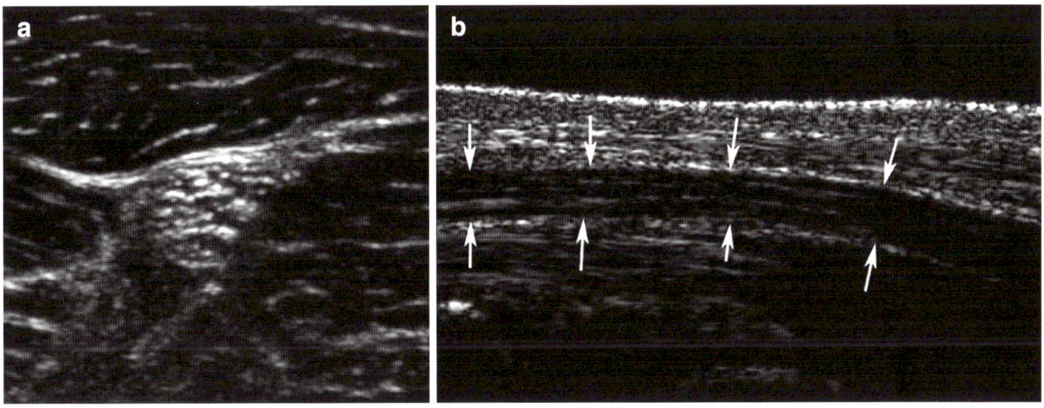

Fig. 17.19 Transverse (**a**) and longitudinal views (**b**) through a peripheral nerve. In the transverse view of the sciatic nerve, the typical honeycomb texture of the echo can be seen clearly. It represents the echo-poor fascicles, surrounded by the echo-rich epineurium and endoneurium. In the longitudinal view of the median nerve, an echo-poor structure (between the *arrows*) is seen containing echo-rich strands Copyright: [Author]

17.6.2 Nerves Which Follow the Course of Leg Veins

The **sciatic nerve** terminates into the **tibial nerve** and the **common peroneal nerve** in the popliteal region. These nerves may run very close to the small saphenous vein and the saphenopopliteal junction (Ricci 2005).

In transverse view the sciatic or tibial nerve, depending on the level at which the common peroneal nerve branches off, lies between the deep popliteal vein and the superficial small saphenous vein. When the small saphenous vein joins the popliteal vein in the popliteal region, it usually runs down deeper and immediately lateral to the nerve (Fig. 17.21). The close relation to this nerve puts it at risk during surgery and endoluminal treatments. Dissection injury or the heat conduction from endothermal procedures may cause damage with consequent neurological deficit (Creton et al. 2004 in Appendix 2). If the small saphenous vein drains into the great saphenous vein or a deep thigh vein further up, then its course may be medial to the sciatic nerve.

Direct examination of the sciatic nerve or its terminal branches may reveal the true cause of a patient's symptoms rather than a venous aetiology. For example, other causes include neurogenic tumours, traumatic lesions or a compressed nerve (Figs. 17.22a, b and 17.23a, b). The not so rare condition of a varicosity causing sciatic nerve irritation has been described in the literature (Ricci et al. 2005).

The **femoral nerve** passes under the inguinal ligament lateral to the femoral artery, while

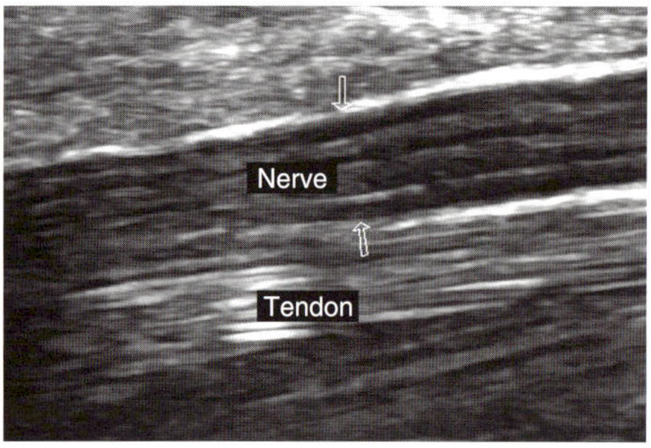

Fig. 17.20 The difference between the nerve ("nerv", between *arrows*), as an echo-poor, cable-like strand with wavy, echo-rich bands, and the tendon ("tendon"), with its strictly parallel, echo-rich, fibrillar texture, can be seen Copyright: [Author]

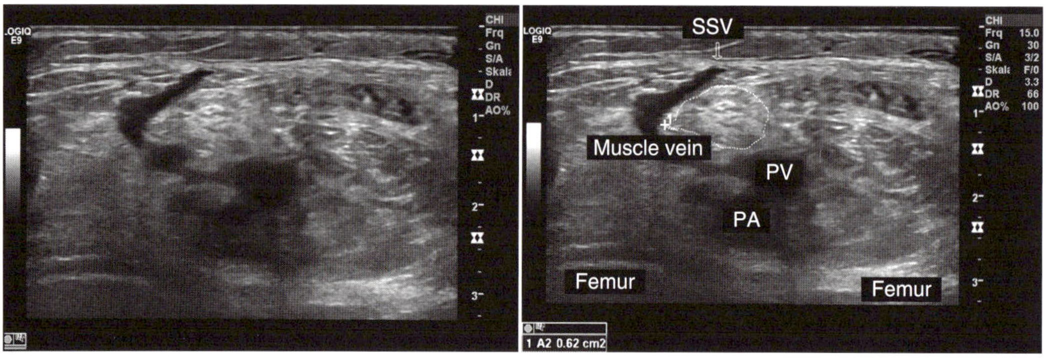

Fig. 17.21 Transverse view above the popliteal skin crease. The popliteal vein (*PV*) is slightly compressed by the probe. In a deeper location, the popliteal artery (*PA*) is seen as a round, echo-poor structure. The tibial nerve, the larger of the two terminal branches of the sciatic nerve, appears as an echo-rich structure (marked with a *dotted line*). It is immediately medial to the small saphenous vein (*SSV*) and a muscle vein (*MV*) as it runs down to join the popliteal vein (see accompanying online material) Copyright: [Author]

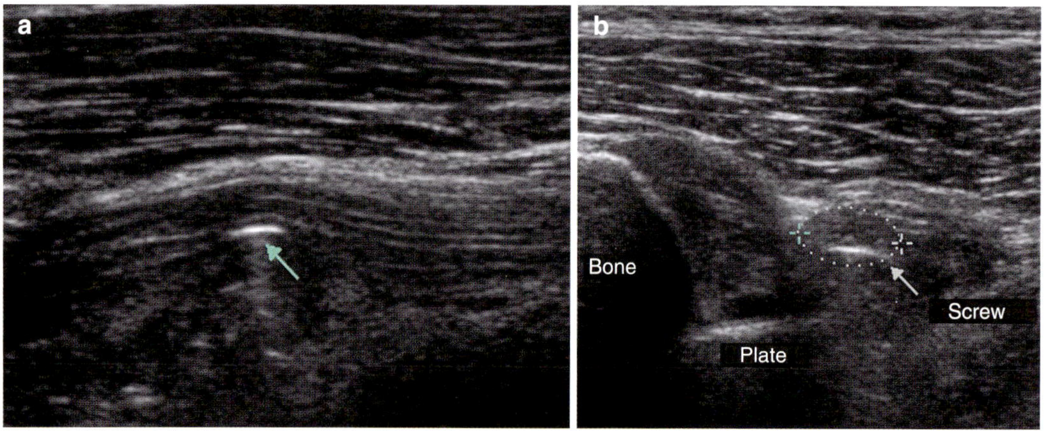

Fig. 17.22 Longitudinal (**a**) and transverse views (**b**) in the gluteal region after fixation of a pelvic ring fracture. The sciatic nerve is seen compressed and deviated by the head of a bone screw (*arrowed*) Copyright: [Author]

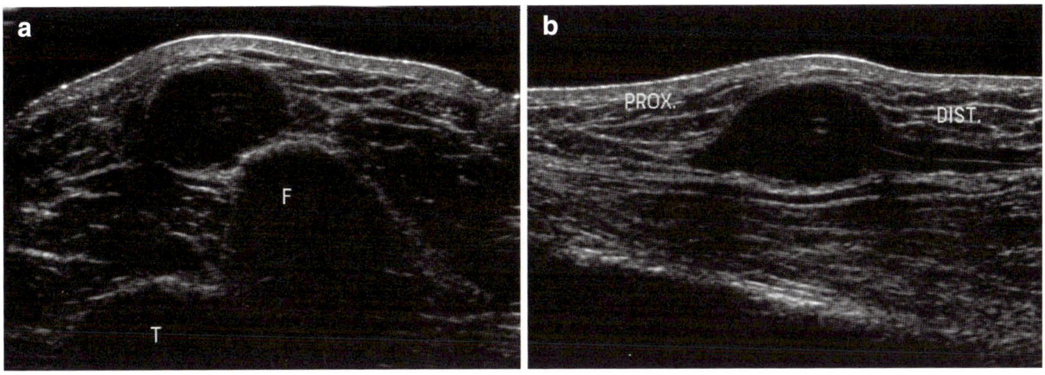

Fig. 17.23 Schwannoma of the common peroneal nerve in transverse (**a**) and longitudinal views (**b**). The hypoechoic schwannoma lies directly against the fibula (*F*) and tibia (*T*) Copyright: [Author]

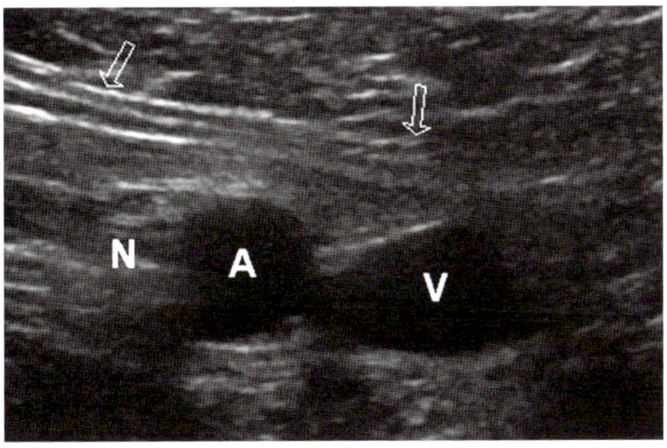

Fig. 17.24 The IVAN mnemonic. Under the inguinal ligament (*arrowed*) the order is the following: **i**nside (medial) the femoral vein (*V*), then the femoral artery (*A*) and finally the femoral nerve (*N*). The femoral nerve is hard to identify from the surrounding connective tissue because of its echo-rich interfascicular epineurium (see accompanying online material) Copyright: [Author]

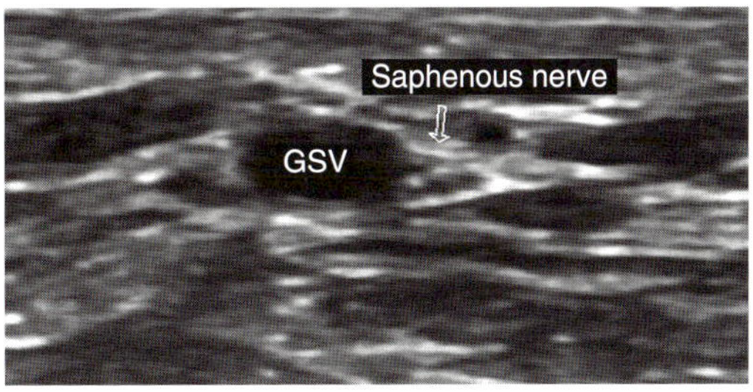

Fig. 17.25 The saphenous nerve (*arrowed*) runs immediately behind the great saphenous vein (*GSV*) in the lower leg. In this case its diameter is approximately half that of the vein. Its fascicular construction and characteristics are best seen using high-resolution ultrasound Copyright: [Author]

the femoral vein lies medial to the artery. This configuration is remembered using the mnemonic IVAN (inside–vein–artery–nerve) and serves to remind the surgeon during a saphenofemoral dissection (Fig. 17.24). Just after emerging from beneath the inguinal ligament, the femoral nerve separates into several terminal branches, most of which are motor nerves for the quadriceps muscles. The sensory end branch of the femoral nerve is the saphenous nerve which is susceptible to injury when it runs close to the great saphenous vein. Injuries to the saphenous nerve and the sural nerve are among the typical surgical complications on primary varicose veins (Hach and Hach-Wunderle 2002).

The **saphenous nerve** runs under the sartorius muscle and then passes between the tendons of the sartorius and gracilis muscles just beyond the knee. It surfaces in the region of the pes anserinus insertion (sartorius, gracilis and semitendinosus). It then joins the great saphenous vein which it accompanies further down along the medial border of the tibia. The common course (Fig. 17.25) makes the saphenous nerve prone to injury during surgery. There is a wide discrepancy in the rates reported of complications involving injury of the saphenous nerve during treatment. In a series of Morrison and Dalsing (2003), 40 % of patients reported symptoms consistent with saphenous nerve injury at some time after operation, but these symptoms affected quality of life in only 6.7 %. Symptoms persisted at further evaluation in 17.8 %, and only one patient (2.3 %) reported any negative effect on quality of life.

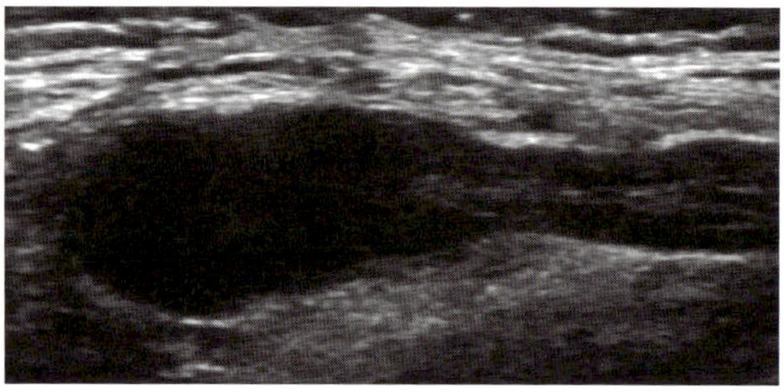

Fig. 17.26 Amputation or stump neuroma after severance of the tibial nerve. The proximal end of the severed nerve develops a bulbous protrusion (*left* in the image) Copyright: [Author]

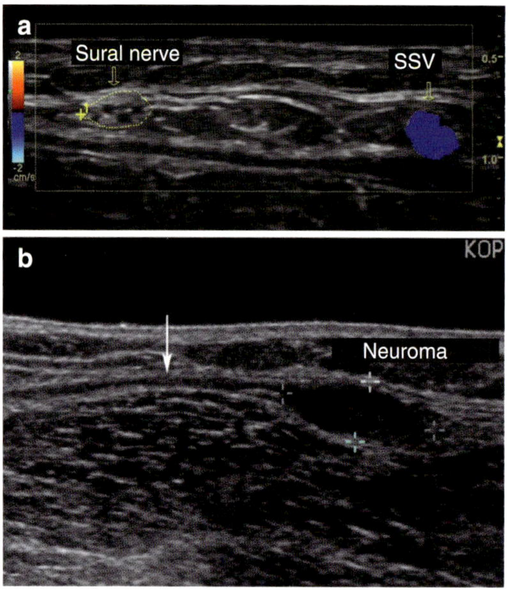

Fig. 17.27 In the upper part of the calf, the sural nerve and small saphenous vein (SSV) lie close together in a channel between the two gastrocnemius heads. Further down (**a**), a small distance frequently separates the sural nerve from the small saphenous vein. Therefore, damage to the sural nerve with neuroma formation (**b**) is less likely during operations in this region than higher up in the calf Copyright: [Author]

Modern pin strippers, inversion stripping and limiting the extent of stripping to the refluxing sections of the great saphenous vein may reduce the rate of injury to the saphenous nerve (Polterauer et al. 2007 in Appendix 2). Despite this, it remains a significant problem.

Saphenous nerve injury results in a loss/alteration of sensation on the medial side of the lower leg. If the nerve is severed, a traumatic neuroma may develop. The newly regenerating axons and Schwann cells bud out of the proximal stump and are unable to find their target. This results in a tangled mass called a neuroma. If the nerve is severed completely and the stumps are sufficiently far apart, an amputation/stump neuroma will develop. On ultrasound this appears as a sharply defined, bulbous, homogeneously echo-poor lesion in continuity with the proximal end of the severed nerve (Fig. 17.26). If the nerve is partially severed, an excrescence may form at the site when it is known as an in-continuity neuroma.

Patients with neuromas frequently suffer severe neuropathic pain with powerful electrifying shocks along the previous supply area of the nerve especially when the neuroma is touched or pressed.

The **sural nerve** can be inadvertently damaged during treatment of, or a varicosity near, the small saphenous vein. It is a very sensitive nerve originating in the popliteal region as a branch of the medial sural cutaneous nerve (branch of the tibial nerve) and the lateral sural cutaneous nerve (branch of the common peroneal nerve). Like the small saphenous vein, it runs in a channel between the two gastrocnemius heads in a caudal direction and then lateral to the Achilles tendon to reach the lateral side of the foot (Fig. 17.27a, b).

Direct damage to the **lateral femoral cutaneous nerve** during treatment of varicose veins is unlikely because this very sensitive nerve runs clear of the saphenous veins in the lateral thigh. However, a positional injury may result if the patient is lying prone and anaesthetised during a popliteal fossa dissection. Pressure on this nerve may be caused at the point where it passes through the inguinal ligament immediately medial to the anterior superior iliac spine. This is a physiological constriction point. If there is a pre-existing impingement syndrome, termed meralgia paraesthetica, it may be exacerbated (Fig. 17.28).

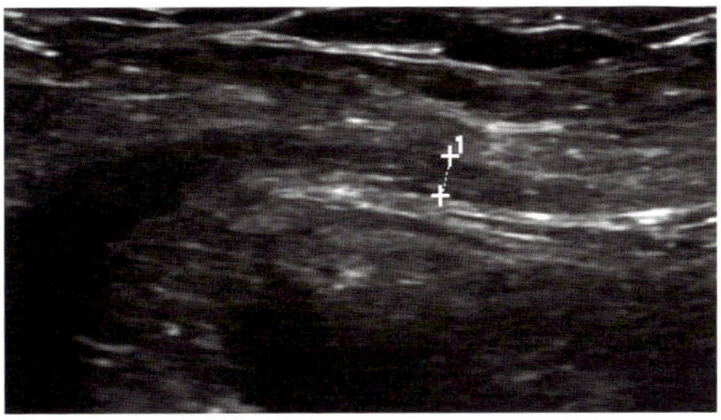

Fig. 17.28 Meralgia paraesthetica. It is useful to recognise how the course of the echo-poor, swollen, lateral femoral cutaneous nerve (marked with 1) changes from horizontal to vertical as it passes through the inguinal ligament medial to the anterior superior iliac spine Copyright: [Author]

References

Hach W, Hach-Wunderle V (2002) Neural lesions in surgical treatment of primary varicose veins. Gefäßchirurgie 7:97–102

Kopf H, Loizides A, Mostbeck GH, Gruber H (2011) Diagnostic sonography of peripheral nerves: indications, examination techniques and pathological findings. Ultraschall Med 32:242–263

Lattimer CR, Azzam M, Kalodiki E, Makris GC, Geroulakos G (2012). Saphenous pulsation on duplex may be a marker of severe chronic superficial venous insufficiency. J Vasc Surg 56:1338–1343

Morrison C, Dalsing MC (2003) Signs and symptoms of saphenous nerve injury after greater saphenous vein stripping: prevalence, severity, and relevance for modern practice. J Vasc Surg 38(5):886–890

Ricci S (2005) Ultrasound observation of the sciatic nerve and its branches at the popliteal fossa: always visible, never seen. Eur J Vasc Endovasc Surg 30:659–663

Silvestri E, Martinoli C, Derchi LE, Bertolotto M, Chiaramondia M, Rosenberg I (1995) Echotexture of peripheral nerves: correlation between US and histologic findings and criteria to differentiate tendons. Radiology 197:291–296

Appendix 1: Further Reading

Debari Iyoob S, Arger PH (2004) Complete guide to vascular ultrasound. Lippincott Raven, Philadelphia. ISBN-10: 0781753465, ISBN-13: 978–0781753463

Dieter RS, Dieter RA, Dieter RA III (2009) Peripheral arterial disease. Mcgraw-Hill Professional, New York. ISBN-10: 0071481796, ISBN-13: 978–0071481793

Gloviczki P, Dalsing MC, Eklöf BG (2008) Handbook of venous disorders: guidelines of the American Venous Forum, 3rd edn. Hodder & Stoughton, London. ISBN-10: 0340938803, ISBN-13: 978–0340938805

Goldmann M (2011) Sclerotherapy, 5th edn. Saunders, Philadelphia. ISBN-10: 0323073670, ISBN-13: 978–0323073677. Textbook with CD

Negus D, Coleridge-Smith PD, Bergan JJ (2005) Leg ulcers diagnosis and management, 3rd edn. Hodder & Stoughton, London. ISBN-10: 0340810130, ISBN-13: 978–0340810132

Polak JF (2004) Peripheral vascular sonography: a practical guide, 2nd edn. Lippincott Williams & Wilkins, Philadelphia. ISBN-10: 0781748712, ISBN-13: 978–0781748711

Polak J, Pellerito JF (2012) Introduction to vascular ultrasonography: expert consult – online and print version, 6th edn. Saunders, London. ISBN-10: 143771417X, ISBN-13: 978–1437714173

Schäberle W, Herwig B (2011) Ultrasonography in vascular diagnosis: a therapy-oriented textbook and atlas. Springer, Heidelberg. ISBN-10: 3642025080, ISBN-13: 978–3642025082

Weiss R, Weiss M, Beasley K (2011) Sclerotherapy and vein treatment, 2nd edn. McGraw-Hill Professional, New York

E. Mendoza et al. (eds.), *Duplex Ultrasound of Superficial Leg Veins*,
DOI 10.1007/978-3-642-40731-4, © Springer-Verlag Berlin Heidelberg 2014

Appendix 2: Literature German Version

Chapter 1

Mendoza E (2002) CHIVA – Ein Handbuch. Arrien, Wunstorf

Weskott HP (2006) Physikalische Grundlagen der Sonographie. In: Gross M (ed) Sonographie, Schritt für Schritt zur Diagnose. Urban & Fischer, Stuttgart

Chapter 2

Askar O (1963) The short saphenous vein. J Cardiovasc Surg 4:126–137

Bailly M (1992) Cartographie CHIVA. Encyclopdie Medico-Chirurgicales, Paris, pp 43–161–B, 1–4

Bergan JJ (1999) Common anatomic patterns of varicose veins. In: Goldmann MP, Weiss RA, Bergan JJ (eds) Varicose veins and telangiectasias. Quality Medical Publishing Inc, St Louis, pp 70–86

Caggiati A (2000) Fascial relations and structure of the tributaries of the saphenous veins. Surg Radiol Anat 22:1–4

Caggiati A (2001) Fascial relationships of the short saphenous vein. J Vasc Surg 34:241–246

Caggiati A, Mendoza E (2004) Segmental hypoplasia of the great saphenous vein and varicose disease. Eur J Vasc Endovasc Surg 28:257–261

Caggiati A, Ricci S (1999) The long saphenous vein compartment. Phlebology 12:107–111

Caggiati A, Ricci S (2000) The caliber of the human long saphenous vein and its congenital variations. Ann Anat 182:1–7

Caggiati A, Macchiarelli G, Familiari G (1998) Topographical structural variations of the human long saphenous vein and its age-related remodelling as revealed by correlated light and scanning electron microscopy. Phlebology 13:156–162

Caggiati A, Bergan JJ, Gloviczki P, Jantet G, Wendell-Smith CP, Partsch H (2002) Nomenclature of the veins of the lower limbs: an international interdisciplinary consensus statement. J Vasc Surg 36:416–422

Cavezzi A, Tabarini C, Collura M, Sigismondi G, Barboni MG, Carigi V (2002) Hemodynamique de la junction sapheno-poplitee: evaluation par echo-doppler couleur. Phlebologie 55:309–316

Coleridge-Smith P, Labropoulos N, Partsch H, Myers K, Nicolaides A, Cavezzi A (2006) Duplex ultrasound investigation of the veins in chronic venous disease of the lower limbs-UIP consensus document, Part I. Basic principles. Eur J Vasc Endovasc Surg 31:1–10

Creton D (2005) Saphenopopliteal junctions are significantly lower when incompetent. Phlebolymphology 48:347–354

Dodd H (1958) Persistent varicose veins with special reference to the varicose tributaries of the superficial femoral and popliteal veins. Proc R Soc Med 51:817–820

Dodd H (1964) The varicose tributaries of the popliteal vein. Proc R Soc Med 57:394–396

Dodd H, Cockett FB (1976) The pathology and surgery of the veins of the lower limb. Churchill Livingstone, Edinburgh/London/New York

Ferner H (1987) Die untere Extremität. In: Ferner H (Hrsg) Eduard Pernkopf: Atlas der topographischen und angewandten Anatomie des

Menschen. Urban & Schwarzenberg, München, S 334–401

Gisel A (2003) Anatomie des Venensystems. In Rabe E (Hrsg) Grundlagen der Phlebologie. Viavital, Köln, S 25–50

Günther B, Heberer G (1987) Chirurgische Anatomie der Venen. In: Heberer G, van Dongen RJAM (Hrsg) Gefäßchirurgie. Springer, Berlin/Heidelberg, S 29–30

Kosinski C (1926) Observations on the superficial venous system of the lower extremities. J Anat 60:131–138

Kubik S (1985) Anatomie des Oberschenkels aus vaskulärer Sicht. In: Brunner U (Hrsg) Aktuelle Probleme der Angiologie: 43. Der Oberschenkel – Diagnostische und therapeutische Aspekte der Arteriologie, Phlebologie und Lymphologie. Hans Huber, Bern Stuttgart Wien, S 15–68

Kubik S (1986) Anatomie der Beinvenen. In: Wuppermann T (Hrsg) Varizen, Ulcus cruris und Thrombose. Springer, Berlin/Heidelberg, S 1–54

Marshall M, Breu FX (2005) Handbuch der Angiologie 13, Erg-Lfg. Ecomed, Landsberg

Mendoza E (2001) Zur topographischen Anatomie der Vena saphena magna – Eine duplexsonographische Studie im Hinblick auf chirurgisch relevante Aspekte. Phlebologie 30:140–144

Mendoza E (2002) CHIVA – Ein Handbuch. Arrien, Wunstorf

Mendoza E, Caggiati A (2003) Anatomie im Dienste der Ultraschalldiagnostik und der Therapie der Varikose. Gefäßchirurgie 8:295–303

Mühlberger D, Morandini L, Brenner E (2007) Frequency and exact position of valves in the saphenofemoral junction. Phlebologie 36:3–7

Müller-Bühl U, Diehm C (1991) Anatomie der Beinvenen. In: Müller-Bühl U, Diehm C (Hrsg) Angiologie – Praxis der Gefäßerkrankungen. Kohlhammer, Stuttgart Berlin Köln, S 193–196

Pernkopf E, Ferner H (1987) Atlas der topographischen und angewandten Anatomie des Menschen. Urban & Schwarzenberg, München/Wien/Baltimore

Ricci S, Caggiati A (1999) Does a double long saphenous vein exist? Phlebology 14:59–64

Sebastiani F (1935) Sullo sviluppo prenatale della fascia superficiale di alcune regioni dell'ipoderma umano. Scritti Biologici 10:3–45

Tillaux P (1897) Trait d'tnatomie topographique avec applications a la chirurgie. In: Neuvime (ed) Asselin et Houzeau, Paris, pp 1011–1073

Chapter 3

Bernardini E et al (2002) Development of primary superficial venous insufficiency: the ascending theory. Observational and hemodynamic data from a 9 year experience. Ann Vasc Surg 24:709–720

Creton D (2005) Saphenopopliteal junctions are significantly lower when incompetent. Phlebolymphology 48:347–354

Dodd H, Cockett FB (1976) The pathology and surgery of the veins of the lower limb. Churchill Livingstone, Edinburgh/London/New York

Evans CJ, Allan PL, Lee AJ, Bradbury AW, Ruckley CV, Fowkes FGR (1998) Prevalence of venous reflux in the general population on duplex scanning: the Edinburgh Vein Study. J Vasc Surg 28:767–776

Franceschi C, Bahnini A (2005) Treatment of lower extremity venous insufficiency due to pelvic leak points in women. Ann Vasc Surg 19:1–6

Hach W, Hach-Wunderle V (1994) Die Rezirkulationskreise der primären Varikose – Pathophysiologische Grundlagen zur chirurgischen Therapie. Springer, Berlin/Heidelberg

Hennies F, Kahle B (2001) Bleibt der Korrelationsindex aus venösem und arteriellen Stromzeitvolumen (VAFI) über einen längeren Messzeitraum stabil? Phlebologie 30:53–59

Huck K (2005) Kursbuch Doppler- und Duplexsonographie. Thieme, Stuttgart/New York

Kahle B, Hummel S, Kirchner P (2001) Quantifizierung des Effektes von Varizenoperationen auf die venöse Hämodynamik mittels des Veno-Arteriellen Flow-Index (VAFI). Phlebologie 30:1–6

Kahle B, Hennies F, Bolz S, Pritsch M (2003) The reproducibility of the ratio of volume flow in the common femoral vein and artery (VAFI) for quantification of the severity of venous insufficiency. Vasa 32:199–203

Labropoulos N, Tiongson J, Pryor L, Tassiopoulos AK, Kang SS, Mansour A, Baker

WH (2003) Definition of venous reflux in lower-extremity veins. J Vasc Surg 38:793–798

Lurie F, Comerota A, Eklof B, Kistner RL, Labropoulos N, Lohr J, Marston W, Meissner M, Moneta G, Neglen P, Neuhardt D, Padberg F, Welsh HJ (2012) Multicenter assessment of venous reflux by duplex ultrasound. J Vasc Surg 55:437–445

Mendoza E (2002) CHIVA – Ein Handbuch. Arrien, Wunstorf

Mendoza E, Berger V, Zollmann C, Bomhoff M, Amsler F (2011) Kaliberreduktion der V. saphena magna und der V. femoralis communis nach CHIVA. Phlebologie 40:73–78

Rouviere H (1974) Anatomie humaine, vol 2, 11th edn. Masson, Paris

Rudolphi P, Hunold P, Kahle B (2012) Quantitative Erfassung desSchweregrads der venösen Insuffizienz anhand der Hämodynamik. Posterpräsentation 54. DGP-Jahrestagung in Lübeck

Silbernagel S, Despopoulos A (1988) Taschenatlas der Physiologie, 3. Aufl. Thieme, Stuttgart/New York

Trendelenburg F (1891) Ueber die Unterbindung der Vena saphena magna bei Unterschenkelvaricen. Beiträge zur Klinischen Chirurgie (Tübingen) 7:195–210

Zamboni P, Marcellino MG, Cappelli M, Feo CV, Bresadola V, Vasquez G, Liboni A (1998) Saphenous vein sparing surgery: principles, techniques and results. J Cardiovasc Surg 39:151–162

Chapter 4

Antignani PL, Cornu-Thnard A, Allegra C, Carpentier PH, Partsch H, Uhl JF (2004) Results of a questionnaire regarding improvement of 'C' in the CEAP classification. Eur J Vasc Endovasc Surg 28:177–181

Caggiati A, Mendoza E (2004) Segmental hypoplasia of the great saphenous vein and varicose disease. Eur J Vasc Endovasc Surg 28:257–261

Cappelli M, Molino Lova R, Ermini S, Turchi A, Bono G, Franceschi C (1996) Comparaison entre Cure C.H.I.V.A. et stripping dans le traitement des veines variqueuses des membres infrieurs: suivi de 3 ans. J Mal Vasc 21:40–46

Eklöf B, Rutherford RB, Bergan JJ, Carpentier PH, Gloviczki P, Kistner RL, Meissner MH, Moneta GL, Myers K, Padberg FT, Perrin M, Ruckley CV, Coleridge-Smith P, Wakefield TW (2004) Revision of CEAP classification for chronic venous disorders (CVD). J Vasc Surg 40:1248–1252

Eklöf B, Rutherford RB, Bergan JJ, Carpentier PH, Gloviczki P, Kistner RL, Meissner MH, Moneta GL, Myers K, Padberg FT, Perrin M, Ruckley CV, Coleridge Smith P, Wakefield TW (2005) Revision der CEAP-Klassifizierung für chronische Venenleiden. Consensus Statement. Phlebologie 34:220–226

Franceschi C (1988) Thorie et pratique de la cure conservatrice et hmodynamique de l'insuffisance veineuse en ambulatoire. Prcy-sous-Thil (Armanon)

Franceschi C (1997) Mesures et interpretation des flux veineux lors des manœvres des stimulation. Compressions manuelles et manœvre de Parana. Indice dynamique de reflux IDR et indice de Psatakis. J Mal Vasc 22:1–5

Franceschi C, Bahnini A (2005) Treatment of lower extremity venous insufficiency due to pelvic leak points in women. Ann Vasc Surg 19:1–6

Hach W, Hach-Wunderle V (1994) Die Rezirkulationskreise der primären Varikose – Pathophysiologische Grundlagen zur chirurgischen Therapie. Springer, Berlin/Heidelberg

Mendoza E (2001) Zur topographischen Anatomie der Vena saphena magna – Eine duplexsonographische Studie im Hinblick auf chirurgisch relevante Aspekte. Phlebologie 30:140–144

Mendoza E (2002a) CHIVA – Ein Handbuch. Arrien, Wunstorf

Mendoza E (2002b) Einteilung der Rezirkulationen im Bein: anatomische und physiologische Grundlagen der CHIVA-Methode. Phlebologie 31:28–35

Mendoza E (2006) Duplexsonographie der oberflächlichen Beinvenen. Steinkopff-Verlag, Darmstadt

Mendoza E, Berger HA (2001) Provokationsmanöver für die duplexsonographische Diagnostik der Varikosis. Gefäßchirurgie 6:43–46

Nicolaides AN (2000) Investigation of chronic venous insufficiency – a consensus statement. Circulation 102:126–163

Rabe E (1994) Chronische Venenkrankheiten: In: Rabe E (Hrsg) Grundlagen der Phlebologie. Kagerer-Kommunikation, Bonn, S 69–86

Trendelenburg F (1891) Ueber die Unterbindung der Vena saphena magna bei Unterschenkelvaricen. Beiträge zur Klinischen Chirurgie (Tübingen) 7:195–210

Zamboni P, Marcellino MG, Cappelli M, Feo CV, Bresadola V, Vasquez G, Liboni A (1998) Saphenous vein sparing surgery: principles, techniques and results. J Cardiovasc Surg 39:151–162

Chapter 5

Coleridge-Smith P, Labropoulos N, Partsch H, Myers K, Nicolaides A, Cavezzi A (2006) Duplex ultrasound investigation of the veins in chronic venous disease of the lower limbs-UIP consensus document, Part I. Basic principles. Eur J Vasc Endovasc Surg 31:1–10

Eklöf B, Rutherford RB, Bergan JJ, Carpentier PH, Gloviczki P, Kistner RL, Meissner MH, Moneta GL, Myers K, Padberg FT, Perrin M, Ruckley CV, Coleridge-Smith P, Wakefield TW (2004) Revision of CEAP classification for chronic venous disorders (CVD). J Vasc Surg 40:1248–1252

Mendoza E (2002) CHIVA – Ein Handbuch. Arrien, Wunstorf

Noppeney T, Nüllen H (2009) REVAT (Recurrent Varices After Treatment) – Definition und Klassifikation der Rezidivvarikose. Phlebologie 38:271–274

Perrin MR, Guex JJ, Ruckley CV, dePalma RG, Royle JP, Eklof B, Nicolini P, Janet G and the REVAS group (2000) Recurrent varices after surgery (REVAS), a consensus document. Cardiovasc Surg 8:233–245

Vasquez MA, Rabe E, McLafferty RB, Shortell CK, Marston W, Gillespie D, Meissner M, Rutherford RB, American Venous Forum Ad Hoc Outcomes Working Group (2010) Revision of the venous clinical severity score: venous outcomes consensus statement: special communication of the American Venous Forum Ad Hoc Outcomes Working Group. J Vasc Surg 52:1387–1396

Chapter 6

Coleridge-Smith P, Labropoulos N, Partsch H, Myers K, Nicolaides A, Cavezzi A (2006) Duplex ultrasound investigation of the veins in chronic venous disease of the lower limbs-UIP consensus document, Part I. Basic principles. Eur J Vasc Endovasc Surg 31:1–10

Mendoza E (2002) CHIVA – Ein Handbuch. Arrien, Wunstorf

Mendoza E, Berger HA (2001) Provokationsmanöver für die duplexsonographische Diagnostik der Varikosis. Gefäßchirurgie 6:43–46

Obermayer A, Garzon K (2010) Sourcing of superficial reflux in venous leg ulcers using duplex ultrasound. J Vasc Surg 52:1255–1261

Sietzen P, Kaiser R, Rendl KH (1997) Vergleich von Valsalva-Manöver und distaler Dekompression zur Refluxprüfung der V. saphena magna. Eine sonographische und phlebographische Untersuchung. Gefäßchirurgie 2:204–207

Chapter 7

Coleridge-Smith P, Labropoulos N, Partsch H, Myers K, Nicolaides A, Cavezzi A (2006) Duplex ultrasound investigation of the veins in chronic venous disease of the lower limbs-UIP consensus document, Part I. Basic principles. Eur J Vasc Endovasc Surg 31:1–10

Lattimer CR, Azzam M, Kalodiki E, Makris G, Geroulakos G (2012) Saphenous pulsation on duplex may be a marker of severe chronic superficial venous insufficiency. J Vasc Surg 56:1338–1343

Mendoza E (2002) CHIVA – Ein Handbuch. Arrien, Wunstorf

Mendoza E (2012) Great saphenous vein diameter at the saphenofemoral junction and proximal thigh as parameters of venous disease class. Eur J Vasc Endovasc Surg. doi:10.1016/j.ejvs.2012.10.014

Mühlberger D, Morandini L, Brenner E (2009) Venous valves and major superficial tributary veins near the saphenofemoral junction. J Vasc Surg 49:1562–1569

Oswald M (2005) Unser blaues Wunder – Sexualhormone und Krampfadern. http://ebook-browse.com/unser-blaues-wunder-pdf-d76330333

Chapter 8

Cockett FB, Jones DE (1953) The ankle blow-out syndrome. Lancet 1:17

Huck K (2005) Kursbuch Doppler- und Duplexsonographie. Thieme, Stuttgart/New York

Recek C (1996) Auswirkung der Krossektomie auf die venöse Zirkulationsstörung bei primärer Varikose. Phlebologie 25:11–18

Zamboni P (ed) (1996) La chirurgie conservativa del sistema venoso superficiale. Gruppo Editoriale Faenza Editrice, Faenza

Chapter 11

Decousus H et al (2010) Superficial venous thrombosis and venous thromboembolism. Ann Intern Med 152:218–224

Kalodiki E, Strvrtinova V, Allegra C, Andreozzi GM, Antignani PL, Avram R, Brkljacic B, Cadariou F, Dzsinich C, Fareed J, Gaspar L, Geroulakos G, Javien A, Kozak M, Lattimer CR, Minar E, Partsch H, Passariello F, Patel M, Pécsvárady Z, Poredos P, Rotocil K, Scuderi A, Sparovec M, Szostek M, Skorski M (2012) Superficial vein thrombosis: a consensus statement. Int Angiol 31:203–216

van Langevelde K, Lijfering WM, Rosendaal FR, Cannegieter SC (2011) Increased risk of venous thrombosis in persons with clinically diagnosed superficial vein thrombosis: results from the MEGA study. Blood 118:4239–4241

Chapter 12

Almeida JI, Min RJ, Raabe R, McLean DJ, Madsen M (2011) Cyanoacrylate adhesive for the closure of truncal veins: 60-day swine model results. Vasc Endovascular Surg 45:631–635

Breu FX, Guggenbichler S, Marshall M (2004) Konsensuskonferenz zur Schaumsklerotherapie. Phlebologie 33:97

Coleridge-Smith P, Labropoulos N, Partsch H, Myers K, Nicolaides A, Cavezzi A (2006) Duplex ultrasound investigation of the veins in chronic venous disease of the lower limbs-UIP consensus document, Part I. Basic principles. Eur J Vasc Endovasc Surg 31:1–10

Elias S, Raines JK (2012) Mechanochemical tumescentless endovenous ablation: final results of the initial clinical trial. Phlebology 27:67–72

Franceschi C (1988) Thorie et pratique de la cure conservatrice et hmodynamique de l'insuffisance veineuse en ambulatoire. Prcy-sous-Thil (Armanon)

Hamel-Desnos C (2003) Evaluation of the efficacy of polidocanol in the form of foam compared with liquid form in sclerotherapy of the greater saphenous vein. Dermatol Surg 29:1170

Marshall M, Breu FX (2005) Handbuch der Angiologie 13, Erg-Lfg. Ecomed, Landsberg

Mendoza E (2002) Einteilung der Rezirkulationen im Bein: anatomische und physiologische Grundlagen der CHIVA-Methode. Phlebologie 31:28–35

Nicolaides AN (2000) Investigation of chronic venous insufficiency – a consensus statement. Circulation 102:126–163

Partsch B (2004) Die Schaumverödung – eine Renaissance der Sklerotherapie. Phlebologie 33:30

Prince EA, Soares GM, Silva M, Taner A, Ahn S, Dubel GJ, Jay BS (2011) Impact of laser fiber design on outcome of endovenous ablation of lower-extremity varicose veins: results from a single practice. Cardiovasc Intervent Radiol 34:536–541

Proebstle TM, Alm J, Göckeritz O, Wenzel C, Noppeney T, Lebard C, Pichot O, Sessa C, Creton D, European Closure Fast Clinical Study Group (2011) Three-year European follow-up of endovenous radiofrequency-powered segmental thermal ablation of the great saphenous vein with or without treatment of calf varicosities. J Vasc Surg 54:146–152

Rabe E, Pannier-Fischer F, Gerlach H, Breu FX, Guggenbichler S, Zabel M (2003) Leitlinien der Sklerosierungsbehandlung der Varikose. Phlebologie 32:101

Ricci S, Caggiati A (1999) Echoanatomical patterns of the long saphenous vein in patients with primary varices and in healthy subjects. Phlebology 14:54–58

Schwarz T, von Hodenberg E, Furtwängler C, Rastan A, Zeller T, Neumann FJ (2010) Endovenous laser ablation of varicose veins with the 1470-nm diode laser. J Vasc Surg 51:1474–1478

Wildenhues B (2005) Endovenöse kathetergestützte Schaumsklerosierung. Phlebologie 34:165

Wollmann JC (2002) Schaum – zwischen Vergangenheit und Zukunft. Vasomed 16:34

Yamaki T, Nozaki M, Sasaki K (2002) Alternative greater saphenous vein-sparing surgery: valvuloplasty combined with axial transposition of a competent tributary vein for the treatment of primary valvular incompetence – 18-month follow-up. Dermatol Surg 28: 162–167

Chapter 13

Carandina S, Mari C, De Palma M, Marcellino MG, Cisno C, Legnaro A, Liboni A, Zamboni P (2008) Varicose vein stripping vs haemodynamic correction (CHIVA): a long term randomised trial. Eur J Vasc Endovasc Surg 35:230–237

de Maeseneer MG, Vandenbroeck CP, Hendriks JM, Lauwers PR, van Schil PE (2005) Accuracy of duplex evaluation one year after varicose vein surgery to predict recurrence at the sapheno-femoral junction after five years. Eur J Vasc Endovasc Surg 29:308–331

Geier B, Mumme A, Kummel T, Marpe B, Freis H, Stücker M, Asciutto G (2008) Validität des Duplex-Ultraschalls bei der Klassifizierung von Leistenrezidiven nach Crossektomie. Phlebologie 37:3–47

Geier B, Stücker M, Hummel T, Burger P, Frings N, Hartmann M, Stenger D, Schwahn-Schreiber C, Schonath M, Mumme A (2008) Residual stumps associated with inguinal varicose vein recurrences: a multicenter study. Eur J Vas Endovasc Surg 36:207–210

Juan J, Escribano JM, Maeso J (2002) Hämodynamik des Varizenrezidivs nach Strippingoperationen. Abstractband Jahreskongress 2002 der DGG: 35 (nachzulesen unter www.chiva.info)

Kaps M, von Reutern GM, Stolz E, von Büdingen HJ (2004) Ultraschall in der Neurologie. Thieme, Stuttgart/New York

Mendoza E (2002) Einteilung der Rezirkulationen im Bein: anatomische und physiologische Grundlagen der CHIVA-Methode. Phlebologie 31:28–35

Mühlberger D, Morandini L, Brenner E (2007) Frequency and exact position of valves in the saphenofemoral junction. Phlebologie 36:3–7

Nicolaides AN (2000) Investigation of chronic venous insufficiency – a consensus statement. Circulation 102:126–163

Perrin MR, Guex JJ, Ruckley CV, dePalma RG, Royle JP, Eklof B, Nicolini P, Janet G and the REVAS group (2000) Recurrent varices after surgery (REVAS), a consensus document. Cardiovasc Surg 8:233–245

Rasmussen LH, Lawaetz M, Bjoern L, Vennits B, Blemings A, Eklof B (2011) Randomized clinical trial comparing endovenous laser ablation, radiofrequency ablation, foam sclerotherapy and surgical stripping for great saphenous varicose veins. Br J Surg 98:1079–1087

Chapter 14

Badgett DK, Comerota MC, Khan MN, Eid IG, Kerr RP, Comerota AJ (2000) Duplex venous imaging: role for a comprehensive lower extremity examination. Ann Vasc Surg 14:73–76

Blättler W, Gerlach H, Hach-Wunderle V, Konstantinides S, Noppeney T, Pillny M, Riess H, Schellong S, Stiegler H, Wildberger JE (2010) Interdisziplinäre S2 Leitlinie: Diagnostik und Therapie der Venenthrombose und der Lungenembolie. Vasa 39(Suppl):78

Caggiati A, Bergan JJ, Gloviczki P, Jantet G, Wendell-Smith CP, Partsch H (2002) Nomenclature of the veins of the lower limbs: an international interdisciplinary consensus statement. J Vasc Surg 36:416–422

Chylarecki C, Hierholzer G, Rudofsky G (1995) Physikalische Thromboseprophylaxe mit motorisierten Sprunggelenkbewegungen. Unfallchirurgie 21:137–147

Hach W, Hach-Wunderle V (1994) Die Rezirkulationskreise der primären Varikose – Pathophysiologische Grundlagen zur chirurgischen Therapie. Springer, Berlin/Heidelberg

Hollerweger A, Macheiner P, Rettenbacher T, Gritzmann N (2000) Sonographische Diagnose von Muskelvenenthrombosen des Unterschenkels und deren Bedeutung als Emboliequelle. Ultraschall Med 21:66–72

Jungius KP, Lenhart M, Jung EM (2004) Digitale Ultraschalldiagnostik der Unterschenkelvenenthrombose mit Harmonic Imaging und Cross Beam Technik. Ultraschall in Med 25 (Abstractband): WS-20–07

Kubik S (1985) Anatomie des Oberschenkels aus vaskulärer Sicht. In: Brunner U (Hrsg) Aktuelle Probleme der Angiologie: 43. Der Oberschenkel – Diagnostische und therapeutische Aspekte der Arteriologie, Phlebologie und Lymphologie. Hans Huber, Bern Stuttgart Wien, S 15–68

Lindhoff-Last E (2011) Risk assessment of recurrence of venous thromboembolism. Hamostaseologie 31:7–12

Schellong S, Gerlach H, Hach-Wunderle V et al (2009) Diagnosis of deep vein thrombosis: adherence to guidelines and outcomes in real-world health care. Thromb Haemost 102:1234–1240

Schwarz T, Schmidt B, Schellong SM (2001) Die Muskelvenenthrombose. Dtsch Med Wschr 126:367–369

Stiegler H, Habscheid W, Ludwig M (2002) Leitlinien zur Diagnostik der tiefen Becken-/Beinvenenthrombose. Ultraschall Med 23:274–278

Strauss AL (1995) Farbduplexsonographie der Arterien und Venen. Springer, Berlin/Heidelberg

Wuppermann T (2002) Die chronisch venöse Insuffizienz. Internist 43:16–26

Chapter 15

Nicolaides AN (2000) Investigation of chronic venous insufficiency – a consensus statement. Circulation 102:126–163

Chapter 16

Cornely M (2011) Das Lipödem an Armen und Beinen. Phlebologie 40:21–25

Marshall M, Breu FX (2005) Handbuch der Angiologie 13, Erg-Lfg. Ecomed, Landsberg

Chapter 17

Creton D, Milleret R, Uhl JF (2004) Comment choisir la meilleure technique d'obliteration endovasculaire: Closure, Laser ou la sclerose à la mousse cur cathter. Phlebologie 57:31–35

Gasser G, Pohl P, Mildner A (1995) Läsionen des N. saphenus in Abhängigkeit von der Technik des Strippings. Phlebologie 24:76–77

Hach W, Hach-Wunderle V (2002) Das aktuelle phlebologische Thema läsionen in der Chirurgie der primären Varikose. Neural lesions in surgical treatment of primary varicose veins. Gefäßchirurgie 7:97–102

Kopf H, Loizides A, Mostbeck GH, Gruber H (2011) Diagnostic sonography of peripheral nerves: indications, examination techniques and pathological findings. Ultraschall Med 32:242–263

Polterauer P, Gollackner B, Nanobachvili J, Domenig C (2007) Evidenzbasierte Therapie des Krampfaderleidens. Z Gefäßmed 4:4–9

Ricci S (2005) Ultrasound observation of the sciatic nerve and its branches at the popliteal fossa: always visible, never seen. Eur J Vasc Endovasc Surg 30:659–663

Silvestri E, Martinoli C, Derchi LE, Bertolotto M, Chiaramondia M, Rosenberg I (1995) Echotexture of peripheral nerves: correlation between US and histologic findings and criteria to differentiate tendons. Radiology 197:291–296

Weber H, Stöhr M, Loeprecht H (2003) N.-peroneus-communis Läsion als Komplikation des V. saphena parva Strippings. Gefäßchirurgie 8:36–39

Appendix 3: Abbreviations Used to Label the Figures

AASV	Anterior accessory saphenous vein
Art	Artery
CFA	Common femoral artery
CFV	Common femoral vein
Fem	Femoral
FV	(superficial) femoral vein
GSV	Great saphenous vein
MV	Muscle vein
PASV	Posterior accessory saphenous vein
Perf	Perforator
SFJ	Saphenofemoral junction
SPJ	Saphenopopliteal junction
SSV	Small saphenous vein
Trib	Tributary

Index

E. Mendoza et al. (eds.), *Duplex Ultrasound of Superficial Leg Veins*,
DOI 10.1007/978-3-642-40731-4, © Springer-Verlag Berlin Heidelberg 2014

I

K

L

M

N

Printing and Binding: Stürtz GmbH, Würzburg